Medical Ethics Today
The BMA's handbook of ethics and law

Second edition

Medical Ethics Today
The BMA's handbook
of ethics and law

Second edition

Project Managers	Veronica English Gillian Romano-Critchley
Head of Medical Ethics	Ann Sommerville
Written by	Veronica English Gillian Romano-Critchley Julian Sheather Ann Sommerville
Editorial Secretariat	Patricia Fraser Fenella Overington
Director of Professional Activities	Vivienne Nathanson

Information about major developments since the publication of this book may be obtained from the BMA's website or by contacting:

Medical Ethics Department
British Medical Association
BMA House
Tavistock Square
London WC1H 9JP
Tel: 020 7383 6286
Fax: 020 7383 6233
Email: ethics@bma.org.uk
Website: http://www.bma.org.uk/ethics

© BMJ Publishing Group 2004
BMJ Books is an imprint of the BMJ Publishing Group
© BMA Medical Ethics Department 1993 (first edition)

First published in 1993
Second impression 1995
Third impression 1996
Fourth impression 1998
Fifth impression 2002
Second edition 2004
by BMJ Books, BMA House, Tavistock Square,
London WC1H 9JR

http://www.bmjbooks.com

British Library Cataloguing in Publication Data

A catalogue record for this book is available from the British Library

ISBN 0 7279 1744 7

Typeset by SIVA Math Setters, Chennai, India
Printed and bound by MPG Books, Bodmin, Cornwall

Contents

Medical Ethics Today CD Rom

Features

Medical Ethics Today PDF eBook

- Bookmarked and hyperlinked for instant access to all headings and topics
- Fully indexed and searchable text – just click the 'Search Text' button

BMJ Books catalogue

- Instant access to BMJ Books full catalogue, including an order form

Instructions for use

The CD Rom should start automatically upon insertion, on all Windows systems. The menu screen will appear and you can then navigate by clicking on the headings. If the CD Rom does not start automatically upon insertion, please browse using "Windows Explorer" and double-click the file "BMJ_Books.exe".

Tips

The viewable area of the PDF ebook can be expanded to fill the full screen width, by hiding the bookmarks. To do this, click the tag labelled 'Bookmarks' on the left of the screen. To make the bookmarks visible simply repeat this procedure.

By clicking once on a page in the PDF ebook window, you 'activate' the window. You can now scroll through pages using the scroll-wheel on your mouse, or by using the cursor keys on your keyboard.

Note: the Medical Ethics Today PDF eBook is for search and reference only and cannot be printed. A printable PDF version can be purchased from http://www.bmjbookshop.com

Troubleshooting

If any problems are experienced with use of the CD Rom, we can give you access to all content via the internet. Please send your CD Rom with proof of purchase to the following address, with a letter advising your email address and the problem you have encountered:

Medical Ethics Today eBook access
BMJ Books
BMA House
Tavistock Square
London
WC1H 9JR

List of statutes and regulations

Page numbers are shown in **bold**

United Kingdom

Non-United Kingdom

List of cases

Page numbers are shown in **bold**

United Kingdom

Non-United Kingdom

Where to find legal references online

UK legislation since 1988, and Northern Irish legislation since 1921, are available on Her Majesty's Stationery Office website at http://www.hmso.gov.uk. Some statutory instruments are also available on this site.

Selected legal judgments are available on the court service website at http://www.courtservice.gov.uk.

Selected judgments from the Civil or Criminal Divisions of the Court of Appeal, or from the Administrative Court, are available from the British and Irish Legal Information Institute (http://www.bailii.org).

House of Lords' judgments delivered since 14 November 1996 are available on the House of Lords website (http://www.parliament.uk).

In addition, a number of commercial companies provide online access to legal judgments.

Medical Ethics Committee

A publication from the BMA's Medical Ethics Committee (MEC). The following people were members of the MEC for one or both of the two committee sessions this book was in preparation:

Dr Ian Bogle	Chairman of Council, BMA
Sir David Carter	President, BMA (2001–2002)
Sir Anthony Grabham	President, BMA (2002–2003)
Dr George Rae	Chairman of the Representative Body, BMA
Dr David Pickersgill	Treasurer, BMA (2002–2003)
Dr Michael Wilks	Chairman. Forensic medical examiner, London
Dr James Appleyard	Children's physician, Kent
Mr Dipak Banerjee	Consultant ophthalmologist, Wigan
Dr Anthony Calland (deputy)	General practitioner, Gwent
Professor Alastair Campbell	Professor of Ethics in Medicine, Bristol
Dr Mary Church	General practitioner, Glasgow
Ms Jennie Ciechan	Medical student, Edinburgh
Dr Peter Dangerfield	Medical academic, Liverpool
Professor Len Doyal	Professor of Medical Ethics, London
Ms Marie Fox	Senior lecturer in law, University of Manchester
Dr Alex Freeman	General practitioner, Southampton
Professor Robin Gill	Professor of Modern Theology, Canterbury
Professor Raanan Gillon	General practitioner and Professor of Medical Ethics, London
Dr Anita Goraya	General practitioner, London
Dr Evan Harris	Member of Parliament and former hospital doctor
Professor John Harris	Sir David Alliance Professor of Bioethics, Manchester
Dr Nick Jenkins (deputy)	SHO in emergency medicine, London
Dr Surendra Kumar	General practitioner, Widnes
Dr Geoffrey Lewis (deputy)	Consultant anaesthetist, Leicester
Professor Sheila McLean	Director of Institute of Law and Ethics, Glasgow
Dr Omer Moghraby	Junior doctor, London
Professor Jonathan Montgomery	Professor of Health Care Law, Southampton
Professor Derek Morgan	Professor in Health Care Law and Jurisprudence, Cardiff
Dr Jane Richards	Retired general practitioner, Exeter

Dr Peter Tiplady (deputy)	Public health physician, Carlisle
Dr Jeremy Wight	Public health physician, Sheffield
Dr M E Jan Wise	Psychiatrist, London

Thanks are due to other BMA committees and staff for providing information and commenting on draft chapters.

Acknowledgements

Thanks are due to the many people and organisations who gave so generously of their time in commenting on earlier drafts and discussing the very difficult medical, legal, and ethical issues with us. Although these contributions helped to inform the BMA's views, it should not be assumed that this guidance necessarily reflects the views of all those who contributed. Particular thanks are due to the following:

Dr Richard Ashcroft, Dr Susan Bewley, Ms Anne Clarke, Professor Angus Clarke, Ms Jane Denton, Professor Colin Drummond, Ms Sarah Elliston, Dr George Fernie, Dr Fleur Fisher, Dr Frances Flinter, Ms Ann Furedi, Professor Sally Glen, Dr Selina F Gray, Dr John Guillebaud, Mr Andrew Hobart, Ms Gillian Howard, Dr George Ikkos, Dr Michael Jarmulowicz, Dr Suzanne Kite, Ms Gerison Lansdown, Dr Graham Laurie, Dr Mhoira Leng, Ms Penny Letts, Ms Penney Lewis, Dr Donald Lyons, Dr Jane Marshall, Professor Kenyon Mason, Dr Alan Mitchell, Dr Ann Orme-Smith, Dr Keith Palmer, Dr Michael Parker, Dr Charles Saunders, Professor James Underwood, Dr Ivan Waddington and Dr Frank Wells.

Alzheimer's Society, Association of Medical Secretaries, Practice Managers, Administrators and Receptionists (AMSPAR), Association of Community Health Councils for England and Wales, British Fertility Society, CancerBACUP, Children and Family Court Advisory and Support Service, Consumers for Ethics in Research, Crown Office and Procurator Fiscal Service, Department of Health – Clinical Ethics and Human Tissue Branch, Department of Health – Information Policy Unit, Department of Health – Prison Health Policy Unit and Task Force, Department of Health – Teenage Pregnancy Unit, Doctor Patient Partnership, General Medical Council, Genetic Interest Group, Human Fertilisation and Embryology Authority, Human Genetics Commission, Marie Curie Centre Liverpool, Medical Foundation for the Care of Victims of Torture, Mental Health Alliance, Medical Protection Society, National Institute for Clinical Excellence, National Prescribing Centre, Northern Ireland Prison Service, Nursing and Midwifery Council, Progress Educational Trust, Royal College of Midwives, Royal College of Nursing, Royal College of Obstetricians and Gynaecologists, Royal College of Surgeons of Edinburgh, Royal Pharmaceutical Society, Sick Doctors Trust, The Medical and Dental Defence Union of Scotland, The Association for Palliative Medicine, The Patients Association.

Bridging the gap between theory and practice: the BMA's approach to medical ethics

> "The central moral objective of medicine – adhered to by doctors and health care workers since Hippocratic times – is to produce net medical benefit for the patient with as little harm as possible. Today we may add to that Hippocratic objective the moral qualifications that we should pursue it in a way that respects people's deliberated choices for themselves and that is just or fair to others (whether in the context of distribution of scarce resources, respect for people's rights, or respect for morally acceptable laws)."[1]

Doctors and medical students are concerned with the ethical practice of medicine; they are confronted with ethical issues, problems or dilemmas virtually every day of their working lives. Most of these issues are not new, and doctors have been responding to ethical challenges for centuries. Although in the past, however, it was acceptable for doctors to base their decisions on conscience, intuition, received wisdom, and codes of practice, changes in the nature of the doctor–patient relationship and in the accountability of doctors have demanded a more formal and explicit approach to medical ethics. Doctors are increasingly required to explain and justify their decisions to patients, other health care workers, the media, regulators, and the courts, and to each other. In order to do so they need skills in ethical reasoning combined with an understanding of the law and knowledge of professional guidance. This book is one part of the BMA's attempt to help doctors to achieve these objectives. In addition, links to useful websites, including organisations mentioned throughout this book, can be found on the BMA's website at: http://www.bma.org.uk.

The BMA and medical ethics

The British Medical Association, as the professional association for doctors in the UK, provides advice and guidance on a wide range of ethical issues. Unlike guidance from the General Medical Council (GMC), which has statutory, regulatory powers, the BMA's guidance is not binding on doctors, although it is intended to help them to practise medicine in an ethical manner and within the boundaries of what is legally and morally acceptable.

The BMA's role and standing in medical ethics has grown exponentially over recent years. Its influence in this area relies on a unique combination of two factors:

its extensive knowledge of the practical ethical dilemmas confronting doctors, through contact with its members, and the interdisciplinary and intellectual rigour provided by the members of its Medical Ethics Committee (MEC), who combine clinical, legal, philosophical, ethical, and theological expertise. These two factors have helped to develop a mechanism that not only provides confidential ethical advice for individual doctors but also ensures that the BMA is able to contribute to the development of public policy on a range of ethical issues. Its guidance and discussion papers have been quoted approvingly by the courts[2] and its views have been influential in Parliament and other policymaking arenas.[3]

Part of the role of the MEC, and the staff of the BMA who work with it, is to look ahead to identify future ethical dilemmas and begin the process of review and critical analysis in order to produce guidance and direction that is ethically robust. It is guided in doing so by the traditions of the medical profession and by policy developed through the BMA's representative framework (its Representative Body). Although the MEC's decisions are taken in the light of societal values, its role is not simply to reflect public opinion but sometimes to help to shape and develop it. An important part of the work of the MEC is to facilitate and encourage rational debate, among health professionals and wider society, about what are frequently very sensitive and emotive issues. This dual approach, of both providing ethical guidance for doctors and contributing to the development of public policy, is reflected in this book. Inevitably this means that the form of individual chapters differs; some chapters focus more on practical advice and others enter into more philosophical debate about aspects of public policy. Both are important for those using the book, whether practising doctors or students, since resolving both day to day questions and major dilemmas involves the same strands of reasoning.

Each chapter of this book centres on ethical questions with which doctors have to deal and on which advice from the BMA is frequently sought. The book, while informed by moral theory and the law, maintains a practical approach that has relevance for doctors' day to day experiences. Since doctors tend to need a quick and workable solution for an immediate case, the guidance focuses on practical responses to these common questions, but this process inevitably brings in reference to philosophy and law. Abortion, embryo research, and euthanasia, for example, raise weighty moral issues that must be explored to some degree, although the actual procedures are regulated by law in such a way that most questions about what is permissible can be answered briefly. Even superficially simple queries, such as how much information to give a patient, or whether children can choose treatment for themselves, cannot be answered fully without mentioning how legal cases and ethical discussions influence medical practice and vice versa. Law and ethics are therefore closely intertwined and, where the courts have provided useful criteria, this is reflected through the inclusion of case summaries. Information about major developments after the publication of this book will be placed on the BMA's website (http://www.bma.org.uk/ethics).

This introductory chapter aims to set out the context within which the BMA's more specific guidance and advice, given in the chapters that follow, can be applied. It discusses what is meant by medical ethics and how this has changed over time. It also gives very practical guidance on how to approach an ethical dilemma, draws attention to the interaction between ethics and law, and highlights the importance of doctors being familiar with both legal and professional guidance. For some readers this will be sufficient to put the rest of the book into context and to provide the guidance needed to resolve day to day dilemmas. Those who are interested in the philosophy and theory that underpin the guidance, however, will find at the end of this chapter a brief thumbnail sketch of the main philosophical approaches to medical ethics and a short illustration of how each of these theories relates to modern day medical practice.

What is medical ethics?

Medical ethics is the application of ethical reasoning to medical decision making. It is a rich and varied discipline often involving appeal to different perspectives and principles as well as taking account of information and guidance of various sorts. It is concerned with critical reflection about "norms or values, good or bad, right or wrong, and what ought or ought not to be done in the context of medical practice".[4] It deals with ordinary everyday practice as well as with the unusual, dramatic, and contentious. Medical ethics often involves a search for morally acceptable and reasoned answers in situations where different moral concerns, interests, or priorities conflict. This involves critical scrutiny of the issues and careful consideration of various options. Here medical ethics may often be as much concerned with the process through which a decision is reached as with the decision itself. As well as referring to critical moral reflection in the context of medical practice, the term "medical ethics" is also used to refer to more traditional views of the subject as "the standards of professional competence and conduct which the medical profession expects of its members".[5] (The shift from "traditional" to "analytical" medical ethics is discussed below.)

Even when principles and agreed moral norms are set out as professional standards in ethical codes or guidance on good practice, the challenge for health professionals is often to extrapolate from those general principles to individual circumstances. This may require a careful assessment of morally relevant concerns and interests that need to be taken into account in reaching a decision. The BMA, through both its written guidance and its individual advice to doctors, aims to facilitate this process, not by telling doctors what to do but rather by helping them to explore the issues thoroughly in order to reach a decision they can justify with soundly reasoned arguments.

As the BMA's role is to provide advice to and guidance for doctors, this book focuses primarily on the tensions and dilemmas that arise in the doctor–patient relationship and on the role of doctors in influencing public policy. Although it refers throughout to "medical ethics", the BMA recognises that this is one subset of the broader discipline of "healthcare ethics". The advice provided is set within the context of an increasingly multidisciplinary working environment in which the emphasis is placed strongly on teamwork and partnership. The practice of medicine does not, of course, involve just doctors and their patients, it also concerns other health professionals, managers, administrators, other healthcare workers, families, and carers. Although specifically written for doctors, this book is of relevance to all those involved in the provision of health care.

The transition from "traditional" to "analytical" medical ethics

Ethics has been a central concern of medicine for at least 2500 years; the Hippocratic Oath and its successors have expressed a fundamental medical duty to pursue patients' best medical interests, to avoid harming or exploiting them, and to maintain their confidences. Until the middle of the twentieth century, paternalism was the norm and "traditional" medical ethics was less concerned with respect for patients' autonomy and with justice. Typically, the clinical interests of individual patients were the doctor's overriding ethical concern. Ethical norms were imparted and enforced in the process of medical socialisation, and reinforced by written codes, typically based on the Hippocratic Oath, without explicit analysis of the issues. In addition to substantive ethical obligations, such as those noted above, such codes contained matters that today would be considered etiquette rather than ethics: consultation procedures; the proper demeanour of doctors to patients and to each other; appropriate attitudes to medical teachers; and limits on advertising, including the size of brass nameplates.

A turning point in medical ethics is widely agreed to have occurred after the Second World War, although explanations for this vary. They include: the medical atrocities of the Nazi doctors; changing social attitudes, including less deference to authority; more assertive attitudes to individual rights and self determination; a shift from the preoccupation of medical ethics with the individual patient at the expense of the community; the increasing plurality of cultural and religious norms within some nations, including the UK; and the development of a system of internationally recognised human rights (see below). As well as all these factors, medicine itself began to develop a wide variety of ever more powerful and expensive technologies, including those with the capacity to prolong life, alter psychological states, impede and enhance reproductive capacity, and, more recently, change our genetic structure.

It is hardly surprising that medical ethics had to develop towards a more analytical approach in response to such changes. This approach has seen a clear shift from the previous reliance on medical paternalism to a doctor–patient partnership approach, adding respect for patients' autonomy and an increasing awareness of justice to the traditional "Hippocratic" concern to provide health benefits with minimal harm. This shift has been reflected in the number, nature, and complexity of the enquiries received by the medical ethics department of the BMA.

Two concepts of medical ethics are now acknowledged: "traditional medical ethics" – seen as the professional norms and standards of medical practice – and "analytical medical ethics" – seen as the critical process through which substantive ethical claims are justified (or criticised) in the light of argument and counterargument. This second type of medical ethics informs the first type and is itself informed by a wide variety of perspectives, including those of our multicultural society and of various academic disciplines such as moral philosophy, law, the social sciences, history, and theology. Thus medical ethics has ceased to be the sole domain of doctors and has become, as Kennedy advocated, "part of the general moral and ethical order by which we live" and increasingly in practice "tested against the ethical principles of society".[6]

Medical ethics and human rights

Modern medical ethics has grown partly from philosophy plus the traditional duties expressed in professional codes and from the concepts of "rights" that became incorporated into many aspects of modern culture in the second part of the twentieth century. Many aspects of the way in which concepts of human rights are reflected in law have implications for medicine (and these are set out in a separate BMA publication[7]). Perhaps even more importantly, the language of human rights and the underlying theory that all people have the same legal rights merely by reason of being human have affected medical ethics.

The United Nations' Universal Declaration of Human Rights[8] of 1948 ushered in an era in which ideas of personal autonomy and "rights" came to be seen as central in many parts of the world, including Britain and Europe. The international and legal concepts about human dignity, self determination, freedom from interference, and welfare protection articulated in the UN Declaration were defined further in international covenants in the 1970s.[9] These detailed two broad categories of human rights: "liberty" rights (freedom from certain things) and "entitlement" or "welfare" rights (to receive certain benefits). Freedom from torture or unfair punishment[10] is a typical example of the former. Rights to a fair wage, education, and "the enjoyment of the highest attainable standard of physical and mental health"[11] exemplify the latter. Some (but not all) of these basic notions of human rights were enacted in European[12] and domestic legislation. In the UK, this was in the form of the Human Rights Act 1998 (see below), which focuses more on being free from interference than the right to receive specific benefits.

For clarity, any discussion of "rights" needs to distinguish between "moral" and legally enforceable rights. In much ethical debate, the rights under discussion are moral ones ("he had a right to know his child was ill"). Human rights, however, are legally enforceable and generally non-negotiable (although some rights are progressively implemented according to resources and some legitimate interference with rights is permitted).

Many of the concepts that feature heavily in modern ethical analysis are either derived from statements of human rights or reflect them closely, but they are couched in terms of moral rights and duties. These rights can seem more vague than "human rights" precisely because they may be debatable; the moral claims of different individuals can clash. A's right to confidentiality can conflict with B's right to know. Ethical concepts are part of a problem solving tool that takes into account the context of the dilemma in order to balance out such conflicts of moral rights. Since they are set out in law, human rights are not dependent upon context in the same way and they are less flexible even though there is scope for legitimate debate concerning their interpretation in some contexts.

Practical approaches to medical ethics

It is not necessary for doctors to be experts in academic law or philosophy in order to address the type of dilemmas that arise in medical practice. Doctors, like everybody else, have their own views – their own philosophy – of what medicine should strive to achieve and how best to achieve that in an individual case or with an individual patient. However, they do not, necessarily intuitively know the action to take in every situation nor, indeed, how most appropriately to respond when their own view of the right action diverges from that of their patient. During their training, medical students learn the art of critical analysis and the basic principles and virtues that should influence their behaviour. These skills need to be honed and practised throughout a doctor's career. The methods used for this critical analysis vary. Some people adopt what has come to be called the "four principles approach"[13] or some modification on this theme. Although people may disagree about their underlying philosophical, religious, cultural, or political beliefs, they probably can agree, at a minimum, that commitments to promoting benefit (beneficence) and avoiding or minimising harms (non-maleficence), to respecting people and their autonomy (respect for autonomy), and to fairness (the principle of justice), provide a sound basis for consideration of moral obligations in health care. Assessing the relevance of each of these principles to a particular situation will not provide "the answer", but such principles can provide a mechanism for analysing the problem in a rigorous manner and for ensuring that all morally relevant concerns have been considered.[14] Another practical approach to ethics is to use narrative or storytelling in order to give the problem context, by looking at the patient's situation as a whole rather than considering a particular dilemma in isolation.[15] Considering the dilemma from different viewpoints provides a way of ensuring that all relevant perspectives and perceptions are considered.

The BMA takes a reasoned eclectic approach to ethical analysis, combining elements of both practical and philosophical approaches (see pages 17–20). The MEC itself also combines people from a variety of moral and occupational backgrounds. When considering ethical problems, the BMA is concerned with the narratives or stories central to particular cases. These are addressed with an awareness of widely accepted general principles, of legal and professional guidelines and obligations, and of previously settled cases, both uncontentious and hotly disputed. Principles and virtues, duties and consequences, community orientated perspectives, and individual or patient orientated perspectives are considered.

In its attempt to provide a very practical and "hands on" approach to medical ethics, the BMA tends to use key concepts that are familiar to practising doctors. All of these concepts can be seen as aspects of the central moral obligation to respect persons; they include: self determination or "autonomy"; honesty, consent, and confidentiality; best interests, benefits, and harms; and fairness, equity, and the avoidance of unfair discrimination. Most of the ethical dilemmas encountered, whether in the questions that doctors ask the BMA to address or in the public policy aspects of its work, tend to concern one or more of these key concepts.

Key concepts in medical ethics

Self determination: the ability to think, choose, decide, and act for oneself, also sometimes referred to as "autonomy". There is a prima facie moral obligation to respect people's self determination insofar as such respect is compatible with equal respect for the self determination of all those potentially affected.

Honesty: the communication of information in ways that are believed to be truthful and that are not intended in any way to deceive the recipient.

Consent: competent patients have the right to give or withhold consent to treatment or invasive procedures irrespective of the outcome.

Confidentiality: patients are entitled to confidentiality, but that right is not absolute; there may be cases where an overriding public interest would justify a breach of confidentiality.

Harm and benefit: the overall aim of medical treatment should be to promote (health) benefit and minimise harm to all parties involved. When patients are competent they are the best judges of benefit and harm for themselves. When they are not competent to give or withhold consent, only treatment and intervention that is in their overall best interests should be provided. With safeguards, certain exceptions may be justified where interventions are of minimal or negligible harm and are of benefit to others, as for example in non-therapeutic research involving minor interventions such as blood tests.

Fairness or equity: individuals should be treated fairly and should not be inappropriately discriminated against in the provision of health services.

Approaching an ethical issue or dilemma

The way in which individuals approach an ethical issue or dilemma varies and depends, at least in part, on the complexity of the question. Many decisions raise ethical issues but can nonetheless be easily and quickly resolved. This could be by reference to the general duties of a doctor, such as the duty of confidentiality, or, in more specific cases, by referral to relevant law or professional guidance, such as to determine who may give consent on behalf of a young child. In more complex cases, particularly where duties to different parties conflict, more detailed consideration is needed to ensure that the dilemma is subject to a thorough and robust critical analysis. Over a number of years the BMA's ethics department has developed its own methodology for helping doctors to analyse and resolve ethical questions. This approach involves up to six separate stages.

Approaching an ethical dilemma

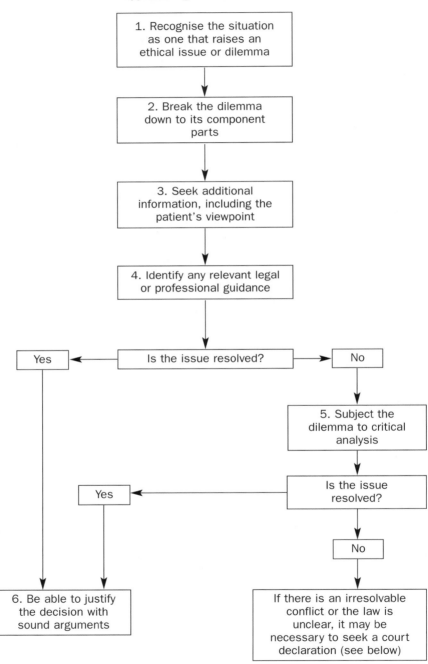

1. Recognise the situation as one that raises an ethical issue or dilemma

2. Break the dilemma down to its component parts

3. Seek additional information, including the patient's viewpoint

4. Identify any relevant legal or professional guidance

Yes ← Is the issue resolved? → No

5. Subject the dilemma to critical analysis

Yes ← Is the issue resolved?

No

6. Be able to justify the decision with sound arguments

If there is an irresolvable conflict or the law is unclear, it may be necessary to seek a court declaration (see below)

1. Recognise the situation as one that raises an ethical issue or dilemma

This may initially appear to be an obvious point, but in practice many difficulties and complaints have arisen because doctors have failed to recognise that there is an ethical issue, or a potential conflict of interest, in their proposed action. Alternatively, they know and understand the principles but fail to apply them to individual circumstances. Responding to a relative's enquiry about a patient's health, without the patient's consent, is an obvious example in which a breach of confidentiality can occur unintentionally as a result of the doctor failing to identify the ethical issues raised by the enquiry.

The fact that a situation raises issues of clinical judgment does not mean that it does not also have an ethical dimension; the two categories of problems are not mutually exclusive and many dilemmas require both clinical knowledge and ethical reasoning to be resolved satisfactorily. Deciding whether to provide a very expensive new treatment, for example, not only depends upon a clinical assessment of the individual patient, but also requires consideration of the opportunity costs for others and the principles of fairness in the allocation of limited resources. In order to recognise that a situation raises ethical issues it is important for health professionals to be constantly aware of the possibility of conflict arising and also to keep up to date with professional and legal guidance. A situation can be seen to raise ethical issues when it appeals to, for example, interests, values, fairness, justice, rights, autonomy, or civil liberties. Where the general principles that would normally be relied upon for dealing with such issues are either of no help or come into conflict with one another, the situation can be seen to raise an ethical problem or dilemma.[16] These are situations where there are good moral reasons to act in two or more different ways, each of which is also in some way morally flawed.

2. Break the dilemma down into its component parts

Many of the ethical enquiries that are referred to the BMA's ethics department are complex and involve long and detailed accounts of the situation. Although it is important to be aware of the full situation in order to consider the dilemma in context, it is also important mentally to clear away some of the excess information in order to identify the key issues raised by the dilemma. For example, are the key issues ones of confidentiality or consent, or balancing benefits and harms to different individuals?

3. Seek additional information, including the patient's viewpoint

Having identified the key issues, the next stage is to build up information to assist with the process of analysing the situation. This may involve identifying whether more facts or information are needed in order to consider the issue. For example, if the enquiry concerns consent for the treatment of a child or young person, a crucial assessment is whether the young person is sufficiently mature to make the decision. It may also be necessary, if the child is very young, to make enquiries about whether the father has parental responsibility and so is legally able to give consent on behalf of the child. The type of information that is needed varies depending on the circumstances; part of the role of this book is to identify the factors that are relevant to take into account.

As medical ethics involves an approach to care that is patient-centred, it is essential that, wherever possible, the patient's viewpoint is taken into account. As part of identifying the facts, therefore, doctors need to find out what the patient thinks rather than relying on their own assumptions. This is a stage that is frequently overlooked. For example, a doctor may seek advice from the BMA's ethics department about whether it would be ethically acceptable to publish an interesting case study provided all identifying information is removed. In many cases, the doctor has not asked the patient whether he or she would be willing to consent to the information being published and, when making such an approach, finds that the patient is very happy to agree. Alternatively, a doctor may be concerned about whether particularly sensitive information should be revealed in response to a request from a patient's solicitor, but has not discussed these concerns with the patient to determine whether the disclosure authorised extends to this information.

In addition to facts about the case, it is also necessary to ensure that the action proposed is not contrary to the law or to guidance issued by the GMC, which is binding on all doctors.

4. Identify any relevant legal or professional guidance

Depending upon the complexity of the issue, it may be necessary to identify and collect information from a range of sources to be taken into account in reaching a decision. This could include:

- any relevant statute or case law about the subject (see pages 12–14)
- any relevant guidance from the GMC (see pages 14–15)
- any relevant guidance from professional bodies, such as the BMA, the Royal Colleges or other organisations such as the Department of Health, the Human Fertilisation and Embryology Authority, or the Human Genetics Commission.

Advice may also be sought from the doctor's defence body and should always be obtained when the situation involves questions of clinical competence.

In addition to providing the BMA's ethical guidance, this book also contains a summary of the relevant statute and case law, GMC guidance, and guidance from other organisations. Further advice, and links to other useful organisations, can be found on the BMA's website or obtained from the BMA's medical ethics department.

With some enquiries, accessing additional information provides a straightforward answer to the question. For example, GPs sometimes ask the BMA whether patients can have access to all of their medical records, including reports prepared by other health professionals. The law, and guidance, are clear that patients have a statutory right of access to the whole of their medical record with only limited exceptions (see chapter 6 on health records). Subject to those limited exceptions, access must be given. Some ethical problems and dilemmas are more complex and require a careful balancing of the competing interests and so the next stage of the process is required.

5. Subject the dilemma to critical analysis

When making difficult ethical decisions, doctors may need to seek and take account of the views of other members of the healthcare team who may have a different perspective or additional information to contribute. Having identified the key issues and collected together the facts and other information relevant to the decision, the information needs to be analysed to consider the competing interests and to reach the most appropriate solution. Doctors frequently have to make such decisions quickly and in very stressful circumstances; they are not expected to be omniscient, but they are expected to act reasonably in the circumstances and to be able to justify their decisions. Keeping up to date with professional guidance on a regular basis and knowing where to find such guidance when it is needed can prepare doctors to confront difficult ethical dilemmas.

Duties owed to different parties often conflict. A common enquiry to the BMA concerns requests from police officers for copies of patients' medical records. There is a duty of confidentiality to patients, but doctors also have to consider their duty to protect others from harm. Legally, the police do not have an automatic right of access to patient records but can obtain a court order that obliges the doctor to comply. The GMC's guidance states that "you should not disclose personal information to a third party such as a solicitor, police officer or officer of a court without the patient's express consent" except in limited specified circumstances.[17] It states that "disclosure of personal information without consent may be justified where failure to do so may expose the patient or others to risk of death or serious harm".[18] Doctors asked by the police for access to a patient's records in connection with a criminal investigation must therefore balance their duty of confidentiality to the patient against their duty to protect people from risk of death or serious harm. Among the factors that need to be taken into account in deciding how to proceed are:

- Is it possible to obtain the patient's consent to disclosure? If not:
- What is the crime and is it sufficiently serious for the public interest to prevail?
- Is the patient, or are others, at risk of death or serious harm?
- Would the task of preventing or detecting the crime be seriously prejudiced by refusing access to the medical record?

- Is the information sought available from another source that would not necessitate a breach of doctor–patient confidentiality?
- What, if any, information on the medical record is relevant and should therefore be considered for disclosure?

Based on an assessment of these types of factors, the doctor needs to decide whether to accede to the request. In some cases disclosure to the police will be justified; in others it will not. Sometimes the police will seek a court order if access is refused; this situation is discussed in chapter 5.

6. Be able to justify the decision with sound arguments

Some doctors may find it helpful in reaching a decision to discuss the dilemma, on an anonymous basis, with a colleague, the BMA, or their defence body. Ultimately, however, the doctor who is responsible for the patient's care must make the decision about how to proceed, be prepared to justify it, and explain his or her reasoning. For example, doctors who decide to withdraw treatment that is prolonging life should be able to demonstrate, from both a clinical and an ethical perspective, on what basis the decision was reached. If the patient was competent, discussions with him or her should be recorded in the medical record. If the patient was not competent, the doctor should be able and willing to explain why providing the treatment was not considered to be in his or her best interests. Information should be recorded on the medical record about any guidance referred to or any additional advice sought.

In some cases, it is not possible for the healthcare team and the patient to resolve the dilemma, either because there is an apparently irresolvable conflict or because the law is unclear. In such cases it may be necessary to seek a court declaration (see below).

The relationship between ethics and law

Problems that doctors refer to the BMA frequently involve aspects of both law and ethics. Current guidance for doctors has sometimes evolved through court judgments on what are both legal issues and complex moral dilemmas. Therefore, some case examples illustrating specific points of law have been included in the following chapters. Almost without exception, the judgments in these cases contain a wealth of knowledge, wisdom, and skill in the art of critical analysis, and some discuss fundamental questions like "when does life begin?" and "what does it mean to be alive?". Increasingly it is recognised that the types of issues addressed by medical law – from control of reproduction and fertility to whether people can claim assistance to die – have important philosophical, ethical, sociological, religious, and political dimensions as well as legal ones.[19] The relationship between ethics and law is a reciprocal one: "law frames the setting within which ethical choices may be practically exercised, but ethics frames the limits within which law is voluntarily obeyed and respected as an expression of the values and aspirations of the society in which it applies".[20] The two are, to a large extent, inseparable: "it is pointless to attempt to disengage the moral from the legal dispute – when we talk about legal rules, we are inevitably drawn into a discussion of moral rules".[21]

Doctors are required to follow the law. In medical matters, doctors are also frequently involved in debates about the law: what the law is, what the law should be, and sometimes seeking to promote changes to the law. In many high profile medicolegal cases, such as those of Re F (see Chapter 7, pages 236–7) or Tony Bland (see Chapter 10, page 359), the role of the court was to consider the facts of the case and issue a declaration about the lawfulness of the proposed action. In this way, the courts provide a protective role for doctors, giving reassurance of the legality of their actions. In such cases, the courts take into account the views of doctors and of bodies like the BMA when deciding what satisfies the necessary legal test of what constitutes a "responsible body of medical opinion" (see Chapter 21, pages 747–8). In many cases, the courts also issue guidance to doctors for future cases. In the chapters that follow, examples are given of the types of cases in which, if agreement cannot be reached between the parties involved or if the law is unclear, a court declaration may be required.

Some law is set out in statute, such as the Abortion Act 1967 or the Human Fertilisation and Embryology Act 1990, while other aspects of law, such as most of the law around consent, is common (judge made) law. In deciding cases, judges follow the precedents set out in previous cases; the common law is formed by the rules that are extracted from those decisions (this is often also referred to as case law). Recognising the difficulty for busy doctors of keeping up to date with changes in the law, this book draws attention to relevant legal provisions. Major developments following its publication will be included on the BMA's website. Where relevant, differences in the law applicable in England and Wales, Scotland and Northern Ireland are highlighted in the text.

The Human Rights Act 1998

The Human Rights Act 1998, which came fully into force in October 2000, incorporated into UK law the bulk of the substantive rights set out in the European Convention for the Protection of Human Rights and Fundamental Freedoms.[22] It is particularly important for doctors to be aware of this piece of legislation because they are required to observe the rights of the Convention (see box below) in reaching decisions and must be able to demonstrate that they have done so. This should not, however, represent a major change in practice for health professionals since the requirements of the Human Rights Act reflect, very closely, existing good practice. Decisions taken by doctors on the basis of current ethical standards are likely to be compliant with the Act. Issues such as human dignity, communication and consultation, and best interests, which are central to good clinical practice, are also pivotal to the Convention rights.

Convention rights with particular relevance to the practice of medicine

Article 2 – right to life
Article 3 – right to freedom from torture or inhuman or degrading treatment or punishment
Article 5 – right to liberty and security
Article 6 – right to a fair trial
Article 8 – right to respect for private and family life
Article 9 – freedom of thought, conscience and religion
Article 10 – freedom of expression
Article 12 – right to marry and found a family
Article 14 – enjoyment of these rights to be secured without discrimination.

In making medical decisions, doctors must consider whether an individual's human rights are affected and, if so, whether it is legitimate to interfere with those rights. Any interference with a Convention right must be proportionate to the intended objective. This means that, even if there is a legitimate reason for interfering with a particular right, the desired outcome must be sufficient to justify the level of interference proposed. Where different rights come into conflict, doctors must be able to justify choosing one over the other in a particular case. The BMA has issued specific guidance on the impact of the Human Rights Act on medical decision making[23] and throughout the following chapters reference is made, where appropriate, to areas of practice that could be open to challenge under the Act. This book also highlights medical cases where a challenge has been made using the Human Rights Act.

The General Medical Council

Guidance issued by the GMC is binding on all doctors and failure to comply with it can result in a finding of serious professional misconduct with a range of sanctions including, ultimately, erasure from the medical register. All registered medical practitioners are sent copies of the GMC's guidance and it is essential that doctors familiarise themselves with it and keep it in a safe place for future reference. The guidance is also available on the GMC's website (http://www.gmc-uk.org). In addition, this book makes reference to relevant GMC guidance and demonstrates how to apply it to specific circumstances. The GMC provides both statements about the general duties of a doctor (see below) and specific advice for particular situations.

The GMC's guidance on the duties of a doctor

"Patients must be able to trust doctors with their lives and wellbeing. To justify that trust, we as a profession have a duty to maintain a good standard of practice and care and to show respect for human life. In particular, as a doctor you must:

- make the care of your patient your first concern
- treat every patient politely and considerately
- respect patients' dignity and privacy
- listen to patients and respect their views
- give patients information in a way they can understand
- respect the rights of patients to be fully involved in decisions about their care
- keep your professional knowledge and skills up to date
- recognise the limits of your professional competence
- be honest and trustworthy
- respect and protect confidential information
- make sure that your personal beliefs do not prejudice your patients' care
- act quickly to protect patients from risk if you have good reason to believe that you or a colleague may not be fit to practise
- avoid abusing your position as a doctor
- work with colleagues in the ways that best serve patients' interests.

In all these matters you must never discriminate unfairly against your patients or colleagues. And you must always be prepared to justify your actions to them."[24]

In the chapters that follow, some examples are given of cases where doctors have failed to meet the standards set by the GMC and have been found guilty of serious professional misconduct. The intention of doing so is not to draw attention to the specific failings of those doctors but to warn others of the type of conduct that could bring their registration into question.

Philosophical approaches to medical ethics

For those who are interested in the theory underpinning much of the ethical discussion in this book, brief and simplified accounts of some of the main philosophical approaches to medical ethics are given below. It is not the role of this book to provide a detailed account of these different approaches; other publications fulfil this role admirably for those who wish to explore them in more detail.[25]

Deontological ethics: focuses primarily on duties ("deontology" comes from the Greek for "duty" or "what is due"). Such theories are based on certain principles, such as respect for persons, which should be followed. Kant, the most significant exponent of this view, held that people should never be treated merely as means to an end but always as ends in themselves and that people should act as if they were legislating for a kingdom of such ends in themselves – variants of Kant's famous "categorical imperative". Kant's views have been influential in the development of medical ethics, perhaps because they fit well with modern day concepts of respect for individuals and their autonomy. It is sometimes not realised, however, that Kant's notion of autonomy is a highly demanding one according to which people are autonomous only insofar as they act in the pursuit of their moral duty. Contemporary accounts of autonomy – literally "self rule" – tend to interpret it as reasoned self determination, rather than reasoned self determination in the pursuit of one's moral duty. A second point about Kantian notions of respect for individuals' autonomy that is sometimes forgotten is that it has to take into account the autonomy of all other potentially affected people in the "kingdom of ends". Many of the moral dilemmas that arise in medical practice are those in which doctors' duties to different people conflict.

Consequentialist ethics: (such as utilitarianism) focuses on consequences, with the basic aim of maximising welfare, or utility, or in some way achieving "the greatest good for the greatest number". It is clearly important for doctors to take account of the consequences of their decisions and to provide the maximum net benefit for their patients. Leaving aside some of the inherent difficulties of deciding what is meant by welfare or happiness and how it should be measured, however, a major criticism of a solely consequentialist approach is that it can result in morally counterintuitive outcomes. Certain moral principles that intuitively seem appropriate to govern our relationships with each other, such as respect for other people and their autonomy or justice and honesty, can be dispensed with when greater overall welfare would derive from ignoring those principles.[26] Some variations of consequentialism, such as rule utilitarianism, attempt to overcome this problem by weighing the consequences of acting according to general moral rules.[27] A more recent variant of utilitarianism attempts to combine adherence to widely accepted intuitive moral principles, such as honesty and fairness, with a readiness to switch to utilitarian "critical reasoning" about overall welfare in cases where it is clear that overall welfare may be seriously undermined by sticking to the intuitive moral principle.[28]

Communitarian ethics: focuses on both the responsibilities and the rights of individuals, and advocates policies based on consensus rather than compromise. It asserts that individual rights need to be balanced against responsibilities to the community and suggests that a concern for others should be taken into account when decisions are made. This approach comes to the fore when considering the health and wellbeing of communities rather than individuals, and so is particularly relevant in relation to the public health dimensions of medical practice, although it is also relevant in other areas of clinical medicine. It has also gained renewed interest in the light of developments in genetics, which emphasise the interrelatedness of individuals and of their interests. Theories based on notions of community, however, tend to have difficulties explaining why practices such as female genital mutilation or sexual abuse would be wrong if a particular community approves of them.[29] They also raise concerns about conflict and discrimination within the group and questions about the extent to which individuals may and should be sacrificed for the good of the community.

Virtue ethics: is derived from Aristotelian ethics and embeds ethics in people's characters rather than in general principles. It is concerned with the character traits of an individual rather than his or her actions; with "what shall I be?" rather than "what shall I do?". Thus, someone who displays characteristics such as kindness, care, respect for others, honesty, and compassion, will be a "model of moral conduct".[30] Such traits clearly form an important part of what it means to be a doctor, and unquestionably help doctors to act in an ethical manner. The benefit of virtue theories to those confronted by ethical dilemmas is that they question what a virtuous person would do in such circumstances. They also highlight what is expected of doctors by society and by their peers. Although theorists who concentrate on moral principles do not deny the importance of virtue and virtues, they argue that the very decision that a character trait is virtuous requires reference to some general moral principle or norm and that both principles and virtues are needed for moral life.

Core values for medical practitioners

In 1994 the BMA called together representatives of a number of other medical bodies to discuss whether and, if so, how the core values of the profession were changing.[31] More than 800 doctors from a range of grades and disciplines were asked to help to define, and rank in order of importance, the values they saw as most relevant to their profession. The core values most doctors saw as enduring and relevant medical principles, combining both skills and virtues, were:

- competence
- caring
- commitment
- integrity
- compassion
- responsibility
- confidentiality
- spirit of enquiry
- advocacy.

Bridging the gap between theory and practice

In the form set out in the previous section, the philosophical theories discussed above can appear abstract and totally unconnected to day to day decision making. In practice, however, the type of ethical decisions made in relation to health care are underpinned to a greater or lesser extent by these philosophical approaches.

Sometimes the law gives clear direction to doctors, such as that a competent adult has the right to refuse life prolonging treatment even if the refusal would result in the patient's death (see chapter 2). This does not mean, however, that this situation is unproblematic from an ethical perspective or that everyone would agree that this is the right approach. People's views on such issues depend upon a range of factors, including their religious, cultural or political beliefs. Some people have views closer to one philosophical approach than another, even though they may not articulate them in that way, and this also affects the way they approach such dilemmas. Thus, a general understanding of different moral theories can help to show how and why ethical problems in medicine are often formulated and resolved in different, and sometimes competing, ways. It also explains why doctors sometimes disagree about the best way to resolve ethical dilemmas raised by specific clinical circumstances. Despite the different approaches that individual doctors may adopt, however, their actions must be consistent with the law and with the expectations of the society in which they practise. In the UK, this means that greater emphasis is generally placed on autonomy relative to other values.

There is general agreement about the basic ethical duties of doctors: to produce net medical benefit to their patients with minimum harm; to respect the autonomy of their patients; and to exercise these duties in a fair and unprejudiced way. Difficulties and dilemmas arise, however, because of the different ways that individual doctors interpret these duties and how they should be applied in individual cases, or because these basic duties come into conflict, requiring judgments to be made about the appropriate weight to be given to each.

Refusal of life prolonging treatment[32]

Ms X is 36 years old. She is married with two children and is part of a closeknit extended family. After a road traffic accident, Ms X is paralysed from the neck down and is unable to breathe unaided. After extensive investigations her doctors have informed her that she is unlikely to develop any movement and will be dependent on the ventilator for the rest of her life. Ms X is competent and is able to speak and interact with her family and friends. Discussions about her prognosis have taken place over a number of weeks, involving all members of the healthcare team, her family and close friends, and, at her request, the local priest. After these discussions Ms X has expressed her wish to have the ventilator disconnected, after she has had time to say goodbye to her family. She knows that this will result in her death and she accepts this. Members of her family are very distressed by her decision and feel that she is letting them down, believing that she should continue with treatment at least until her children are old enough to understand. They ask the doctors to continue treatment contrary to her wishes. The doctors explain that the patient is competent and thus is legally entitled to make this decision for herself and that they cannot continue to provide treatment without her consent. Although there is a clear legal solution to this situation, views within the healthcare team and the family are mixed about the ethical position.

Some doctors believe that their actions should be primarily focused on maximising the health and welfare of their patients, rather than their practice being hindered by following what they perceive to be the unwise and harmful wishes of an individual patient. This focus on the consequences of intervention may lead the doctor to believe it would be morally wrong to follow the wishes of Ms X, which would, in the view of these doctors, clearly be harmful to her because it would result in her death. Clinicians who take this approach – who focus primarily on the consequences of their action – are embracing one interpretation of utilitarian moral reasoning. These doctors, despite being aware that continuing to provide the treatment would be unlawful, would not personally wish to be involved in its withdrawal because such action offends their own moral views.

Other doctors may place more moral emphasis on the right of patients to be autonomous: the right of Ms X to plan her own life and make her own decisions about what represents a harm and what represents a benefit for herself, even if these choices are deemed by others to be irrational or harmful. According to this view, to do otherwise would be an affront to those very attributes that underscore human dignity: reason and choice. Those who take this position – who believe that their primary duty is to respect the views of the patient, even though this may lead to harmful consequences – could be seen as endorsing a deontological approach to ethics, one more concerned with duty than with the consequences of what might happen through doing one's duty.

It would be misleading, however, to imply that a doctor adopting a consequentialist approach would inevitably be morally opposed to withdrawing treatment. Another doctor may focus on the consequences of ignoring individuals' wishes and argue, also on utilitarian grounds, that more satisfaction would be produced for more people by following individuals' wishes. Similarly, a third doctor may argue, on deontological grounds, that the primary duty of a doctor is not to respect autonomy but to save and protect human life.

Although personal autonomy and individual decision making generally take precedence in modern liberal democracies, this is not always or necessarily the case. Those who adopt a more communitarian approach to ethics focus less on the individual's personal wishes and more on the views and needs of the community as a whole. More weight could therefore be given to the views of members of Ms X's family and friends, and on the needs and future welfare of her children. Rather than focusing solely on her right to make the decision, Ms X could be encouraged to consider her duty to make a decision that promotes the wellbeing of her family. Some doctors would consider that she has a moral obligation to continue treatment for the sake of her children or the rest of her family. The fact that individuals are perceived to have moral obligations, however, does not mean that they necessarily can or should be forced to fulfil them, still less that the law should be used to enforce those obligations or even morality more generally.

Another important moral perspective that informs our understanding of good clinical practice focuses on the moral character of doctors, arguing that the virtues they exhibit in their professional lives are as important in ensuring good clinical practice as specific moral beliefs. This is because the ability to do what is right – however this may be defined – still demands attitudes and personal skills that cannot in themselves be reduced to moral beliefs about what is right. For example, decisions about how to break bad news to patients like Ms X, and to discuss openly with them the nature and severity of their condition, are indeed influenced by the degree to which clinicians take the rights of patients seriously. However, believing that information of a certain kind should be communicated is not the same as having, say, the courage to do so in the face of the patient's distress or the prudence not overly to burden patients with detailed explanations that they clearly do not want. Similarly, knowing and believing that Ms X's wishes should be followed still requires doctors to have the strength of character and compassion to carry out her wishes in a professional and sensitive manner. Courage, prudence and compassion are examples of the virtues emphasised by those who argue that it is just as important to build moral character in medical students and young doctors as it is to teach them philosophical theories about the moral basis of good clinical practice. (The concern that moral virtues are sometimes overlooked in the pursuit of scientific excellence is discussed in chapter 1.)

As has been demonstrated, it is not the case that a particular philosophical approach will lead inevitably to a particular outcome in any given scenario, and this message is reinforced throughout this book. By recognising the moral approach underpinning their views, however, doctors can be clearer about what their beliefs are and why, and will be better able to articulate their reasons for advocating one course of moral action rather than another. Ultimately, however, doctors must be able to reconcile their own approach with both the expectations of society and the requirements of the law and their regulatory body.

The approach taken in this book

In all societies, some values are given prominence over others. In the UK, it is thought that the law now generally gives greater weight to autonomy compared with other values; this is reflected both within the practice of medicine generally and in the discussion throughout this book. Patients are, nonetheless, encouraged in all situations to consider the impact of their decisions on others. We also emphasise that patients have certain responsibilities as well as rights, although the extent to which these responsibilities can be enforced varies depending on the circumstances. In addition, there are some specialties in which personal autonomy inevitably gives way to a more communitarian approach. A clear example is in discussion about public health dimensions of medical practice, where individual wishes may need to yield to the greater good of the community. Similarly, developments in genetics can be seen to exemplify the interrelatedness of people's interests and this represents an area in which the notion of a truly autonomous and personal decision is questionable.

In providing practical advice and guidance, the BMA considers and balances a range of different philosophical approaches to address different situations. We take account of duties as well as consequences, autonomy as well as the needs of the community, and throughout we reflect the principles and virtues that make a good doctor. We provide information on the law and on the professional guidance available, as well as exploring why, in some cases, doctors can, equally vehemently, adopt opposing views about what is "right" and "wrong" in relation to a particular issue. In doing so, our aim is to help health professionals to engage in the practice of analytical medical ethics in order to promote and facilitate the ethical practice of medicine.

References

1 Gillon R. Patients in the persistent vegetative state: a response to Dr Andrews. *BMJ* 1993;**306**:1602–3.
2 See, for example, the statement from Lord Goff about the BMA's discussion paper on treatment of patients in persistent vegetative state in: Airedale NHS Trust v Bland [1993] 1 All ER 821.
3 See, for example, the statement about the BMA's work on advance statements in: Lord Chancellor's Department. *Making decisions: the Government's proposals for making decisions on behalf of mentally incapacitated adults.* London: The Stationery Office, 1999: para 14 (Cm 4465).
4 Gillon R. *Philosophical medical ethics.* Chichester: Wiley, 1985:2.
5 Boyd KM, Higgs R, Pinching AJ, eds. *The new dictionary of medical ethics.* London: BMJ Publishing Group, 1997:157.
6 Kennedy I. *The unmasking of medicine.* London: George, Allen and Unwin, 1981:78–9.
7 British Medical Association. *The impact of the Human Rights Act 1998 on medical decision making.* London: BMA, 2000.
8 Universal Declaration of Human Rights, adopted and proclaimed by the United Nations General Assembly resolution 217 A (III) on 10 December 1948.
9 The International Covenant on Economic, Social and Cultural Rights and the International Covenant on Civil and Political Rights were both adopted in 1966 and entered into force in 1976.
10 Articles 7 and 9 of the Covenant on Civil and Political Rights.
11 Articles 7, 12 and 13 of the Covenant on Economic, Social and Cultural Rights.
12 *Convention for the Protection of Human Rights and Fundamental Freedoms.* (4. ix. 1950; TS 71; Cmnd 8969.)
13 Beauchamp T, Childress J. *Principles of biomedical ethics, 5th ed.* New York: Oxford University Press, 2001.
14 Gillon R. *Philosophical medical ethics. Op cit:* p. viii.
15 Greenhalgh T, Hurwitz B, eds. *Narrative based medicine.* London: BMJ Books, 1998.
16 Campbell AV. *Moral dilemmas in medicine, 2nd ed.* London: Churchill Livingstone, 1975:3.
17 General Medical Council. *Confidentiality: protecting and providing information.* London: GMC, 2000: para 45.
18 *Ibid:* para 36.
19 Morgan DM. *Issues in medical law and ethics.* London: Cavendish, 2001:5.
20 Dickens B. Ethical issues in health. In: Shenfield F, Sureau C, eds. *Ethical dilemmas in assisted reproduction.* Carnforth: Parthenon, 1997:77.
21 Mason JK, McCall Smith RA, Laurie GT. *Law and medical ethics, 6th ed.* Edinburgh: Butterworths, 2002:5.
22 *Convention for the Protection of Human Rights and Fundamental Freedoms. Op cit.*
23 British Medical Association. *The impact of the Human Rights Act 1998 on medical decision making. Op cit.*
24 General Medical Council. The duties of a doctor registered with the General Medical Council. In: General Medical Council. *Good medical practice.* London: GMC, 2001 (inside front cover).
25 See, for example: Campbell A, Gillett G, Jones G. *Medical ethics, 3rd ed.* Oxford: Oxford University Press, 2001. Gillon R. *Philosophical medical ethics. Op cit.* Harris J. *Bioethics.* Oxford: Oxford University Press, 2001. Chantler C, Doyal L. Medical ethics: the duties of care in principle and practice. In: Powers M, Harris N, eds. *Clinical negligence, 3rd ed.* London: Butterworths, 2000.
26 Gillon R. *Philosophical medical ethics. Op cit:* p. 25.
27 Boyd KM, *et al.,* eds. *The new dictionary of medical ethics. Op cit:* p. 267.
28 Hare RM. *Moral thinking: its levels, method and point.* Oxford: Clarendon Press, 1981.

29   Parker M, ed. *Ethics and community in the health care professions.* London: Routledge, 1999:8.

30   Campbell A, *et al. Medical ethics. Op cit:* pp. 8–9.

31   British Medical Association, General Medical Council, Joint Consultants Committee, Committee of Postgraduate Medical Deans, Council of Deans of UK Medical Schools and Faculties, Conference of Medical Royal Colleges and their Faculties in the UK. *Core values for the medical profession in the 21st century: report of a conference held on 3–4 November 1994.* London: BMA, 1995.

32   This is a hypothetical case used to illustrate different theoretical approaches to a particular dilemma.

1: The doctor–patient relationship

The questions covered in this chapter include the following.

- Do doctors in different types of relationship with patients have very different obligations?
- Can doctors choose which patients they accept in the same way as patients choose their doctor?
- When does the "duty of care" start and end?
- What kind of responsibilities do patients have?
- Can patients choose not to have any information about their treatment?
- What happens when the doctor–patient relationship breaks down?

Themes for discussion

Increasingly, health care is provided by a team within which the contribution of each person is an important part of the overall package. Most of this book, therefore, has a patient–health team relationship in mind and, although we focus particularly on the medical role, we do not envisage doctors working in an isolated manner. Chapter 19 in particular considers the implications and dilemmas associated with team working. Nevertheless, there is merit in looking also at some aspects of relationships specifically between doctors and patients because expectations on both sides have changed. This chapter also discusses some of the most common ethical enquiries received by the BMA. It covers seven broad themes central to the evolving relationship between patients and their doctors:

- general principles pertinent to the relationship
- historical background and changing expectations
- the search for balance in the relationship
- the importance of communication
- trust and reciprocity, including what happens when relationships break down
- respective responsibilities
- doctor–patient relationships of the future.

General principles

The general principles that doctors must observe have already been discussed in the introductory chapter, where the General Medical Council's (GMC) guidance is quoted. In this chapter we focus more closely on the reciprocal nature of those principles and some of the practical implications of the GMC's requirement that doctors be "honest and trustworthy", that they "respect patients' dignity", and "treat every patient politely". The following principles apply to the doctor–patient relationship.

- Doctors owe special duties of care to their patients, but all interactions involving doctors and patients should be characterised by honesty, politeness, and respect on both sides.
- Doctors have the main duty to make the relationship work, but patients also have responsibilities to it.
- Establishing appropriate boundaries is essential.
- Effective communication requires both parties to listen as well as talk and to query anything that seems unclear.

How such principles can be implemented in practice is discussed later in this chapter (pages 31–65).

Changing expectations of the doctor–patient relationship

What patients now expect from doctors is quite different from the expectations of their parents and grandparents. Much of this is due to societal change and differing views about how, for example, fundamental concepts such as benefit, harm, and best interests should be interpreted. Whereas, in the past, judgments were made mainly by doctors and usually in terms of clinical criteria, patients now frequently take the lead in assessing what constitutes a benefit for them and how their overall best interests can be promoted. Doctors' expectations of their role have also changed. All ethical codes and statements from organisations such as the World Medical Association continue to emphasise doctors' traditional duty of beneficence, but what counts as benevolent behaviour has undergone reappraisal. In addition, the growing focus on patient rights has influenced public perceptions. At the start of 2001, for example, the Lord Chief Justice of England and Wales summed up what he perceived as a radical shift in public attitudes, noting that medical litigation was rising and that society was focusing more on individuals' enforceable rights.[1] He referred to a general "move to a rights-based society" in which the courts rather than doctors would increasingly be the ultimate arbiters on questions of medical ethics and judges would no longer automatically make the presumptions about medical beneficence that they had done in the past.

Medicine is often defined as being both an art and a science, although it can be argued that the science side has gradually become more pre-eminent. Although acknowledging the vital importance of technical expertise and a sound evidence base, the BMA also emphasises the need to develop the personal characteristics of "a good doctor" (see the introductory chapter and Chapter 18 on education and training). Anxieties about a perceived focus solely on technical competence rather than also on the human side of medical practice have been expressed by some analysts in the USA. Cassell, for example, argues that "what doctors had long done out of kindness, sympathy, patience and personal interest – attentions directed solely at the person rather than the disease" have been "derogated as hand-holding or bedside manner".[2] He warns that "scientific medicine" and evidence-based outcomes have created a risk that the focus of medicine is on the disease rather than the whole person being treated. A former BMA President says that:

Two hundred years ago, when little effective treatment was possible, the ability to comfort and help a patient to accept illness and death – in other words the art of medicine – was paramount. Today, when many patients with previously fatal diseases can expect from medicine an almost normal life span, science is vital. Even now, however, common complaints cause much misery, there is no cure for many serious diseases and the death rate for us all is one hundred percent in the end. So the old art is still a vital characteristic of the good doctor.[3]

Historical context

There is a widespread perception that patient expectations underwent a radical change in the second half of the twentieth century as part of a broad cultural shift that fundamentally altered the relationship between doctor and patient. To set this in context, it may be useful to look back briefly at the prior history of that relationship and the expectations that shaped it. Physicians initially applied the term "patient" to their paying clientele in the upper classes, distinguishing "patients" from the non-paying "sick poor" treated in hospitals. Thomas Percival's 1803 text on medical ethics was innovative and influential in that it erased the distinction by calling all sick people "patients" and assuming that all, regardless of their status, would be entitled to the same respect.[4] The same ethical obligations were owed to all. Percival's text also looked at the personal character traits that made a good doctor. Believing that these should be a balance of compassion and authority, he urged doctors "to unite tenderness with steadiness".[5] There is a modern resonance in his expectation that doctors should be sensitive to patients' feelings and emotions and aware of their fears and anxieties. The focus was on caring for the sick in a rather holistic way, rather than on simply treating their ailments. Although well intentioned and reflecting contemporary expectations, many of these early ethics texts now appear rather patronising or condescending. Percival talked, for example, about how doctors should develop a "familiar confidence" with their patients and act as a "friendly monitor"[6] to nudge patients into making proper provision for their families in the event of their demise. He also expected that patients would be shielded from difficult information. For generations, doctors were taught that they should keep up patients' hopes and spirits, soothing their mental anguish by withholding bad news. Doctors were advised that

> the life of a sick person can be shortened not only by the acts, but also by the words or manner of a physician. It is, therefore, a sacred duty … to avoid all things which have a tendency to discourage the patient and to depress his spirits.[7]

Such ethical advice led doctors to believe that it was primarily their responsibility to sort out what would be best for patients without necessarily involving them in the choices. From today's perspective, such guidance can be seen as embodying the best and worst aspects of paternalism in that doctors were expected to be thoughtful and caring of their patients but without engaging with them as equals.

It is interesting that Percival's text was particularly taken up by the country that has subsequently come to epitomise the rights of individuals to self determination. It formed the basis of the 1847 code of ethics of the American Medical Association, in which the first chapter gave equal attention to the "duties of physicians to their patients" and the "obligations of patients to their physicians".[8] It may also be worth noting that patient responsibilities have continued to be discussed in the American Medical Association's codes of medical ethics, although the same has not been true in the past in the UK. A possible marker of changing trends was a consultation document published in 2003 by the Scottish Consumer Council on *Patient rights and responsibilities*.[9] As well as setting out the practical benefits that patients ought to be able to expect in terms of access to a second medical opinion, translation services, and access to accurate information about waiting times, it also lists patients' duties (see section on "Patients' duty to treat health professionals reasonably" later in this chapter).

In the introductory chapter, we discussed the ethical obligation to maximise benefit and minimise harm for patients. For over a century after Percival, this duty of beneficence was widely interpreted as giving doctors leeway to withhold frightening information from patients and effectively make decisions on their behalf. From the 1950s, this interpretation became increasingly discredited and by the 1980s such paternalism was seen as completely outmoded. Although paternalistic attitudes often had a benevolent goal and were motivated by a perceived need to protect the vulnerabilities of sick people, they infantilised patients and removed their choices. All current ethical guidance, including that from the BMA, sees patients themselves as the most suitable arbiters of their own best interests. This entails them being given all the relevant information about their condition. Throughout this book, we emphasise the key importance of patient autonomy and the need for health professionals to help patients to make the decisions that are best for them rather than assuming that all patients necessarily have similar goals or values. Such advice focuses on the majority of patients who are willing and able to know about the options open to them. Clearly, however, not everyone falls into this category. Very frail and seriously ill patients, for example, may have other expectations of the doctor–patient relationship more akin to the caring engagement described by Percival. They may not want full information or a list of options. Some patients do not want to feel that they alone are responsible for making decisions, for example. Therefore, among the issues discussed in this chapter are: the sort of support patients can expect, whether they can opt out of decisions or refuse to receive information, and whether there are any circumstances in which doctors may not offer such details.

The changing roles of GPs and hospital consultants leave some concerned that they will increasingly become more technicians than real partners in their relationships with patients. They object to what Cassell terms "cafeteria medicine",[10] which appears to require doctors simply to offer patients a menu of choices in a routine and inflexible manner regardless of the context. A common enquiry to the BMA, for example, concerns whether or not there is a duty to discuss cardiopulmonary resuscitation (CPR) with all patients, including those who are terminally ill. Some doctors say that there is an expectation that they should automatically raise the issue of CPR even with patients who are clearly and inexorably dying because they have rights to such information even though it also causes distress. Although there must be a presumption that patients are informed about decisions being made in relation to their treatment, the fear of being seen as paternalistic or disrespectful of patient autonomy should not mean that doctors automatically apply the same checklist in all cases. As is made clear in the discussion on caring for patients at the end of life (Chapter 10), the BMA does not see a duty to discuss treatments that could confer no benefit to that individual. Rather, it emphasises looking at patients as individuals and assessing the needs of the person in each case. Although it is wrong to discriminate solely on factors such as the patient's age, other criteria such as the likelihood of success are relevant to whether or not an option is offered.

Types of relationships in modern medicine

All health professionals have moral and legal duties for people in their care, so those duties are of a different order in the usual therapeutic relationship compared with the obligations of an independent medical assessor. Two broad categories of professional relationship can be defined.

The therapeutic relationship and duties to the patient

When we talk about the doctor–patient relationship or partnership, the therapeutic model is the one we mean, whether it takes place in a primary care or hospital setting. Here the doctor is seen as having a firm commitment to the patient even though other professionals may manage specific episodes of care. What distinguishes this from other models of care is that the doctor is responsible to the patient, whose best interests are the key concern. In exceptional cases, however, the doctor may have to act contrary to the patient's wishes where these conflict seriously with a wider duty to society and put other people's health at risk.

Independent assessors and duties to the commissioning agent

Doctors also act as impartial examiners accountable to a third party who commissions their services. Common examples include pre-employment or insurance examiners and experts providing reports to the courts or immigration authorities. Patients often have no choice about which doctor is approached by the agency commissioning the report. Promoting patients' own health interests and protecting their confidentiality are not the goals of this interaction, as they are in the case of a therapeutic relationship. Therefore the exact nature of the doctor's role must be clearly explained to patients. They should be aware that any tests and the information derived from the examination are not for the purposes of health care. Reports such as those for insurance and employment are undertaken either by the patient's own GP acting temporarily in a non-therapeutic capacity or by a doctor who has no other relationship with the patient. In this context, the patient's own GP can be seen as having "dual obligations" whereas other independent examiners have no continuing obligations to the patient and do not become involved in treatment. Acting in an independent capacity can create some dilemmas and a lack of openness. Patients may try to limit or conceal some information because the goal of examination is unrelated to their health care and the party commissioning the report may instruct doctors to keep their findings secret from the patient. Despite such instructions, however, patients may have a right of access to the report under the Data Protection Act 1998 (see Chapter 6 on health records). Also, in the BMA's view, doctors who do not have a clinical relationship with such patients still have some responsibilities to them. If doctors discover information significant to the management of the patient's health, they should bring it to the attention of the patient's GP or the patient. How such eventualities will be handled should be discussed with the patient in advance. It can also be discussed with the agency commissioning the report so that it is aware that appropriate steps are taken to inform the patient.

In addition to these two categories, there are also some doctors, such as those who work in prisons, who have a split responsibility to the patient and another party. They have enhanced responsibilities to their employer, but they also have clear duties to the detainees who are their regular patients and who may have no real choice of doctor. Unlike the independent medical assessor, doctors with dual loyalties have a therapeutic relationship with their patients but usually have to work within additional constraints in comparison with other doctors in the community. Nevertheless, ethical responsibilities and the duty of care are the same for all patients. That is to say that the obligations are not any less just because a patient happens to be a prisoner or a detained asylum seeker. (This is discussed in detail in Chapter 16 on dual obligations.)

Choice and duty

Can patients choose their doctor?

In the primary care setting, patients may be able to choose their GP but, in practice, where local lists are full they may have to be allocated by the primary care organisation to any practice with capacity to accept new patients. The BMA receives many enquiries from members of the public who have difficulty registering with the practice of their choice owing to full lists or who are unaware that they have a right to be registered with a GP within the NHS. In custodial settings, patients generally have no choice of doctor, although, if they are already registered with a local doctor, remand prisoners and people held in police stations can request a visit from their own GP. (Whether or not the GP will attend, however, depends to some extent on the circumstances of the case: see Chapter 17.) For hospital treatment, patients are referred to the consultant who is considered most appropriate by the GP, but NHS hospital trusts may transfer patients from the long waiting list of one consultant to the shorter list of another. Patients should be given information about this and have the option of waiting to see the specific person to whom they were referred. If, however, the patient's condition is urgent, the priority within the NHS is to arrange treatment by any appropriately trained doctor and the patient's preference may not be a feasible option. In the private sector, patients have more choice, but, if their care is funded by their insurer, the latter may specify where treatment is provided and designate a consultant.

Can doctors choose their patients?

Sometimes doctors providing standard therapeutic services would like to select the patients they see. Within the NHS, however, doctors must provide care on an equitable basis according to their capacity to take on new patients. That is to say they cannot be selective simply to reduce their workload by excluding people whose condition requires a lot of attention, while taking on other patients. Factors such as the patient's age, lifestyle, or the cost of providing care for that person should not be grounds for acceptance or refusal. It is unacceptable for GPs, for example, to specify that they register only English speakers, refuse to accept asylum seekers,[11] or exclude all patients in nursing homes when their lists still have vacancies. The BMA hears of complaints from patients who find it very difficult to change their GP because practices seem to assume that a person wishing to leave another surgery list is probably difficult or demanding. Where vacancies exist, patients should not be refused without good reason (but those with a history of threatening behaviour are likely to have problems and may need to be allocated). In the private sector, too, doctors should not act in an arbitrary or unfairly discriminatory manner in terms of taking on new patients.

Similarly, in the hospital setting, doctors are expected to treat all patients equitably and in a non-judgmental manner. It is not, for example, the role of hospital doctors to verify the immigration status of patients presenting for care. It is quite another matter, however, if the doctor–patient relationship has broken down and either the doctor or the patient considers a change to be essential (see also later section on violent patients). In some cases, based on their past experience of an individual patient, consultants know that they will not be able to achieve a constructive relationship with that person. Even when there is a justifiable reason for recommending that the patient be seen by another doctor, the consultant still has a duty to identify a suitably qualified colleague. Junior doctors and non-consultant career grade doctors may find themselves in a situation in which they lack sufficient experience to attend a particular patient, in which case they must ask the consultant to make appropriate arrangements.

Who has a duty of care?

In the BMA's view, a duty exists whenever a doctor interacts with a patient in a professional capacity, but questions sometimes arise about when precisely the duty of care begins and ends. Doctors may question, for example, the duty owed to patients who continually transfer between the NHS and private practice, or the duty they have to patients who consult them by email or the internet. (These issues are discussed in Chapters 13 and 19.) Also, although it is clear that consultants have a duty to patients seen by them or by their team and accepted on to their waiting list, doctors may question the extent of any duty they have for patients referred but not yet seen by them. In some non-urgent situations, for example, patients are booked by GPs referring them to a consultant prior to the latter becoming aware of the patient at all. Consultants generally vet incoming referral letters in order to prioritise them according to clinical urgency. Once doctors have accepted a patient – either by examining that person or having studied the clinical details of an individual referred to them for treatment – some moral responsibility exists. It is then generally the role of that consultant to deal with the patient's problems at an appropriate time, according to their urgency, or to recommend that treatment be sought elsewhere if waiting times are inappropriate for that patient's condition. Similar duties exist for consultants such as radiologists or endoscopists, who are involved only with some aspect of a patient's investigation. In no cases can patients be "abandoned", but another practitioner willing to take over the duty of care should be identified as promptly as possible.

When a patient has been assessed as non-urgent and placed on a list, consultants need periodically to review the assessment if that patient's condition is likely to deteriorate during the waiting time. If the consultant's clinics are overbooked and a new patient's condition is such that it would be inappropriate to add him or her to a waiting list, the referring GP should be informed and asked to make an alternative arrangement appropriate to the patient's need. This also means that consultants should be generally aware of the waiting times for specific medical conditions in their area and draw managers' attention to the problem if urgent cases are not being seen fast enough in their locality. Consultants may also be asked by patients about waiting times and they obviously need to be careful and accurate in their response. (In Chapter 19, for example, the case is quoted of a consultant disciplined by the GMC for deliberately misleading patients about potential waiting times in order to promote private treatment.)

The BMA also occasionally receives enquiries about disagreements between doctors concerning who should be providing care for a specific patient. In private facilities, for example, a patient may be referred to one consultant but be seen initially by another, who may begin treatment. In the past, when the concept of "poaching" patients was current, doctors had almost a sense of ownership of "their" patients in a way that is now outdated, especially as teams rather than individuals now generally provide care. In some cases, patients may prefer to wait to see the specific private consultant to whom they were referred. Their choice should be respected. This may not be possible in the NHS if their preferred consultant already has a long waiting list. Once an episode of care has been commenced, the doctor who initiated it has a responsibility to ensure that it is completed unless all agree to an alternative arrangement, such as when doctor–patient trust breaks down and transfer is required.

A common area in which residual notions of "ownership" of patients still exist concerns doctors working on a sessional basis in private clinics that are often owned by non-medical managers. In such situations doctors leaving the practice may wish to take "their" patients with them, although the latter have contracted with the clinic rather than an individual practitioner. Doctors may also express concerns that confidential medical records should remain in medical ownership in the absence of any new incoming practitioner. Clearly, employment contracts need to make clear the rights and responsibilities of doctors and the rights of the patients they treat. Patients need to have information about how transfer of care and of records will be handled, and the choices they have in those matters (see also Chapter 6 on health records). Similar situations may arise if doctors work on a sessional basis in nurse-led practices in the NHS. Doctors employed in such settings need to assure themselves that adequate arrangements are in place for continuity of care, and inform the nurse manager and the commissioning agency if this seems problematic. Clearly, patients need to be aware of the arrangements for continuity of their treatment.

Summary – the changing relationship

- Doctors should involve patients closely in any decisions.
- This needs to be done in a supportive way and not presented as merely a menu of options.
- Efforts should be made to accommodate patients' preferences, but doctors also need to be realistic in explaining the practical limitations in choice.

The search for balance

Patients consult doctors for a variety of health and related social purposes. This contact is somehow perceived as special. It gives doctors privileged access to anxious or sick people, to their bodies, their stories, their families, and their secrets. It requires special moral safeguards. The responsibilities that doctors owe are therefore perceived to be of a different order to the responsibilities of other service providers to their clients. This is partly because these encounters concern the very stuff of life. Although much regular contact between doctors and patients is about relatively mundane matters, medicine also deals with the most intimate and basic aspects of survival. "Medicine means life and death, deliverance and despair, hope and fright, mystery and mechanics. It is a microscope trained upon life's fundamentals".[12] For such reasons, the relationship between doctors and patients is seen as particularly important and doctors are continually urged to improve their understanding of the patient's perspective.

By urging doctors to see things from the patient's viewpoint, ethical guidance attempts to bring balance into an inherently asymmetrical relationship. Doctors have more information and influence within the medical domain than patients, but also, because they have those advantages, all of the long articulated duties fall to them and all the newly articulated rights belong with the patient. Differing power levels remain even though patients have more access to information about treatment options than ever before. In the primary care setting, doctors probably know more than ever about the details of their patients' lives since they deal not only with their illnesses and stresses but also with social issues such as insurance applications, sick notes, housing problems, and disability benefits. Although the notion of a family doctor providing care to succeeding generations is increasingly out of step with reality, many GPs still see themselves as the holder of families' histories. Hospital doctors often have indepth knowledge of the patients and families that they see repeatedly or for prolonged periods of inpatient care. As discussed in the introductory chapter, the GMC sets out a series of ethical obligations that doctors must observe to create successful relationships with patients. Doctors are seen as having particular responsibilities for making these relationships work. The GMC makes clear that they must show respect for patients' views, their privacy and dignity, and involve them fully in decisions about their care.[13] The BMA strongly supports this advice but one of the issues we examine in this chapter is whether patients too have duties and responsibilities and, if so, what those could be.

Patient autonomy

Relationships between doctors and patients are based on the concept of partnership and collaboration. Ideally, decisions are made through frank discussion, in which clinical expertise seeks to match the available options to the patient's individual needs and preferences. The patient's consent is the trigger that allows the interchange to take place. Patients of all ages and abilities are encouraged to be actively engaged in health decisions that affect them. This includes the option of requesting specific interventions (see, for example, the discussion of elective caesarean section in Chapter 7) or declining some medical advice without prejudicing the doctor–patient relationship. The main role of doctors in such situations is to provide information, explain the available options and their implications, and address any misunderstandings that may exist. (Aspects of refusal are discussed in detail in Chapter 2.)

Doctors' autonomy

Consent and autonomy are not the sole prerogatives of patients. Doctors offer treatment, not simply because it is requested but because in their view it is clinically appropriate. Their advice should be evidence based and reflect best practice guidelines that may not necessarily fit in with patient expectations, for example, when patients ask for antibiotics. Doctors recommend interventions that they think best for individual patients, having regard to patients' own views and available resources. In a therapeutic relationship, the principal responsibility must be to the patient rather than to issues of resource management, but difficult questions can still arise if a patient rejects a low cost remedy in favour of a more costly alternative. Religious groups such as Jehovah's Witnesses, for example, may feel able to accept only certain options and, wherever possible, a solution acceptable to the patient should be the goal. Obviously, it is always important to discuss the options and avoid making assumptions in order properly to understand individual patients' reasons and the values that underlie their choices. In other cases, doctors are unable to give patients treatments that would be harmful. Everyday examples concern patient demand for amphetamine-type appetite suppressants or athletes' and bodybuilders' requests for steroids. Sports medicine is discussed in Chapter 16 on dual obligations.

In practice, the doctor–patient partnership functions best when the doctor's skills are tailored to meet the patient's requirements and the patient's requests do not exceed what the doctor is able legally, ethically, and practically to provide. Doctors have some responsibilities to society beyond their duty to particular patients, although individual patients must be the focus of attention. Doctors also have considerable power, not to decide the patient's treatment but effectively to influence the range of options from which the patient chooses.

The importance of communication

A growing and complex literature has developed about aspects of doctor–patient communication, particularly about how to communicate risks to patients.[14] In simple terms, however, effective communication is not only about conveying information, it is also about establishing positive interpersonal relationships.[15] In 2000, when the BMA was looking specifically at future developments in primary care,[16] patient and research organisations were asked to summarise the main aspects of care that patients most valued. Many identified effective communication and continuity of the relationship as key issues. The Institute for Public Policy Research, for example, reported that, when people were asked what they meant by a good relationship with their doctor, they mentioned time to talk, a willingness to listen, and continuity of the relationship, but it also said that many older people still felt inhibited about questioning doctors.[17] In terms of secondary care, too, the importance of hearing and understanding patients' views is similarly highly valued. Describing a surgical procedure he had undergone, for example, the Vice Chairman of the UK Coalition of People Living with HIV and AIDS said that his experience of health care had been much better when doctors listened to his requests and understood that he was the expert on his own body. "The surgeon may have performed a thousand of these procedures," he said, "but I doubt if he'd ever had one".[18]

The GMC advises that all doctors must take appropriate steps to find out what patients want to know and ought to know about their condition and its treatment.[19] They should also try to identify patients' individual needs and priorities because factors such as their beliefs, culture, or occupation may have a bearing on the information they need to make a decision.[20] Chronic diseases impact on patients' lives in various ways and so it is important that they have relevant information to manage their condition in ways compatible with their own wishes and lifestyle. As much of the balance of control in decision making passes to patients, doctors still need to do more than simply provide a list of options. Most patients also want an informed opinion about what is likely to be most appropriate and efficacious in their own case. As well as the available evidence to support the doctor's recommendation, they are likely to want to know the limits of what is proved, including disputed science and the doctor's own uncertainties.

There is wide recognition that written information for patients can be very valuable because it:

- increases satisfaction and reduces complaints
- increases adherence to treatment
- increases self care and self management activity
- promotes active coping
- reduces psychological distress and anxiety.[21]

Nevertheless, some problems have been highlighted that are general to the way information is given. For example, attention has been drawn to the fact that it is questionable whether there is an ultimate truth that can be conveyed because much "health care information and medical knowledge is contested knowledge" even if based on statistical probability.[22] It is produced by health professionals who may assume that patients want to know more about the medical aspects of their condition than about the experience of living with it. Leaflets sometimes gloss over the fact that a test or treatment may be uncomfortable or even painful. Some people have proposed, therefore, that patient groups should take the lead in producing information leaflets,[23] although others argue that such groups often have their own perspective and political agenda.[24] Talking in depth to patients with a serious condition indicates that, in their experience, the messages they receive verbally from health professionals can be at complete variance with the information provided by the standardised patient leaflets for their condition.[25] Also, as in face to face discussions, individual patients vary in how much honesty and detail they want displayed in leaflets, especially those discussing conditions that are likely to be fatal. In the BMA's view, there are good arguments for a range of materials to be available that reflect both the clinical aspects of various conditions and the experience of other patients coping with them. It seems clear that patients would benefit from descriptions that place more emphasis on how treatments feel to the recipient, but there is also a role for more research into how patients generally would like healthcare information to be conveyed.

A basic issue that often needs to be discussed with patients being admitted to hospital is whether they want other people to be kept informed of their condition or actually involved in decisions if they become incapable of communicating for some reason. All competent adults are asked formally to nominate their next of kin on admission to hospital and they should be advised that this does not necessarily have to be a blood relative; nor is it simply a contact number, but rather someone who could be involved, if necessary, in decisions (see Chapter 3). Often, but not invariably, it will be obvious who should be consulted, but health professionals must be careful not to make assumptions. Appropriate people close to the patient may well be non-relatives, such as unmarried partners or same sex partners. NHS trusts should provide a short information leaflet for patients, explaining why it could be important to nominate someone to help in decision making and to check that their nominee is willing to do that. Leaflets may also need to remind patients that, if they do nominate someone to be consulted, they need to keep that person informed of their preferences.

There is a difference between doctors providing clinical advice and discussing moral views. Doctors are obviously entitled to their own moral opinions, but should not share these with patients unless asked to do so. If doctors feel that their own beliefs are likely to affect their advice or treatment in particular cases, they should tell the patients and explain that they can see another doctor.[26] Furthermore, the GMC emphasises that doctors must not allow their personal views about factors such as patients' lifestyle, culture, beliefs, race, colour, gender, sexuality, age, or social or economic status to affect treatment.[27] The fact that patients' actions have contributed to their condition should not be a reason for delaying or refusing treatment. (Nevertheless, in some cases aspects of the patient's lifestyle, such as smoking or drug or alcohol addiction, may have implications for the effectiveness of the treatment, in which case, those aspects would have to be taken into account and discussed with the individual.)

Can patients refuse to receive information?

Patients generally want to have their views heard and, although each one is different, most do want to be closely involved in decisions. They may want more or less information at different stages of their treatment, especially as assimilating difficult or painful news takes time and appropriate support (see Chapter 10). Not everyone necessarily wants the same amount of detail. If individuals make it clear that they want very little information, it cannot be forced upon them but, in order for their consent to be valid, they should know the core facts about what is proposed. Patients may agree in general terms to a procedure whose purpose they understand but without wanting to know every aspect of it. Nevertheless, competent patients should be encouraged to know information that is essential to maintaining their own health, as well as that relevant to the treatment in question and its potential side effects, although they may opt out of other details if that is their preference. Patients can also choose to delegate some decisions to others and the information needed to make these decisions. Health teams need to be sensitive to individuals' wishes while ensuring that core information is communicated effectively. Relatives sometimes ask for information to be withheld from patients, but the importance of listening to patients' own views about what they want to know cannot be overemphasised. (This issue is also discussed in Chapter 10.)

Failing to *offer* sufficient information could invalidate the patient's consent (see Chapter 2, pages 78–9). In particular, when innovative or risky procedures are proposed, patients need to be aware that there are risks involved. Nevertheless, effective communication about risks, their probability and magnitude, is often difficult even when patients are keen to understand. It is liable to be more so if patients are reluctant to acknowledge them. A recommendation in 2001, in *Learning from Bristol: the report of the public inquiry into children's heart surgery at the Bristol Royal Infirmary 1984–1995* (the Bristol report), was that patients should always be given a chance to ask questions, seek clarification, and ask for more information.[28] The Bristol report emphasised that the working arrangements of health professionals need to be adjusted if the necessary time slots are not available.

The kind of information patients need to make valid and informed decisions is discussed in detail in Chapter 2 on consent and refusal. The basic information includes:

- the evidence base for the diagnosis and prognosis, including the limits of what is known
- available treatment options, including those that may not be available on the NHS
- the implications, drawbacks, and likely side effects of those treatments
- the main alternatives, including non-treatment, and their implications
- if possible, sources of further information and relevant patient support groups.

Truth telling by doctors

Part of the doctor's role is to ensure that decision making is returned as much as possible to the patient, rather than pre-empting the choice by withholding potentially important information. Although in the past it was felt that some information was potentially so distressing that it would demoralise patients, ruin their quality of life, or undermine the doctor–patient relationship, this view erroneously assumed that most people could not cope with the truth. In our own society, which prizes openness, it should not be forgotten that frankness is a relatively recent expectation. In the past, doctors concealed the truth

> not because they were morally defective but because, in their eyes, all they had to offer was an attitude of optimism. Especially since at that time, personal matters that might arise from these illnesses and the doctors' lies – lost hopes, unhappiness, anxieties, sadness, suffering, death and grief – were personal matters kept from the view of others.[29]

Clearly, much has changed and patients expect to have honest answers and support for the anxieties that may flow from them. One of the important recommendations arising from the Bristol report was that "patients should be supported in dealing with the additional anxiety sometimes created by greater knowledge".[30]

Patients often have their own goals as well as matters to put in order and so need to have as accurate information as possible about what is achievable. Clearly, the clinical limitations need to be discussed but doctors also need to be open about any other factors that are likely to affect treatment decisions or their timing. The need to meet externally set targets for treatment, for example, may impinge on the scheduling of certain procedures. This should not be concealed from those affected by it. Health professionals provide information in order to empower patients to exercise informed choice and this is equally important when the options are very limited. Obviously, difficult information has to be given with extreme sensitivity. Patients rightly expect both information and support. Traditionally, doctors were discouraged from confessing any doubts or uncertainties because this could undermine patients' morale. Now, it is recognised that patients face stress and anxiety precisely when they feel information is being concealed.

Giving information can raise anxiety in the recipients and it is never easy to deliver bad news. Therefore the BMA strongly emphasises the importance of all health professionals being properly trained to do this in a manner that is supportive of patients and relatives. There is particular ambivalence about giving bad news or distressing information where there is little that the patient or health team can do to alter the situation, such as when there is no effective intervention. In 2000, complaints were voiced in Parliament about the manner in which some older patients were being asked to give a view on whether or not they wished resuscitation to be attempted in the event of cardiac arrest.[31] Some found it unacceptable that such emotive issues were being raised with vulnerable patients. Others found it unacceptable not to discuss them. In the BMA's view, health professionals should ensure that there are adequate opportunities for discussion and be willing to talk about such matters. When individuals are unwilling to consider them or when such an intervention would clearly be futile, health professionals are not obliged to raise the issue (see Chapter 10 on caring for patients at the end of life). Similar debates have occurred regarding the difficulties of obtaining parental consent to innovative treatment and research on sick neonates (see Chapter 14 on research and innovative treatment) and seeking relatives' consent to the retention of tissue after postmortem examination (see Chapter 12 on responsibilities after a patient's death). Despite the very real difficulties of raising such subjects, patients need to be given the opportunity of talking about them if they wish.

Doctors' duty to acknowledge mistakes

Doctors should be open with patients about the uncertainties involved in treatment. They should be equally honest in retrospectively acknowledging mistaken diagnoses. The GMC says that, when patients suffer harm, doctors should act immediately to put matters right if that is possible.[32] They should explain fully and promptly to the patient (or to the family or carer of incapacitated adults and young children) what has happened and the likely long term and short term implications. This may include giving the information necessary for patients to make a complaint. Clearly, where appropriate, an apology should be offered promptly.

The BMA receives queries about the handling of very difficult and sensitive cases where clinicians believe that previously responsible doctors have either missed important signs of a serious condition or laboratory tests have been misinterpreted in a manner that is not easily rectifiable. In any situation where it seems that substandard practice may have occurred, there is an obligation to do something about it. An important consideration must also be whether the error was likely to have been a one off occurrence or part of a pattern of mistakes that may mean an ongoing risk of harm. Whistleblowing involves drawing mistakes to the attention of the person or organisation who can remedy them as well as to those who have suffered from them. (This is discussed in detail in Chapter 21.) Where there is a pattern of error in hospital care, it is normal for the trust to set up a system for contacting patients and informing them. Doctors should be auditing their performance so that they can spot their own errors and address the implications.

Difficulties in acknowledging mistakes

A patient's breast biopsy was confused with someone else's sample by the histopathologist, with the result that, although completely healthy, the patient had undergone an unnecessary mastectomy. Both she and her family suffered great distress, believing her to be at serious risk of premature death. The mistake was subsequently suspected by a consultant oncologist who then contacted the consultant histopathologist and asked him to review the slides. He did so and found that they showed normal tissue without any evidence of malignancy. The patient's GP was informed of this and, after discussion, it was decided that the whole situation should be explained to the patient at the hospital by the surgeon who had operated on her, together with two nurses to provide support. Telling patients that they have undergone unnecessary distress and a superfluous operation is clearly difficult. In this case, the patient said that "it was easier to accept the mastectomy when I thought I had cancer because I believed that it was necessary to save my life and I actually felt worse once I knew that it has all been a mistake and unnecessary. I felt very depressed. I was always breaking down and crying and I thought constantly about the operation".[33] Despite extensive reconstructive surgery to try and restore her former appearance, the patient developed a serious psychiatric disorder which some psychiatrists believed was unlikely to improve since she had been "wounded both physically and psychiatrically".[34] In December 2002 the case went to the High Court, which awarded the patient £350 000 damages. Her husband and son were awarded £5000 and £1000 respectively for the trauma they had undergone as a result of what happened to her.

Froggatt v Chesterfield and North Derbyshire NHS Trust[35]

Such mistakes are clearly difficult to acknowledge and potentially traumatic for patients to learn about. Even when sensitively done, there may be a sense that the patient's situation is being made even worse rather than better by disclosing an error. We acknowledge, therefore, that disclosure can be costly in terms of human suffering as well as financial expense for the defendants if litigation results, but these are not valid reasons for secrecy. Factual information should not be withheld but patients need expert support and counselling to cope with it. There is obviously a significant difference between a previous clinician misinterpreting a biopsy or confusing it with that of another patient – errors that should have been detected earlier – and legitimate differences of clinical opinion in interpreting any such signs. In some cases in which doctors contact the BMA it is unclear whether warning signs of serious illness were actually missed or wrongly interpreted, or whether the diagnosis was quite reasonably made on the currently available evidence. Clearly, it is important not to impose the knowledge gained by hindsight on the information available to the diagnosing clinician when the original decision was made. When there is ambiguity, it is important for health professionals who are involved later to obtain a clear view of the facts before talking to the patient or putting their suspicions into the medical notes. Clarifying what has occurred in the past is likely to involve contacting the previous clinician and reviewing any samples taken and records made at the time of diagnosis. A specialist interpretation of the evidence may be needed. If it is obvious that an error was made, there should be discussion about how the patient can sensitively be prepared for that information and who should take responsibility for doing so.

When a doctor is aware that a mistake may have been instrumental in causing a death, people close to that individual need to be informed sensitively and the events formally investigated. The GMC says that, in relation to the deaths of children, the circumstances should be explained to the best of the doctor's knowledge to parents or people with parental responsibility. The partner or close relatives of adults should be similarly informed.[36] If the cause of death is misadventure or is not fully known, the coroner or procurator fiscal must be involved. (This is discussed further in Chapter 12 on responsibilities after a patient's death.) Even when there is no evidence of error, an elective (or hospital) postmortem examination may be requested by the doctor of the deceased to verify the accuracy of the diagnosis and to assess whether the best treatment was provided or if important signs were missed. Information gained from such investigations should be shared, as appropriate, with people close to the patient. When information is discovered that the patient is likely to have wanted to be kept confidential, there needs to be discussion about how to keep a balance between the interests of natural justice, the rights of the family, and the confidentiality owed to the deceased.

Should doctors tell patients about unfunded treatments?

The candour that is now accepted practice in relation to medical information does not automatically extend to other categories of information that have a direct bearing on patient choice. A particular area of enquiry to the BMA concerns the range of options that patients should be told about when there is little or no likelihood of some of those options being made available to them. Anecdotal evidence bears out the view that doctors sometimes base their judgments about discussion of possible options on their assessment of the patient's potential ability to access those treatments privately. Although it is not doctors' place to make any assumptions about their patients' financial resources, they feel embarrassed about having to tell patients that some treatments are available only in the private sector. In some cases, they fear that the knowledge of unfunded but potentially beneficial options may only cause greater distress.

It is important to provide the highest degree of transparency possible concerning NHS decisions about rationing. Unrealistic expectations can damage the doctor–patient relationship. In cases where the treatment cannot be funded, patients should have access to information about the factors leading to the rationing decision. The issue becomes more complicated when there is no clinical agreement about the efficacy of the treatments or where only a small improvement can be expected but the financial cost is great. While their budgets are healthy, some purchasers are willing to pay for innovative and as yet unproven treatments for patients who are devoid of other options, but these are the first categories of treatment to be dropped when finances are tight. With this background awareness of what is available locally, doctors have to make clinical decisions about which treatments are potentially beneficial to individual patients and which would be futile. In the BMA's view, there is no ethical obligation to tell patients about treatments that would clearly be futile. All questions should be answered frankly, however, and wherever possible patients should be offered a second opinion if they require reassurance about the likely outcome of a particular option.

Although it could be argued that patients should be protected from the distress of receiving information about treatment options that are not publicly funded, this undermines the increasingly accepted concept of a partnership in decision making between patients and health professionals. It must be recognised that knowing a possible, even if unproven, treatment exists may make some families feel pressured to incur debts to buy it. On the other hand, however, patients and their families increasingly want to have the choice of making even difficult decisions of this type for themselves. In the BMA's view, doctors must be as open and frank as possible about potentially beneficial procedures or drugs. Patients increasingly seek out information themselves from sources such as the internet and can lose trust in their medical advisers if they discover belatedly that information about potential options has been withheld. (Issues about openness with patients and the movement of patients in and out of the NHS are discussed in more detail in Chapters 13 and 19.)

Being open about employment disputes

Another problematic area in which the BMA's advice is sometimes sought concerns what patients should be told when doctors are in dispute with their employers. For example, consultants sometimes want to inform their own patients why they are temporarily suspended, without undermining confidence in the service or in past or future care provision. Clearly, this can be immensely tricky and there may also be implications under data protection legislation if patient information – including names and addresses – is used by a clinician who is no longer providing care to those patients (see also Chapter 5 on confidentiality). Communicating the facts about patients being allocated to another clinician should be handled by the relevant trust. The GMC says that, when doctors are suspended by an employer or have restrictions placed on their practice because of concerns about their performance or conduct, they need to inform any other organisations for whom they work so that cover arrangements can be made. The GMC also says that doctors need to inform any patients whom they see independently of such organisations if the treatment being given to those patients falls within the area of concern to which the suspension or restriction relates.[37] Further advice can be sought from local BMA employment advisers. Among the principles that need to be borne in mind is that patient data, including names and addresses, are provided for the provision of health care and so doctors need to be wary of retaining or using such data if they are no longer providing care. Any information doctors give to their patients about a dispute — whether in a hospital setting or in a GP partnership — must not cast aspersions on the standards of care provided by the unit or by colleagues. If there are concerns about care standards, these need to be raised through the appropriate channels, as is discussed in Chapter 21 (see pages 754–8).

Truth telling by patients

The importance of health professionals being truthful is often emphasised in ethical and legal guidelines, but the obligation of patients to be equally frank is less discussed. An exception is found in the codes of patient duties set by the American Medical Association. This states that

> patients have a responsibility to be truthful and to express their concerns clearly to their physicians. Patients have a responsibility to provide a complete medical history, to the extent possible, including information about past illnesses, medications, hospitalizations, family history of illness and other matters relating to present health.[38]

In the BMA's view, a relationship of trust depends upon reciprocal honesty. Health professionals are frustrated when patients withhold relevant information that can affect treatment decisions. For example, sometimes patients feel awkward about telling their doctor that they are using medication such as weight reduction drugs prescribed by a private clinic. Clearly, doctors need to emphasise to patients the importance of disclosing any factors that could seriously affect treatment decisions or expose them to the adverse effects of clashing medication. Sometimes patients deliberately conceal information owing to anxiety about its further disclosure to employers, insurers or other third parties. Although the law and ethics require that disclosure in such cases only occurs with patient consent, patients are well aware that they have little option but to agree if they genuinely want the job or the insurance. This can lead to the concealment from doctors of important information about sensitive matters such as mental health problems, sexually transmitted infections, addiction, and stress related illnesses. Many doctors see this as problematic and consider that the best solution would be for health records to be used only for the provision of health care and related purposes such as clinical audit or research, but with a prohibition on other social functions that currently require medical records. Reports for insurance, employment, and the like would then have to be done by independent medical examiners who do not have access to the patient's health record, rather than by doctors who know the patient. The BMA has argued, however, that there are often advantages for patients in having reports made by their own doctor, who can point out if a particular test result appears inconsistent in relation to the patient's overall health record. From the patient's perspective, this is also generally the most convenient solution. (The use of information for insurance is discussed further in Chapter 16.)

Communication and intimate examinations

The importance of good communication both in advance and after an intimate examination cannot be overemphasised. The GMC constantly receives complaints from patients who feel that doctors have behaved improperly during intimate examinations and some of these are partly the result of very poor communication. Providing a full explanation of what is intended and why, and then gaining patient consent are obviously essential prerequisites (see also the section on chaperones on pages 48–9). Ideally, there should also be appropriate opportunities for patients to raise the issue promptly with the practice or clinic if they feel a doctor's behaviour has been untoward. The "challenge is to create a climate of trust and honesty within which patients who may be confused or upset about events occurring in the surgery are able to articulate their concerns and obtain explanation and reassurance where appropriate".[39] Health facilities could display notices, for example, encouraging patients to talk about their complaints or anxieties with staff. This could help to identify when genuine abuse is being perpetrated as well as reducing the number of unjustified complaints.

Communication, interpretation, and translation

Inevitably in some cases, a third party is needed to aid communication. In many health facilities, information given in a range of languages encourages patients to give advance notice if they need language or signing assistance. Patient information leaflets are also increasingly available in a range of languages (including those, for example, inviting patients to participate in research; see Chapter 14). Patients often come accompanied by people who they want to translate for them or it may be their expectation that other family members will actually make the decision in question. Children should not generally be expected to interpret for adults, especially when very sensitive subjects are discussed. Health professionals need to make clear that individual patients are entitled to privacy, while recognising that not all patients wish to exercise that right.[40] If the patient is not accompanied, interpretation and translation should be provided, wherever possible, by professionals rather than staff such as hospital porters. Translators and interpreters, including those who provide sign language, can be found through the National Register of Interpreters.

Summary – the importance of communication

- Patients should be offered information but are not obliged to receive all the details.
- Efforts must be made to convey information in a manner in which patients can understand; this may include translation.
- Questions should be answered as honestly as possible.
- Frankness should extend to funding and rationing decisions as well as treatment.

Trust and reciprocity

The kind of reciprocal respect that should ideally exist in this relationship has been described as "the doctor–patient mutual investment company".[41] As this implies, both parties invest effort in making the relationship work and both also strive to maximise the patient's health.

Covert medication

The concept of covert medication for a competent person is clearly at variance with our emphasis on informed patient consent and mutual trust. Furthermore, as is shown by the case of WP described below, covert medication can still be contentious when the patient could be treated under mental health legislation. Nevertheless, the BMA continues to receive queries about whether it is ever ethically acceptable to administer medication to a competent person without first explaining the implications and gaining the individual's cooperation. In our view, it is not, other than as a last resort in the kind of circumstances where a competent patient is violent or threatening people's safety and when covert medication would avoid the risks of harm possibly associated with the use of physical restraint. (The use of restraint in custodial settings, for example, is discussed in Chapter 17.) Refusal of treatment by competent patients is discussed in detail in Chapter 2, where it is made clear that treatment refusal by a competent and informed adult is legally and ethically binding on health professionals. The only exception is compulsory treatment authorised under mental health legislation when patients – sometimes despite retaining mental capacity – are considered a danger to themselves or others (see Chapter 3).

Contexts in which this question arises commonly involve the residential care of older people, people with learning disabilities, or patients with challenging behaviour. In many cases, medication is not exactly administered secretly, but rather provided in a routine and mechanical way without explanation. As a general principle, it is not ethically acceptable to omit to explain their medication to competent patients solely on grounds of convenience, lack of time, or the complexities of communication. The BMA emphasises that "although some older people might have difficulty communicating, hearing or understanding, this does not lessen health professionals' obligation to consult older patients and to gain their consent to care and treatment programmes".[42] Direct questions from any patient concerning the purpose and effects of medication should be answered truthfully. In emergencies and exceptional cases, such as where violence is threatened, the primary aim must be to avoid harm to people. Nevertheless, interventions without explanation should not be a routine or automatic response to patients with whom communication is difficult.

Covert medication may be acceptable in cases where the individual is not competent to give valid consent or refusal, or where compulsory treatment under mental health legislation is justified. The latter allows for certain treatments to be given without consent to patients who could be detained compulsorily. In such cases, if some form of chemical restraint is required and the patient is unwilling to accept it, health professionals have the choice of attempting to administer it by force or covertly. When patient consent is not legally required, it seems sensible that medication should be administered in a manner least likely to cause harm and with the least amount of interference, although health professionals still need to consider the likely impact on patients' willingness to trust them in future. Therefore, although deceit is normally unacceptable, in these limited cases it may be permissible although still controversial.

Administering covert medication to a violent person

WP was a 91-year-old widower, resident in an old people's home, who occasionally showed unpredictable aggression. He attended a day hospital for older people where, on one particular occasion, he was subject to extreme changes of mood but refused to be admitted as an inpatient or to take a tranquilliser. The team considered him to be hypomanic and unsafe to return to the residence without treatment. Compulsory admission under section 2 of the Mental Health Act 1983 was therefore discussed, but in the meantime efforts were made to persuade him to accept medication, which he continued to refuse. The consultant thought that there were two feasible options. One was to give WP an injection of haloperidol by force, risking injury to him and undermining both his rapport with the team and his self respect. The other option was to give him liquid haloperidol disguised in a cup of tea. The ward sister was told to do this. After the crisis had passed, WP subsequently agreed to electroencephalography and was found to need anticonvulsant drugs. The covert medication was discussed with him and he strongly supported the action that had been taken, as did WP's nephew. In this instance, the patient's relationship with the health staff did not appear to suffer. The Mental Health Act Commission agreed that the consultant had acted correctly but it was subsequently reported that the hospital sister who had put the medication in WP's tea on the consultant's instructions was suspended and given a formal warning, indicating that such action is still seen as controversial, even in these circumstances.[43]

Some of the cases concerning covert medication raised with the BMA are far from straightforward but fall within a grey area where the patient is thought to suffer from some degree of mental illness or impairment but, unlike WP, not to an extent sufficient to warrant compulsory medication under mental health legislation. For example, a continuing problem concerns patients with a history of psychotic episodes whose insight about their illness wanes, so that, believing themselves well, they decline the medication that would prevent a crisis occurring. Health professionals are then faced with the dilemma of either effectively provoking a mental health crisis by stopping treatment until the patient deteriorates to the extent that the compulsory treatment criteria are met or illegally treating the patient without proper consent. The law is clear that people who do not fall within the remit of mental health legislation and have sufficient competence and understanding to make a valid decision should not be treated against their will. Health professionals can offer support and counselling to try to restore the patient's insight and voluntary compliance. Nevertheless, if the patient continues to reject medication, there is a tension for doctors between two conflicting imperatives: that of maintaining the patient's health and that of following that person's express wishes.

One mechanism occasionally proposed for such situations is a form of advance statement. Patients with such a history of illness can be asked, when at their most lucid and insightful, to agree in advance a treatment plan that would be triggered at the very start of a decline in mental capacity, rather than allowing the patient to reach crisis point and compulsory treatment. Although such a mechanism appears more respectful of patient autonomy, it is fraught with practical difficulties. Not least of these is the fact that, legally and ethically, patients are not required to demonstrate profound insight but rather need a grasp of the core information in order to decline treatment and override their previously given consent. A patient's current decision, if backed by information and an understanding of the implications, effectively trumps any earlier agreement. Nevertheless, an agreed treatment plan that has involved the patient in advance planning may be the best option available.

Trust and covert surveillance

People using health care facilities should generally be made aware by notices if surveillance cameras are in use for purposes such as security. There are few occasions in which covert video surveillance is acceptable. It is occasionally used to monitor children who are receiving inpatient care when there are grounds to suspect relatives or carers of causing injury to the child. Such surveillance without the knowledge and consent of families occurs in cases where the child would otherwise be placed at unacceptable risk of harm and as an aid to the diagnosis of Munchausen's syndrome by proxy. The law recognises that, when a minor is likely to be at risk of significant harm, a compulsory intervention in family life in the child's interests is justified.[44] A body of guidance exists on this subject as a result of a report in 2000 on research in North Staffordshire NHS Trust,[45] which called for the development of guidelines to assist in identifying children who have illnesses fabricated or induced by carers. In 2001, the Royal College of Paediatrics and Child Health issued a report[46] setting out the role of paediatricians and other health professionals with recommendations about liaison with other agencies. In 2002, the Department of Health and Welsh Assembly published detailed guidance on the subject.[47] This guidance is intended to provide a national framework as a basis for agencies and professionals to use in drawing up local work plans. Although surveillance to protect a child is justifiable, more controversial is the continued use of such surveillance primarily to gather evidence to bring legal proceedings. This could expose children to a continuing risk of harm after the problem has been identified sufficiently for diagnostic purposes. In 2001, the BMA expressed strong reservations about surveillance of patients solely for legal purposes.[48]

The use of measures such as covert surveillance, including secret video filming, is covered by legislation in the UK.[49] The purpose of this legislation is to ensure that investigatory powers are used in accordance with fundamental concepts of human rights.

Covert filming for medicolegal purposes

In 2003, the Court of Appeal considered a case in which an insurer arranged for the secret filming of an insurance claimant. Jean Jones suffered a small cut to her hand at work and claimed in excess of £135 000 for what she said was a continuing disability. An investigator hired by the insurers went twice to her house, posing as a researcher, and filmed her using a hidden camera. A medical expert retained by the insurer who saw the film concluded that the claimant had the full function of her hand, but the expert retained by Jean Jones reached the opposite conclusion. The Appeal Court case focused on the use of secret surveillance rather than the substance of the claim. If the secret film was inadmissible, it could not be used in court and new medical experts would have to be found. Lord Woolf said that the significance of video evidence would vary from case to case, as would the gravity of a breach of the right to privacy under human rights legislation. He said that, in this case, the behaviour by the insurers was not sufficiently outrageous to rule out the evidence, but it was still a contravention of the privacy of Jean Jones. He said it would be undesirable for the insurers to go uncensured as this could encourage others to infringe people's privacy in an unacceptable way. Therefore the insurers had to pay the costs of all the proceedings before the district judge, circuit judge and Court of Appeal to resolve the issue of the video.

Jones v University of Warwick[50]

The BMA and the GMC have particular concerns about the use of covert surveillance cameras on medical premises by doctors and medical firms providing independent reports for the assessment of patients' disability as part of a compensation claim. The GMC states that doctors "must obtain permission to make, and consent to use, any recording made for reasons other than the patient's treatment or assessment".[51] It acknowledges as an exception the use of covert surveillance to detect illness induced in children by carers, noting that in exceptional circumstances, you may judge that it is in the patient's best interests to make an identifiable recording of a patient without first seeking permission, and to disclose the recording to others without [the patient's] knowledge. Before proceeding you should discuss the recording with an experienced colleague. You must be prepared to justify your decision to the patient and, if necessary, to others. If the recording will involve covert video surveillance of a patient, it is likely to be within the scope of the Regulation of Investigatory Powers Act and you should seek advice before proceeding. A decision to use covert video surveillance, for example in cases of suspected induced illness in children, will normally be based on discussions amongst all the agencies involved, and the surveillance itself should be undertaken by the police.[52]

In connection with compensation claims, the purpose of covert monitoring is to verify whether patients are indeed as disabled as they claim and identify those who may be acting fraudulently. The GMC says that, even when doctors are acting as expert witnesses or producing a medicolegal report and therefore have a primary duty to the court or another third party, this does not negate all duties to the individual being examined.[53] That person is not a "patient" and hence the usual obligations of doctors to patients do not arise. Nevertheless, in the GMC's view, medical expert witnesses are exercising their professional knowledge and judgment as doctors and are bound by the duties set out in GMC guidance. This says that doctors must respect the privacy and dignity of the individuals they see. Both the GMC and the BMA advise that doctors should not collude with covert recordings except where it is in the patient's interest. Doctors should not arrange such secret surveillance on the premises where they work. They should take legal advice if they believe that filmed material that they have been asked to view or comment on is likely to have been improperly obtained.

Trust and declaring a financial interest

Patients trust that doctors will base their advice on an assessment of patients' best interests rather than on any other consideration, such as a possible advantage for the doctor in recommending one treatment, medical device or health care facility over another. Both the BMA and the GMC emphasise the importance of doctors being open with patients and families in situations where the doctor or people close to the doctor stand to benefit financially from the patient accepting a particular course of action. The most common situation in which this is likely to occur is that in which a doctor has invested in a residential nursing home or similar facility and would like to refer some patients to it. Even if it is the doctor's spouse or partner that stands to benefit, rather than the doctor personally, it is generally best to be open about such investments. Other cases brought to the BMA concern instances where doctors have substantial investments in a particular pharmaceutical company and wish to change their patients' existing medication to one produced by that company. Despite the fact that the link may be relatively distant and the sums gained in terms of investment revenue relatively small, such practices can undermine patient trust if not declared. It is partly for this reason that the BMA generally advises doctors not to hold investments in such companies if they are likely to want to prescribe its products for their patients. This subject is also discussed in Chapter 13 on prescribing and administering medication.

Receiving payment for referrals or recommendations

The GMC says that doctors must not accept or offer payment for a referral.[54] Accepting any inducement, gift, or hospitality as a reward from another practitioner for referring patients or arranging their care is unacceptable. Payment for endorsing other practitioners to patients is also likely to fall within this prohibition. Any measure that seems to be a variation on the theme of payment in exchange for recommendation or endorsement should be avoided. Payment for referral to solicitors or other non-health professionals is discussed in Chapter 19 (page 700).

Need for a chaperone

Situations arise in which either the doctor or the patient feels more comfortable if a chaperone is present. For example, the GMC[55] and medical defence bodies recommend that the option of a chaperone should be offered for intimate examinations, whenever possible. In 1997 the Royal College of Obstetricians and Gynaecologists (RCOG) published a detailed report about intimate examinations,[56] which also emphasised the importance of having a chaperone available for such procedures, regardless of the gender of the doctor. In one study, teenagers of both sexes seemed to prefer to have a family member with them for intimate examinations[57] and being accompanied may also be part of the general social or cultural expectations of some patients. Chaperones can be important for difficult psychiatric interviews and doctors may also require them if there is a risk of a patient becoming violent.[58] Patients undergoing an examination in connection with an insurance or litigation claim may want to bring a witness such as a lawyer or trade union representative to the consultation. The same applies to people being examined for forensic purposes by a police surgeon (see Chapter 17 on custodial settings). The 1997 RCOG report drew attention to a wide range of potential benefits for patients in having a chaperone present. These included providing reassurance to an anxious patient and physically assisting an infirm person, as well as maintaining communication and eye contact while the doctor's attention is focused on procedures such as colposcopy or hysteroscopy. The main disadvantages include the practical problems sometimes involved in arranging a suitable chaperone and the reduced opportunity for one to one communication about particularly sensitive issues such as past sexual abuse or domestic violence.

It is sometimes suggested that, in the primary care setting, a receptionist or practice manager could act as a chaperone in the absence of a practice nurse or other health professional. These options, however, raise issues of privacy and confidentiality that need to be agreed in advance between the doctor and the patient. Alternatives, such as leaving an intercom switched on or the surgery door ajar, are generally unacceptable. In secondary care, it is also sometimes the case that appropriate chaperones are not available in urgent situations unless other people have accompanied the patient. In the medical literature, the perceived need for a chaperone has traditionally focused on the doctor, typically male, being protected against unfounded allegations of impropriety by the patient, typically female.[59] In reality, however, complaints of indecent assault have been made by patients of both sexes and are not restricted to allegations against a doctor of the opposite sex. Providing an appropriate male chaperone for men in clinics where most health staff are female can be particularly difficult and in some situations there may be little option but to proceed without one, as long as the patient agrees. Wherever possible, however, such a need should be foreseen and planned for.

BMA advice on chaperones

- Although the stereotypical situations requiring chaperones are intimate examinations of female patients by male doctors, they need to be considered in any situation where a doctor proposes to carry out an intimate examination of patients of either gender.
- Situations requiring particular care also include occasions when it is necessary to darken the room for retinoscopy or similar procedures.
- Ideally, the option of having a chaperone should be discussed with patients in advance, particularly when patients need to be invited to bring a relative or friend (this is what the GMC advises for intimate examinations).
- When patients request a chaperone, this wish should be respected.
- In non-urgent situations where a chaperone is desirable but unavailable, the examination could be rescheduled.
- Health facilities should consider who would be appropriate to be a chaperone in the context of the services they provide.

Ensuring that staff are safe and reliable

When doctors employ colleagues or other staff or accept volunteers to do specific tasks, they should take appropriate steps to ensure that these people are safe and reliable, especially those working with children or vulnerable adults. Traditionally, in the primary care setting, it has been left to each practice to decide what checks to make. Since 2002, however, published guidance has been available regarding pre- and postappointment checks for anyone working in the NHS in England, whether as an employee, volunteer or contracted service provider.[60] This guidance includes reference to checking with the Criminal Records Bureau.

When offering employment to a fellow doctor, for example in a locum post, GPs routinely check that colleague's insurance and registration details. For any other information, they generally rely heavily on references provided. The importance of providing accurate testimonials is discussed in Chapter 21 (see pages 758–9), where attention is drawn to a GMC decision in which a doctor was found guilty of serious professional misconduct for failing to give a truthful account, in a reference, of a colleague's problems. Trusts carry out health screening and pre-employment checks on all staff and it is obviously important that similar checks are made in relation to volunteer workers. In addition, all staff, volunteers, and people such as students doing work observation[61] must be aware of the obligation to maintain patient confidentiality.

Requests for a second opinion

Patient requests for a second opinion[62] can appear as a symptom of mistrust in a doctor's clinical judgment. Patient advisory groups emphasise that patients always have a right to *ask* and, if reasonable, such requests are likely to be met.[63] The BMA supports this, stressing that requests for a second opinion need to be sensitively handled and should be met where feasible. It does not consider, however, that patients have an automatic "right" to obtain a second opinion unless treatment is being provided within the private sector and financed by the patient. Within the NHS, referral for a second opinion is dependent upon agreement between patient and doctor. The BMA's advice is that patients must not be made to feel uncomfortable or a nuisance. Such requests sometimes reflect a previous breakdown in communication. The responsibility for identifying a suitable doctor to give a further opinion rests with the referring GP, although consultants are often happy to suggest names. If a second specialist opinion concurs with the advice already provided, the question of who should provide care should reflect the patient's preferences. If the second specialist's opinion differs from the first, the original consultant should discuss these conflicting views with the patient. If the patient prefers to follow the advice provided in the second opinion, it is appropriate for the original specialist to suspend treatment and refer the patient on to the second consultant. Nevertheless, the first doctor may retain a duty of care if urgent treatment is needed and cannot be provided by the other doctor or if the person is currently an inpatient.

Recording of consultations by patients

Doctors sometimes feel that a patient's request to tape record a consultation is symptomatic of a lack of trust or an intention to bring a complaint later if any of the doctor's opinions are subsequently proved to be erroneous. In the enquiries raised by doctors with the BMA, most anxiety is expressed about patients attempting to tape record the interview clandestinely, apparently for the purposes of potential litigation at a later stage. In 1997 the BMA issued advice that doctors should not seek to prohibit recording but should encourage patients to do it openly rather than secretly.[64] The BMA was also concerned that recording risked reducing the opportunity for consultations in which doctors felt able to admit to uncertainty, but outlined the likely treatment choices patients would face later. Fear of possible litigation could result in health professionals becoming far more reserved and unwilling to discuss possible scenarios prior to having concrete data. On the other hand, however, tape recording has increasingly come to be seen as a way in which patients can remember important advice provided during a consultation. Any mechanism likely to assist patients to remember and cooperate actively with medical advice should be supported. In addition, one of the recommendations concerning patient consent that arose in 2001 from the Bristol report was that: "tape recording facilities should be provided by the NHS to enable patients, should they so wish, to make a tape recording of a discussion with a health care professional when a diagnosis, course of treatment, or prognosis is being discussed".[65]

Recording of consultations by doctors

The audio or video recording of consultations by doctors is mainly undertaken for the purposes of training or audit. Any recording of competent people for such purposes should have their consent or, for young children, the permission of parents. Clearly, any recording, whether done for the patient's or the doctor's purposes, can affect the nature of the consultation. These issues are considered in more detail in Chapter 6 (pages 205–7).

Patients who fail to attend appointments

Although considerable resources are lost through some patients failing to attend for an NHS appointment without any notice, the BMA is opposed to the proposal that they should be fined. It is believed that this could damage the doctor–patient relationship and subsequently make those patients reluctant to see their doctor when it is essential to do so. Clearly, the cost of missed appointments should be brought to patients' attention and the consequences for their own health (and their place on a waiting list, for example) as a result of repeated defaulting should be discussed.

Breakdown of the doctor–patient relationship

When the doctor–patient relationship breaks down irretrievably, patients generally transfer to another doctor, although, as mentioned earlier, they may encounter some difficulties in so doing. In the hospital setting, a consultant can either request a colleague to take on the care of the patient or ask the patient's GP to make an alternative referral. In cases other than violence and abuse, the BMA recommends that the decision to refer or transfer a patient elsewhere should be made only after careful consideration and not in the heat of the moment. Patients who are misusing services or failing to attend appointments may alter their behaviour if this is brought to their attention. If all else fails, however, the BMA believes that it is not in the best interests of either patient or doctor for an unsatisfactory relationship to continue. It is obviously important for doctors to maintain a high standard of professionalism even in circumstances where patients are difficult. Furthermore, explaining to patients how their behaviour has affected the doctor or the practice may help them in forming a better relationship with their next doctor or in making more appropriate use of services.

In general practice, patients can apply direct to another GP or be allocated by the local primary care organisation. GPs should not remove patients from their list because their treatment is too costly. Where the costs of treating an individual patient are higher than anticipated, adequate mechanisms exist to enable doctors to seek and be granted an increase in their prescribing budget. Nor should they remove patients on grounds of age. Looking after patients "from the cradle to the grave" is the essence of general practice. Some, but by no means all, elderly patients may have an increased need for medical attention. This is recognised in higher capitation fees for older patients and normally also in the formula for allocating prescribing budgets. Sometimes it is not the patients themselves but carers, particularly staff of private nursing and residential homes, who can generate excessive and inappropriate demands for services from the doctor or the practice. In these cases, the practice should attempt to resolve any problems through discussion. If the behaviour of one member of a household has led to his or her removal from a GP's list, this does not mean that the removal of other family members should automatically follow. Bearing in mind the need for patient confidentiality and prior discussion with the individual concerned, an explicit discussion with other family members about the problem can obviate the need for any further action. In rare cases, however, because of the possible need to visit patients at home, it may be necessary to terminate responsibility for other members of the family or the entire household. The prospect of visiting patients where a relative resides who is no longer a patient of the practice by virtue of this person's unacceptable behaviour, or being regularly confronted by such a patient, may make it too difficult for the GP to continue to look after the whole family. This is particularly likely when the patient has been removed from the GP's list because of violence or threatening behaviour and continuing to treat the other family members could put doctors or their staff at risk. (Violent patients are discussed on pages 58–60.)

Complaints

NHS GPs and hospitals must make information generally available about their complaints procedure. Private practitioners should also ensure that their patients are aware of how to register a complaint. Such information should make clear that patients are not disadvantaged simply for complaining because, if made in a reasonable and constructive manner, complaints can help to improve services. The complaints procedure can also provide opportunities to discuss instances where a patient or a doctor is felt to be behaving inappropriately. Early notification of a possible problem in their relationship can give doctors and patients an opportunity to discuss ways of preventing future difficulties. Persistent or demonstrably unfounded complaints, however, are usually indicative of a serious breakdown of the patient–doctor relationship. It is a breakdown of the relationship rather than a complaint *per se* that must form the basis of any decision to transfer the patient to a colleague.

Summary – trust and reciprocity

- Covert measures such as filming or giving medication without consent are generally unacceptable and should be considered only in very exceptional circumstances.
- Doctors must be open about any financial affairs that could be seen as influencing them.
- It is good practice to offer a chaperone for intimate examinations.
- Doctors have duties to ensure that their staff are safe and reliable.
- If the relationship breaks down irretrievably, transferring the patient to another practitioner is in the interests of all.

Recognising responsibilities and boundaries

Despite the emphasis given to the special caring relationship between doctors and patients, some clear boundaries must be maintained. There are various ways in which boundaries can be transgressed. The main responsibility for ensuring that proper limits are observed lies with doctors.

Boundaries in treatment

Self diagnosis and treatment

All doctors, as well as all patients, should be registered with their own GP. In the past, doctors often fell into the habit of treating themselves or informally asking a colleague to provide treatment. The BMA strongly advises against this. Although they must reasonably monitor their own health, especially in terms of whether they may pose any health risk to others, doctors should not self medicate. If self treating, doctors may lose insight into the potential risk they pose to others. Where they suspect that they may have been exposed to a communicable disease, doctors must seek and follow professional advice without delay and must not rely on their own assessment of the risks they pose to patients.[66] This is discussed further in Chapter 13 (page 478). General advice about sick doctors is given in Chapter 21.

Treating family, friends, or colleagues

Doctors are sometimes asked to treat their families or other people close to them. Although it may appear convenient to do so, this is inadvisable. A confusion of roles can develop and doctors can find it hard to keep the right emotional distance. They may fail to notice symptoms that a dispassionate observer would note and, if treating a relative at home, may not be able to carry out all the tests that would be done in a formal consultation. They may have conflicts of interest or be erroneously perceived as having such conflicts.

Doctors may be suspected of neglect or facilitating harm, for example, when they stand to inherit or otherwise benefit from a relative's death. Supplying controlled drugs to an addicted friend or relative is obviously unacceptable and to comply with such requests is mistaken loyalty. Sometimes the request for treatment does not come from the relative, but rather doctors assume that they should treat their own spouse or children, for example. This can have disadvantages for those who may find that, as treatment progresses, they do not have the same rights to privacy as other patients.

Staff who are also patients

It would be unfair to discount potential applicants for jobs in general practice surgeries simply because they are registered with the practice. The BMA's Equal Opportunities Committee has produced general guidance on how doctors can avoid discrimination against any employee, which emphasises commonsense precautions such as ensuring that selection for a job is based on the requirements previously set out in the job description.[67] It is clearly not ideal, however, for an individual's doctor to also be that person's employer. Conflicts and difficulties often arise, particularly in terms of patient confidentiality. The risk of this occurring can be diminished if the issues are discussed in advance. Therefore, if a position is offered to someone who is also a patient of the practice, that person should be offered the opportunity to register with another practice. If, however, the individual wishes to remain with the practice, that decision should be accommodated. In rural areas there may be no reasonable alternative. Advance thought should be given by both parties, however, to the potential difficulties that could arise, for example, if the patient were to need a lot of sick leave and the practice needed verification of illness. In addition, if disciplinary procedures should be invoked, the patient/employee's health record may hold relevant information that is known only to the employer by virtue of being the employee's doctor. In such circumstances, the record should not be used for purposes unrelated to the provision of health care without the individual's consent. In some exceptional cases raised with the BMA, it seems that some individuals have probably sought jobs in a surgery with a view to altering aspects of their own or their family's medical records, by removing reference to child protection proceedings, for example. Clearly, the practice needs to be alert to that possibility.

All staff must be advised about confidentiality and, specifically, that it is totally inappropriate for them to look at the medical records of relatives, neighbours, or friends. All information is confidential and available only to those working in the practice on a strict "need to know" basis. If the employee's relatives themselves are unhappy about the individual potentially having access to their records, they should also have the option of moving to another practice. In terms of the GP's access to the records of an employee's relatives, this should be on the same basis as for any other records and should be on grounds of needing to know. It would clearly be inappropriate for a GP to look at the records of an employee's relatives simply to obtain information about the employee.

Managing patient expectations

Patients sometimes expect their doctor to assist them to obtain various social goals, such as by providing references, signing passport applications, or supporting requests for special housing on health grounds. It is important that doctors put their signature only to documents that they have verified because they may be liable if they countersign something that is untrue. It is unethical for a doctor to advocate a course of action on a patient's behalf when there is no evidence to justify it. For example, GPs are sometimes asked by families to provide a report advocating that a child should attend a particular school on medical grounds when there is no record of any medical problem. Clearly, it can be a difficult balance to maintain patient trust in such situations, but it would be wrong to assist patients to manipulate the education or state benefit systems.

Managing relatives' expectations

Patients and their families are vulnerable at times of illness and anxiety. Doctors must ensure that inappropriate attachments or dependence are not allowed to develop. The BMA is occasionally contacted by doctors who, having acted completely properly, are, nevertheless, concerned that during the progress of a long illness the spouse or close relative of a patient has become inappropriately dependent upon them. This can occur in the course of an acute or terminal illness when the doctor can become the main focus for an otherwise socially isolated carer. Such situations are delicate and relatives may be particularly emotional, anticipating bereavement. Nevertheless, it is essential that an emotional distance is maintained. Wherever possible, other health and social care professionals should be involved and it may assist relatives to be put in touch with patient support groups. In the case of terminal illness, other members of the primary health care team and hospice outreach services may be able to share in providing support.

Managing personal relationships

Any form of intimate personal contact between doctors and patients is at risk of being viewed as a potential case of professional misconduct. The GMC tells doctors that they must not use their "professional position to pursue a sexual or improper emotional relationship with a patient or someone close to them".[68] Therefore, as a general principle, sexual relationships or emotional dependence between doctors and their patients or the close relatives of patients must be discouraged. Doctors have access to past health information about their patients and see them when they are feeling ill and vulnerable, all of which puts patients at a disadvantage. Although, in theory, it is the use of their "position" to pursue the relationship that is prohibited, in practice it may be hard to distinguish whether or not this is the case. Intimate personal relationships can arise in good faith when doctors and patients initially meet in a purely social setting but, even so, the doctor can be very vulnerable to complaint if the relationship ends acrimoniously. Doctors who discover that a person with whom they are developing a personal or sexual relationship is also their patient should immediately cease the relationship or take steps to ensure that medical care is provided by another practitioner. In some circumstances, this may be difficult. GPs practising in remote and isolated areas, for example, may find that any eligible person in the area is already on their practice list and finding an alternative doctor involves some difficulty for the patient. Nevertheless, all reasonable steps must be taken to ensure this. In a secondary care setting, doctors should not embark on a personal relationship with a patient or a person close to a patient while they are responsible for an episode of care. Doctors also sometimes ask for advice on how to handle a situation in which they feel attracted to a patient or the close relative of a patient and therefore need to ask that person to transfer to another doctor before it is clear whether or not a personal relationship is likely to grow. It can seem very presumptuous to ask patients to transfer, but this is advisable at an early stage if a personal relationship is intended.

Abusive behaviour by doctors

Questions of misconduct can arise in any situation where there is an imbalance of power. There are various ways in which doctors may improperly use their position. The GMC, for example, emphasises that doctors must not put pressure on patients to accept private treatment or encourage them to make loans, gifts, or donations to any organisation or individual.[69] Nor should they exploit patients' lack of knowledge when making charges for treatment or, indeed, in any other aspect of care. Patients are often accustomed to following their doctor's instructions in relation to physical examinations, for example, even if they themselves feel unsure about the necessity for them. Patients are, therefore, often initially reluctant to question their doctor's behaviour, even when it is inappropriate.

Abusive behaviour

In 2002 a male GP locum was found guilty by the GMC of serious professional misconduct in relation to his inappropriate behaviour towards two female patients. As a locum in Nottingham, he had carried out, without explanation, an unnecessary breast examination of a patient complaining of earache and attempted to persuade her to consent to an unnecessary internal examination. He had also asked the patient irrelevant questions of an explicitly sexual nature and refused her request for a chaperone to be present for any intimate examination. A few months later, as a locum in Manchester, he asked another female patient who had a sore throat to remove her blouse and inappropriately touched her breast. The GMC also strongly criticised the fact that the doctor sent both women Christmas cards at their homes when he knew he was subject to disciplinary proceedings at which they would be witnesses. In its judgment, the GMC emphasised how seriously it views inappropriate or indecent behaviour by doctors since such acts undermine public trust, offend patients' rights, damage the reputation of the profession, and constitute an abuse of the doctor's position.[70]

The BMA and the GMC strongly condemn any inappropriate contact between doctors and patients. Situations in which there is an imbalance of power, sufficient to vitiate consent or where the patient has impaired competence, are covered by the law on consent. Doctors who abuse or exploit patients are liable to disciplinary action by the GMC as well as prosecution under the criminal law. They are likely to be struck off the medical register if it is shown that they have used their position to establish an improper relationship with a patient or a patient's close relative. Health professionals who have grounds to suspect that a colleague is abusing or exploiting patients should take steps to have the matter properly investigated. Some circumstances invariably give cause for particular concern. Among the most obvious examples are patients who are consulting a psychiatrist for emotional difficulties or visiting a GP after a loss or bereavement. In such circumstances, even if doctors and patients do not themselves perceive it as such, a personal relationship will inevitably be seen as potentially exploitative and a cause for disciplinary proceedings.

Patients' duty to treat health professionals reasonably

Most patients are considerate and certainly do not need to be advised on how to behave reasonably. Nevertheless, in 2003 the Scottish Consumer Council published for consultation a booklet for patients setting out the rights and responsibilities for everyone who uses the health service in Scotland.[71] It listed the duties of patients as the obligation to:

- be on time
- be polite
- follow the advice given by health professionals
- give doctors, dentists, and hospitals up to date contact details
- finish any medicine prescribed, avoid taking any out of date medicine and return unused medicine to a pharmacist for disposal
- keep oneself healthy
- call emergency services only in a real emergency
- cooperate with surveys and requests for feedback.

It also told patients how to be a blood donor and how to be an organ donor without implying that these were obligations, but rather things they could consider. As yet, other consumer bodies do not appear to have adopted a similar approach, but the BMA supports the provision of such information booklets to patients. Ideally, these should not only clarify their own rights but also give attention to patients' responsibilities to use health services appropriately.

The BMA occasionally receives enquiries from doctors or commissioning bodies about how to respond to patients who persistently make unreasonable demands on health services. In some cases, this may involve repeated but unfounded complaints, excessive or unjustified demands for home visits, misuse of emergency services, or persistently telephoning a GP's surgery or hospital switchboard for long periods, blocking calls from other patients. Such activities can disrupt the provision of care and waste resources. Eventually, healthcare staff become reluctant to see or talk to such patients, although it is clear that in some of these cases the individuals concerned are mentally ill and lacking insight into the effects of their behaviour. In other cases, patients regard the health facility as a general source of social support for a range of medical and non-medical problems. Offering counselling or arranging for the patient to have an advocate can help to modify or rechannel some of the excessive or inappropriate demands, as can information about other possible sources of support and advice, including NHS Direct or the Samaritans. Alternatively, healthcare staff may arrange a meeting or case conference with the patient (and an advocate or friend) to establish a reasonable agreement about how the patient's problems can be handled. Establishing clear boundaries about the regularity of contact, case review, and the limits to what can be provided by the health service may be the only feasible way forward.

Payment for services

Obviously, patients who request private treatment ought to be prompt in paying for the care provided. Doctors sometimes enquire whether they have any obligation to continue to provide care for private patients who have failed to pay for past private treatment. When emergency care is required and no alternative doctor is available, all doctors are ethically obliged to provide essential care (see Chapter 15, pages 549–52). If a patient has neglected to pay for private care, but is subsequently seen by the same doctor in an NHS setting, the fact of past non-payment must never interfere with the obligations owed by that doctor. In situations where doctors decide to pursue patients for payment that is owed, they need to be careful not to infringe patients' confidentiality by disclosing any information to third parties about the care provided.

Can violent people expect to receive medical care?

Violence in this context includes verbal abuse and threats as well as physical assaults, all of which have been addressed by the government's zero tolerance campaigns since 2000. Whether or not doctors are obliged to treat violent people depends on the reason for the behaviour and the urgency of the patient's need. Unexpectedly aggressive behaviour can be caused by patients' medical condition or their medication. Identifying whether there is an organic cause is essential when patients appear to be acting out of character. In cases where violent behaviour is a facet of mental illness, the patient may have to be restrained and possibly admitted to hospital for assessment (see discussion of WP on page 44). In 1998 the Royal College of Psychiatrists published detailed advice on the management of violence in such situations.[72] In facilities providing care for people with mental illness, it is essential that all staff have appropriate training in conflict avoidance and management of aggression. It is essential that physical restraint and sedation are limited to situations where they are necessary to prevent harm to the patient or to other people. Detailed guidance on restraint is given in Chapter 17.

When it is not a symptom of their illness, patients who are threatening or racially abusive should not be denied urgent treatment or necessary immediate care, if this can be provided safely. In some trusts and GP premises, however, it has proved necessary, as a last resort, to withhold treatment from some patients, although this raises dilemmas for clinicians. In 2001 the Department of Health issued advice to GPs[73] and provided general guidelines to help trusts[74] to develop their own local policies on withholding treatment in these circumstances. This was made available throughout the UK and the BMA strongly supported the campaign for "zero tolerance" of violence against NHS staff. In Northern Ireland, for example, the BMA called upon all candidates for the Northern Ireland Assembly to support the full implementation of zero tolerance at a local level. The NHS guidance advised that withholding treatment is appropriate only when abusive behaviour is likely to:

- prejudice any benefit for the patient
- prejudice the safety of people providing treatment
- lead staff to believe that they cannot undertake their duties properly
- result in damage to property
- prejudice the safety of other patients.

If a violent patient does not need treatment urgently, or when treatment is impossible because of the patient's extreme behaviour, the police can be called to remove the patient, either from hospital or GP premises. If the patient is detained, a police surgeon may supervise him or her until appropriate treatment can be given. (Care in custodial settings is discussed in Chapter 17.) Doctors and health facility personnel may need to take legal advice if they intend to ban from medical premises patients or their relatives who have been violent in the past. (In some cases, as a result of an assault, bail conditions may specify a prohibition on returning.) GPs can also request the immediate removal from their lists of any patient who is threatening or violent. In some primary care premises and hospital settings, special segregated areas or after hours clinics deal with persistently aggressive patients in a secure environment with police or security officers on hand. This system was piloted in South Wales where it met with such success that the National Assembly called for the widespread use of it in police stations or secure surgeries.[75] Many of the patients treated during the pilot study were addicts demanding prescription drugs and some were able to return to normal surgeries when their behaviour changed after a year of segregation.

Patient confidentiality and violent patient markers

All healthcare premises should have clear policies on the handling of violent people and these can be publicised in leaflets or posters. Patients should be made aware that there are limits to their rights to treatment and to confidentiality. They should know that violent or threatening behaviour can result in them being removed from healthcare premises, and information about them passed on to other healthcare providers and possibly the police. Violent patient markers are a mechanism used in primary care and NHS hospital trusts for tagging the paper or electronic health records of certain patients and alerting healthcare professionals who come into contact with them. The marker must be removable and regularly reviewed. In the healthcare setting, its meaning should be obvious to the health team but not to other people such as patients who may inadvertently catch sight of records. Advice from the Information Commissioner is that:

> To comply with the fairness element of the first data protection principle, as soon as the decision is made data controllers should inform individuals who are identified as being potentially violent that their records will indicate this. They should also be informed of the incident which led to them being so identified, to whom this information may be passed, and when the decision to identify them as potentially violent will be removed or examined with a view to removal.[76]

In hospitals, senior staff and managers should be closely involved in establishing policies and making decisions about the treatment of aggressive individuals. Such decisions should not be left to unsupported junior doctors and nurses. In addition to advice from the Department of Health, a range of guidance covers aspects of conflict management and dealing with aggression.[77]

Stalkers

Health professionals can be very vulnerable. In the BMA's experience, emotional pressure can come from patients. The Association has received anecdotal reports of both male and female patients who initially appear engaging and personable but end up stalking doctors and subjecting them to intense emotional pressure by, for example, threats of self harm. Doctors in such situations need to take advice and support from professional colleagues and take steps to pass on care of the patient to another health team. If the behaviour persists, they may well need to involve the police and should make this clear to the individual.

Gifts and bequests

NHS guidance on gifts and bequests

In 1993 NHS guidance specified that NHS employees should not accept substantial gifts from patients or others. Nevertheless, it also noted that:

> Casual gifts offered by contractors or others, e.g. at Christmas time, may not be in any way connected with the performance of duties so as to constitute an offence under the Prevention of Corruption Acts 1906 and 1916. Such gifts should nevertheless be politely but firmly declined. Articles of low intrinsic value such as diaries or calendars, or small tokens of gratitude from patients or their relatives, need not necessarily be refused. In cases of doubt, staff should either consult their line manager or politely decline acceptance.[78]

Patients or their relatives often wish to show their gratitude to the health professionals who have looked after them by a gift or bequest. Health professionals employed by the NHS, however, are subject to restrictions regarding the acceptance of gifts from patients and their families. Doctors who are not NHS employees, such as private doctors and GPs should also be aware of this advice. Non-NHS employees can accept unsolicited gifts, although the GMC makes clear that it is a disciplinary offence for doctors to demand them or exert any pressure to obtain a donation.[79] They should make clear to the patient that the quality of care is not influenced by the provision or absence of gifts. In England and Wales, the Health and Social Care Act 2001 made provision for a reporting and recording system for gifts over a particular level; at the time of writing this had not been implemented. In some cases, the donor intends the gift for the institution – either the GP practice or the hospital trust – which may have special arrangements to manage such funds. GPs, for example, often use unsolicited gifts to improve the practice or buy new equipment. Many hospitals also have endowment funds with charitable status that can accept gifts.

Most gifts do not involve significant sums and are a genuine reflection of gratitude. Nevertheless, doctors also need to be aware that in some rare cases gifts or loans may be offered by patients as a means of establishing an improper sense of closeness within the doctor–patient relationship. Without appearing dismissive, it is advisable to avoid accepting such gifts. Doctors are also sometimes aware that a gift is part of a strategy by donors to send a message to their relatives. It may, for example, be a means of expressing frustration at neglect by family members. The responsibility of talking to patients about the implications of their choices sometimes falls to doctors. Problems can arise if the patient's family challenges either the gift or questions the mental capacity of the patient at the time of making the gift or bequest. The BMA advises doctors that they should not become involved in carrying out assessments of mental capacity for patients who may wish to leave them money or other gifts. In such cases, it is advisable that any assessment of mental capacity should be entrusted to an independent doctor who does not stand to benefit in any way from the outcome of the assessment. Joint BMA and Law Society guidance[80] on assessment of mental capacity includes details of the legal tests that patients must meet in order to be seen as competent to make a gift or make or revise a will.

Doctors as witnesses to wills and legal documents

A common enquiry concerns the implications of doctors acting as witnesses to a patient's will or advance directive ("living will"). The courts have seen it as being highly desirable that a doctor should witness legal documents in situations where the drafter's mental capacity may later be questioned. The BMA's advice is that doctors so doing need to be aware that they will be assumed to have verified the patient's mental capacity and so they are not seen to be just witnessing the authenticity of the signature. Nevertheless, when they are confident that the patient is clearly competent, this should not be problematic. It means, however, that doctors should not witness documents for patients whom they have not examined recently without considering whether an assessment of mental capacity is needed.[81] Doctors are also sometimes asked to assume powers of attorney for patients who may be elderly and at risk of losing their capacity to direct their own affairs. Clearly, the full implications of accepting such a task need to be looked into by any doctor so approached. The question of possible remuneration or other reward for taking on such a task also needs to be considered, since this may raise a conflict of interest, as may the transfer of such a patient into a nursing home in which the doctor has a financial interest. It is the responsibility of the doctor considering such a role to investigate any other potential conflicts of interest before accepting.

Responsibilities of doctors: a "duty to pursue"?

A very common question raised with the BMA concerns the extent and limits of doctors' duties to pursue patients who are likely to need further treatment. Both GPs and hospital doctors are concerned when patients fail to keep follow up appointments or do not collect the results of laboratory tests. The BMA's advice is generally to examine all reasonable options, including writing to or telephoning the patient. When the information to be conveyed to the patient is particularly sensitive or there are reasons to suppose that the patient would not wish to be contacted in the usual way, an arrangement should be made in advance as to how test results will be communicated. Clearly, issues of confidentiality may arise if the patient is a minor or a person who does not wish to be contacted at home. Teenagers awaiting the results of a test for pregnancy or a sexually transmitted infection, for example, can be asked to specify how they wish to receive the results in order to ensure their privacy.

When patients fail to attend for hospital appointments, the GP should be informed. Some hospital trusts are reluctant to allow consultants to offer follow up appointments to patients who have previously missed one or more without any explanation. Where it is clinically important for the patient to be seen, however, consultants should have the right to offer a new appointment and it may be helpful for them to liaise with the GP so that patients can be made aware of the importance for their health. Inevitably, however, difficulties arise when a particular consultant has a long waiting list for new patients and those who have previously defaulted on their appointments also need to be fitted in. The extent to which doctors should attempt to accommodate such patients partly depends upon the gravity of the condition in question, the availability of an effective therapy for it, the likelihood of these patients persisting with treatment, and the practicalities or obstacles involved in making contact with them. Ultimately, a balance must be sought between attempting to encourage non-attenders to accept an opportunity that could be vital to their health, respecting the fact that some of them choose not to and ensuring that new patients who are keen to receive care are not kept waiting longer than necessary by repeated non-attendance.

Responsibilities of patients to safeguard health

Patients are no longer seen as just recipients of health care but as active partners in disease prevention and management. Most patients are keen to take steps to maintain their own health and protect people close to them. They need information about how best to do that. Clearly, however, this does not mean that doctors can oblige patients to receive information that they do not want or lecture them about their responsibilities. As discussed above, patients can decline some details but need to be generally aware of the implications of their condition, including the likely consequences for other people. Clear information needs to be available to patients about the potential actions they could take to preserve their own and other people's health, including the importance of taking prescribed medication (see Chapter 13, pages 454–5). Health professionals cannot impose their own values and preferences on their patients, nor is rudeness ever acceptable. However, any deliberate misuse of the healthcare system should be pointed out. Most patients, however, are well aware of the pressures on health care and of the need to use resources wisely. Patient obligations in this respect have not traditionally been given attention in professional codes in the UK, although they have a long tradition in the USA.

American code of medical ethics – patient responsibilities

"Once patients and physicians agree upon the goals of therapy, patients have a responsibility to co-operate with the treatment plan. Patients also have a responsibility to disclose whether previously agreed upon treatments are being followed and to indicate when they would like to reconsider the treatment plan."[82]

"Patients should be committed to health maintenance through health-enhancing behaviour. Patients must take personal responsibility when they are able to avert the development of disease. Patients should also have an active interest in the effects of their conduct on others and refrain from behaviour that unreasonably places the health of others at risk. Patients should enquire as to the means and likelihood of infectious disease transmissions and act upon that information which can best prevent further transmission."[83]

Obvious difficulties arise when patients perceive themselves as having rights of access to care and medication without taking the concomitant obligations into account. In some common cases raised with the BMA, patients urgently and repeatedly request extensions of their prescriptions from their GP but fail to attend the practice for the necessary examination that should accompany renewal of the prescription. In such cases doctors should consider writing in a detailed way to these patients, explaining the risks incurred if they do not attend for a checkup and the fact that the doctor cannot simply go on renewing the prescription. For the doctor there is likely to be a point at which the risks of extending a prescription yet again without having examined the patient exceed the risks of the patient not having the medication. GPs need to make patients aware that for them to prescribe repeatedly without carrying out an examination may be considered negligent and contrary to their duty to ensure that their prescribing is appropriate and justifiable.

Reciprocity: do doctors still owe duties when patients refuse medical advice?

If the doctor–patient partnership is seen as one of mutual trust and respect, the refusal of one partner to follow advice may lead the other to feel absolved from all further responsibilities. In the BMA's view, however, it is important that doctors should continue to encourage their patients to take control of their own health in a positive and responsible way, without lecturing or appearing to abandon them.

Refusal of advice and hospital treatment

BMA advice is that, even when patients refuse treatment, the usual ethical principles apply for health professionals. Patients have a right to veto treatment providing they understand the implications and are mentally competent. Doctors have a duty to offer to treat, but cannot oblige competent patients to accept their advice. If the patient requires medication that can be self administered and which is felt to be essential, this should be explained to the patient, who should be offered the drugs. Failure to offer discharge drugs or a follow up appointment may seem like abandoning the patient and vulnerable people may slip through the net. Although adults have a right to make unwise choices, they should also have a chance to change their mind. Health professionals should try to make clear precisely why they recommend the treatment, the medication, or the need for follow up appointments, but competent people cannot be forced to accept medication or return. Health professionals should be able to demonstrate that they have acted reasonably and it may therefore be desirable for the patient to sign a disclaimer or treatment waiver, noting the reasons for the medical advice and the patient's decision. (This is discussed further in Chapter 2, page 87) If the patient was referred by a GP, it is important to keep the GP informed of what has happened and what drugs are recommended. If the patient refuses permission for the hospital to contact the GP, this refusal too should be documented. Doctors should ensure that the notes are fully written up at the time of discharge and a note made that the doctor believes the patient to be capable of making a valid decision.

Summary – recognising responsibilities and boundaries

- Doctors and patients need to fulfil their respective responsibilities.
- Doctors and patients each have obligations in terms of maximising patients' health.

- Close personal relationships between doctors and their patients or their patients' close relatives must be avoided.
- Patients and doctors need to be unambiguously aware that aggressive or rude behaviour is unacceptable.

The doctor–patient relationship of the future

Continuity of care

Expectations of the doctor–patient relationship continue to change and evolve. Facets such as continuity of care, which patients seem to value,[84] are increasingly difficult to provide. In primary care, out of hours services are increasingly provided by doctors other than the patient's own GP. In the short term at least, the shortage of doctors in both primary and secondary care may entail more patients being sent abroad so that their treatment and aftercare are shared between health professionals abroad and in the UK. Also, as many as a third of doctors working in the UK originally qualified overseas.[85] There is a continuing need to recruit such overseas trained health professionals who are perfectly competent, but may have a different attitude and approach to the relationship. (Differing attitudes to truth telling in different cultures, for example, is discussed in Chapter 10, pages 368–9.) This highlights the importance of including ethics teaching and an awareness of patient expectations in continuing training for qualified health professionals.

Multidisciplinary practice

More services are provided by extended teams in which the doctor is one participant. As we discuss in Chapter 19, care increasingly involves a range of practitioners and therapists, with a consequent blurring of some of the traditional professional boundaries. Limited formularies to be prescribed by other health professionals are developing. The trend for informed self medication by patients is likely to continue, advised by pharmacists.

Telemedicine and other forms of care at a distance

With the growth of technology, it is increasingly feasible for doctor–patient consultations to be conducted at a distance. Telemedicine is medicine practised at a distance. It incorporates tools such as videoconferencing, multimedia communications, internet, and intranet for a range of clinical purposes including diagnosis, treatment, and clinical education. Telemedicine includes both live and time delayed consultations. Live telemedicine involves some combination of patients, GPs, and specialists communicating by means of a realtime live audiovisual link. At its best, live telemedicine can improve communication because the patient and the GP who knows the patient's history can be present together when a specialist is consulted by videoconferencing. GPs can also begin treatment following the advice of the specialist via the video link. Time delayed telemedicine involves the electronic transmission of a previously recorded visual image of the patient, consisting either of a visual sequence such as a video clip of an echocardiogram or single pictures, for example of a skin abnormality. Among its advantages are cost reduction, the speeding up of referral for the patient, avoidance of unnecessary referrals, greater consistency in health care and improved contact between doctors. The number of broken appointments can be reduced and one pathologist, for example, can provide services to a number of different locations.

Regarding the ethical considerations, the principal concerns are accuracy of the image or text, security, and confidentiality. Mistakes can be made and an erroneous diagnosis given by video link as in any other consultation, and teleconsultation cannot convey the same information as a physical examination. The accountability of doctors and their ethical duties remain the same. Clearly, research needs to compare the diagnostic accuracy of results obtained by telemedicine with those obtained using traditional methods. In 2001 the BMA's General Practitioners Committee published advice on the limitations of telemedicine and other forms of consulting at a distance, such as online text messages.[86] Some international standards have been set by organisations such as the Standing Committee of European Doctors.[87] The BMA advises that patient identifiable data should be encrypted when transmitted electronically (see Chapter 6, pages 212–3). Prescribing drugs electronically and over the internet are discussed in Chapter 13 (see pages 479–80).

Routine telephone communications may also replace some face to face consultations. In the USA, it has been shown that regular telephone review of certain patient groups has the potential to reduce morbidity, drug use, and use of health services by patients with a range of chronic disorders.[88] In primary care in the UK, there have been initiatives to provide systematic monitoring of certain patient groups by telephone. In 2003, for example, the management of asthma patients by telephone consultations was shown to be as effective as and less time consuming than face to face consultations in the surgery.[89] This particular review was undertaken by practice nurses who believed that telephone consultations were more focused and more flexible in terms of time needed to talk to the patient than surgery consultations. Among patients there was no apparent loss of satisfaction.

Better informed patients

Greater patient awareness of healthcare information is likely to continue to impact on the nature of the doctor–patient relationship. Media such as the internet can have immense benefits for patients but also can pose difficulties in terms of assessing the accuracy of the information provided. In 2000 the BMA's General Practitioners Committee published brief advice for patients using the internet.[90] The BMA's ethical guidelines and some of its books on specific medicolegal issues, such as advance directives, are available to the public as well as to doctors on the BMA website.

The overlap between medicine and politics

In the 1980s, attention was drawn to the "medicalisation" of many aspects of life and the fact that some issues that required social and political debate were often portrayed and perceived as being medical.[91] Kennedy argued that many of the decisions taken in health care were issues for society as a whole. Since then, Parliament and the courts have indeed debated and regulated many of the most contentious areas of healthcare provision and treatment withdrawal in legislation such as the Human Fertilisation and Embryology Act 1990 (see Chapter 8) and legal cases, such as that of Tony Bland (see Chapter 10). Nevertheless, the boundaries between medical and political decision making continue to be blurred, particularly on issues such as the management of patient waiting lists and determining priorities for treatment. The BMA continues to receive expressions of concern from hospital doctors in particular about the fact that political priorities and targets seem to be much more influential than clinical criteria in some cases. This is an issue touched on in Chapters 19 on team working and 20 on public health, but it is also a subject requiring greater public debate.

Rights-based expectations

At the start of this chapter, we noted Lord Woolf's comment that medical practice is one of the facets of society likely to become more litigious and focused on patients' enforceable rights. He predicted an increasingly rights-based society in which the courts would continue to be highly influential in establishing ethical boundaries. This seems a trend that is likely to continue and in most chapters of this book we have noted important legal cases that have either set or reinforced ethical standards.

Another facet of a rights-based culture is the potential growth in patient demand for either pharmaceutical products or medical interventions as a "right". Arguably, the demand for so-called "lifestyle" drugs contributes to the perception that medicine is not there only to respond to patient need but also to patients' desires for a different quality of life. (Lifestyle drugs are discussed on pages 458–9.) Parallel to this trend, we also need to note the potential for "medical tourism", whereby individuals seek to bypass the prohibition on, or scarcity of, certain services in one country by seeking treatment overseas. Amongst the examples in this book are fertility services, surrogacy arrangements, and the purchase of human organs. In some cases, however, the NHS has to provide aftercare or remedial treatment if the service purchased elsewhere goes wrong. These kinds of issues need wide public debate and clarification about the acceptability to society of such arrangements.

Some doctors are concerned that health care may be overtaken by consumerist language and attitudes so that medicine comes to be seen as just a job like any other, involving clients who expect to select their preferred options from technicians who provide them. The disadvantages of such a view would be considerable if, as a result, doctors and other health professionals see themselves simply as service providers. Throughout this book we seek to emphasise reasons why doctors should continue to be seen to have special responsibilities over and above those of other citizens.

References

1   Woolf LCJ. Are the courts excessively deferential to the medical profession? http://www.medneg.com/texts/text.cfm?textMaterials_ID=3 (accessed 13 August 2003)
2   Cassell EJ. The principles of the Belmont Report revisited. *Hastings Cent Rep* 2000;**30**(4):12–21: 14.
3   Paine C. Il dissoluto punito: medicine in the age of blame. *Med Leg J* 2002;**70**:161–75: 163.
4   Baker R, Emanuel L. The efficacy of professional ethics. *Hastings Cent Rep* 2000;**30**(4 suppl):S13–S17: S14.
5   Leake CD, ed. *Percival's medical ethics*. Baltimore, MD: Williams and Wilkins, 1927:71.
6   *Ibid:* p. 74.
7   Code of ethics of the American Medical Association, adopted May 1847, reproduced as Appendix III in: Leake CD, ed. *Percival's medical ethics. Op cit:* p. 221.
8   *Ibid:* pp. 219, 221.
9   Scottish Consumer Council. *Patient rights and responsibilities: a draft for consultation.* Edinburgh: SCC, 2003.
10 Cassell EJ. The principles of the Belmont Report revisited. *Op cit:* p. 15.
11 The BMA has specific advice on the implications for medicine of the Human Rights Act 1998 and access to care by asylum seekers in: British Medical Association. *The impact of the Human Rights Act 1998 on medical decision making.* London: BMA, 2000. British Medical Association. *Access to health care for asylum seekers.* London: BMA, 2001.
12 Gordon R, ed. *The literary companion to medicine.* London: Sinclair Stevenson, 1993:2.
13 General Medical Council. *Good medical practice.* London: GMC, 2001: paras 17–19.
14 British Medical Association Board of Medical Education. *Communication skills education for doctors: a discussion paper.* London: BMA, 2003.
15 Tannenbaum SJ. Say the right thing: communication and physician accountability in the era of medical outcomes. In: Boyle P, ed. *Getting doctors to listen.* Georgetown: Georgetown University Press, 2000.
16 Mihill C. *Shaping tomorrow: issues facing general practice in the new millennium.* London: BMA, 2000.
17 *Ibid:* p. 93.
18 Macdonald S. Doctors are servants of patients, says chief medical officer. *BMJ* 2003;**326**:569.
19 General Medical Council. *Seeking patients' consent: the ethical considerations.* London: GMC, 1998: para 3.
20 *Ibid:* para 6.
21 Payne SA. Balancing information needs: dilemmas in producing patient information leaflets. *Health Informatics J* 2002;**8**:174–9: 175.
22 *Ibid:* p. 175.
23 Dixon-Woods M. Writing wrongs? An analysis of published discourses about the use of patient information leaflets. *Soc Sci Med* 2001;**52**:1417–32.
24 Payne SA. Balancing information needs: dilemmas in producing patient information leaflets. *Op cit:* p. 176.
25 *Ibid:* p. 177. Payne conducted studies involving cancer patients to evaluate written materials.
26 General Medical Council. *Good medical practice. Op cit:* para 6.
27 *Ibid:* para 5.
28 The Bristol Royal Infirmary Inquiry. *Learning from Bristol: the report of the public inquiry into children's heart surgery at the Bristol Royal Infirmary 1984–1995.* London: The Stationery Office, 2001: recommendation 11. (Cm 5207 (II).)
29 Cassell EJ. The principles of the Belmont Report revisited. *Op cit:* p. 16.
30 The Bristol Royal Infirmary Inquiry. *Learning from Bristol: the report of the public inquiry into children's heart surgery at the Bristol Royal Infirmary 1984–1995. Op cit:* recommendation 14.
31 Hutton J, Burstow P. *House of Commons official report (Hansard).* 2000 May 15: col 124.
32 General Medical Council. *Good medical practice. Op cit:* para 22.
33 Froggatt v Chesterfield and North Derbyshire NHS Trust, 2002 WL 31676323: para 25.
34 *Ibid:* para 44.
35 *Ibid.*
36 General Medical Council. *Good medical practice. Op cit:* para 23.
37 *Ibid:* para 31.
38 American Medical Association. *Code of medical ethics.* Chicago, IL: AMA, 2002: sect. E-10·02 (1–2).
39 Jones R. The need for chaperones. *BMJ* 1993;**307**:951–2: 952.
40 See also: British Medical Association. *Asylum seekers: meeting their healthcare needs.* London: BMA, 2002.
41 Mihill C. *Shaping tomorrow: issues facing general practice in the new millennium. Op cit:* p. 97.

42 British Medical Association. *The older person: consent and care.* London: BMA, 1995:51.
43 Kellett JM. A nurse is suspended. *BMJ* 1996;**313**:1249–51.
44 The Children Act 1989 s31 introduced the concept of significant harm as the threshold justifying compulsory intervention in family life. See also The Children (Northern Ireland) Order 1995 art 50(3) and the Children (Scotland) Act 1995 s57.
45 NHS Executive, West Midlands. *Report of a review of the research framework in North Staffordshire NHS Trust (Griffiths inquiry).* Birmingham: NHS Executive, 2000.
46 Royal College of Paediatrics and Child Health. *Fabricated or induced illness by carers.* London: RCPCH, 2001.
47 Department of Health, Home Office, Department for Education and Skills, Welsh Assembly Government. *Safeguarding children in whom illness is fabricated or induced.* London: DoH, 2002. (At the time of writing, there is no separate guidance for Northern Ireland and Scotland.)
48 British Medical Association. *Consent, rights and choices in health care for children and young people.* London: BMJ Books, 2001.
49 Regulation of Investigatory Powers Act 2000. Regulation of Investigatory Powers (Scotland) Act 2000.
50 Jones v University of Warwick [2003] 1 WLR 954.
51 General Medical Council. *Making and using visual and audio recordings of patients.* London: GMC, 2002: para 12.
52 *Ibid:* para 11.
53 General Medical Council. Covert video recording is unacceptable. *GMC News* 2003;**17**:8.
54 General Medical Council. *Good medical practice. Op cit:* para 55.
55 General Medical Council. *Intimate examinations.* London: GMC, 2001.
56 Royal College of Obstetricians and Gynaecologists. *Intimate examinations.* London: RCOG, 1997.
57 Phillips S, Friedman SB, Seidenberg M, Heald FP. Teenagers' preferences regarding the presence of family members, peers and chaperones during examination of genitalia. *Pediatrics* 1981;**68**:665–9.
58 See: British Medical Association. *Provision of care to violent and racially abusive patients.* London: BMA, 2000.
59 Jones R. The need for chaperones. *Op cit.*
60 NHS Employment Policy Branch. *Pre-employment checks for NHS staff [extract taken from HSG 98/064].* Leeds: NHS Employment Policy Branch, re-issued 2001. For advice in Wales, see: National Assembly for Wales. *Pre and post-employment checks for all persons working in the NHS in Wales.* Cardiff: National Assembly for Wales, 2003. (WHC (2003) 007.) In Scotland and Northern Ireland, at the time of writing, the need for guidance for pre-employment checks was under review.
61 See: British Medical Association. *Work observation guidelines.* London: BMA, 1999.
62 A guidance note on this subject has been drawn up by the British Medical Association's consultants' and GPs' committees and the ethics department. British Medical Association. *Patients requesting a second opinion: guidance for consultants.* London: BMA, 2000.
63 See, for example: Scottish Consumer Council. *Patient rights and responsibilities: a draft for consultation. Op cit:* p. 7.
64 British Medical Association. *Trust in the doctor/patient relationship: guidance for doctors and patients on professional boundaries.* London: BMA, 1997.
65 The Bristol Royal Infirmary Inquiry. *Learning from Bristol: the report of the public inquiry into children's heart surgery at the Bristol Royal Infirmary 1984–1995. Op cit:* recommendation 10.
66 General Medical Council. *Serious communicable diseases.* London: GMC, 1997.
67 British Medical Association. *Equal opportunities: guidelines for BMA members.* London: BMA, 2003.
68 General Medical Council. *Good medical practice. Op cit:* para 20.
69 *Ibid:* para 53.
70 General Medical Council Professional Conduct Committee hearing, 11–15 March 2002.
71 Scottish Consumer Council. *Patient rights and responsibilities: a draft for consultation. Op cit.*
72 Royal College of Psychiatrists. *Management of imminent violence: clinical practice guidelines to support mental health services.* London: RCPsych, 1998.
73 National Health Service Executive. *Tackling violence towards GPs and their staff.* Leeds: NHSE, 2000. (HSC 2000/001.)
74 National Health Service. *Withholding treatment from violent and abusive patients in NHS trusts.* London: DoH, 2002. For more information see: http://www.nhs.uk/zerotolerance.
75 Brindley M. GPs in fear find a safe haven near cells. *Western Mail* 2002 Aug 19:1.
76 Information Commissioner. *Data Protection Act 1998 compliance advice. Violent warning markers: use in the public sector.* Wilmslow: Information Commissioner, 2002:2.
77 See, for example: British Medical Association. *Combating violence in general practice: guidance for GPs.* London: BMA, 1996. Health and Safety Executive. *Violence and aggression to staff in the health service:*

guidance on assessment and management. London: HSE Books, 1997. Poyner B, Warne C. *Preventing violence to staff*. London: HSE Books/Tavistock Institute of Human Relations, 1988.

78 National Health Service Executive. *Standards of business conduct for NHS staff*. Leeds: NHS, 1993. (HSG(93)5.)

79 General Medical Council. *Good medical practice. Op cit:* para 53.

80 British Medical Association, The Law Society. *Assessment of mental capacity: guidance for doctors and lawyers, 2nd ed*. London: BMJ Books, in press. This book covers the law in England and Wales.

81 *Ibid.*

82 American Medical Association. *Code of medical ethics. Op cit:* section E-10·02.

83 *Ibid.*

84 Mihill C. *Shaping tomorrow: issues facing general practice in the new millennium. Op cit.*

85 Prentice G. *House of Commons official report (Hansard)*. 2001 Dec 10: col 722.

86 General Practitioners Committee. *Consulting in the modern world*. London: British Medical Association, 2001.

87 Standing Committee of European Doctors. *CPME guidelines for telemedicine*. Brussels: CPME, 2002.

88 Wasson J, Gaudette C, Whaley F, Sauvigne A, Baribeau P, Welch HG. Telephone care as a substitute for routine clinic follow up. *JAMA* 1992;**267**:1788–93.

89 Pinnock H, Bawden R, Proctor S, *et al*. Accessibility, acceptability and effectiveness in primary care of routine telephone review of asthma: pragmatic, randomised controlled trial. *BMJ* 2003;**326**:477–9.

90 General Practitioners Committee. *Searching the internet for medical information – tips for patients*. London: British Medical Association, 2000.

91 Kennedy I. *The unmasking of medicine*. London: George Allen and Unwin, 1981.

2: Consent and refusal: competent adults

The questions covered in this chapter include the following.

- What is the purpose of seeking consent from patients?
- Who should seek consent?
- When is a signed consent form needed?
- May patients refuse treatment?
- Are there limits to a patient's consent?

The nature and purpose of consent

Decisions about medical treatment are ideally made through discussion, with the doctor's clinical expertise and the patient's individual needs and preferences being shared in order to select the best treatment option. The patient's consent is then the trigger that allows treatment or examination to take place. Seeking consent from patients therefore forms a crucial part of the partnership between doctors and patients discussed in Chapter 1, and of the everyday practice of almost every doctor. It is central to good medical practice.

Legal and ethical requirements often overlap in medicine and this is particularly true with issues of consent. Many medical and surgical interventions could be harmful, but are acceptable because the expected benefits outweigh the harms. Patients agree to the invasive procedures of medicine, which, under any other circumstances, could well lead to criminal charges. Doctors must be aware that if they fail to seek consent they too could be vulnerable to legal challenge for battery, negligence, or breach of human rights.

The purpose of consent is not, of course, purely to protect doctors from legal challenge. Seeking consent is a moral requirement, and the BMA believes that respect for others and their rights lies at the heart of this issue. Society emphasises the value and dignity of the individual. Competent adult patients have both an ethical and a legal right to self determination and to respect for their autonomy. This entails their having choice about what happens to their bodies. In addition to the moral and symbolic importance, the need for patient cooperation with examination and treatment is a very practical reason for seeking patient consent.

It would be wrong to assume that consent is relevant only when initiating an examination or treatment. Consent is a process and not an event, and it is important that there is continuing discussion to reflect the evolving nature of treatment. Clearly, the opportunity to consent to treatment is counterbalanced by a right to refuse it. This chapter therefore covers issues of competent patients' refusal of treatment as well as their consent.

General principles

Consent is patients' voluntary agreement to treatment, examination or other aspects of health care. When they know what is proposed, patients may indicate that they give consent orally, in writing, or simply by cooperating.

- For consent to be valid the patient must:

  - be able to understand in broad terms the nature and purpose of the procedure
  - be offered sufficient information to make an informed decision
  - believe the information and be able to weigh it in the balance to arrive at a decision
  - be acting voluntarily and free from pressure
  - be aware that he or she can refuse.

- Before examining or treating competent adult patients, consent must be obtained.
- Adults are always assumed to be competent unless demonstrated otherwise. If there are doubts about their competence, the question to ask is: "can this patient understand and weigh up the information needed to make this decision?" Unexpected decisions do not mean the patient is incompetent, but may indicate a need for further information or explanation.
- Patients may be competent to make some healthcare decisions, even if they are not competent to make others.
- Giving and obtaining consent is usually a process, not a one-off event. Patients can change their minds and withdraw consent at any time. If there is any doubt, doctors should always check that the patient still consents to the care or treatment.
- It is always best for the person actually treating the patient to seek the patient's consent.
- Patients need sufficient information before they can decide whether to give their consent: for example, information about the benefits and risks of the proposed treatment, and alternative treatments, and about the implications of having no treatment. If patients are not offered as much information as they reasonably need to make their decision, and in a form they can understand, their consent may not be valid.
- Consent must be given voluntarily: not under any form of duress or undue influence from health professionals, family, or friends.
- Consent may be given in various ways. It can be written, oral or non-verbal. A signature on a consent form does not itself prove the consent is valid; the point of the form is to record the patient's decision, and also the discussions that have taken place.
- Competent adult patients are entitled to refuse treatment, even where treatment would clearly benefit their health. The only exception to this rule is where the treatment is for a mental disorder and the patient is detained under mental health legislation (see Chapter 3, pages 123–6).[1]

Standards and good practice guidance

There is a considerable amount of written guidance on consent, from regulatory, professional, and indemnifying bodies as well as government departments.[2] Despite this, the BMA has been concerned for some time about the way in which consent has been sought in practice. In 2001 a BMA working party report concluded that: "the whole process of obtaining patient consent must be thoroughly re-assessed. Greater emphasis needs to be placed on the initial explanation given to the patient, with provision for continuing opportunity for discussion in order that the patient can raise any concerns and/or questions".[3]

It is hoped that initiatives such as the Department of Health's "Good practice in consent initiative" will achieve their aims of improving practice in the way patients are asked to give consent to treatment, care, or research. Part of its work involved publishing a reference guide,[4] a series of booklets dealing with consent in specific situations,[5] leaflets for patients,[6] and an implementation guide that includes a model consent policy and consent forms.[7] The health departments in Wales[8] and Northern Ireland[9] published similar documentation and, at the time of writing, the Scottish Executive Health Department is also intending to produce guidance for health professionals.

The process of seeking consent

Consent is not a one-off event, but involves a process of information giving and explanation that facilitates informed decision making. It is essential that informing and involving patients is not seen as "additional" to medical practice, but as an integral part of it. When the Department of Health brought out its documentation on consent and the accompanying forms in 2001, there was fear amongst some doctors that an additional administrative burden was being brought to the health service, which would eat into time that should be spent on patient care.[10] A proper process of seeking consent was seen by some as a dispensable luxury. Detailed explanations of complex procedures can, of course, be time consuming, but usually decisions about treatment emerge during discussions about care and should not put an additional burden on health professionals' time.

In much of health care, patients indicate their consent through actions such as opening their mouth for examination, offering an arm for blood pressure to be taken, or attending a doctor and giving information about an illness. Consent that is indicated in this way is often termed "implied consent" and applies only to the immediate procedure, and not necessarily to subsequent tests or treatment that flow from it. Acquiescence when a patient does not know what the intervention entails or that there is an option of refusing is not "consent".

In contrast, consent that is given orally, in writing, or via other means of communication available to the patient is known as "explicit", or "express", consent. A signed consent form, which is often seen as the ultimate form of consent, is simply evidence that the process of information giving and explanation has taken place. It is the quality and clarity of the information provided, rather than the signature on a piece of paper, that determines the validity of the consent (see pages 81–2).

Capacity to give valid consent

In order for patients to be able to make choices about care, they must have the mental capacity to make a decision. (The terms mental "capacity" and "competence" are often used interchangeably, although the former is most often used in law.) Adult patients are presumed to have the capacity to make treatment decisions unless there is evidence to the contrary. They can decide on whatever basis they wish, and decisions can still be valid even if they appear irrational. Irrational decisions that are based on a misperception of reality, on the other hand, such as believing that blood is poisoned because it is red,[11] may indicate a lack of capacity and it will be necessary to consider further whether the patient has the capacity to make a decision.

To have capacity to make decisions about medical treatment patients should be able to:

- understand what the medical treatment is, its nature and purpose and why it is being proposed for them
- understand its principal benefits, risks, and alternatives
- understand in broad terms what will be the consequences of not receiving the proposed treatment
- retain the information for long enough to make an effective decision
- weigh the information, balancing the risks and benefits, to arrive at a choice.

Assessing capacity and decision making for people who are unable to decide are discussed in Chapter 3, where it is explained how capacity is not something that patients either definitively have or lack, but that the boundary may be less certain. People's abilities fluctuate, often in response to temporary factors such as confusion, shock, fatigue, pain, or medication, and since capacity is judged according to the particular decision that has to be made, patients who are not able to make complex choices may be capable of making simpler decisions. It is important that health professionals give patients who need it practical assistance to maximise their decision making capacity. Patients should not be regarded as incapable of making or communicating a decision unless all practical steps have been taken to maximise their ability to do so.[12] There is further advice on enhancing capacity in Chapter 3 (pages 107–8).

Who should seek consent?

A concern identified in the BMA's 2001 report on consent was that seeking consent was often delegated to less experienced members of the healthcare team.[13] It emerged from the BMA's enquiries that preregistration house officers were frequently required to seek consent for surgery and anaesthesia, even though they had little knowledge or training on how the operation would proceed or why it was clinically indicated for that particular patient. Such practice is clearly at odds with the emphasis in all published guidance on the importance of providing adequate information and giving patients an ongoing opportunity to ask questions and raise concerns. It also represents a failure to recognise the importance of consent.

The BMA believes that the doctor recommending the treatment or intervention has responsibility for providing an explanation to the patient about what the procedure involves – including a discussion of the various treatment options, the alternatives available, the prognosis, and the risks associated with the intervention – and for obtaining the patient's consent.

Responsibility in law rests with the doctor who is in overall charge of the care, usually a consultant or GP. Once a GP has referred patients to a specialist, responsibility passes to the specialist. Additionally, doctors who take responsibility for a particular aspect of care, for example anaesthesia, should ensure that they seek consent before proceeding.

The General Medical Council (GMC) allows doctors to delegate explanation, discussion, and seeking consent to their colleagues in certain circumstances, but it does not permit doctors to delegate the process of seeking consent to other doctors who are unfamiliar with the procedure. It states:

> If you are the doctor providing treatment or undertaking an investigation, it is your responsibility to discuss it with the patient and obtain consent, as you will have a comprehensive understanding of the procedure or treatment, how it is carried out, and the risks attached to it. Where this is not practicable, you may delegate these tasks provided you ensure that the person to whom you delegate:
>
> - is suitably trained and qualified
> - has sufficient knowledge of the proposed investigation or treatment, and understands the risks involved
> - acts in accordance with the guidance in this booklet.
>
> You will remain responsible for ensuring that, before you start any treatment, the patient has been given sufficient time and information to make an informed decision, and has given consent to the procedure or investigation.[14]

Health professionals are also reminded that when they are providing information as part of seeking consent, they "must be competent to do so: either because they themselves carry out the procedure, or because they have received specialist training in advising patients about this procedure, have been assessed, are aware of their own knowledge limitations and are subject to audit".[15]

If there has been a significant time lapse between consent being given and the procedure being carried out, it is crucial to reaffirm the patient's agreement. Clinical circumstances may have changed by the time the patient is due to undergo the procedure and the risks associated with it could have altered significantly if, for example, the patient's condition has deteriorated. This further discussion of the patient's wishes should usually be undertaken either by the clinician who originally proposed the procedure or by the clinician who is due to undertake the intervention. It may, however, be delegated to another member of the team provided that person is suitably trained and qualified and is familiar with the procedure. Crucially, the delegated person must possess the necessary communication skills and should know where to seek help if he or she is unable to respond to the patient's questions.

In addition to the more formal part of the consent process in which the patient indicates a decision about treatment, throughout the process other members of the healthcare team are involved. Patients often find it easier to communicate with nurses and junior doctors than with more senior clinicians, and these professionals have an important role in clarifying the information the patient has been given and answering questions. Senior clinicians should provide information and support for their junior colleagues in this process.

Providing information

Providing patients with sufficient information to enable them to make an informed choice is both an ethical and a legal requirement. Without the offer of such information, any "consent" obtained is invalid. Perceptions of what constitutes "sufficient" information have changed over the last 20 years, with increased patient expectations for more, and more detailed, information. The courts, too, are requiring greater amounts of information to be provided.[16] Consequently, information giving and communication skills have become pivotal to the medical profession. Developing strategies for improving the quality of information available to patients is a crucial aspect of improving patient care.

Generally, patients need information about their condition, options for treatment, what the treatment and aftercare would entail, risks and expected benefits, and the consequences of doing nothing. They may also need to know other aspects, such as where treatment can be given, whether it will involve a stay in hospital, and how long they can expect to take to recover.

Accessibility of information

Information is useful only if it is provided in a manner that is accessible and intelligible to the patient, and is given at a pace at which the recipient can understand. The use of clear, well written patient information leaflets and audiovisual materials can be a useful aid to discussion, but should not be seen as a substitute for a personal consultation. The advantage of these types of information provision is that patients can use them at their leisure and share them with friends and family. The BMA has recommended that the health departments should fund the development and evaluation of high quality patient information materials covering common clinical problems.[17] *The report of the public inquiry into children's heart surgery at the Bristol Royal Infirmary 1984–1995* (the Bristol report) recommended that the NHS Modernisation Agency should make the improvement of the quality of information for patients a priority and should identify and promote good practice throughout the NHS.[18]

In some types of case, for example, patients who are very ill, hard of hearing, or have difficulty communicating, there is sometimes a tendency to discuss the patient's care primarily with relatives simply because it is quicker and easier. Occasionally, when communication difficulties are so severe that only family members are able to communicate with the patient, this may be the only option. Usually, however, patients can be helped to express their views by being given appropriate aids, such as hearing aids or communicators. Taking the patient to a quiet room and minimising distractions may also help him or her to concentrate and express what he or she wants. Patients may also respond better to the approaches of particular staff or relatives.

Translation for patients who need it is discussed in Chapter 1 (pages 42–3).

Type of information to be given

The GMC provides helpful guidance on the type of information that patients want or ought to know before deciding about treatment:

- details of the diagnosis, and prognosis, and the likely prognosis if the condition is left untreated;
- uncertainties about the diagnosis including options for further investigation prior to treatment;
- options for treatment or management of the condition, including the option not to treat;
- the purpose of a proposed investigation or treatment; details of the procedures or therapies involved, including subsidiary treatment such as methods of pain relief; how the patient should prepare for the procedure; and details of what the patient might experience during or after the procedure including common and serious side-effects;
- for each option, explanations of the likely benefits and the probabilities of success; and discussion of any serious or frequently occurring risks, and of any lifestyle changes which may be caused by, or necessitated by, the treatment;
- advice about whether a proposed treatment is experimental;
- how and when the patient's condition and any side-effects will be monitored or re-assessed;
- the name of the doctor who will have overall responsibility for the treatment and, where appropriate, names of the senior members of his or her team;
- whether doctors in training will be involved, and the extent to which students may be involved in an investigation or treatment;
- a reminder that patients can change their minds about a decision at any time;
- a reminder that patients have a right to seek a second opinion;
- where applicable details of costs or charges which patients may have to meet.[19]

It is not sufficient for doctors simply to provide patients with a list of alternatives from which to select their preferred option. In seeking treatment, patients are generally looking for their doctor's advice about which procedure is likely to be the most effective or appropriate for them from a clinical perspective. Failing to give this advice can be as unhelpful as failing to offer any information about possible alternatives to the treatment proposed.

Amount of information to be given

Patients vary in how much information they want about their diagnosis, prognosis, and care. Doctors should presume that patients want to be well informed, and should volunteer information of the type that is necessary for patients to make informed choices. In addition, doctors should always be prepared to answer patients' questions truthfully, and to refer them to other sources of specialist advice if necessary.

There are no hard and fast rules about the amount and nature of information doctors should provide to patients, nor about the type of risk factors they should mention, since this varies according to the individual circumstances of the patient. Factors such as the nature of the condition, the complexity of the treatment, the risks associated with the treatment or procedure, and the patient's own wishes all affect how much information should be given. Doctors must take steps to find out what patients want to know about their condition and its treatment. A careful balance must be struck between listening to what patients want and providing enough information in order that their decisions are informed.

The legal duty to inform patients, as part of the doctor's duty to exercise reasonable care and skill, was established by the House of Lords in 1985.[20] This classic judgment is still often quoted.

Duty to warn about risks

Mrs Sidaway had been suffering from a recurrent pain in her neck, right shoulder, and arms. She had an operation in 1974, which was performed by a senior neurosurgeon at the Bethlem Royal Hospital. The operation, even if performed with proper care and skill, carried an inherent risk of about 2% of damage to the nerve roots and a less than 1% risk of damage to the spinal cord, which had more serious implications. The surgeon reportedly warned Mrs Sidaway of the risk of damage to the nerve root but not of the risk to the spinal cord (although the surgeon died before the case was taken to court and so was unable to confirm this). Mrs Sidaway had the operation, during which her spinal cord was damaged and as a result she was severely disabled. She claimed damages for negligence against the hospital and the estate of the deceased surgeon on the grounds that the surgeon had failed to disclose or explain to her the risks inherent in the operation he had recommended. The case was taken to the House of Lords. Mrs Sidaway's claim was rejected at all levels.

Sidaway v Board of Governors of the Bethlem Royal Hospital[21]

Despite giving different reasons for rejecting Mrs Sidaway's claim that she should have been warned about the risk of damage to her spinal cord, there was a general reliance amongst the judges on the approach that had been taken in the earlier case of Bolam,[22] which had determined that a doctor would not be considered negligent if his or her practice conformed to that of a responsible body of medical opinion held by practitioners skilled in the field in question (see Chapter 21, pages 747–8).

Lord Scarman's reasoning for rejecting Mrs Sidaway's appeal is held by many to encapsulate the true ethical position. It was not shared by the other judges at the time, but was later adopted by the Court of Appeal.[23] In his view, the standard for the amount of information to be given is not what the medical profession thinks appropriate, but ideally what the individual patient requires and, failing that, what the average "prudent patient" would want to know.

The prudent patient

"If one considers the scope of the doctor's duty by beginning with the right of the patient to make his own decision whether he will or will not undergo the treatment proposed, the right to be informed of significant risk and the doctor's corresponding duty are easy to understand: for the proper implementation of the right requires that the doctor be under a duty to inform his patient of the material risks inherent in the treatment. And it is plainly right that a doctor may avoid liability for failure to warn of a material risk if he can show that he reasonably believed that communication to the patient of the existence of the risk would be detrimental to the health (including, of course, the mental health) of his patient.

Ideally, the court should ask itself whether in the particular circumstances the risk was such that this particular patient would think it significant if he was told it existed. I would think that, as a matter of ethics, this is the test of the doctor's duty. The law, however, operates not in Utopia but in the world as it is: and such an inquiry would prove in practice to be frustrated by the subjectivity of its aim and purpose. The law can, however, do the next best thing, and require the court to answer the question, what would a reasonably prudent patient think significant if in the situation of this patient. The "prudent patient" cannot, however, always provide the answer for the obvious reason that he is a norm (like the man on the Clapham omnibus), not a real person: and certainly not the patient himself."[24]

Sidaway v Board of Governors of the Bethlem Royal Hospital[24]

The legal and ethical issues should both inform how doctors act. Doctors' actions will meet the ethical and legal requirements if they inform patients about the general risks inherent in the treatment, and also any risks that may be particularly important to the individual patient. The risks and benefits of alternatives and of non-treatment need also to be explained.

There is inevitably a degree of selectivity about the amount of information patients are given. It would be overly burdensome on both patients and health services for every detail to be explained, and patients are extremely unlikely to want this. It is, however, important that patients can be confident that the information they will be given is that which is likely to be relevant to them, and understand that they may always ask for more details or explanation if they wish.

Withholding information

In the past, concern to avoid worrying patients was seen as a reason for not telling them the full implications of either their condition or different options for treatment. Sometimes only their relatives were told about the likely outcome of treatment (presenting problems of confidentiality as well as consent; see Chapter 5). Generally, however, patients do want to know, and even those who do not, need to have the option. Withholding relevant information in an effort to prevent patients from worrying is not a defensible reason for failing to provide them with all the material and relevant facts about their health and care. As Kennedy and Grubb argue:

> Despite all the anecdotes about patients who committed suicide, suffered heart attacks, or plunged into prolonged depression upon being told "bad news", little documentation exists for claims that informing patients is more dangerous to their health than not informing them, particularly when the informing is done in a sensitive and tactful manner ... in light of the values at stake, the burden of justification should fall upon those who allege that the informing process is dangerous to patient health, and information should be withheld on therapeutic grounds only when the harm of its disclosure is both highly probable and seriously disproportionate to the affront to self determination.[25]

The GMC advises that, in the rare event that a doctor decides to withhold information on the basis that providing it would have a deleterious effect on the patient's health, this view, and the reasons for it, should be recorded in the patient's notes and the doctor must be prepared to justify that decision.[26] Advice from the health departments suggests that in an individual case the courts may accept such a justification, but would examine it with great care, and confirms that "the mere fact that the patient might become upset by hearing the information, or might refuse treatment, is **not** sufficient to act as a justification".[27]

Refusing to receive information

In most cases, doctors and patients decide together which treatment option would be the most appropriate. Doctors contribute their clinical knowledge and experience and patients bring their personal needs, preferences, and values to the decision making process.

In some cases, however, patients do not want to know and ask their doctor to make the decision on their behalf. When this happens, doctors should explain to patients the importance of knowing the options open to them and what the treatment will involve. Even if they continue to refuse, the GMC[28] and the BMA[29] consider that basic information must be provided before treatment can be properly given. Without basic information, patients cannot make a valid choice to delegate responsibility for treatment decisions to the doctor. The amount of basic information needed depends upon the individual circumstances, the severity of the condition, and the risks associated with the treatment. Doctors must seek to strike a balance between giving the patient sufficient information for a valid decision, while at the same time respecting the patient's wish not to know. Doctors may find it helpful to discuss the situation, on an anonymous basis, with colleagues.

When patients refuse to receive information, this should not be seen as total abnegation of choice or as relinquishing choice on other issues. Nevertheless, although information and uncertainties should not be forced upon patients at a time when they are particularly vulnerable and clearly unready, most people are able to deal with very difficult choices, despite their anxieties, if they are given support. It must be clear to patients that they may change their mind about how much information they want at any point.

Details that are not wanted by a patient at one stage of treatment may be sought at another. Patients must be in control not only of the amount of information being given but also of the speed and flow of that information. Busy doctors sometimes point out the apparent impracticality of attempting to give information in stages to suit the patient. Sometimes written material or advice about specific patient support groups or voluntary organisations can help patients to inform themselves at their own speed. Contact with group members can show how others in the same position have managed. Such solutions, however, are not a substitute for appropriate discussion between the doctor and the patient.

Some doctors ask patients to sign a form confirming that they were offered information but declined it, both in order to emphasise the importance of the decision the patient is taking and to protect the doctor against future charges of failing to provide sufficient information. Others record each discussion that takes place in the medical notes. Either way, it is important to have a thorough documentation of the refusal of information, and to do so in a form that is easily accessible to others providing care for the patient.

Summary – providing information

- Patients must be offered sufficient information to allow them to make informed decisions about their care.
- When patients have additional questions about their care, these must be answered truthfully.
- Patients may refuse information, but basic information about their condition and treatment should be provided.
- Doctors should document patients' refusals to receive information.

Documenting consent

Doctors should always make a note of discussions with patients about the nature and purpose of a procedure when seeking consent. This is usually by recording in the health record that information has been provided and a discussion has taken place.

In most cases, there is no need for patients to indicate their agreement in writing. Where complex procedures are proposed, however, or there are significant risks associated with the procedure, consent forms are used to document the patient's agreement. They are common, for example, in surgery. A signed consent form is evidence of a process, not the process itself. The form simply documents that some discussion about the procedure or investigation has taken place but it is the quality and clarity of the information given, rather than a signature on a form, that is important.

The GMC recommends that written consent should be obtained in cases where:

- the treatment or procedure is complex, or involves significant risks and/or side effects
- providing clinical care is not the primary purpose of the investigation or examination
- there may be significant consequences for the patient's employment, social or personal life
- the treatment is part of a research programme.[30]

In addition, consent forms are a legal requirement under certain parts of mental health legislation[31] and of the Human Fertilisation and Embryology Act 1990.[32]

In England and Northern Ireland, NHS trusts are required to use their health department's model consent forms. There are separate forms for patients who will remain conscious throughout and for patients who will be unable to communicate during the procedure. There is also information for patients, both about the forms themselves and about consent more generally. All documentation is available in a number of languages.[33] At the time of writing, there are no standard forms for use in Wales or Scotland, although these are planned for Scotland. The BMA does not publish any standard forms for consent to treatment.

The scope of consent

Duration

Doctors sometimes query the length of time for which consent is valid. In usual practice, this is not a question because patients' continued participation in treatment is an indication that they still agree and have not changed their minds. Occasionally, however, if treatment involves a number of invasive or complex procedures over a period of time, for example a course of electroconvulsive therapy, it would be appropriate to ask for explicit, or even written, consent for each intervention.

Sometimes there is a long period between the original consent being sought and the procedure being undertaken, during which time the patient's condition or wishes may have changed. It is then important to reaffirm that the patient is still happy to go ahead with the procedure, even if no new information or explanations are needed. Competent patients also have the option to make advance decisions in case there comes a time when they lose the capacity to choose. This is discussed in Chapter 3 (pages 113–5).

Exceeding consent

Consent is valid only insofar as it applies to the treatment in question; so, for example, when a patient agrees to a surgical procedure, the surgeon cannot simply change his or her mind and perform a different or additional operation. If it becomes clear that the original proposed procedure is no longer indicated, patients generally need to have the opportunity to decide about alternatives. It follows that, when seeking consent, doctors should discuss beforehand with patients any foreseeable problems that could arise when the patient is unconscious. The purpose of such discussion is to ascertain the patient's views about additional or alternative procedures. The only time when doctors are justified in proceeding without prior authority is when it is essential to do so immediately in order to save the life or prevent permanent disability and it is not possible to obtain that person's consent.

Exceeding the scope of consent

Chapter 7 (page 235) discusses a case in which a surgeon continued with a hysterectomy despite discovering that the woman was pregnant. There are many complaints from patients about the scope of their consent being exceeded. On one occasion, a doctor who was removing under local anaesthetic two wisdom teeth from a patient also removed a mole. The patient complained to the GMC, alleging that the doctor did not have consent to do so.[34] Even when doctors act in good faith, believing their actions to be in the patient's interests, they must have consent, although in rare cases proceeding without consent in an emergency in order to save life may be appropriate (see Chapter 15). Doctors should note, however, that a doctor has been successfully sued for removing a patient's mole without consent.[35]

Summary – the scope of consent

- Consent generally remains valid unless the patient indicates otherwise, although consent should be reaffirmed if there has been a significant lapse of time between the initial agreement and the actual procedure.
- If treatment involves a number of invasive or complex procedures over a period of time, explicit, or written, consent should be sought for each intervention.
- Consent covers only those procedures to which the patient has actually agreed.

Pressures on consent

Patients' choices can be influenced by their relationships with people who are close to them, and many people factor into their decision making the effects of their actions on others. Sometimes, however, the pressures are so great as to bring into question the extent to which the patient is making a competent decision about his or her care. In a case involving a 20-year-old woman who had been brought up as a Jehovah's Witness, for example, the Court of Appeal did not uphold her refusal of a blood transfusion because she had been unduly influenced by her mother (see Chapter 3, page 106).[36] Doctors should be alert to the susceptibility of some patients to decide in a way that pleases others, sometimes even the medical staff. They must ensure that they do not put undue pressure on patients to decide in a particular way. Giving patients the opportunity to decide when away from their family and friends can also help to ensure that the patient's decision is a true indication of his or her wishes.

Refusal of treatment

The right to refuse

Competent adult patients have the right to refuse any medical treatment, contemporaneously or in advance, even if that refusal results in their permanent physical injury or death.[37] (They do not generally have a concomitant right to request procedures that have the same result; see pages 88–96, and also Chapter 11 on euthanasia and physician assisted suicide.) The right to refuse also extends to decisions where a woman is carrying a viable fetus, although it has been suggested that this is an area that could be affected by the Human Rights Act 1998, if the right to have one's life protected is extended to the unborn. This issue is discussed in more detail in Chapter 7 (page 227), although the BMA considers it unlikely that the UK courts would consider that a fetus has such rights.

Despite finding some patients' decisions difficult, because they see that medical care could prolong or improve their life, or save the life of a fetus, doctors must respect a competent refusal. The courts have said that it is irrelevant that other people think it is in the patient's best interests to agree to the treatment.[38] When patients are suffering from mental illness, there are rare occasions in which treatment for mental disorder may be provided even against competent refusal of treatment (see Chapter 3, pages 123–6).

There are also rare cases in which the GMC advises doctors that they may take action even if a patient refuses, where the aim is to provide significant benefit to others.[39] If a healthcare worker has suffered a needlestick injury or other occupational exposure to body fluids, and there is reason to believe that the patient may have a condition such as HIV infection for which prophylactic measures are available, the GMC advises that doctors may test an existing blood sample even if the patient refuses. The patient must be informed about the testing at the earliest opportunity. Confidentiality of the result is paramount. Taking blood from a patient who refuses for this purpose, however, could lead to criminal charges and legal advice should always be sought.

Respecting patients' choices is reinforced by the Human Rights Act, which is rooted in respect for the dignity of the person. Although there is a primary duty to protect life in Article 2, this must be balanced against people's right to security of the person in Article 5 and the right to respect for privacy in Article 8. If there is doubt about a person's capacity to refuse, it is important to resolve that doubt as quickly as possible, and meanwhile the patient must be cared for according to the treating doctors' judgment about best interests (see Chapter 3 on incapacitated adults).

Refusal of treatment by a competent adult

Ms B was a 43-year-old woman who, in the summer of 1999, suffered a haemorrhage of the spinal cord in her neck. She was admitted to hospital and a cavernoma was diagnosed, a condition caused by a malformation of blood vessels in the spinal cord. Shortly after her diagnosis she made an advance directive stating that, if she became unable to give instructions, she wished for treatment to be withdrawn if she was suffering from a life threatening condition, permanent mental impairment or permanent unconsciousness.

After a few weeks her condition improved and she was able to leave hospital and return to work. In February 2001, Ms B suffered further damage to her spinal cord, as a result of which she became tetraplegic, suffering complete paralysis from the neck down. She was treated in the intensive care unit of the hospital where, after experiencing respiratory problems, she was placed on a ventilator. In March 2001 Ms B asked for the first time for her ventilator to be switched off. This request was repeated on a number of occasions and in April formal instructions were given to the hospital by her solicitor to withdraw artificial ventilation. According to the medical evidence, without artificial ventilation Ms B would have a less than 1% chance of breathing independently and death would almost certainly follow. The clinicians were not willing to switch off the ventilator but offered the option of a programme of weaning whereby ventilation would be gradually reduced over a period of time with the aim of allowing the body to breathe again on its own. Ms B rejected this on the grounds that it would lead to a painful death over a period of weeks. She had also rejected rehabilitation because it offered her no chance of recovery and because she had no guarantee that the ventilator would be removed in the future at her request.

Ms B was assessed by a number of consultant psychiatrists and in August an independent assessment was conducted, which concluded that she was not depressed and that she had the capacity to make the decision to discontinue treatment. Despite her refusal of treatment, ventilation was continued and Ms B applied to the High Court for a declaration that the artificial ventilation being provided represented unlawful trespass. The trust argued that Ms B did not have the competence to make the decision to stop treatment.

In clarifying her role in the case the judge, Dame Elizabeth Butler-Sloss, said, "I am not asked directly to decide whether Ms B lives or dies but whether she, herself, is legally competent to make that decision. It is also important to recognise that this case is not about the best interests of the patient but about her mental capacity".[40] In his evidence, one of the doctors expressed the view that Ms B was

unable to give informed consent, not because of a lack of capacity in general but her specific lack of knowledge and experience of exposure

(Continued)

> to a spinal rehabilitation unit and thereafter to readjustment to life in the community. Without that opportunity … Ms B did not have the requisite information to give informed consent.[41]
>
> The judge rejected this view, which, she said, was not the law.
>
> The court held that Ms B was competent to make all relevant decisions about her medical treatment, including the decision whether to seek withdrawal of artificial ventilation. The judge also found that Ms B had been treated unlawfully by the trust.
>
> Ms B died in her sleep a month later when her ventilation was withdrawn.
>
> *Re B (adult: refusal of medical treatment)*[42]

In the case of Ms B, the hospital trust had received clear legal advice that if Ms B was competent she should not be treated against her wishes. When the case went to court, the trust was criticised for not following that advice. In making some general comments about refusal of treatment, the judge reminded hospitals that they must take steps to resolve dilemmas of this nature and not allow the situation to continue without resolution. Ultimately, if there is doubt about the legality of complying with a refusal of treatment, it should be assessed as a matter of priority. If doubt still remains, an application to court may be needed, or advice should be sought from the Official Solicitor for England and Wales, the Official Solicitor for Northern Ireland, or the Scottish Office Solicitors. Such steps are pointless, however, if it is clear that the patient has the capacity to make the decision.

Although patients may choose to refuse treatment even if that results in their death, the BMA supports the widely held view that valid treatment refusal by a patient is not in itself suicide. This is an issue that generates moral and legal debate, however. When considered by the House of Lords as part of its deliberations during the case of Tony Bland (see Chapter 10, page 359), Lord Goff said:

> in cases of this kind, there is no question of the patient having committed suicide, nor therefore of the doctor having aided or abetted him in doing so. It is simply that the patient has, as he is entitled to do, declined to consent to treatment which might or would have the effect of prolonging his life, and the doctor has, in accordance with his duty, complied with his patient's wishes.[43]

Of course, some patients who genuinely do attempt suicide may also refuse resuscitation or other forms of potentially life prolonging treatment. Treatment of patients who have attempted suicide is discussed in Chapter 15 (pages 537–9).

Informed refusal

Patients are not obliged to justify their decisions to refuse treatment, but the health team needs to be sure that patients base their decisions on accurate information and that they have corrected any misunderstandings. In the same way as patients giving consent should have sufficient accurate information, those refusing should ideally have an awareness of their condition, the proposed treatment, any significant risks or side effects, the probability of a successful recovery, the consequences of not having the treatment, and alternative forms of treatment. Doctors must not put pressure on patients to decide in a particular way, but should allow them time to consider a decision with potentially serious consequences.

Continuing care

A refusal of a particular treatment does not imply a refusal of all treatment or all facets of care. When a patient has refused treatment, alternative treatments and procedures intended to keep the patient comfortable and free from severe pain or discomfort should still be offered. (Refusal of treatment at the end of life is discussed in more detail in Chapter 10 (pages 354–5), and advance refusals are discussed in Chapter 3 (pages 113–5)) In addition, patients are entitled to change their minds, although if there are circumstances in which not providing treatment at a given time would limit the options for providing treatment in the future, this should be made clear to them. For example, a cancer may be operable at the time a patient presents for treatment. If the patient refuses and then changes his or her mind a month later, the cancer might have progressed to a stage that is inoperable.

Documenting refusal

Patients are sometimes asked to sign a declaration to document that they have refused a particular treatment and that they accept responsibility for declining medical advice. The courts have said that, for their own protection, hospital authorities should seek unequivocal assurances from the patient (to be recorded in writing) that the refusal represents an informed decision, that is, that the patient understands the nature of and the reasons for the proposed treatment, and the risks and likely prognosis involved in the decision to refuse or accept it.[44] If the patient is unwilling to sign a written indication of this refusal, it is likely to be unhelpful, or even counterproductive, to force the issue. Instead, the fact should be noted in the health records. Like consent forms, this documentation acts as evidence that some discussion has taken place between the doctor and the patient about the implications of refusing treatment. They are not "disclaimers". It is important that patients understand that they may still change their mind even after signing a form.

Refusal of blood products by Jehovah's Witnesses

Jehovah's Witnesses have a conscientiously held religious opposition to the use of blood products, and adults' competent refusals of treatment must be respected.

They are, however, generally very anxious to cooperate in every way with alternative options. Most Witnesses do not accept their own blood donated in advance (predeposit), but many are willing to accept the use of blood salvage equipment that serves to recycle their blood in a continuous circuit. "Bloodless" medical procedures are now becoming commonplace, including successful organ transplants. Lists of centres of excellence in bloodless surgery and of doctors experienced in working constructively with Jehovah's Witnesses are held by the Jehovah's Witness hospital liaison committees. Hospital Information Services for Jehovah's Witnesses, a department of their coordinating body, the Watch Tower Society, has published a summary of alternative therapies and references to the medical research that supports these.[45]

Summary – refusal of treatment

- Competent adult patients have the right to refuse any medical treatment, even if that refusal results in their permanent physical injury or death or the permanent physical injury or death of a viable fetus.
- Patients should be offered the following information on which to base their decisions:
  - awareness of their condition
  - knowledge of the proposed treatment
  - information about significant risks or side effects
  - probability of a successful recovery
  - consequences of not having the treatment
  - alternative forms of treatment.
- Patients who refuse treatment may be prepared to accept alternatives and should be offered care and symptom management appropriate to their needs.
- Refusal should be documented in health records, and patients may be asked to sign a form or declaration confirming their refusal.

Are there limits to an individual's consent?

There are limits on patients' choices not only because of legal constraints about what options are allowed but also because of the professional judgment of doctors. Doctors provide treatment not simply because it is requested but because in their view it is clinically appropriate. They recommend the treatment that is best for an individual patient, having regard to that patient's needs and the treatments and resources available. Society thus places doctors in the role of gatekeepers of access to treatment. Difficult questions arise when patients reject low cost remedies in favour of costly alternatives that divert resources from others. Yet, if the patient is a Jehovah's Witness, for example, and the choice is an expensive alternative to blood products or allowing the patient to die, doctors make every effort to accommodate the patient's choice. This example highlights the difficult question of the comparative weight given to different value systems that underlie patient choice.

It is not only resource considerations that impose limitations on the patient. Doctors also refuse to give patients treatments that are "bad for them" or for others. Examples include the excessive use of medication to control weight (see Chapter 13, pages 458–9) and the more extreme cases discussed on pages 89–96. Doctors cannot be required to provide treatment contrary to their professional judgment.

Occasionally, healthy people seek medical assistance to do something that leaves them less physically healthy or even disabled. Some requests aim to help others, such as donating bone marrow or a kidney. Others come from patients with body dysmorphia who ask to have healthy limbs amputated. Society allows a certain amount of risk taking, from driving cars to participating in dangerous sports, but the medical profession, with its public health responsibilities, occasionally seeks to prohibit or discourage certain risky activities. Boxing and smoking are examples of actions the BMA has consistently opposed because of the health risks involved.

Distinctions can be drawn, however, between activities that doctors consider should generally be discouraged because they are likely to affect the overall public health and the equally risk laden activities that individual patients want to undertake to achieve some particular goal. The World Health Organization believes that part of the purpose of medicine is to help individuals to achieve overall wellbeing, not just an absence of disease.[46] Achieving wellbeing obviously takes different forms for different people. A dilemma for doctors is that helping healthy people to follow a course of action that most people would consider leaves them less healthy or even disabled seems paradoxical, even when this is at the patient's request.

In the remainder of this chapter we explore some areas where this dilemma occurs.

Consent to procedures carried out for the benefit of others

Altruism is an important concept in medicine; the UK health service depends heavily on the regular altruistic donation of blood. People are often moved by the plight of others to donate bone marrow, gametes, or embryos. Consent for donating where there are no (or only minimal) risks or discomfort for the donor, blood or sperm for example, is unproblematic and the BMA supports the concept of the altruistic gift relationship. Doctors can, however, be faced with difficult choices about whether to facilitate interventions in which a healthy person undergoes a risk of physical or psychological harm to benefit someone else. For many years, for example, the Association had reservations about facilitating the practice of surrogate motherhood, partly because of its implications for children but also because of the potential psychological and physical risks for the woman undergoing a pregnancy on behalf of someone else.[47] Its eventual position on this particular subject, however, has been that the best way forward is to ensure that people who do undergo such risks are given the maximum information about the implications for themselves and their existing families of what they propose to do (see Chapter 8, pages 298–302).

Organ donation from live donors

There are two different types of living donor. In the first, an organ becomes available as a result of a procedure carried out primarily for the benefit of the donor. The most common scenario is what is known as a "domino" transplant, in which a patient needing new lungs has heart and lungs removed and replaced by organs from a cadaveric donor. The patient's own heart is then available for transplantation to another person. Recipients are asked to consent both to the clinical procedure itself and to the donation of other organs removed in the course of the treatment.

The second type of live donation — altruistic donations from healthy donors — raises more concerns about consent. Such donations have traditionally formed only a very small part of the overall transplant programme in the UK, although the numbers are increasing. These donations are almost exclusively restricted to kidneys. Segments of liver and lung have been transplanted from healthy living donors, but at the time of writing these procedures have not been carried out routinely.

Risks and benefits The main objection to living donation from healthy volunteers is that it exposes donors to the risks inherent in major surgery and, in the case of kidney donors, to the health risks of having only one kidney (although evidence from overseas suggests that these risks are small[48]). Living donation does, however, carry significant advantages for recipients. Donation from a healthy volunteer — both related and unrelated — carries a higher chance of success for the recipient compared with cadaveric donors.[49] Living donation has other advantages: it facilitates pre-emptive transplantation for someone with progressive renal failure, so avoiding the need for dialysis; it allows the transplant to proceed at the optimal time for the recipient; and it allows those with end stage renal failure to escape the long wait for a kidney from a cadaveric donor. Although the physical benefit is all for the recipient, those who donate to people close to them may achieve psychological and practical benefits from the recipient's recovery.

What level of risk is acceptable? Many medical interventions carry a risk of harm, but this is outweighed by the anticipated benefit. In the examples discussed here and on pages 94–6, however, the risk is one of significant harm and the anticipated benefit for the individual undergoing it is solely (or mainly) psychological. Nevertheless, it has long been accepted that competent adults are entitled to put themselves at risk to help other people. Bone marrow and oocyte donation, for example, are accepted even though they put the donor at some degree of risk with no personal physical benefit. The BMA has considered the arguments for and against live donation and concludes that living donation is acceptable provided that donors are properly informed and that safeguards are in place to ensure that they are not subjected to any coercion, whether financial or emotional.[50]

Having accepted that, as a general principle, people may expose themselves to risk for the benefit of another person, are there limits to the extent of that risk? If a surgeon removed, for donation, an individual's heart, resulting in the patient's inevitable death, "any consent would be invalid since the surgeon would commit murder".[51] Apart from such extremes, however, there is no legal restriction on the extent of risk to which individuals may expose themselves in the process of donating organs. Arguably, it is for the competent individual, who has sufficient information and is acting voluntarily, to establish what level of risk he or she is willing to take. Of course, there are also some external controls over such matters. There are independent checks for those who are not genetically related (see below). In addition, surgeons cannot be forced to act contrary to their clinical judgment and any surgeon asked to undertake the operation would need to be satisfied not only that the potential donor was truly competent, informed and acting voluntarily, but also that the overall benefits of carrying out the procedure outweighed the harms.

Surgeon's refusal to meet a patient's request

Mr P had two sons, aged 33 and 29. Both sons had Alport's syndrome, an inherited condition that causes kidney failure. Mr P successfully donated a kidney to his younger son. His older son, R, received a cadaveric kidney, but the transplant failed. As it had been a poor match, R developed antibodies that made him incompatible with 96% of the population. Finding a suitable kidney was therefore extremely unlikely, unless his parents were suitable donors. Mrs P was told that she was not suitable. Mr P wanted to donate his second kidney to R.

Mr P argued it would be better for him to be on dialysis rather than his son. He was retired and prepared for the lifestyle change that dialysis would bring. Despite finding support from some doctors, Mr P's request was turned down by three transplant teams. Some of the deliberations of the third were filmed and shown on television.[52]

Members of the transplant team had mixed views about Mr P's request. Some understood and felt they would want to do the same for their own children. Although some believed that the benefits were one sided, others agreed that there could be emotional benefits for Mr and Mrs P if the transplant was a success for R. There were also concerns about the impact on the family (the younger brother was opposed to the operation) and about how R in particular would feel about the effects on his father's length and quality of life. The resource implications of ending up with two people on dialysis rather than one if the transplant was not successful were also discussed.

The decision rested with the transplant surgeon. Although he knew that Mr P understood the nature and implications of his request, and that he could see ethical and rational justifications for the operation taking place, he knew that ultimately he would feel unable to perform the operation. Mr P was therefore turned down.

As a last resort, Mrs P was tested again to see if she might be a match. Although she had been rejected several times in the past, she was found to be a match.

The BMA believes it is right that the level of harm to which people can give consent is limited but, as in other areas, resists the imposition of inflexible rules. Each case needs to be considered individually and, if the health professionals concerned believe that the risks are too great, the decision and the reasons for it should be sensitively explained to both the potential donor and the recipient.

Safeguards for living organ donation   Any use of healthy living donors must be subject to strict safeguards to ensure that the fundamental principles of consent – competence, information, and voluntariness – are met. In 1989 legislation was introduced restricting the live donation of non-regenerative organs.[53] Under that legislation, people who are closely genetically related must provide evidence of that genetic relationship before proceeding. Donations between people who are not genetically related, including spouses or long term partners, must be approved by the Unrelated Live Transplant Regulatory Authority (ULTRA). In 2002 a consultation exercise was conducted about whether these restrictions should continue to apply.[54] An update on the outcome of this exercise can be obtained from the Department of Health, the Welsh Office or the BMA. These areas of law are also under review in Scotland and Northern Ireland.

Conditions for live unrelated organ donation

Before ULTRA approves an application for donation by a living unrelated donor, it must be satisfied that:

- no payment has been, or is to be, made
- the person referring the case for consideration is the doctor with clinical responsibility for the donor
- a doctor has explained to the donor the nature of the procedure and the risks involved in the removal of the organ in question
- the donor's consent was not obtained by coercion or the offer of an inducement
- the donor understands that his or her consent can be withdrawn at any time
- the donor and the recipient have been interviewed separately by a suitably qualified independent person who is not part of the transplant team, and that person is satisfied that the above conditions have been met.[55]

ULTRA's conditions are required to be met only in the case of unrelated donors. This, however, ignores the very real pressures that could be placed on individuals to donate to a relative. In the BMA's view, there do not appear to be legitimate grounds for making a distinction between related and unrelated donors. It believes that the conditions are equally important whether the donation is from a relative or from an unrelated donor. All live donations should be subject to the same rigorous assessment, either by ULTRA or via some other mechanism, to ensure that the potential donation is truly voluntary and free from pressure. Without wishing to increase the time taken for approval to be given, the BMA would support the introduction of a streamlined approval process for *all* live donors to ensure that they have sufficient information and are not subject to any coercion, whether financial or emotional. This has been discussed as part of the review of the law on organ donation in England and Wales.[56]

In addition to the legislative framework, professional guidance has also been issued by the British Transplantation Society and the Renal Association.[57] This states that living donor kidney transplantation should be undertaken only if four essential conditions are met:

- the risk to the donor is low
- the donor is fully informed
- the decision to donate is entirely voluntary and not due to coercion or the offer of an inducement
- the transplant procedure has a good chance of providing a successful outcome for the recipient.

The BMA believes as a matter of principle that only competent adults should be considered as live organ donors. There should, however, be scope for children[58] or incompetent adults (see Chapter 3, pages 118–20) to be considered as donors in truly exceptional cases with the authorisation of a court.

Live donation from strangers   Donation of blood or bone marrow by strangers is commonplace, and occasionally people offer to donate an organ to a stranger. Such donation is not prohibited by law in the UK, but ULTRA had not accepted any such applications at the time of writing.[59] In 2002 the Department of Health and Welsh Assembly sought views on whether it should be permitted, as part of its broader review of the legislation on human organs and tissues, including organ donation.[60]

Live donation by strangers

In 1999 Mr Ron Johnson, from Northampton, flew to Missouri in order to donate a lung lobe to 10-year-old Lisa Ostrovsky, whom he had never met. Lisa had cystic fibrosis and would die without the operation; even with the operation she had only a 50:50 chance of survival. Mr Johnson had volunteered to help Lisa after being touched by an appeal for donors in a Jewish newspaper. Lisa died a few weeks after the operation.[61]

The motives of such people are sometimes questioned. It is, of course, essential to consider whether the potential donor has the capacity to give consent, but it is equally important to recognise acts of genuine altruism. The lengths to which some people go in order to help others, even people they do not know, can be quite astounding. Some people are moved by the plight of others and genuinely want to do what they can to help. It is also increasingly recognised that donation can bring personal benefits to the donor in terms of improved self esteem and personal satisfaction.

The number of people offering to donate a kidney to a stranger is likely to be small. Many of those who volunteer do so without realising the true nature of the procedure or the risks involved, and some may decide not to proceed once that information has been received. For those who are informed and competent, however, the BMA has no objection in principle to them donating to strangers and would like to see this issue explored further.

Requests for amputation of healthy limbs

Doctors sometimes ask the BMA for advice about patients with a psychological condition known as body dysmorphia. These patients have what they perceive to be an extraneous limb (or limbs) that they want removed. There was considerable public disquiet when it was announced in February 2000 that a surgeon in Scotland had removed healthy limbs from two such patients. The hospital subsequently withdrew its permission for any further operations of that nature to be undertaken on its premises.[62] The BMA has profound reservations about the ethical and legal acceptability of such operations. Of course, having a psychiatric disorder does not, of itself, render a person unable to give valid consent, but it may affect the individual's decision making capacity in relation to issues connected with the disorder. Consent for amputation would have to be carefully scrutinised.

Amputation of a healthy limb

In 2000, 55-year-old Gregg Furth, a psychoanalyst from New York, travelled to the UK to see psychiatrists and the surgeon who had previously amputated the healthy legs of two men with body dysmorphic disorder. Since before he was 10 years old, Mr Furth could recall feeling that the lower part of his right leg was not part of his body. Since then he constantly thought about being without that part of his leg and had searched for many years to find a surgeon willing to amputate it. Mr Furth had undergone many years of therapy but had not been able to repress the feelings he had about his leg. He was assessed by two psychiatrists in the UK, both of whom confirmed that he was competent to make the decision and was suffering from body dysmorphic disorder. Both psychiatrists recommended him for amputation and the surgeon agreed to carry out the procedure. Shortly before the operation was due to take place, however, the hospital withdrew its permission for any more operations of this type to be undertaken on its premises.[63]

Legal issues

There is debate about whether amputating a healthy limb in these circumstances is lawful. Discussion focuses on the ancient common law offence of maim, which grew up in relation to the duty of all males to fight for their sovereign and country, if required. Maim is therefore defined as "bodily harm whereby a man is deprived of the use of any member of his body, or of any sense which he can use in fighting, or by the loss of which he is generally and permanently weakened".[64] It has also been suggested that "were a patient to consent to having his limbs amputated, for no good reason, his consent would not prevent the amputation from amounting to the offence of battery".[65] This, of course, invites the question of what would be "good reason".

Much discussion about the limits of consent followed the 1993 House of Lords' judgment in a case about men practising consensual sadomasochistic activities involving maltreatment of the genitals, ritualistic beating, and branding.[66] The men were convicted and imprisoned, despite the fact that the "victims" gave consent. Although the two scenarios are different, the latter case highlighted the legal limits of consent as a defence when a person carries out a potentially harmful procedure at the request of another person. The Law Commission's subsequent consultation on consent in the criminal law considered the extent to which an individual's apparently valid consent to "injury" removes the act from the remit of the criminal law. It recommended that "the intentional causing of seriously disabling injury [including injuries that involve the loss of a bodily member] to another person should continue to be criminal, even if the person injured consents to such injury or to the risk of such injury".[67] It went on to make an exception for cases in which the injury is caused during the course of proper medical treatment, in which it included the surgical aspects of gender reassignment, which, some could argue, is a similar use of a surgical procedure to make a healthy body conform to its owner's body image. The Law Commission did not specifically consider, however, amputation as treatment for body dysmorphia and the legality of this practice has not been tested in the courts. Extreme caution should, therefore, be exercised and specific legal advice is essential before proceeding with such a case.

Ethical issues

In addition to the potential legal issues, there are also ethical difficulties with acceding to patients' requests for amputation. One of the goals of medicine is to enable patients to live as "normal" and independent a life as possible. Mutilating surgical procedures are usually seen as a last resort in cases where a physical disease has been identified. Therefore most doctors have an intuitive aversion to the notion of deliberately removing healthy tissue in the absence of physical disease, even at the patient's request. Part of this reluctance is due to the permanent disabling effect for the patient. Whereas doctors may disagree with patients' views about the need for interventions like cosmetic surgery, patients are not deliberately disabled by them. Similarly, as a treatment for gender identity dysphoria, surgery is a major step but is not intrinsically disabling and the psychological benefits are recognised. Amputation, on the other hand, is disabling and in some cases may render the patient dependent upon support from society, raising questions about whether people have duties to society as well as rights.

Some people accept amputation as an effective form of treatment for body dysmorphia in extreme cases where other forms of treatment such as medication or psychotherapy have failed. In order for this to be convincing, it would have to be shown that all other less invasive alternatives had been exhausted and that the patient is expected to suffer even more serious harm if the procedure is not carried out. Some patients with body dysmorphia have tried to injure themselves by gunshot wounds or lying across rail tracks to make amputation a medical necessity; others are reported to have committed suicide as a result of their inability to rid themselves of their obsession.[68] There is no doubt that this condition can have very serious consequences and that the needs of these patients require further exploration and debate.

Summary – are there limits to an individual's consent?

- Society limits the things that competent people are allowed to consent to – people cannot consent to being killed, for example.
- The BMA believes that procedures that are primarily for the physical benefit of another person are acceptable in some circumstances, but that there should be safeguards in place to ensure that consent is valid and freely given.
- When physically healthy patients seek procedures that are disabling, legal advice will be needed before proceeding.

From the everyday to the extreme

The advice in this chapter is the keystone for all doctors interacting with patients. Consent is central to everyday practice, and this chapter gives general guidance on the everyday issues faced by all doctors.

It also highlights some particular areas of difficulty. It shows that there are complex questions about where the boundaries of acceptable practice lie, whether to allow requests for mutilating procedures, for example. These are ultimately for society to debate and may be matters for consideration by Parliament if further regulation is needed.

References

1   Based on: Department of Health. *12 key points on consent*. London: DoH, 2001.
2   See for example: General Medical Council. *Seeking patients' consent: the ethical considerations*. London: GMC, 1998. Department of Health. *Reference guide to consent for examination or treatment*. London: DoH, 2001. The Medical Defence Union. *Consent to treatment*. London: MDU, 1999.
3   British Medical Association. *Report of the Consent Working Party: incorporating consent toolkit*. London: BMA, 2001: recommendation 2.
4   Department of Health. *Reference guide to consent for examination or treatment. Op cit.*
5   Examples relevant to the patient group considered in this chapter include: Department of Health. *Seeking consent: working with people with learning disabilities*. London: DoH, 2001. Department of Health. *Seeking consent: working with older people*. London: DoH, 2001.
6   Examples relevant to the patient group considered in this chapter include: Department of Health. *Consent – what you have a right to expect: a guide for adults*. London: DoH, 2001. Department of Health. *Consent – what you have a right to expect: a guide for people with learning disabilities*. London: DoH, 2001. Department of Health. *Consent – what you have a right to expect: a guide for relatives and carers*. London: DoH, 2001.
7   Department of Health. *Reference guide to consent for examination or treatment. Op cit.*
8   Welsh Assembly Government. *Reference guide for consent to examination or treatment*. Cardiff: Welsh Assembly Government, 2002. Welsh Assembly Government. *Consent – what you have a right to expect*. Cardiff: Welsh Assembly Government, 2002.
9   Department of Health, Social Services and Public Safety. *Reference guide to consent for examination, treatment or care*. Belfast: DHSSPS, 2003. Department of Health, Social Services and Public Safety. *Good practice in consent. Consent for examination, treatment or care*. Belfast: DHSSPS, 2003.

10 Pritchard L. New consent forms dubbed "charter for patients to sue". *BMA News* 2001;(Nov 3):2.
11 Re MB (medical treatment) [1997] 2 FLR 426.
12 British Medical Association, The Law Society. *Assessment of mental capacity: guidance for doctors and lawyers, 2nd ed.* London: BMJ Books, in press.
13 British Medical Association. *Report of the Consent Working Party: incorporating consent toolkit. Op cit:* p. 9.
14 General Medical Council. *Seeking patients' consent: the ethical considerations. Op cit:* para 14.
15 Department of Health. *Good practice in consent implementation guide.* London: DoH, 2001:20. Department of Health, Social Services and Public Safety. *Good practice in consent. Consent for examination, treatment or care. Op cit:* p. 20.
16 Pearce v United Bristol HC NHS Trust [1999] 48 BMLR 118.
17 British Medical Association. *Report of the Consent Working Party: incorporating consent toolkit. Op cit:* recommendation 4.
18 The Bristol Royal Infirmary Inquiry. *Learning from Bristol: the report of the public inquiry into children's heart surgery at the Bristol Royal Infirmary 1984–1995.* London: The Stationery Office, 2001: recommendation 8. (Cm 5207 (II).)
19 General Medical Council. *Seeking patients' consent: the ethical considerations. Op cit:* para 5.
20 Sidaway v Board of Governors of the Bethlem Royal Hospital [1985] AC 871.
21 *Ibid.*
22 Bolam v Friern Hospital Management Committee [1957] 2 All ER 118.
23 Pearce v United Bristol HC NHS Trust [1999]. *Op cit.*
24 Sidaway v Board of Governors of the Bethlem Royal Hospital [1985]. *Op cit:* pp. 888–9.
25 Kennedy I, Grubb A. *Medical law, 3rd ed.* London: Butterworths, 2000:702.
26 General Medical Council. *Seeking patients' consent: the ethical considerations. Op cit:* para 12.
27 Department of Health. *Reference guide to consent for examination or treatment. Op cit:* para 5·5. Welsh Assembly Government. *Reference guide for consent to examination or treatment. Op cit:* para 5·5. Department of Health, Social Services and Public Safety. *Reference guide to consent for examination, treatment or care. Op cit:* para 4·8.
28 General Medical Council. *Seeking patients' consent: the ethical considerations. Op cit:* para 11.
29 British Medical Association. *Consent tool kit.* London: BMA, 2001: card 3.
30 General Medical Council. *Seeking patients' consent: the ethical considerations. Op cit:* para 28.
31 Mental Health Act 1983. Mental Health (Care and Treatment) (Scotland) Act 2003. Mental Health (Northern Ireland) Order 1986.
32 For example, Schedule 3 of the Human Fertilisation and Embryology Act 1990 requires that a donor of genetic material should give written consent to its future use. For further reading, see: Lee RG, Morgan D. *Human fertilisation and embryology: regulating the reproductive revolution.* London: Blackstone, 2001.
33 All of the Department of Health's consent publications are available at http://www.doh.gov.uk/ consent.
34 GMC Professional Conduct Committee hearing, 14–15 and 17 August 2000.
35 Medical Defence Union. *Additional treatment whilst anaesthetised.* http://www.the-mdu.com (accessed 28 March 2003).
36 Re T (adult: refusal of medical treatment) [1992] 4 All ER 649.
37 *Ibid.*
38 Re B (adult: refusal of medical treatment) [2002] 2 All ER 449.
39 General Medical Council. *Serious communicable diseases.* London: GMC, 1997: paras 9–10.
40 Re B (adult: refusal of medical treatment) [2002]. *Op cit:* p. 455.
41 *Ibid:* p. 465.
42 *Ibid.*
43 Airedale NHS Trust v Bland [1993] 1 All ER 821: 864.
44 St George's Healthcare NHS Trust v S, R v Collins and others, ex parte S [1998] 3 All ER 673.
45 Watch Tower Bible and Tract Society of Pennsylvania. *Family care and medical management for Jehovah's Witnesses.* New York: Watch Tower Bible and Tract Society of New York, 1995.
46 Preamble to the Constitution of the World Health Organization as adopted by the International Health Conference, New York, 19–22 June, 1946; signed on 22 July 1946 by the representatives of 61 States (Official Records of the World Health Organization, no. 2:100) and entered into force on 7 April 1948.
47 British Medical Association. *Changing conceptions of motherhood. The practice of surrogacy in Britain.* London: BMA, 1996.
48 Major complications for the kidney donors are rare and the mortality rate is around 0·03%. See, for example: Nicholson ML, Bradley JA. Renal transplantation from living donors should be seriously considered to help overcome the shortfall in organs [editorial]. *BMJ* 1999;**318**:409–10.

49 See, for example: Cecka JM. Results of more than 1,000 recent living-unrelated donor transplants in the United States. *Transplant Proc* 1999;**31**:234. Also: Terasaki PI, Cecka JM, Gjertson DW, Takemoto S. High survival rates of kidney transplants from spousal and living unrelated donors. *N Engl J Med* 1995;**333**:333–6.

50 For a legal exploration of these arguments, see: Law Commission. *Consultation paper no. 139 – consent in the criminal law*. London: HMSO, 1995. For comment on the Law Commission report see: Alldridge P. Consent to medical and surgical treatment – the Law Commission's recommendations. *Med Law Rev* 1996;**4**:129–43.

51 Kennedy I, *et al. Medical law, 3rd ed. Op cit:* p. 1758.

52 *The decision*, "Whose kidney is it anyway?" Channel 4, 1996 Feb 20.

53 Human Organ Transplants Act 1989. Human Organ Transplants (Northern Ireland) Order 1989.

54 Department of Health, Welsh Assembly Government. *Human bodies, human choices. The law on human organs and tissue in England and Wales*. London: DoH, 2002.

55 Department of Health. *Unrelated Live Transplant Regulatory Authority report 1995–1998*. London: DoH, 1999.

56 Department of Health, *et al. Human bodies, human choices. The law on human organs and tissue in England and Wales. Op cit.*

57 British Transplantation Society, The Renal Association. *United Kingdom guidelines for living donor kidney transplantation*. London: BTS, 2000.

58 For further discussion of children as potential donors see: British Medical Association. *Consent, rights and choices in health care for children and young people*. London: BMJ Books, 2001.

59 Department of Health, *et al. Human bodies, human choices. The law on human organs and tissue in England and Wales. Op cit:* para 14·29.

60 *Ibid*: pp. 130–2.

61 Anonymous. Lung donor girl dies. *BBC online* 2000 Jan 3. http://news.bbc.co.uk (accessed 12 March 2003).

62 Anonymous. "Healthy" amputation rejected. *BBC online* 2002 Aug 25. http://news.bbc.co.uk (accessed 12 March 2003).

63 This case was covered in a documentary on body dysmorphia: *Horizon*, "Complete Obsession," BBC2, 2000 Feb 17.

64 Kennedy I, *et al. Medical law, 3rd ed. Op cit:* p. 771.

65 Skegg PDG. *Law, ethics and medicine*. Oxford: Clarendon, 1984:38.

66 R v Brown [1993] 2 All ER 75.

67 Law Commission. *Consultation paper no 139 – consent in the criminal law. Op cit:* p. 46.

68 *Horizon*, "Complete Obsession." *Op cit.*

3: Treatment without consent: incapacitated adults and compulsory treatment

The questions covered in this chapter include the following.

- What is capacity?
- How should capacity be assessed?
- How can a person's "best interests" be determined?
- Who may give consent to treatment on behalf of an incapacitated adult?
- Are advance decisions legally binding?
- When is compulsory treatment an option?

Consent and the alternatives

As was discussed in Chapter 2, the partnership between doctors and patients allows patients to express their needs and preferences, and to make decisions about their care with medical support. Except for the rare circumstances in which the law allows compulsory treatment (see pages 123–6), consent from a competent adult is the trigger that allows treatment or examination to take place. Treatment of children is covered in Chapter 4.

The first part of this chapter deals with the medical treatment of patients who lack capacity to give consent to treatment. When patients lack the capacity to express their wishes or to make decisions, others clearly need to decide on their behalf. Families often feel that they are the natural decision makers, but in law they are entitled to give consent for treatment on behalf of an incapacitated adult only when they have been appointed as the patient's proxy decision maker. At the time of writing, in the UK the appointment of a proxy to make medical decisions is an option only in Scotland, although there are proposals for law reform for England and Wales, and the issues are being discussed in Northern Ireland (see pages 126–7). In all other cases, relatives have no right to give consent for treatment; responsibility usually falls to the doctor in charge, who decides based on what is necessary and what is in the patient's best interests. Despite this, families of adults who have lost their capacity play an essential role. This chapter looks at the scope and limits of that role. It describes the nature of decision making capacity, the importance of involving incapacitated patients to the fullest extent possible in decision making, and how decisions about the medical care of incapacitated adults are made. The chapter primarily concerns patients who have reached the age of majority: 18 years in England, Wales and Northern Ireland, 16 years in Scotland. Decisions about involving incapacitated adults in medical research are covered in Chapter 14.

The second part of this chapter sets out the circumstances in which the law allows compulsory treatment of adults without consent, and even against their wishes. These situations are rare.

General principles

The following general principles should be taken into account when considering the medical treatment of a patient lacking capacity. Patients are entitled to the following.

- **Liberty:** Patients should be free from interventions that inhibit liberty or the capacity to enjoy life unless such intervention is necessary to prevent a greater harm to the patient or to others. Treatment options should be the least restrictive effective option. Appropriate justification must be shown for the use of restraints and it is inappropriate for restrictive measures to be used as an alternative to adequate staffing levels.
- **Autonomy:** Patients' autonomy should be promoted in a manner that is consistent with their needs and wishes.
- **Dignity:** Patients should be treated with respect and courtesy, and their social and cultural values should be respected.
- **Having their views taken into account** even when they are considered legally incapable of determining what happens.
- **Privacy:** Patients should be free from any medical procedures unless there are good therapeutic reasons for them.
- **Confidentiality:** Personal health information should be treated confidentially.
- **Having their health needs met:** These should be met as fully as practicable, while recognising that the availability of resources may limit treatment options.
- **Being free from unfair discrimination:** Treatment options should be considered on the basis of the patient's need and patients should not be treated differently solely because of the condition that gives rise to the incapacity.
- **Having the views of people close to them taken into account:** This applies even when they are not entitled in law to make decisions on behalf of the patient.

In complex cases, for example where the benefits and burdens of the treatment are finely balanced, it is advisable to obtain a second opinion from another doctor. This can both assure the doctor proposing to treat the patient that the patient does lack capacity to decide and that the treatment is in the patient's best interests. The following steps are intended as a guide.

- Consider whether there are alternative ways of treating the patient, particularly equally effective measures that may be less invasive, keep future options open, and promote independence.
- Consider whether the proposals impact on the patient's human rights.
- Discuss the treatment with the healthcare team.
- Discuss the treatment with the patient insofar as this is possible.

- Consult relatives, carers and any proxy decision makers.
- Consider any anticipatory statement of the patient's views.
- Consult other appropriate professionals involved with the patient's care in the hospital or community.
- Consider the need to obtain a second opinion from a doctor skilled in the proposed treatment.
- Ensure that a record is made of the discussions.

When can treatment be given to adults who lack capacity?

Best interests, benefit, and necessity

When patients cannot make a valid choice, ethical principles require doctors to act in patients' best interests (see pages 108–9). Under the Adults with Incapacity (Scotland) Act 2000, the term "benefit" is used to mean the same thing. Similarly, the law allows doctors to treat incapacitated patients when there is some necessity to act and it is in the best interests of the person concerned. The overall effect must be to benefit the patient. In Scotland, this is known as the "general authority to treat" and a certificate of incapacity must be issued before this authority can be used to treat a patient.

Throughout the UK, the ability to treat people who cannot give consent is not generally limited to emergencies, but applies equally to routine health care procedures. The House of Lords has indicated that doctors' actions in the care of incapacitated adults "may well transcend such measures as surgical operation or substantial medical treatment and may extend to include such humdrum matters as routine medical or dental treatment, even simple care such as dressing and undressing and putting to bed".[1] If the incapacity is temporary because of anaesthetic, sedation, intoxication, or temporary unconsciousness, however, doctors should not proceed beyond what is essential to preserve the person's life or prevent deterioration in health.

Emergencies

Doctors should also provide treatment necessary to preserve life in an emergency when consent cannot be obtained, unless the person has registered a prior objection. The range of action that may be taken in an emergency is not limited to preventing immediate deterioration. It may also include steps to prepare for recovery to become an option. Non-urgent decisions should generally wait, however, in the hope that the patient will participate later or people close to the patient will indicate the patient's views.

If, in an emergency, a patient refuses treatment and there is doubt about his or her capacity to do so validly, doctors should take whatever steps are necessary to prevent deterioration of the patient's condition and then consider matters of capacity and consent. The processes are the same in Scotland, even when a proxy refuses to give consent but the doctor in charge judges that treatment is in the patient's best interests. Once essential treatment has been given, the procedures for resolving disagreement between doctors and proxies must be followed (see pages 111–2). When it is clear that a patient is competent to refuse treatment, however, or has a valid advance directive that is applicable to the circumstances, doctors may not provide treatment against the patient's wishes (unless the treatment is provided under mental health legislation, see pages 123–6).

General issues in emergency care are covered in Chapter 15.

Compulsory treatment

Mental health legislation, and to a very limited extent public health legislation, permit the use of compulsion to provide treatment in limited circumstances. The use of compulsion is rare, and most incapacitated adults are treated in accordance with the principles set out at the beginning of this section. This chapter contains a short discussion of the issues around compulsory treatment on pages 123–6.

What constitutes capacity?

Mental "capacity" and "competence" are often used interchangeably, but the former is the term most often used in law. People aged over 16 are presumed to have the capacity to make decisions until the contrary is shown. Capacity often fluctuates over time, and many people who lack capacity to take complex decisions are able to make other choices.

The level of capacity the law requires a person to have in order for a decision to be valid depends upon the decision. The complexity of the decision, the person's ability to understand at the time the decision is made, the nature of the decision required, and its implications are all features. Ultimately, capacity is a legal concept, and if there is doubt or disagreement, the courts may have to decide, taking into account evidence from doctors. Doctors are involved in assessing capacity not only for deciding about medical treatment but they also may become concerned in assessing people's capacity to make other decisions, for example making a will. Different tests of capacity apply to different tasks. When doctors are asked to assess somebody's capacity they must therefore ensure that they understand the legal function of the assessment and the level of capacity necessary in law to be competent in the particular area in question. This is often referred to as the "functional" nature of capacity. The BMA publishes, jointly with the Law Society, advice on assessing capacity in a range of situations.[2]

Two legal cases have been especially significant in setting out the test of capacity to make a decision about medical treatment. In the first, a mentally ill patient was found to have the capacity to refuse treatment for a physical condition.

Refusal of treatment for a physical condition by a mentally ill patient

C was a 68-year-old patient suffering from paranoid schizophrenia. In 1993 he developed gangrene in a foot during his confinement in a secure hospital to which he had been transferred under mental health legislation while serving a 7-year-term of imprisonment. He was removed to a general hospital, where the consultant surgeon diagnosed that there was an 85% chance that he would die imminently if the leg was not amputated below the knee. C refused to consider amputation. He said that he would rather die with two feet than live with one.

C had grandiose and persecutory delusions, including that he had an international career in medicine during the course of which he had never lost a patient. He expressed complete confidence in his ability to survive aided by God, the good doctors, and the good nurses, but acknowledged the possibility of death as a consequence of retaining his limb. He was content to follow medical advice and cooperate with treatment provided his rejection of amputation was respected. Conservative treatment was progressing well at the time of the hearing.

The High Court identified three necessary components of capacity to give consent to medical treatment. The patient must be able to:

- understand and retain the information relevant to the decision in question
- believe that information and
- weigh that information in the balance to arrive at a choice.

The court found that C's schizophrenia did impact on his general capacity, but what was relevant to the decision about amputation was that he had understood and retained the relevant treatment information, that in his own way he believed it, and in the same fashion arrived at a choice. The hospital was therefore not entitled to amputate his leg without his express written consent, nor could it do so in the future, even if his mental capacity deteriorated.

Re C (adult: refusal of treatment)[3]

In a second case, the Court of Appeal dismissed a 23-year-old woman's appeal against a decision to administer medical procedures necessary as part of a caesarean section.[4] This case is also discussed in Chapter 7 (page 226).

Refusal of treatment due to phobia

MB was 40 weeks pregnant. The fetus was in the breech position. MB had a needle phobia and would not agree to a caesarean section because of the venepuncture involved. The Court of Appeal considered whether she had the capacity to decide about the procedure. Noting that adults are presumed to be competent unless the contrary is proven, and that a competent woman may for religious reasons, other reasons, rational or irrational reasons, or no reason at all, choose not to have medical intervention, even though the consequences may be the death or serious handicap of the child she bears or her own death, the court set out the relevant test of capacity:

(Continued)

A person lacks capacity if some impairment or disturbance of mental functioning renders the person unable to make a decision whether to consent to or to refuse treatment. That inability to make a decision occurs when:

- the patient is unable to comprehend and retain the information that is material to the decision, especially as to the likely consequences of having or not having the treatment in question; or
- the patient is unable to use the information and weigh it in the balance as part of the process of arriving at a decision.

The court found that MB's fear of needles dominated her thinking, and "made her quite unable to consider anything else". She was found to lack the capacity to refuse treatment and it was therefore lawful for the doctors to administer anaesthetic in an emergency if it was in MB's best interests to do so. The court also noted that it was obvious that MB was more likely to suffer significant long term harm from death or injury to the baby than from receiving the anaesthetic against her wishes. It was likely, therefore, that should anaesthetic become necessary, it would be in her best interests to administer it.

Re MB (medical treatment)[5]

In addition, in Scotland, incapacity has a statutory definition in the Adults with Incapacity (Scotland) Act. When the provisions of the Act are being used (see pages 110–2) a person is defined as being incapacitated if he or she is incapable of:

- acting or
- making decisions or
- communicating decisions or
- understanding decisions or
- retaining the memory of decisions
- by reason of mental disorder or of inability to communicate because of physical disability.

The legislation also notes that a person does not fall within this definition by reason only of a lack or deficiency in a faculty of communication if that lack or deficiency can be made good by human or mechanical aid.[6]

Throughout the UK, the key principles for doctors that arise from the law are that, in order to demonstrate capacity to give or withhold consent for medical treatment, individuals should be able to:

- understand in simple language what the medical treatment is, its purpose and nature and why it is being proposed
- understand its principal benefits, risks and alternatives
- understand in broad terms what will be the consequences of not receiving the proposed treatment
- retain the information for long enough to make an effective decision
- weigh the information in the balance
- make a free choice (i.e. free from pressure).

Although knowledge and experience may improve people's abilities to make decisions, lack of these does not necessarily mean a person lacks capacity. In a High Court case of a patient who refused artificial ventilation, one of the doctors caring for the patient, Ms B, said that she was

> unable to give informed consent, not because of a lack of capacity in general but her specific lack of knowledge and experience of exposure to a spinal rehabilitation unit and thereafter to readjustment to life in the community. Without that opportunity ... Ms B did not have the requisite opportunity to give informed consent.[7]

The judge rejected this view, which, she said, was not the law. The emphasis is on understanding and ability, not knowledge and experience. The case of Ms B is discussed in more detail in Chapter 2 (pages 85–6).

Capacity to refuse

As mentioned above, the more serious the decision, the higher the test of capacity. Generally, the measures that doctors propose are in the best medical interests of patients, and deciding not to follow medical advice can have serious implications. Therefore, although consent and refusal are opposite sides of a coin, the courts have shown themselves more reluctant to accept weak evidence on capacity when refusal is at stake. This has sometimes meant, in practice, that patients are more likely to be regarded as lacking capacity when they refuse treatment than when they accept it.

Capacity being commensurate with the gravity of the decision

In a case involving a Jehovah's Witness who refused a blood transfusion, the Master of the Rolls said:

> Doctors faced with a refusal of consent have to give very careful and detailed consideration to the patient's capacity to decide at the time when the decision was made. It may not be the simple case of the patient having no capacity because, for example, at that time he had hallucinations. It may be the more difficult case of a temporarily reduced capacity at the time when his decision was made. What matters is that the doctors should consider whether at that time he had a capacity which was commensurate with the gravity of the decision which he purported to make. The more serious the decision, the greater the capacity required. If the patient had the requisite capacity, they are bound by his decision. If not, they are free to treat him in what they believe to be his best interests.

Re T (adult: refusal of medical treatment)[8]

People are entitled to choose an option that is contradictory to that which most people would choose, but where their choice also appears to be a very reckless choice or contradict their previously expressed attitudes, health professionals would be justified in questioning in greater detail their capacity to make a valid refusal in order to eliminate the possibility of a depressive illness or a delusional state. A specialist psychiatric opinion may be required.

Refusal rendered invalid by misinformation and undue influence

T was 20 years old when she was injured in a road traffic accident. She was 34 weeks pregnant. She had been brought up as a Jehovah's Witness and, on admission to hospital, twice refused a blood transfusion after having spent a period of time alone with her mother. A caesarean section was carried out, but the baby was stillborn. T's condition deteriorated and, had it not been for her advance refusal, the anaesthetist would have given her a blood transfusion. On the following day T's father and boyfriend decided to go to court to challenge the validity of the advance refusal. The challenge was upheld and the blood transfusion was given. The basis for this decision was that T had been acting under the influence of her mother and the refusal did not represent a legitimate expression of T's free will. There were also serious doubts about whether T had intended her refusal to apply to a situation that was life threatening.

The Court of Appeal held that doctors should accept that a refusal is valid only after considering whether capacity is diminished by illness, medication, false assumptions, or misinformation, or whether the patient's will had been overborne by another's influence. In T's situation, it was held that the effect of her condition, together with misinformation and her mother's influence, rendered her refusal of consent ineffective.

Re T (adult: refusal of medical treatment)[9]

Assessing capacity

The assessment of adult patients' capacity to make a decision about their own medical treatment is a matter for clinical judgment guided by professional practice and subject to legal requirements. It is the personal responsibility of any doctor proposing to treat a patient to judge whether the patient has the capacity to give valid consent. Indeed, doctors constantly assess whether patients have the capacity to make the decision with which they are faced.

Mental abilities can be influenced by both physical and psychiatric conditions. All doctors involved with direct patient care, whatever their specialty, should be able to take a psychiatric history and conduct a basic mental state examination in order to define straightforward abnormalities, irrespective of their cause. GPs are often well placed to judge capacity, especially if they have a close, long term acquaintance with the person being assessed. Where the person's capacity is uncertain or unclear, however, or the treating doctor does not feel able to make an objective assessment, specialist advice should be sought.

Capacity is assessed in relation to a particular decision that needs to be made. An assessment of capacity is not based on the test "would a rational person decide as this person has decided?" The fact that a person acts in a way that an ordinary prudent person would not is not in itself evidence of impaired capacity. Rather, the thought processes behind the decision are relevant.

In cases where patients have borderline or fluctuating capacity, it can be difficult to assess whether the individual can make valid decisions on very serious issues. Doctors should be aware that capacity can be influenced by many things, including medical condition, medication, pain, fatigue, time of day, and mood. Mental disorder and impairment may affect capacity, although these things do not necessarily prevent patients from making a valid choice. A very wide spectrum of ability is found within the group of patients whose competence to decide is permanently or temporarily affected. Doctors should aim to minimise the effects of factors that affect capacity, and allow patients to make choices when they are best able to do so.

The BMA publishes detailed practical advice about assessing capacity.[10] In many cases there is, of course, no doubt about a person's capacity. When there is, however, a comprehensive psychological investigation may be needed and any elective, non-urgent treatment should be postponed until the issues of capacity are resolved. Emergencies should be dealt with in accordance with the guidance on pages 101–2. The psychological investigation would seek to determine whether the adult:

- is capable of making a choice
- understands the nature of what is being asked
- understands why a choice is needed
- has memory abilities that allow the retention of information
- is aware of any alternatives
- has knowledge of the risks and benefits involved
- is aware of the decision's personal relevance to him or herself
- is aware of his or her right to refuse, as well as the consequences of refusal
- is aware of how to refuse
- is capable of communicating his or her choice
- has ever expressed wishes relevant to the issue when greater capacity existed
- is expressing views consistent with previously preferred moral, cultural, family, and experiential background.[11]

Assessing capacity to give consent to medical treatment is somewhat different from other capacity assessments since the assessor may also be the person proposing the treatment. If the procedure proposed is risky or involves innovative techniques or if there is a divergence of opinion as to its benefits for the patient, additional safeguards are likely to be needed (see pages 116–20).

Factors affecting capacity and how to enhance capacity

Barriers to achieving competent decisions can sometimes be overcome by providing the best opportunity for patients to participate. Doctors have a general ethical duty to enhance capacity when it is possible to do so, and should seek to engage patients in decision making when they are best able to participate. The venue should be non-threatening and welcoming. GPs in particular may find that the patient's own home is a good choice because anxiety about unfamiliar surroundings may be inhibiting. Capacity and simply the ability to participate can be enhanced with treatment or symptom management. For example, management of pain or treatment of encephalopathy can mean a patient is more able to take part in decision making. Similarly, the effects of medication, for example euphoria induced by systemic corticosteroids, can affect capacity. Whenever possible, patients should be given the opportunity to express their views when any detrimental effects of medication are absent or at a minimum. The effects of some medications take a long time to diminish, and doctors should consider whether it would be appropriate to allow time for these long term effects to dissipate before assessing capacity. Similarly, depression and anxiety can be difficult to recognise, but may also interfere with capacity. Where there is doubt about mental state, a psychiatric opinion is often needed.

It may also help if decisions are broken down into a series of smaller choices. Vulnerability to coercive influences should be acknowledged and minimised. It is important that people are not judged to be incapable of making decisions just because they have communication difficulties. Communication support must be offered if appropriate. Speech and language therapy may be helpful. Written and other forms of recorded information can also be used to enhance communication.

Summary – capacity: defining, assessing, enhancing

- A person has capacity to decide if he or she can:
    - understand in simple language what the medical treatment is, its purpose and nature and why it is being proposed
    - understand its principal benefits, risks and alternatives
    - understand in broad terms what will be the consequences of not receiving the proposed treatment
    - retain the information for long enough to make an effective decision
    - weigh the information in the balance
    - make a free choice (i.e. free from pressure).

- Capacity is often assessed by the doctor who proposes treatment. Specialist advice should be sought if there is any doubt.
- Doctors should seek to enhance patients' capacity to participate in decision making.

Best interests and benefiting patients

When patients are competent and have access to information, they are the best judge of what is in their interests and whether the expected benefits of a proposed treatment outweigh the burdens. When patients lack the capacity to decide, many factors are important in deciding what may benefit them or be in their best interests:

- the patient's own wishes and values (where these can be ascertained), including any advance statement
- clinical judgment about the effectiveness of the proposed treatment, particularly in relation to other options
- when there is more than one effective option, which option is least restrictive of the patient's future choices
- the likelihood and extent of any degree of improvement in the patient's condition if treatment is provided
- the views of people close to the patient, especially close relatives, partners, carers, or proxy decision makers about what the patient is likely to see as beneficial
- any knowledge of the patient's religious, cultural, and other non-medical views that may have an impact on the patient's wishes.

Screening and preventive measures

General issues around screening and immunisation are discussed in Chapter 20, which stresses that screening programmes must be based on a robust body of evidence. Chapter 20 also notes that one of the benefits of screening is peace of mind for those with negative findings, and there are questions about whether this is a benefit that incapacitated adults are likely to experience. When considering involving incapacitated adults in screening programmes, it is important to judge the programme according to the needs of this particular group of patients, and not to assume that the considerations are necessarily the same as for competent adults.

It is, however, important that mentally incapacitated patients are not deprived of the benefits of screening or immunisation, provided those benefits outweigh the burdens of the procedures involved. Incapacitated elderly people who could benefit from immunisation against influenza, for example, should have the same opportunity to receive it as others. Whether it will ultimately be given depends on the individual circumstances: whether for the particular patient the benefit outweighs any potential harm.

Offering cervical screening to women who are unable to give consent, particularly those with learning difficulties who have never had capacity, raises questions about whether health professionals know if the woman is, or has ever been, sexually active. Knowing who is, or has been, sexually active is not always simple. Some women can give a different impression each time they are asked.[12] Staff working on one cervical screening programme found that it was helpful to have the local sex education team on hand to provide reassurance for both staff and patients. Information about the sex education service was made available during the screening programme and referrals to it made, if appropriate.

Although mentally incapacitated patients should be encouraged to access services that may benefit them, women in this group may find cervical or breast screening distressing, and it is equally important to balance this distress against the potential benefits for them. Having a relative or carer accompanying the woman may help to provide reassurance. If she becomes unduly distressed, or resists the intervention, health professionals should stop.

In summary, screening services should be offered to patients with learning difficulties or who are unable to give consent for another reason, if they are likely to experience some benefit from being screened. As with all decisions about medical interventions, the benefits and burdens for the individual patient must be assessed.

Involving people close to the patient

At present, nobody can give consent to treatment on behalf of another adult (except in Scotland if a health care proxy has been appointed, see below). Even when their views have no legal status, however, it is often good practice to involve people close to patients in decisions, bearing in mind the duty of confidentiality to the patient (see Chapter 5). Taking account of the views of people who are close to the patient is a legal requirement in some circumstances under the Adults with Incapacity (Scotland) Act.[13] There may also be practical benefits for patients in terms of improved clinical outcomes when people close to them are able to help and meet their care needs.

As far as possible, patients should be offered a choice about whom they want to be told about their health and condition, and whom they would like to be involved in decisions about their care. If patients are able to decide about involving people close to them, their agreement should be sought. It may also be helpful to ask competent patients whom they want, or do not want, to be involved in decision making if they become incapacitated. When a patient's wishes are not known, decisions about disclosure to close friends and family should be made according to the patient's best interests, including the need to maximise the patient's future choices. This is particularly important when a patient's incapacity is temporary.

It is important to be clear that the information sought from people close to patients is to help to ascertain what the patient would have wanted in these circumstances, as opposed to what those consulted would like for the patient or what they would want for themselves if they were in the same situation.

The role of people close to the patient

Adults with Incapacity (Scotland) Act

In Scotland there is an additional statutory framework that regulates decision making on behalf of incapacitated adults (people over 16 years). The Adults with Incapacity (Scotland) Act 2000 allows patients to appoint a proxy to make decisions about medical treatment on their behalf when they become incapacitated. The sheriff may appoint a proxy on behalf of an incapacitated adult. Where there is no proxy, treatment is provided under the "general authority to treat" (see page 101), but this may not be used when there is a proxy decision maker or if an application to be a proxy is pending.

The Act sets out general principles that must underpin any intervention in the affairs of an incapacitated adult. Interventions must:

- benefit the adult
- take account of the adult's wishes, as far as these can be ascertained
- take account of the views of relevant others, as far as it is reasonable and practical to do so
- restrict the adult's freedom as little as possible while still achieving the desired benefit.

Proxy consent

The roles and responsibilities of proxies are set out in codes of practice.[14] Proxies have a duty of care to the adult on whose behalf they act, and a duty to abide by the general principles set out in the Act. When an adult lacks the capacity to make a decision, a proxy who has been granted the relevant power may give consent to medical treatment on behalf of the adult. When a doctor is aware that a proxy decision maker has been appointed, and it is reasonable and practicable to obtain the proxy's consent for treatment, this must be sought. Wherever possible, doctors should postpone treatment until a proxy has been consulted. In all cases, however, it is important to ensure that discussion with a proxy does not introduce delays that jeopardise the patient's care. Proxies may also refuse medical treatment, provided they are fulfilling their duty of care to the adult and are abiding by the general principles in the Act. If doctors have concerns about the ability of a proxy to fulfil his or her role, they should take legal advice.

Disputes

It is always best to proceed with consensus on medical treatment. When everybody is in agreement over the proposed treatment, generally it may proceed with a proxy's consent or, where there is no proxy, under the doctor's general authority to treat. Disagreement about treatment should be rare. Discussion and ongoing consultation can help doctors to understand the patient's priorities, and help proxies and others close to the patient to understand the reasoning behind clinical decisions. If agreement cannot be reached, however, the Act puts in place procedures for resolving disputes.

If the doctor and proxy disagree about a treatment (or non-treatment) decision, the doctor must obtain a second opinion from a medical practitioner nominated by the Mental Welfare Commission.[15] The nominated medical practitioner must consult the proxy and anybody else nominated by the proxy (as far as is reasonable and practicable). If the nominated medical practitioner agrees with the treating doctor, the treatment may be given or withheld notwithstanding the proxy's objection, unless the proxy or another person with a personal interest in the patient's welfare applies to the Court of Session.

If the nominated medical practitioner disagrees with the treating doctor, legal advice should be sought. An appeal may be made to the Court of Session by the treating doctor to determine whether the treatment should be given or not. In the interim, only emergency treatment may be provided (see pages 101–2).

Summary – proxy decision making in Scotland

- A proxy decision maker may be appointed by or on behalf of an incapacitated adult in Scotland but not in the rest of the UK.
- A proxy may give consent to, or refuse, medical treatment on behalf of the adult provided that the decision:
  - benefits the adult
  - takes account of the adult's wishes, as far as these can be ascertained
  - takes account of the views of relevant others, as far as it is reasonable and practical to do so
  - restricts the adult's freedom as little as possible while still achieving the desired benefit.

If there is disagreement about an adult's treatment, there are procedures that must be followed, including obtaining a second medical opinion. If disagreement persists, an application may be made to court.

England, Wales, and Northern Ireland

In England, Wales, and Northern Ireland patients can hope to make their views known at a later stage by appointing, in advance, another person to speak for them. Decisions expressed by such a proxy can be useful in the same way that an advance statement of the patient's general views and preferences is helpful (see pages 113–6). These proxy decisions do not, however, currently have legal force in the way that decisions of proxies in Scotland do. The BMA has been pressing for legislation to allow for proxy decision making in all parts of the UK. Despite government consultations on the issue since the early 1990s, Scotland is, at the time of writing, the only part of the UK that has enacted legislation (see pages 126–7).

Patient advocates

Patient advocates have no formal decision making powers, but can help the decision making process by facilitating communication with the patient and explaining the patient's views. The BMA supports the provision of independent, integrated advocacy services for all patients who require them, in order to support and assist the decision making process. Services need to be efficiently run, and advocates must be properly trained and have access to necessary advice and support.

Part of the role of the advocate is to facilitate communication between incapacitated patients and health professionals, but it is essential that doctors aim to communicate directly with the patient wherever possible. Some patients who have advocates, or who have been accompanied to hospital by carers, report feeling excluded when health professionals do not speak directly to them.

Health professionals need to understand the scope and limits of the powers of advocates in order that professionals and advocates do not infringe the boundaries of their respective responsibilities. Although friends and family have an important role to play, there are times when an independent advocate with no emotional investment in the situation is the most appropriate person to support a person making difficult decisions. An advocate can be crucial for ensuring that people's needs, rights, and wishes are met. Doctors should work with advocates whenever possible. There is, however, potential for conflict when roles are not properly defined.

Advance statements

Advance statements provide a mechanism whereby competent people can give instructions about what they wish to be done if they should subsequently lose the capacity to decide for themselves. Their purpose is to provide a means for patients to continue to exercise autonomy and shape the treatment they receive when they become incapable of expressing their wishes. Advance statements are likely to be particularly useful to those who have some form of advance warning by age or illness of impending mental incapacity. The later stages of dementia always lead to mental incompetence, but by means of an advance statement an individual may be able to control the provision of treatment as far as this can be foreseen. In 1995 the BMA produced a code of practice for health professionals, giving advice and guidance on advance statements covering:

- refusals of treatment (often called advance directives)
- requests for treatment
- statements of general wishes or values
- statements that name someone to be consulted when health care decisions are needed.[16]

The BMA does not actively encourage people to make advance statements, but believes that people should have the opportunity to plan for their future care if they so wish. Although making decisions in advance may help to ensure that the care individuals receive is what they would want in the circumstances, there are disadvantages. The way healthy people feel about illness before they have experienced it may be quite different to how they feel when it happens. It is also possible that a badly worded statement may be misinterpreted or implemented in circumstances the patient had not foreseen. Health professionals should ensure that patients are aware of the advantages and disadvantages before deciding to make an advance statement.

The legal position

There is currently no legislation covering advance statements. It is clear from legal cases heard in England, however, that competent, informed adults have a legal right to refuse medical procedures in advance. An unambiguous and informed advance refusal of treatment (advance directive) is as valid as a contemporaneous decision. Although the decisions of courts in England are not necessarily binding on courts in other parts of the UK, it is likely that the courts in Scotland and Northern Ireland would take a similar approach, and doctors are advised to follow the advice in this section until cases are heard in their own jurisdiction.

The following principles emerge from the legal cases:[17]

- An advance refusal of treatment is legally binding if:
  - the patient is an adult and was competent when the directive was made and
  - the patient has been offered sufficient, accurate information to make an informed decision and
  - the circumstances that have arisen are those that were envisaged by the patient and
  - the patient was not subjected to undue influence in making the decision.
- Adults are presumed to be competent to make decisions, unless the contrary is shown. As with all decision making, the test of capacity to make an advance refusal of treatment is functional and the understanding required depends on the gravity of the decision.
- A refusal of treatment does not need to be a wise decision and the fact that a decision is contrary to what would be expected of the vast majority of adults does not affect its validity.
- In cases of genuine doubt about the validity of an advance refusal, the presumption is in favour of providing lifesaving treatment. When there is doubt, and time permits, a declaration should be sought from a court.
- Any persons, including health professionals and carers trained in providing treatment such as cardiopulmonary resuscitation, who knowingly provide treatment in the face of a valid advance refusal may be liable to legal action for battery or assault.
- Advance "consent" or requests for treatment are not legally binding, although they may be helpful in assessing a patient's likely wishes and preferences.

Whether these principles should be enshrined in statute has been a matter of considerable debate. Some people believe that statute is required to clarify the law, particularly in relation to the potential liability of doctors and the ability of patients to refuse "basic care" (see page 115), while others believe that the law is already clear and that the greater flexibility provided by the common law is preferable to rigid statutory provision. In proposals for reforming the law on decision making for incapacitated adults in England and Wales, the government announced in October 1999 that it did not consider it appropriate to legislate on advance directives at that time because "the guidance contained in case law, together with the Code of Practice, *Advance Statements about Medical Treatment*, published by the BMA, provides sufficient clarity and flexibility to enable the validity and applicability of advance statements to be decided on a case by case basis".[18]

Women of childbearing age should consider the fact that an advance statement may be implemented at a time when they are pregnant. Such women should consider including their wishes regarding treatment during pregnancy. Unless an advance statement makes unambiguously clear that it is intended to apply during pregnancy, even if that would endanger the life or health of a fetus, the courts are likely to assume that the woman had not intended the directive to apply during pregnancy and rule it invalid. If an incapacitated pregnant woman presents with an apparently valid advance directive refusing treatment, legal advice should be sought.

Scope of advance statements

Whatever wishes people express while they are competent should be given serious consideration. Nevertheless, people cannot authorise or refuse in advance procedures that they could not authorise or refuse contemporaneously. For example, they cannot authorise unlawful procedures, such as euthanasia, nor can they insist upon futile or inappropriate treatment. The BMA also believes that people should not be able to refuse, in advance, the provision of "basic care". This includes the administration of medication or the performance of any procedure that is solely or primarily designed to provide comfort to the patient or alleviate that person's pain, symptoms, or distress.

Provision of information

In order to make informed choices about advance statements, patients have a legitimate expectation of being provided with information in an accessible form. Thus, doctors should ensure that the foreseeable options and implications are adequately explained, admit to uncertainty when this is the case, and make reasonable efforts to discover if there is more specialised information available to pass on to the patient.

Format of advance statements

Oral statements are likely to be legally valid if supported by appropriate evidence, but there are clear advantages to recording general views and specific refusals in writing. Advance statements are an aid to, rather than a substitute for, open dialogue between patients and health professionals. There are no specific legal requirements concerning the format of advance statements but it is recommended that the following information is included as a minimum:

- full name
- address

- name and address of GP
- whether advice was sought from health professionals
- a clear statement of wishes or the name, address and telephone number of a person to be consulted
- signature and the date the document was written and reviewed.

It is recommended that the statement is reviewed on a regular basis and at least every five years. More frequent review is likely to be appropriate for people with a progressive, degenerative condition. The validity of an advance statement may be questioned if significant time has elapsed without review, especially if major changes have occurred either in the patient's general health or in treatment options.

There is no requirement for advance statements to be witnessed, but if doctors are asked to do so they should consider whether there are any reasons to doubt the patient's capacity to make the decisions in question. The signature of a doctor, or other health professional, as a witness may well imply that an assessment of capacity has taken place.[19]

Storage of advance statements

Storage of an advance statement, and notification of its existence, is primarily the responsibility of the patient. A copy of any written advance statement should be given to the GP to keep with the patient's medical record and, where possible, the patient should draw it to the attention of hospital staff before any episode of hospital care. Patients should also be encouraged to inform their friends and relatives or advocate about the existence of the advance statement, its general content, and where it can be found. This would enable those close to the patient to bring it to the attention of the healthcare team if a situation arises in which the statement may be invoked.

Summary – advance statements

- Patients who understand the implications of their choices can state in advance how they wish to be treated if they suffer loss of capacity.
- Competently made advance refusals, that are applicable to the circumstances, are legally binding.
- General statements of preferences can be helpful in assessing best interests and should be respected, but are not legally binding.

Treatment safeguards and procedures

For most everyday or uncontroversial healthcare decisions, such as taking blood samples for anaemia or lithium levels, providing a mild analgesic for a headache, or providing antibiotics for an infection in an otherwise fit person, the procedures for making decisions outlined in the early sections of this chapter are sufficient. The aim is agreement about treatment between health professionals, people close to the patient, and the incapacitated person (insofar as he or she can express a view).

Some decisions, however, require additional safeguards. The most difficult and complex must be taken to court. Other decisions require second opinions or formal clinical review. The rules about which category a particular treatment decision falls into come from statute, case law, and best practice guidance. The rules are slightly different in Scotland so, for ease of reference, there are separate summary boxes for Scotland in this section.

Clinical review and second opinions

Some procedures, such as withdrawing or withholding artificial nutrition and hydration from a patient who is not imminently dying (see Chapter 10, pages 360–1), give rise to special concern about the best interests and rights of a person who lacks capacity, particularly when the patient has never expressed wishes or preferences about the issue. In such cases it is always good practice to involve a specialist in the area of the patient's incapacity, and where there is doubt or disagreement about the patient's best interests, legal advice may be necessary. Some cases need to be considered by a court (see pages 118–20). As with all procedures, less invasive or reversible options should always be considered. It is essential that the focus remains on the patient's needs and best interests, not on the needs of carers or relatives. Safeguards for protecting the rights of incapacitated adults taking part in research are covered in Chapter 14.

Second opinions are also necessary when the primary aim of an intervention is not the incapacitated patient's benefit, but benefit to a third party. When a health professional has suffered needlestick injury or other occupational exposure to blood or body fluids, for example, it is likely to be appropriate to test an existing blood sample for HIV or other serious communicable disease without consent. Doctors considering doing so should always consult an experienced colleague first. The General Medical Council offers detailed advice.[20]

In the BMA's view, formal clinical review, or second opinions should be sought in the following cases:

- restricting the movements of incapacitated adults to prevent them from self harming, for example, by applying a temporary soft splint to the teeth or using arm splints to prevent self injury
- medical treatment that, as a side effect renders a person infertile, for example surgical intervention for a gynaecological cancer, although court approval is necessary when the aim of the intervention is sterilisation[21]
- termination of pregnancy when there is no doubt that it is the most appropriate therapeutic response[22]
- electroconvulsive therapy

- testing existing blood samples for serious communicable diseases after occupational exposure to body fluids
- withdrawing or withholding artificial nutrition and hydration from a patient who is not imminently dying
- withdrawing artificial nutrition and hydration from a patient in a persistent vegetative state (a court declaration may also be required by law, see Chapter 10, pages 358–60).

Additionally, in Scotland it is a legal requirement for the following procedures to have approval from a practitioner appointed by the Mental Welfare Commission:

- drug treatment for the purpose of reducing sex drive, other than surgical implantation of hormones
- electroconvulsive therapy for mental disorder
- abortion (in addition to meeting the provisions of the Abortion Act 1967)
- any medical treatment that is considered likely by the medical practitioner primarily responsible for that treatment to lead to sterilisation as an unavoidable result.[23]

Doctors treating patients under mental health legislation should also be aware that the law requires second opinions in certain circumstances.[24]

If there is any doubt about the patient's interests, or the legality of a proposed intervention, legal advice must be sought. If the patient is receiving compulsory treatment under mental health legislation, different considerations may apply (see pages 123–6).

Court review

As the cases highlighted in this chapter make clear, the courts may become involved when there is doubt about a person's capacity to refuse. The courts may issue a declaration that the patient lacks capacity to make the decision in question and that, despite the patient's refusal, providing treatment would be lawful. If doctors are in doubt about whether a person has the capacity to refuse treatment, they should approach their lawyers for advice, and meanwhile provide only emergency treatment (see pages 101–2). When necessary, the courts will give rulings at all hours and very quickly.

In addition, there are some decisions that are so serious that each case must be brought before the courts for independent review. The rules differ throughout the UK, and are summarised at the end of this section.

Court review – bone marrow donation

A woman was suffering from a bone marrow disorder that was expected to progress to acute myeloid leukaemia within three months. Her only realistic

(Continued)

prospect of recovery was a bone marrow transplant. Two of her three sisters were not suitable as donors, although preliminary investigation showed that the third sister, Y, may be a possible match. Y had been severely mentally and physically handicapped from birth and lived in a community home. A declaration was sought from the High Court that it would be lawful for Y to donate bone marrow (and be subjected to associated tests).

It was argued that donation would be in Y's best interests. The family was close and regularly visited Y in her community home. If her sister died, it was argued, the adverse effect on the mother would jeopardise her ability to visit Y, who would be harmed by the lack of contact. The court found that it would be to the emotional, psychological, and social benefit of Y to act as a donor because in this way her positive relationship with her mother was likely to be prolonged. The burdens associated with harvesting were described as "very small".

The court also stated that it was appropriate for any case where there was a need or wish to perform a bone marrow harvesting procedure on an incapacitated adult to be brought before a court before the procedure took place.

Re Y (mental incapacity: bone marrow transplant)[25]

In any case where organ or tissue donation is being considered, it is essential that legal advice is obtained. Although the courts authorised donation in the case described above, the circumstances of the case were very specific, and the judge went to lengths to point out that the decision was based on the direct benefits to the incapacitated adult that would accrue from the treatment for her sister. Benefit to the sister alone would not be sufficient reason to subject an incapacitated adult to such procedures.

The courts also hear cases in which a patient's family members want treatment to be provided, but the medical opinion is that treatment would be inappropriate. In such cases, although the courts could rule that providing treatment would not be unlawful, they cannot compel doctors to provide treatment contrary to their professional judgment.

The following boxes list those procedures for which, at the time of writing, court review is essential. It should be noted, however, that the courts may add or remove procedures in the future.

Court review – England, Wales and Northern Ireland

Court approval is essential in the following cases:

- non-therapeutic sterilisation
- withdrawing artificial nutrition and hydration from a patient who is in a persistent vegetative state
- organ or tissue donation
- where there is doubt about a person's capacity and the proposed intervention is controversial or sensitive.

Court review – Scotland

Court approval is essential in the following cases:

- non-therapeutic sterilisation
- organ or tissue donation
- surgical implantation of hormones for the purpose of reducing sex drive
- where there is doubt about a person's capacity and the proposed intervention is controversial or sensitive.

Physical restraints and other measures of control

Patients sometimes behave in such a way as to pose a risk to themselves or others. Individual care plans for patients should address how to handle challenging behaviour, and hospitals should take steps to ensure that the risks are minimised in wards and other places where patients spend time. Giving each patient a defined personal space and a place for the safe keeping of personal possessions, ensuring access to open space, and providing quiet areas on the ward, recreation rooms, single sex areas, and visitors' rooms, can all help.[26]

Controlling behaviour by the use of restraints should be a matter of last resort.[27] These measures should never be used routinely. Restraining measures may be required to prevent violent patients from hurting themselves or other people, but restraint should be used only when immediately necessary and must always be the minimum possible in the circumstances. Restraints or physical support may also be used, with the patient's consent, in connection with provision of treatment. For example, an anorexic patient had her arms encased in plaster, with her consent, to prevent her from injuring herself.[28]

Particular concerns have been expressed that in residential care sometimes the main reason for restraint is to forestall behaviour that may be potentially disruptive to the smooth running of the home, so that the objective is institutional compliance rather than protection of individuals.[29] A wide range of measures have been used in the past, including locking people in, placing them in special chairs that restrict movement, treating them with inappropriate sedation, or simply arranging seating at a height or angle that makes it difficult for the sitter to rise unaided. These are inappropriate. Measures that are sometimes put forward as alternatives to such restraints are electronic tagging or surveillance cameras. The purpose of these measures should be to allow people the maximum amount of freedom and privacy compatible with their own safety. They should also respect patients' dignity and be compatible with their human rights, in particular the right to be free from inhuman or degrading treatment, and the right to liberty and security.

When any form of restraint is proposed to protect mentally incapacitated people from hurting themselves, this should be used only to the extent of preventing risk beyond that which would normally be taken by a similarly frail, mentally alert person. Restraint that involves either tying or attaching a patient to some part of a building or to its fixtures or fittings must not be used. Staff must have specific training and make a balanced judgment between the need to promote individuals' autonomy by allowing them to move around at will and the duty to protect them from likely harm. In every case where the physical freedom of an individual is curtailed, staff should record the decision and the reasons for it, and state explicitly in a care plan under what circumstances restraint will be used, what form the restraint will take, and how it will be reviewed. Every episode of restraint should be fully documented and reviewed. Restraint should not be used as a substitute for adequate staffing or as a punishment, and can be justified only when it contributes to the individual's quality of life or prevents risk to others.

Doctors who are considering using restraint or other forms of control should consult advice from government departments about patients who present particular management problems.[30]

Summary – restraint

- Restraints may be used when essential to contain patients who endanger themselves or others and when less restrictive measures have failed.
- Staff should have training in conflict avoidance and the safe use of restraints.
- Institutions should have formal policies that should be monitored and regularly reviewed.
- Such policies should encourage the exploration of alternatives to restraint.
- The healthcare team should record the use of restraints and this record should be reviewed regularly.
- Restraints should never be used as a substitute for adequate staffing.
- Staff should identify and report to managers any improper uses of restraint.

Treatment in hospital

Most incapacitated patients agree to being admitted to hospital for care. It has been established by the House of Lords that it is lawful to treat people who lack capacity to agree to admission without recourse to mental health legislation.[31] When patients object, however, it may be necessary to detain them compulsorily under mental health legislation (see pages 123–6). Such legislation contains clear safeguards for detained patients, including external review of the need for compulsion, second opinions from approved doctors to authorise patient treatment plans, and oversight by an independent body.[32] The House of Lords has drawn attention to the fact that compliant incapacitated patients who are being treated under common law provisions do not benefit from the safeguards in mental health legislation.

"Detention" of informal patients

L was a 48-year-old man with autism and complex disabilities. He was unable to express a preference about where he lived. After being resident for 30 years

(Continued)

121

at Bournewood Hospital he went to live with a family of carers. During a visit to a local day centre, L became agitated and was taken to the emergency department of the local hospital. From there he was taken to the mental health behavioural unit at Bournewood Hospital where, in spite of requests from his carers for him to return home, he remained as an inpatient. As L was compliant and made no attempts to run away, he was admitted as an informal patient, although his clinical supervisor made it clear that, had he attempted to run away, he would have been admitted under the Mental Health Act 1983.

A case was taken to court on behalf of L. The courts were called upon to establish a number of issues crucial to the position of informal patients who do not possess the capacity to consent or refuse. First, as they are theoretically free to leave, are such patients actually detained? Secondly, if they are, is their detention justified by the common law doctrine of necessity that justifies the giving of treatment to incapacitated adults in their own best interests?

The Court of first instance and the Court of Appeal both found L was "*de facto*" detained. In the House of Lords, however, the majority view was that L was not in fact detained but that, even if he had been, detention would not have been unlawful if it could be justified according to the common law doctrine of necessity. The trust would have had to show that detention was in accordance with its duty of care to the patient and was in the patient's best interests.

R v Bournewood Community and Mental Health NHS Trust[33]

Doctors should consider carefully whether informal admission or use of mental health legislation is the best route for patients who cannot give consent, but nevertheless comply with treatment. The Department of Health and Welsh Office recommend that informal admission should be used if, at the time of admission, the patient is mentally incapable of consent but does not object to entering hospital and receiving care or treatment.[34] The specific purpose of the intervention needs to be evaluated with regard to the patient's best interests and the doctrine of necessity. All relevant factors need to be taken into account, such as the duration of the treatment, the seriousness of the illness, and whether the patient is, in fact, compliant. The decision about whether to use mental health legislation must reflect patients' needs and preferences, wherever possible. If patients show any signs of resistance, for example through disturbed behaviour or becoming uncharacteristically withdrawn, their "compliance" must be reassessed.

Although the Bournewood case highlighted the difficulties facing some informal patients and defined the limits of the common law in their treatment, the House of Lords did not have the power to resolve the original problem. Subsequent review of mental health legislation in England addressed itself to introducing safeguards for patients who lack capacity to consent, but who do not resist treatment, patients who had hitherto fallen through "the Bournewood gap".

In Scotland, some safeguards are available to informal patients being treated under the Adults with Incapacity (Scotland) Act (see pages 110–2). It is also anticipated that the code of practice to accompany the Mental Health (Care and Treatment) (Scotland) Act 2003 will address this issue and give advice. At the time of writing, the situation in Northern Ireland is uncertain. Doctors who are in doubt should seek legal advice.

Summary – detention

- Decisions about detention, restraint or other forms of control must balance the patient's right to be free to move around with the duty to protect them, or sometimes others, from harm.
- Doctors must consider whether mental health legislation should be used when incapacitated patients are effectively detained in hospital, even when the patient complies with treatment.

Compulsion: mental health

Mental health legislation provides a legal structure for the compulsory psychiatric care and treatment of people suffering from mental disorders. At the time of writing, mental health legislation throughout the UK is undergoing review (see pages 127–9). We therefore avoid detailed descriptions of the legislation, with which doctors practising in the field will already be familiar, but discuss some of the ethical principles that apply in relation to compulsory treatment.

The use of compulsion is clearly a sensitive issue and one that raises questions about human rights. The Human Rights Act 1998 guarantees the right to be free from inhuman or degrading treatment (Article 3), to liberty and security (Article 5), to a fair trial (Article 6), and to respect for family and private life (Article 8). In addition to meeting the requirements of mental health legislation, all decisions relating to compulsory treatment must be compatible with patients' rights.

Clearly the goal of psychiatric interventions is therapeutic. They aim to return people, as far as possible, to a condition in which they are once again able to manage their mental distress effectively without presenting a danger to themselves or other people. Although for some patients severe mental illness is associated with a corollary lack of capacity, mental disorder does not automatically diminish patients' legal capacity. In these cases, balancing the need for compulsion with respect for autonomy is an important part of care.

Compulsory treatment under mental health legislation applies only to treatment for the patient's mental disorder. In the past, this distinction has not been properly understood, leading to some inappropriate use of mental health legislation, such as in the case of S (see box below). When patients are detained and are unable to give consent to treatment for physical conditions, the procedures set out earlier in this chapter apply.

Inappropriate use of mental health legislation

S was a competent 29-year-old woman with pre-eclampsia. The condition threatened both her life and the life of her unborn child. She fully understood the potential risks but refused the offer of treatment. Her GP arranged an assessment by an approved social worker and two psychiatrists. On the basis that she was depressed, that the depression affected her judgment, and that the state of her health entailed a risk both to herself and to her child, she was forcibly treated under mental health legislation and was delivered of a child by caesarean section. S applied for a judicial review of the decision.

The Court of Appeal found that the grounds in mental health legislation that permit detention for the purposes of treatment had not been met. Her detention was therefore unlawful. The court also considered whether mental health legislation could be used to compel treatment of this nature. It ruled that

In the final analysis, a woman detained under the Act for mental disorder cannot be forced into medical procedures unconnected with her mental condition unless her capacity to consent to such treatment is diminished. When she retains her capacity, her consent remains an essential prerequisite and whether she does, or not, must be decided on the basis of the evidence in each individual case.

St George's Healthcare NHS Trust v S[35]

The case of S (also discussed in Chapter 7, pages 263–4) makes clear that compulsory treatment under the legislation applies only to treatment for the mental disorder for which compulsion has been invoked, and not for physical illness. The separation of physical and mental illness is not always clear cut, however. Mental health legislation does not give powers to treat people for a physical disorder unconnected with their mental disorder, but the courts have given a wide interpretation to "treatment for mental disorder". For example, it has been accepted that feeding without the patient's consent may form part of a programme of treatment for a mental disorder.[36] Thus, where an anorexic patient refuses lifesaving treatment such as nasogastric nutrition, this could be provided under mental health legislation. The Mental Health Act Commission issues guidance on this matter.[37]

Alleviating physical symptoms under mental health legislation

B was a 24-year-old woman with a psychopathic disorder characterised by a compulsion to self harm. Having been compulsorily detained under the legislation and thus having the means to cut and burn herself removed, her self harm took the form of food refusal. As a result she was force fed by nasogastric tube. When invited to pass judgment on the legality of the force feeding, the Court of Appeal stated that medical treatment given for a mental disorder includes "treatment given to alleviate the symptoms of the disorder as well as treatment to remedy its underlying cause". Although the psychopathic disorder was the "underlying cause", the food refusal was a direct symptom of

(Continued)

the disorder and, according to the court, it was legitimate to treat it under the legislation. Thus the court made a clear distinction between the treatment in this case and the treatment proposed for C's gangrenous foot (see page 103).

B v Croydon Health Authority[38]

Ethical principles governing treatment

Generally speaking, the same basic ethical principles (see pages 100–1) that govern physical health care should also govern mental health care, whether or not it is given under compulsory powers. As in other spheres of treatment, it is important to seek to establish a collaborative, trusting relationship with the patient. When compulsory treatment is required, it is important to discuss the reasons for this, as far as is practicable, with the patient. Health professionals also have an obligation to encourage patients to be as involved as possible in decisions relating to their care, and to use their decision making capacity as fully as possible. As this chapter has discussed, just because patients are unable to make a valid decision in relation to one aspect of care or treatment, it does not follow that they cannot make other valid treatment decisions. As with physical health care, treatment should be the least invasive possible, the least restrictive of the individual's freedom, and be based on evidence of efficacy. Even when compulsory treatment has been authorised, health professionals should attempt to work with the patient to find the regimen that is most acceptable to him or her, taking account of any views expressed in an advance statement. Generally speaking it is important that healthcare workers should listen to the concerns of their patients and, where possible, discuss treatment preferences with them.

It is worth noting that mental health legislation authorises mental health treatment for patients of any age. For further advice and information about compulsory mental health treatment of children, see the BMA's publication *Consent, rights and choices in health care for children and young people.*[39]

Additional advice relating to treatment for mental disorder can be found in publications from government departments on the implementation of mental health legislation.[40]

Summary – mental health care

- The general principles governing mental health care are the same as those that govern physical health care.
- Patients who are being treated under mental health legislation do not necessarily lack decision making capacity.
- Patients should be involved as far as is practicable in decisions relating to their care.

- Usually, treatment and support are provided without recourse to compulsion, although the potential benefits of compulsion for some patients, such as compliant incapacitated patients, should be considered.
- Compulsory treatment may extend only to treatment for mental disorder; compulsion cannot be used to provide treatment for physical illness unrelated to the mental disorder.

Compulsion: public health

In addition to mental health legislation, there are limited legal powers permitting compulsory medical treatment or examination in public health (see Chapter 20) and national assistance[41] legislation. In stark contrast to the comprehensive safeguards of mental health legislation, laws giving powers to control people's activities in their own interests, or in the interests of public health, have changed little since they were first introduced in the nineteenth century. They are rarely used in practice.

Public health legislation is concerned with the imposition of treatment in the interests of the health of other citizens (see Chapter 20). As with mental health legislation, any use of compulsory powers must meet human rights requirements because any power to restrict the freedom of citizens to act as they wish is a prima facie breach of their rights. The protection of the public health is one of the limits on freedoms recognised in the articles of the European Convention on Human Rights, including the right to private and family life (Article 8). Detention for the purpose of preventing the spread of infectious diseases is legitimate under Article 5. Any restriction must be proportionate and carried out in pursuance of a legitimate aim.

For many years, there has been discussion about the need to review the National Assistance Act 1948, which allows the removal to suitable premises of persons in need of care and attention without their consent. The provisions can be used when a person is unable to devote proper care and attention to himself or herself, and is not receiving it from others. The person must either be suffering from grave chronic disease or be old, infirm, or physically incapacitated and living in insanitary conditions. The Act only allows the person to be removed. It includes no powers for compulsory medical treatment, which is therefore subject to the usual common law rules. There are detailed procedures that must be followed.[42]

Proposals for law reform

Mental incapacity

In 1995, the Law Commission described the law relating to mental incapacity in England and Wales as being:

unsystematic and full of glaring gaps. It does not rest on clear or modern foundations of principle. It has failed to keep up with social and demographic changes. It has also failed to keep up with developments in our understanding of the rights and needs of those with mental disability.[43]

By the early years of the twenty-first century, there was widespread agreement that law reform was needed to protect incapacitated adults and those who care for them. For example, the BMA supported the introduction of a system of proxy decision makers who could make decisions about medical treatment on behalf of incapacitated adults. Although law reform was under consideration throughout the 1990s and early 2000s,[44] by 2003 Scotland was the only UK jurisdiction to have enacted legislation to address these problems (see pages 110–2). At the same time, the BMA was involved with other professional and representative organisations to press for legislation to put on a statutory footing the authority of doctors to provide treatment to incapacitated adults who cannot give consent, and to allow the appointment of proxies to take decisions on behalf of these patients. At the time of writing, the Lord Chancellor's Department is working on draft legislation, based on the Law Commission's 1995 draft bill.[45] Although there was no indication of the timeframe for its publication, law reform for England, Wales, and Northern Ireland is expected during the lifespan of this book. Information about changes relevant to health care will be made available on the BMA's website. In addition, with the implementation of the European Union Directive on Clinical Trials,[46] a system of personal and proxy decision makers – solely for drug research – was devised (see Chapter 14).

Mental health

At the time of writing, mental health legislation in England and the devolved administrations is also going through a period of uncertainty and review. In England and Wales, for example, a draft bill to replace the Mental Health Act 1983 was published for consultation in 2002 but, largely as a result of criticisms from service provider and user groups, its introduction was delayed for redrafting. In Northern Ireland, a review of the Mental Health (Northern Ireland) Order 1986 was announced in October 2002, a process that was expected to take at least two years to complete. Again, only Scotland had reformed its mental health legislation, with the Mental Health (Care and Treatment) (Scotland) Act 2003.

The reviews have been accompanied by much uncertainty. They have been motivated by a range of factors, including changing patterns of treatment, difficulties with reconciling an enhanced concern for patient autonomy with the occasional need for compulsion, and, in England and Wales, they have been accompanied by unease about the political motivation behind some of the proposed changes. Of particular concern with the English review were provisions for the treatment of individuals with personality disorder. For example, the BMA regarded the suggested removal of the "treatability" criterion from the 1983 Act – which dictated that any intervention was justifiable only in the light of an anticipated therapeutic outcome – as threatening civil liberties and, potentially, turning therapeutic legislation into a vehicle for social control.[47] Furthermore, whereas the Scottish Act incorporated the bulk of the recommendations from its review committee (the Millan Committee),[48] the rejected draft English bill was in some ways at odds with the recommendations of its counterpart (the Richardson Committee).[49] For example the English bill rejected the Richardson Committee's suggestion that any new Act should be prefixed by an explicit statement of principles.

Mental Health (Care and Treatment) (Scotland) Act 2003

This book has not aimed to explain in detail the complex provisions of mental health legislation. Practitioners working with the legislation will be familiar with its scope and application. The 2003 Scottish legislation is of particular interest, however, in articulating a general ethical approach to the provision of treatment for mentally disordered people. Some key areas are mentioned below.

In accordance with the recommendations of the Millan Committee, the Scottish legislation sets out at the start a series of principles intended to guide those exercising its authority.[50] The principles reflect the Act's overarching commitment to ensuring that the therapeutic goal of any intervention is safeguarded, and are given below.

- **Non-discrimination:** people with mental disorder should retain, as far as possible, the same rights as those with other health needs.
- **Equality:** treatment should be provided without discrimination.
- **Informal care:** wherever possible, care and treatment should be provided without recourse to compulsion.
- **Participation:** service users should be as fully involved as possible in their care.
- **Least restrictive alternative:** treatment should be provided in the least restrictive manner compatible with safe and effective care, taking into account the safety of others.

As mentioned above, one of the reasons behind reviewing mental health legislation throughout the UK was the need to bring the law up to date with changing treatment methods, including the extension of treatment in the community. Unlike previous Acts across the UK, the 2003 Scottish Act permits the provision of appropriate compulsory care and treatment in the community in cases in which compulsory treatment in a hospital would be unnecessarily restrictive. It is expected that revised legislation in England, Wales, and Northern Ireland will also contain such provisions.

One interesting development is the new emphasis the Scottish Act gives to the rights and therefore, by extension, to the interests, of carers. The Act contains provisions for carers to request an assessment of the service user's needs by the local authority or health board. If the assessment is not undertaken, the reasons for this must be explained to the carer. This right of request could be particularly useful when, for example, the condition of a patient being cared for in the community is deteriorating rapidly and urgent intervention could be beneficial, both for the patient and the carer.[51]

At the time of writing, the legislation has only just received Royal assent and no code of practice has been published. Without the practical guidance on implementation, and doctors' experience in working within its provisions, it is not possible to comment on the Act's actual impact on patient care, but the BMA is generally supportive of its aims and approach.

References

1   Re F (mental patient: sterilisation) sub nom F v West Berkshire Health Authority [1989] 2 All ER 545: 566.
2   British Medical Association, The Law Society. *Assessment of mental capacity: guidance for doctors and lawyers, 2nd ed.* London: BMJ Books, in press. The book covers the law in England and Wales.
3   Re C (adult: refusal of medical treatment) [1994] 1 All ER 819.
4   Re MB (medical treatment) [1997] 2 FLR 426.
5   *Ibid:* p. 431.
6   Adults with Incapacity (Scotland) Act 2000 s1(6).
7   Re B (adult: refusal of medical treatment) [2002] 2 All ER 449: 465.
8   Re T (adult: refusal of medical treatment) [1992] 4 All ER 649: 661h–662a.
9   *Ibid.*
10 British Medical Association, *et al. Assessment of mental capacity: guidance for doctors and lawyers, 2nd ed. Op cit.* The legal sections of the book address only England and Wales but the practical aspects of assessment of capacity are also relevant to the rest of the UK.
11 Based on: Scottish Executive Health Department. *Code of practice for persons authorised to carry out medical treatment or research under Part 5 of the Act.* Edinburgh: SEHD, 2002: para 1·6.
12 Haire AR, Bambrick M, Jones J. Cervical screening for women with mental handicap. *Br J Fam Plann* 1992;**17**:120–1.
13 The BMA publishes detailed advice on the Act. British Medical Association. *Medical treatment for adults with incapacity. Guidance on ethical and medico-legal issues in Scotland.* London: BMA, 2002.
14 Scottish Executive Health Department. *Code of practice for continuing and welfare attorneys.* Edinburgh: SEHD, 2001. (SE/2001/90.) Scottish Executive Health Department. *Code of practice for persons authorised under intervention orders and guardians.* Edinburgh: SEHD, 2002. (SE/2002/65.)
15 The nominated medical practitioner's fees are paid by the Mental Welfare Commission.
16 British Medical Association. *Advance statements about medical treatment.* London: BMA, 1995.
17 Airedale NHS Trust v Bland [1993] 1 All ER 821. Re C (adult: refusal of medical treatment) [1994] *Op cit.* Re T (adult: refusal of medical treatment) [1992] *Op cit.*
18 Lord Chancellor's Department. *Making decisions: the government's proposals for making decisions on behalf of mentally incapacitated adults.* London: The Stationery Office, 1999.
19 Further advice about witnessing documents is given in: British Medical Association, *et al. Assessment of mental capacity: guidance for doctors and lawyers, 2nd ed. Op cit.*
20 General Medical Council. *Serious communicable diseases.* London: GMC, 1997.
21 Re GF (medical treatment), sub noms Re G (termination of pregnancy), Re GF (a patient) [1992] 1 FLR 293.
22 Re SG (adult mental patient: abortion) [1991] 2 FLR 329.
23 The Adults with Incapacity (Specified Medical Treatments) (Scotland) Regulations 2002. (SSI 2002 No. 275.)
24 Mental health legislation is under review throughout the UK at the time of writing. Advice should be sought from the Mental Health Act Commission (England and Wales), Mental Welfare Commission (Scotland), and Mental Health Commission (Northern Ireland).
25 Re Y (mental incapacity: bone marrow transplant) [1997] 2 WLR 556.
26 Some detailed suggestions are given in: Department of Health, Welsh Office. *Mental Health Act code of practice.* London: The Stationery Office, 1999: ch 19.
27 This is a statutory requirement in Scotland. Section 47(7) of the Adults with Incapacity (Scotland) Act 2000 prohibits the use of force or detention, unless it is immediately necessary and only for so long as is necessary in the circumstances.
28 Re W (a minor) (medical treatment: court's jurisdiction) [1992] 4 All ER 627.
29 Counsel and Care. *Report: what if they hurt themselves?* London: Counsel and Care, 1992.

30 Department of Health, Welsh Office. *Mental Health Act code of practice. Op cit:* ch 19. Mental Welfare Commission for Scotland. *Rights, risks and limits to freedom. Principles and guidance on good practice in caring for residents with dementia and related disorders and residents with learning disabilities where consideration is being given to the use of physical restraint and other limits to freedom.* Edinburgh: MWC Scotland, 2002. Department of Health and Social Service. *Mental Health (Northern Ireland) Order 1986 code of practice.* Belfast: HMSO, 1992:58–66.

31 R v Bournewood Community and Mental Health NHS Trust, ex parte L [1998] 3 All ER 289.

32 Bodies overseeing the welfare of people treated under mental health legislation are the Mental Health Act Commission (England and Wales), Mental Welfare Commission (Scotland), and Mental Health Commission (Northern Ireland).

33 R v Bournewood Community and Mental Health NHS Trust. *Op cit.*

34 Department of Health, Welsh Office. *Mental Health Act code of practice. Op cit:* para 2·8.

35 St George's Healthcare NHS Trust v S, R v Collins and others, ex parte S [1998] 3 All ER 673: 693.

36 B v Croydon Health Authority [1995] 1 All ER 683.

37 Mental Health Act Commission. *Guidance note 3: guidance on the treatment of anorexia nervosa under the Mental Health Act 1983.* Nottingham: MHAC, 1999:6.

38 B v Croydon Health Authority [1995]. *Op cit:* p. 689.

39 British Medical Association. *Consent, rights and choices in health care for children and young people.* London: BMJ Books, 2001.

40 Department of Health, Welsh Office. *Mental Health Act code of practice. Op cit.* Scottish Home and Health Department. *Mental Health (Scotland) Act 1984 code of practice.* London: HMSO, 1990. (A new code of practice is expected to accompany the Mental Health (Care and Treatment) (Scotland) Act 2003.) Department of Health and Social Service. *Mental Health (Northern Ireland) Order 1986 code of practice. Op cit.*

41 National Assistance Act 1948.

42 For detailed advice about national assistance legislation, see: Montgomery J. *Health care law, 2nd ed.* New York: Oxford University Press, 2003.

43 Law Commission. *Mental incapacity.* London: HMSO, 1995:2. (Law Com No. 231.)

44 The Government consulted on law reform in England and Wales in 1997: Lord Chancellor's Department. *Who decides? Making decisions on behalf of mentally incapacitated adults.* London: The Stationery Office, 1997. It subsequently made proposals in 1999: Lord Chancellor's Department. *Making decisions: the Government's proposals for making decisions on behalf of mentally incapacitated adults.* London: The Stationery Office, 1999.

45 Law Commission. *Mental incapacity. Op cit:* pp. 219–84.

46 Directive 2001/20/EC of the European Parliament and of the Council on the approximation of the laws, Regulations and administrative provisions of the Member States relating to implementation of good clinical practice in the conduct of clinical trials on medicinal products for human use, published in the *Official Journal of the European Communities,* No. L121, 2001;(May 1):34–44.

47 British Medical Association press release. *BMA claims new draft mental health bill will bring mental health services to a standstill.* 2002 Sep 18.

48 Scottish Executive. *New directions: report on the review of the Mental Health (Scotland) Act.* Edinburgh: SE, 2001. (SE 2001 No. 56.)

49 Department of Health. *Report of the expert committee: review of the Mental Health Act 1983.* London: DoH, 1999.

50 Mental Health (Care and Treatment) (Scotland) Act 2003 s1.

51 *Ibid:* s227–8.

4: Consent and refusal: children and young people

The questions covered in this chapter include the following.

- Who can give consent for the medical treatment of children?
- When do young people become competent to make their own decisions?
- Are there differences between consent and refusal?
- When do the courts need to be involved in decisions?
- What are doctors' responsibilities with respect to child protection?

Combining respect for autonomy with best interests

During childhood and adolescence, most people attain the maturity that eventually allows them to take responsibility for their own lives. In this phase of development, young people sometimes seek to exercise their autonomy in a way that conflicts with other people's views of their best interests. Doctors, parents, and others who care for young people are torn between respecting the values of developing individuals and protecting those same individuals from the possibly adverse effects of their inexperience. This raises questions of who is best able to judge what is in an individual's interests. In other sections of this book, while recognising that autonomy has some limits, and that many patients involve people close to them in decision making, we have strongly supported the view that judgments should be made by competent patients about their own situation. From an ethical viewpoint, therefore, a decision by a competent young person that is based on an appreciation of the facts demands respect. Both law and ethics stress that the views of children and young people must be heard. In some cases, however, their views alone do not determine what eventually happens.

Combining respect for autonomy with support for minors encourages children and young people to make all those decisions that they feel comfortable and able to make. This is the message of the Children Act 1989 and its equivalents in Scotland and Northern Ireland,[1] which stress that children's views should be heard in decisions that affect them. Children sometimes refuse medical treatment because they lack the maturity and understanding to consider the long term implications of their choices. Their anxieties may be focused on the short term effects, such as fear of injections, in which case they may not be expressing a considered choice in favour of non-treatment. On the other hand, a child's refusal of treatment that is based on awareness of the long term consequences, and is compatible with the child's view of his or her best interests beyond the short term, is likely to be a valid expression of choice. Adults who are responsible for providing care retain a duty to intervene if the child appears to be exploited and/or abused, or if decision making seems seriously awry by the usual standards of what a reasonably prudent person in the patient's position would choose. In the former case, it may mean contacting social services. In the latter, as a starting point it should mean further discussion with the child and family. In cases of decision making for immature children, there must be a reasonable presumption that the parents have the child's best interests at heart. Such a presumption cannot be taken for granted, however, and, when there seem to be grounds for doubt, decisions should be evaluated carefully.

Has human rights changed things for children?

Over recent decades, society has paid increasing attention to the rights of groups of individuals who have been previously ignored. For example, societal attitudes towards the civil liberties of mentally disordered and elderly people have changed, with a consequent emphasis on the rights of individuals to self determination and to receive assistance or services to maximise their liberty. The rights of children and young people have also been the focus of reappraisal. In 1989 the UN General Assembly adopted the Convention on the Rights of the Child, and this was ratified by the UK in 1992.[2] The Convention set internationally accepted minimum standards on issues such as freedom from discrimination on grounds of disability (Articles 2 and 5), privacy (Article 16), and the child's right to have his or her views accorded due weight in relation to the child's maturity (Article 12). The Human Rights Act 1998 gave further weight to legally enforceable rights. The rights particularly relevant in the care of children include: the right to life (Article 2), the right not to be subjected to inhuman or degrading treatment (Article 3), the right to liberty and security (Article 5), the right to a fair hearing (Article 6), the right to respect for private and family life (Article 8), and the right not to suffer discrimination in relation to any of the other basic rights (Article 14). How the rights will be used in practice will become clearer as case law develops, but it is possible that young people will seek to use these rights to demand that their competent choices are respected. It is also possible that parents will seek to use their right to respect for family life to be involved in important decisions concerning their children if they believe they are being prevented from doing so.[3]

Discussion of children's rights is complex because much of the normal focus on patient rights is directed at issues of choice, autonomy, and self determination. Health professionals have come to associate the notion of patient rights with the legally binding power of competent adult patients to refuse or limit certain treatments. Logically, the closer a young person is to achieving similar competence, the more the moral weight should shift towards prioritising that person's right of self determination. However, legal cases where competent young people have sought to exercise such a right have shown the great difficulty society has in dealing with the emerging autonomy of young people (see pages 140–4). Their rights to choose are often limited if their health would be seriously jeopardised as a result of their choices.

Rights are not only possessed by young people who are able to express their views; the human rights of babies and young children are equally important, although protection rather than promoting autonomy may be the principal consideration. It falls to the healthcare team, parents, and others involved in caring for the child to ensure that his or her rights are not breached. Rights must be protected from the moment of birth, and decisions about treatment, or non-treatment, of neonates made on the same basis as decisions about older children who cannot express a view.

Scope of this chapter

This chapter covers the examination and treatment of people in England, Wales, and Northern Ireland who are aged under 18 years, and under 16 years in Scotland. It covers people who completely lack capacity to make decisions (babies) right through to young people who are competent to make complex decisions for themselves. Because the decision making process for babies and very young children is usually straightforward, with people who have parental responsibility (see pages 144–5) deciding for their children based on advice from the healthcare team, much of the focus of this chapter is on situations in which children and young people are able to express their own wishes. We also seek to answer questions such as how to assess children's best interests, what to do when agreement cannot be reached, and how the decision making rights of parents are limited. Some specific areas of health care are covered towards the end of this chapter, and issues relating to contraception are discussed in Chapter 7. The term "children" is used for people who are probably not mature enough to make important decisions for themselves, and "young people" for those who may be.

General principles

Basic principles have been established regarding the manner in which the treatment of children and young people should be approached. These reflect standards of good practice,[4] which are underpinned by domestic and international law.

The welfare of children and young people is the paramount consideration in decisions about their care. They should:

- be kept as fully informed as possible about their care and treatment
- be able to expect health professionals to act as their advocates
- have their views and wishes sought and taken into account as part of promoting their welfare in the widest sense
- be presumed able to make their own treatment decisions when they have sufficient "understanding and intelligence"
- be encouraged to take decisions in collaboration with other family members, especially parents, if this is feasible.

Communication

The development of a trusting relationship and good communication between health professionals and their patients are fundamental aspects of good practice. A good relationship between a health team and a child patient should establish a lifelong pattern of mutual trust and candour. As soon as they are able to communicate and participate in the decisions that affect them, children should be encouraged to express their views, ask questions, and discuss their health worries. Nevertheless, young patients themselves should be able to set the pace for discussion. Sensitivity is required to ensure that they are not overwhelmed with information but given the time they need to absorb it.

Some children may not want to have full information, or they may need time to adjust to one aspect of the situation before receiving more details. Each patient is an individual and is entitled to be given information in a manner that is accessible and appropriate according to his or her level of understanding. Parents may try to insist on secrecy in order to protect their children from painful facts.[5] This situation poses difficult dilemmas that need to be carefully worked through with the family in the light of the circumstances of the case. On the whole, the BMA is against the withholding of information if the child seems willing to know it, even when parents request secrecy. The Association advises against telling children lies in response to a clear question. Questions should always be answered as frankly and as sensitively as possible; where there is uncertainty about the diagnosis, treatment or likely outcome, this should be acknowledged.

Involving children

When medical advice or treatment is sought by children and parents together, health professionals should remember their role as the patient's advocate and ensure that children and young people are not excluded from decision making. Including them should be seen as the norm. If children are excluded from decision making, there must be justification for that stance.

Children who want to participate in decisions should be helped and encouraged to do so. They need information about their condition and options, and doctors should take steps to enhance their ability to make decisions by providing information in a way the child finds most accessible. They should also give the child options about having parents or other third parties present, and talk to the child at a time when he or she is relatively relaxed, comfortable, and free from medication that may affect the ability to choose. Children should not simply be considered incompetent to decide if they are unwilling to participate in decisions or agree to treatment, and should be able to change their minds later if they so wish. In practical terms, although small children may not be asked to make major decisions such as whether to undergo surgery, they should be given a voice on all the lesser points, such as whether parents accompany them to the anaesthetic room. In this way, many of the child's views can be respected and it can be feasible to offer alternatives, even to young children.

Competence to make decisions

In addition to involving all children, it is important to recognise when a young person is able to make a valid choice about a proposed medical intervention. In order for the consent of any person to be valid it must be based on competence, information, and voluntariness. This can be broken down into several fundamental points:

- the ability to understand that there is a choice and that choices have consequences
- the ability to weigh the information in the balance and arrive at a decision
- a willingness to make a choice (including the choice that someone else should make the decision)
- an understanding of the nature and purpose of the proposed procedure
- an understanding of the proposed procedure's risks and side effects
- an understanding of the alternatives to the proposed procedure, and the risks attached to them
- freedom from undue pressure.

Whether a child has the competence to decide is a legal concept, but invariably medical or psychiatric tests are involved in the assessment. There are various ways of testing whether children are competent; no magical definition or "right" method exists, but the "functional" approach has the greatest support.[6] This approach relates the individual ability of the patient to the particular decision to be made. The nature and complexity of the decision or task, and the person's ability to understand at the time the decision is made, the nature of the decision required and its implications, are all relevant. Thus, the graver the impact of the decision, the commensurately greater the competence needed to make it. In short, as with adults, children and young people are competent to give consent to medical treatment if they are able to understand the nature and purpose of the proposed treatment, and to retain the information and weigh it in the balance to arrive at a decision. Although some children clearly lack competence due to immaturity, doctors should not judge the ability of a particular child solely on the basis of his or her age.[7]

Growth of competence

Mental abilities, social understanding, and emotional appreciation increase greatly during childhood development. Young people become more able to consider the long term consequences of their own actions and of what happens to them. They also tend to think about such consequences more in terms of their own sense of responsibility and to have a better awareness of the effects of what they do on other people. Some generalisations can undoubtedly be made about the time at which children develop particular traits, but individuals differ and development is a continuous but uneven process.

Health professionals who work with seriously ill children often comment that those who have undergone suffering and discomfort develop the ability to understand the

135

implications of choices in the light of past experiences at an earlier stage than other children. Children who have already undergone treatment have a greater imaginative perception of what is being proposed when treatment options are put forward. They are also influenced by the level of support, information, and encouragement from key adults around them: parents, nurses, and doctors. There is, therefore, some obligation on clinical staff to create environments in which children are enabled to engage in decisions to the optimum level of their competence.

Children of the same age differ significantly in their ability and willingness to participate. Some believe that, since it is their life that is being affected, they should decide. Others want to share the process with parents, or want parents to decide for them. It is important not to approach young patients with preconceptions about ability.[8]

Confidentiality and involving parents

Young people are becoming increasingly aware of their rights to seek medical advice and treatment without involving their parents. Information provided in schools, on websites, and in the media explains that young people may approach their GP for advice about any health issues, including topics that teenagers are typically reticent about discussing with adults: contraception, smoking, alcohol, and other drugs, for example.[9] Ideally, treatment decisions involve people close to the patient. In the case of an immature child, the parents, or parents and child together, will decide. Unless there are convincing reasons to the contrary, because of an increased risk of harm, for example, doctors should try to persuade the patient to allow parents to be informed of the consultation, but should not override the patient's refusal to do so. In the BMA's view, even when the doctor considers the young person is too immature to consent to the treatment requested, confidentiality should still generally be maintained concerning the consultation. The BMA considers that doctors' duty of confidentiality is not dependent upon the capacity of the patient and, unless there are very convincing reasons to the contrary, for instance if abuse is suspected, the doctor should keep confidential a minor's request for treatment such as contraception, even if the doctor believes the minor to be insufficiently mature for the request to be fulfilled. Further advice should be taken if there is any doubt. For more detailed advice on confidentiality and the situations in which it may be breached, see Chapter 5.

Best interests

A fundamental ethical obligation in the provision of treatment is that of focusing on the interests of the patient and providing benefit for that person. Competent adults are allowed to define their own concept of "best interests", even if their views are very different from those of the rest of society. They can refuse treatment when they feel they have had enough or choose to take some risks with their own health (see Chapter 2). Children and young people have not generally been given the same options. Traditionally, other people – usually their parents – have chosen for them. Increasingly, however, it is being recognised that children and young people have a lot to contribute to decision making. Although children are best cared for in the family, and parents are generally the best decision makers for young children, it is acknowledged that the interests of children and those of the parents are not automatically synonymous. Doctors should try to identify situations in which parents' decisions appear to be contrary to their child's interests.

Regarding the definition of best interests, it is customary to assume that a person's interests are usually best served by measures that offer the hope of prolonging life or preventing damage to health. Health professionals are accustomed to measuring benefit primarily in terms of physical gains. Thus, when medical treatment carries low risk and offers substantial benefit to the patient, it is clearly perceived as being in the person's interests. This is the situation in many of the day to day decisions involving children, although not all choices are that simple. The side effects and other burdens of treatment may not be matched by a genuine prospect of significant and sustained improvement. Alternatively, the promise of physical improvement may necessarily involve compromises that the patient considers unacceptable, such as the administration of blood products to a Jehovah's Witness. In all cases, it is increasingly recognised that an assessment of best interests must involve far more complex matters than physical criteria alone. The following factors are relevant:

- the patient's own wishes and values (where these can be ascertained)
- clinical judgment about the effectiveness of the proposed treatment, particularly in relation to other options
- where there is more than one option, which option is least restrictive of the patient's future choices
- the likelihood and extent of any degree of improvement in the patient's condition if treatment is provided
- risks and side effects of the treatment
- the views of parents and others who are close to the patient about what is likely to benefit the patient.

Preventing harm

Harm is often seen as being an actual injury or impairment, but patients may also be wronged if their own values are denied, regardless of whether they are physically or psychologically damaged by that denial. Arguably, by imposing treatment contrary to the will of a competent young person, physical harm may be prevented, but the individual is nevertheless wronged. The degree to which this is acceptable is dependent upon the scale of the potential harm in comparison with that of the wrong.

Most people would agree, for example, that it would be ethically justifiable to provide treatment contrary to a minor's wishes if this has a very good chance of saving the individual's life or preventing serious deterioration in health.

M's refusal of a heart transplant

M was a 15 year old who refused to consent to a heart transplant operation in 1999 when her own heart failed. Her mother gave legal consent on her behalf, but health professionals were unwilling to proceed without M's agreement. M said she did not want to die but neither did she wish to have the transplant because this would make her feel different from other people.

> I understand what a heart transplant means, procedure explained … checkups … tablets for the rest of your life. I feel depressed about that. I am only 15 and don't want to take tablets for the rest of my life … I don't want to die. It's hard to take it all in … If I had children … I would not let them die … I don't want to die, but I would rather die than have the transplant … I would feel different with someone else's heart, that's a good enough reason not to have a heart transplant, even if it saved my life.[10]

The case was heard in the High Court, and after listening to her views, Mr Justice Johnson decided that M was not capable of making the decision herself and he authorised the operation to go ahead despite her reluctance. "Events have overtaken her so swiftly that she has not been able to come to terms with her situation", he said.[11] Once that decision had been made on her behalf, M agreed to comply with treatment.

Re M (child: refusal of medical treatment)[10]

Prevention of suicide and treatment for drug addiction, depression, or anorexia nervosa exemplify circumstances in which denying the wishes of an apparently competent minor do not usually raise profound ethical dilemmas. Chemotherapy for leukaemia is an example of a treatment that carries particularly unpleasant side effects. Children who have previously undergone this therapy and therefore understand what is involved may be reluctant to accept further treatment. Nevertheless, the chances of treating the condition successfully may be such that some pressure on the child to agree would be justifiable, with the parents' consent, and in England, Wales, and Northern Ireland the courts may overrule even a competent child's opinion if the anticipated benefits in the individual case are good (see pages 140–2).

On the other hand, the imposition of treatments that are either likely to bring only minimal improvement or which involve distressing side effects and have only a dubious chance of success cannot be easily justified if refused by a minor who understands the implications. The treatment proposed may not involve a question of life and death, but gradations of foreseeable improvement. Children with chronic illnesses who have undergone many medical and surgical interventions may be able to weigh for themselves whether the anticipated improvement is worth another period in hospital and it may be appropriate to defer to their opinions. Parents may find it hard to accept this, and doctors need to treat such situations with great care and sensitivity to the needs of all family members.

Emergencies

When consent is not obtainable, for example, in an emergency when the patient is unable to communicate his or her wishes and nobody with parental responsibility is available, it is legally and ethically appropriate for health professionals to proceed with treatment necessary to preserve the life, health, or wellbeing of the patient. An emergency is best described as a situation in which the requirement for treatment is so pressing that there is not time to refer the matter to court.

If such an emergency involves a treatment to which the child or family are known to object, for example, the administration of blood to a Jehovah's Witness, viable alternatives should be explored if time allows. In extreme situations, however, health professionals are advised to accommodate the family's wishes as far as possible, but to take any essential steps to stabilise the child, even against the family's wishes. Legal advice should be sought as a matter of urgency. Although there is some suggestion from the Scottish courts that a competent young person's refusal of treatment may not be overridden (see pages 142–3), in the absence of a clear ruling that this includes lifesaving treatment, the BMA advises that emergency lifesaving treatment should be given and an application made to a court as a matter of urgency. Emergency care is discussed further in Chapter 15.

Consent for examination and treatment

Ideally, medical decisions are made in partnership between the patient, the family, and the health team, with the parental role gradually fading as the child develops in maturity. Ordinarily, it is valid consent from somebody legally entitled to give it that affords doctors the legal authority to provide treatment. In the case of children, consent can come from any one of a number of sources: a competent young person, people with parental responsibility (and in some circumstances other carers such as grandparents or childminders[12]), or the courts. In Scotland it appears that the legal rights of parents, carers, and the courts to give consent may be extinguished when a young person is competent to decide for himself or herself.[13]

If consent is required in writing, which may be the case when treatment involves sedation or general anaesthesia, for example, there are model consent forms produced by the health departments.[14]

Consent from competent young people

People aged over 16 are presumed to be competent to give consent to medical treatment, unless the contrary is shown.[15] Young people under this age who have sufficient understanding and intelligence to comprehend fully what is proposed may also give consent to treatment, regardless of their age[16]; consent from their parents, although always desirable, is not legally necessary. Young people should always be encouraged to involve their parents, but nevertheless treatment may proceed without their knowledge or against their wishes if the young person is competent to decide and cannot be persuaded to include them.

The BMA welcomes this recognition of young people's autonomy, seeing it as productive of better relationships between doctors and young patients. Trust in the doctor–patient relationship is a matter upon which the Association lays great emphasis and such trust should be established as early as possible.

Refusal by competent young people

England, Wales and Northern Ireland

When the views of competent young people come into conflict with those of doctors and other people responsible for the minor, the law may intervene as a last resort. People under 18 can and do regularly give consent to complex and risky procedures, but there is some legal distinction between a young person's consent and refusal, at least in England, Wales, and Northern Ireland. When giving consent to proposed treatment, the patient is accepting the advice of a qualified professional. Deciding not to follow medical advice can have serious implications, in terms of both the immediate physical effects of non-treatment and the possible closing down of options for future treatment. The courts have shown themselves more reluctant to accept weak evidence on capacity when refusal is at stake.

The message from legal cases is that a young person's decision about a very serious matter is valid only when it concurs with the views of the doctor who proposes it. In these cases the courts have said that children and young people have a right to consent to what is proposed, but not to refuse it if this would put their health in serious jeopardy. Consent has been described as a legal "flak jacket" protecting the doctor from litigation. A doctor needs only one flak jacket (i.e. consent), and in England, Wales, and Northern Ireland, when a patient is under 18 it could come from a competent young person, a person with parental responsibility, or a court. Thus, consent from a person with parental responsibility may override a young person's refusal.

The power to override a competent refusal

W was 16 years old and living in a specialist adolescent residential unit under local authority care. Her physical condition due to anorexia nervosa deteriorated to the extent that the authority wished to transfer her to a specialist hospital for treatment. W refused, wanting instead to stay where she was and to cure herself when she decided it was right to do so. The local authority applied to court to be allowed to move W and for authorisation that she could be given medical treatment without her consent if necessary.

The judge in the Family Division of the High Court concluded that W was competent to make a decision to refuse treatment, but that the court could, in exercising its inherent jurisdiction, override a refusal of medical treatment by a competent young person if that was in her best interests.

(Continued)

W appealed against the decision. Her condition deteriorated significantly, and the Court of Appeal made an emergency order enabling her to be taken to and treated at a specialist hospital notwithstanding her lack of consent. In delivering its judgment, the Court of Appeal held that the Family Division judge had been wrong to conclude that W was competent because a desire not to be treated was symptomatic of anorexia nervosa. The court also said that its inherent powers were theoretically limitless and that there was no doubt that it had power to override the refusal of a minor, whether over the age of 16 or under that age but competent to make the decision.

Re W (a minor) (medical treatment: court's jurisdiction)[17]

Thus the law in England, Wales, and Northern Ireland is clear that, in the last resort, medical treatment can be imposed upon competent minors who refuse it if the overall intended effect is to benefit them. Doctors are often unhappy with such a view and the BMA hopes that all possibilities of a compromise solution would be explored first, including bringing in independent advocates to work out measures that the young person may feel able to accept, without having to compromise too far, lose face, or argue through the courts.

If the expected outcome of a proposed procedure is relatively insignificant for the patient it is unlikely to be justifiable to override his or her wishes. When a competent young person refuses treatment, doctors should consider the impact of complying on his or her long term chances of survival, recovery or improvement. For example, an informed refusal of a procedure with a purely cosmetic outcome, or repeated chemotherapy that has not led to significant improvement in the past, is highly influential. It is difficult to envisage a situation in which it is ethically acceptable to provide elective treatment when a competent, informed young person consistently refuses it. There has been no guidance from the courts on this matter because there has been no reported legal case dealing with refusal of elective or prophylactic intervention. This is likely to be because of the reluctance of doctors to impose non-essential treatment on unwilling competent patients.

On the other hand, when non-treatment threatens life, or postponement would lead to serious and permanent injury, the ethical arguments for providing treatment against a young person's wishes are stronger. Doctors must act within the law and balance the harm caused by violating a young person's choice against the harm caused by failing to treat. In cases of doubt, legal advice should be sought.

Refusal of blood products by Jehovah's Witnesses

As explained in Chapter 2, Jehovah's Witnesses have a conscientiously held religious opposition to the use of blood products for themselves. Parents often hold the same view regarding blood products in the medical treatment of their children. It is essential that doctors make every effort to accommodate beliefs rather than resorting to the most obvious medical option that is contrary to the patient's wish or looking to the courts as a first option. Nevertheless, when discussion, negotiation, and consideration of other options fail to resolve the situation and a child's life is at risk, it is likely that the courts will be involved. Courts have indicated that the administration of blood transfusions to Jehovah's Witness children against the wishes of their parents should not be carried out without the approval of a court,[18] although in an emergency doctors are unlikely to be criticised for intervening if this is the only option to save a child's life.

Clearly, whenever time allows, attempts should be made to negotiate with the family to try to find an acceptable solution. Invariably, family members are anxious to save the child's life if this can be done in a way that does not contravene their beliefs. Sometimes this may be possible by referral to a specialist centre where techniques such as bloodless surgery are practised (see pages 87–8).

When faced with a refusal of blood products by or on behalf of a young patient, the following must be borne in mind.

- It is important that health professionals should ensure that the situation is truly life threatening and that there are no other feasible alternatives to the use of blood.
- The child and the parents should be given an opportunity to put forward their views and have these considered.
- The local hospital liaison committee for Jehovah's Witnesses, which may be able to advise on possible alternatives, can be contacted as long as the family or the competent young person agrees.
- If health professionals involved in the case consider blood products to be the only solution they can offer to save the life of the child, the patient or the patient's family may request that treatment be transferred to another facility where bloodless treatment is practised; such wishes should be accommodated where possible.
- When there is no alternative, legal advice should be sought and it may be necessary for the matter to be considered by a court.

As with all refusals of treatment, if patients are competent, informed, and sure of their decision to refuse blood, there are significant ethical arguments for respecting that decision. The imperative to comply with refusal by parents is necessarily weaker than when children themselves make informed decisions; treatment may be given with consent from a competent young person even if the parents refuse. Whenever time allows, there should be careful discussion with the young person and the family to ensure that the situation is fully understood. Legal advice should be taken. It is advisable for health professionals to discuss the implications with the young person separately to ensure that a valid decision has been reached without any pressure.

Scotland

In Scotland, if a competent young person refuses treatment it is probable that its administration would be unlawful, even if that treatment was necessary to save or prolong life. There has been just one reported legal case, in which the sheriff ruled that, once children of any age are judged to be competent, they can consent to or refuse treatment. This follows the situation for competent adult patients (see Chapter 2). Despite there being grounds for maintaining some distinction between consent and refusal (see page 140) some commentators argue that the Scottish position is the more logical.[19] The Scottish courts have not, however, made a definitive ruling on this matter and any doctor faced with a refusal of treatment by a competent young person should seek legal advice.

Competent young person's refusal of treatment

In the only reported Scottish case to deal with refusal of treatment and the scope of the medical treatment provisions of the Age of Legal Capacity (Scotland) Act 1991, an application was made to Glasgow Sheriff Court in respect of a 15-year-old patient. The patient had symptoms of a psychotic illness. He would not consent to treatment and also refused to remain in hospital. The doctors believed that he was capable of understanding the nature and possible consequences of treatment and was therefore legally competent to make decisions on these matters. The doctors also believed that the right to consent carried with it the right to refuse, and that his consent could not be overridden by his mother's consent. Treatment would therefore be lawful only if it fell within the scope of the Mental Health (Scotland) Act 1984, section 18 of which permitted detention on the approval of a sheriff. The doctors were reluctant to use the mental health legislation because of the stigma attached to a detention order.

The patient's mother was prepared to give consent to his treatment and detention in hospital. It was argued on her behalf that, since she was prepared to consent, the proposed order was unnecessary. The sheriff, however, took the view that the decision of a competent young person could not be overruled by a parent. He concluded that logic demanded that, when a young person was declared competent, the young person's decision took precedence over that of a parent. Furthermore, he considered that the Age of Legal Capacity (Scotland) Act covered refusal as well as consent to treatment.

In the circumstances, the sheriff granted the detention order with the observation that, despite the stigma, the patient's serious illness and its treatment were the paramount considerations.

Houston (applicant)[13]

This judgment is taken by some to suggest that a competent young person's refusal may not be overridden by a parent or a court. In fact, the sheriff was able to avoid the issue of whether a court could override a competent refusal because there was an alternative way of dealing with the patient and treatment was given under mental health legislation. A case concerning proposed treatment falling outwith the provisions of mental health law has, at the time of writing, yet to be decided. When doctors are faced with a competent young person's refusal of lifesaving treatment, legal advice is essential.

Advance decision making

In UK jurisdictions where a young person's contemporaneous refusal of treatment may not be determinative, it follows that advance directives, or living wills (see pages 113–6), made by young people cannot be legally binding on health professionals. Young people may wish to express their wishes in advance, however, so that these can be given proper consideration in decision making and assessment of their best interests.

Summary – consent and refusal by competent young people

- Competent young people may give valid consent to medical treatment.
- Competent young people should be encouraged to involve their parents, but are entitled to confidentiality.
- Competent young people must be given the opportunity to have their views heard, even if their refusal of treatment is not determinative.
- Doctors should seek legal advice if a competent young person refuses essential medical treatment, although emergency treatment should not be delayed.

Decision making by people with parental responsibility

Parental responsibility

Parental responsibility is a legal concept that consists of the rights, duties, powers, responsibilities, and authority that most parents have in respect of their children. It includes the right to give consent to medical treatment. Parental responsibility is afforded not only to parents, however, and not all parents have parental responsibility, despite arguably having equal moral rights to make decisions for their children where they have been equally involved in their care. It is possible that these parents could use the Human Rights Act to claim a right to be involved in any important decisions about their child's life, including decisions about medical treatment.

Both of a child's parents have parental responsibility if they were married at the time of the child's conception or at some time thereafter. Neither parent loses parental responsibility if they divorce, and responsibility endures if the child is in care or custody. It is lost, however, if the child is adopted. If the parents have never married, at the time of writing, only the mother automatically has parental responsibility. The father may acquire it in various ways, including by entering into a parental responsibility agreement with the mother, or through a parental responsibility order made by a court. Additionally in Northern Ireland, fathers who are named on the child's birth certificate (from 15 April 2002 onwards) automatically have parental responsibility. Similar arrangements will apply in England and Wales once the relevant provisions of the Adoption and Children Act 2002 come into force. At the time of writing, there is no definite timescale for this. Scotland has also indicated its intention to introduce these arrangements. Information about any changes will be put on the BMA's website.

A person other than a child's biological parents can acquire parental responsibility by being appointed as the child's guardian (an appointment that usually takes effect on the death of the parents) or by having a residence order made in his or her favour, in which case parental responsibility lasts for the duration of the order. A local authority acquires parental responsibility (shared with the parents) while a child is the subject of a care order.

In England, Wales, and Northern Ireland, parental responsibilities may be exercised until a young person reaches 18 years. In Scotland, only the aspect of parental responsibility concerned with the giving of guidance endures until 18 years; the rest is lost when the young person reaches 16 years. Doctors who are treating people over 16 years in Scotland should refer to Chapter 2.

Consent from people with parental responsibility

People with parental responsibilities are entitled to give consent on behalf of their children. Usually, parents make the right decision about their young child's best interests, and most decision making is, rightly, left to children and parents with appropriate input from the clinical team. In cases of serious or chronic illness, parents may need time, respite facilities, possibly counselling, and certainly support from health professionals, but in most cases they are best placed to judge their young child's interests and decide about serious treatment.

There are limits on what parents are entitled to decide, however, and they cannot demand inappropriate treatment for their children.

Parents requesting treatment

C was a 16-month-old girl suffering from spinal muscular atrophy, a progressive disease that causes severe emaciation and disability. She was dependent on intermittent positive pressure ventilation. Her doctors sought authority from the High Court to withdraw the ventilation, and not to reinstate it or resuscitate C if she suffered further respiratory relapse. They maintained that further treatment would cause her increasing distress, could cause medical complications, and could do little more than delay death without significant alleviation of suffering.

The judge described C's parents as highly responsible orthodox Jews, who loved their daughter, but who were unable to "bring themselves to face the inevitable future". The parents' religious beliefs prevented them from standing aside and watching a person die when an intervention could prolong that life. The mother's affidavit, which the judge described as very moving, said that "in such a case the person that stands by will subsequently be punished by God".[20]

(Continued)

145

> The doctor's treatment plan of withholding resuscitation and ventilation and providing palliative care was endorsed by the judge to "ease the suffering of this little girl to allow her life to end peacefully".
>
> *Re C (a minor) (medical treatment)*[21]

Refusal by people with parental responsibility

Notwithstanding the importance of the parental role, if it appears that parents are following a course of action that is contrary to their child's interests, it may be necessary to seek a view from the courts, meanwhile providing only emergency treatment (see page 139) that is essential to preserve life or prevent serious deterioration. When asked to decide about treatment, the courts recognise their duty to protect children and have almost invariably said that serious treatment should be given against the wishes of parents where there is a good chance of it succeeding or providing significant benefit to the child. The courts are required, in their decision making, to have regard to the rights given force by the Human Rights Act and to have the child's welfare as the paramount consideration.[22]

Disagreements between people with parental responsibility

Generally, the law requires doctors to have consent from only one person in order lawfully to provide treatment. In practice, however, parents sometimes disagree and doctors are reluctant to override a parent's strongly held views, particularly when the benefits and burdens of the treatment are finely balanced and it is not clear what is best for the child. Disputes between parents can be difficult for everybody involved in the child's care. Health professionals need to be able to distinguish between the genuine concern of the dissenting parent and an objection that is based on grounds other than the child's welfare, such as a marital dispute. Discussion aimed at reaching consensus should be attempted. If this fails, a decision must be made by the clinician in charge whether to go ahead despite the disagreement. The onus is then on the parent who refuses treatment to take steps to stop it. If the dispute is over an irreversible, controversial, elective procedure, for example male infant circumcision for religious purposes (see pages 150–2), doctors must not proceed without the authority of a court.[23]

A common enquiry to the BMA concerns parents who do not communicate with each other but both want to be involved in their child's health care. For example, GPs are frequently asked to tell the parent with whom the child is not resident when the other parent brings the child to the surgery. Such situations are dealt with in Chapter 6 (page 219).

Summary – consent and refusal by people with parental responsibility

- People with parental responsibility:

  - are entitled to give consent to medical treatment on behalf of their child
  - may refuse medical treatment, when this is consistent with their child's best interests
  - may not insist that doctors provide treatment contrary to their clinical judgment.

- Agreement between everybody who is involved in decision making is the aim.

The courts

In England, Wales, and Northern Ireland, the courts have the power to give consent to treatment on behalf of a person aged under 18. This power endures even if the young person is competent to make decisions for himself or herself. Thus the courts are an ultimate arbiter because consent from a court can override a child's refusal or parents' refusal of a particular treatment if there is evidence that it would provide significant benefit. The courts cannot, however, require doctors to treat contrary to their professional judgment.

In Scotland, the courts have the same powers to give consent to treatment on behalf of people aged under 16 when the child is not competent to give valid consent for himself or herself. It is unclear whether a Scottish court may override the decision of a child if the medical practitioner believes the child is competent, although it is thought that this is unlikely (see pages 142–3). Again, the courts cannot require doctors to treat contrary to their professional judgment.

Court involvement is necessary in only a minority of cases; most decisions are of the type doctors and families are entitled to make and usually agreement is reached by the child, the people with parental responsibility, and the healthcare team. Their goal is the same – to benefit the child – and in the vast majority of cases it is possible to agree on the best route to achieve this. If, however, agreement cannot be reached in a reasonable period of time, which will depend on the nature and likely course of the patient's condition, lawyers may advise that it is necessary to seek a court order. The courts have also indicated that interventions of certain types, for example, decisions about sterilisation, organ donation and, if the parents disagree, religious circumcision, must be referred to court. Detailed advice about the situations in which the courts may become involved is given in the BMA's *Consent, rights and choices in health care for children and young people.*[24] Doctors must take legal advice if there may be a need to involve the courts. In any case in which a court is involved, the Children and Family Court Advisory and Support Service (in England and Wales), the Official Solicitor of the Supreme Court for Northern Ireland, and the Scottish Executive Solicitors' Office look after the interests of the child by working with families and advising the courts on what it considers to be in the child's best interests.

147

Going to court can be distressing for those concerned and it is essential that ongoing support is provided for the child, the parents, other relatives and carers, and the healthcare team. In general, less confrontational means of problem solving are preferable. There are great benefits, however, in a legal system that can give rulings very quickly when necessary. This is an important safeguard for young people and their carers.

Summary – the courts

- When agreement cannot be reached about treatment, doctors should approach their lawyers for advice.
- The courts may become involved and make a decision about treatment.
- The courts cannot require doctors to provide treatment contrary to their professional judgment.

Providing treatment against a child's wishes

Just because consent from a child's parents, or from a court, makes providing treatment lawful does not mean that it inevitably has to be given. Doctors must look at whether the harms associated with imposing treatment on a patient who refuses, whether competently or not, should play a part in the decision about proceeding. How critical the treatment is, whether alternative less invasive treatments are available, and whether it is possible to allow time for further discussion with the patient, are all factors to be weighed. As much time as is practicable should be taken for discussion, and treatment delayed if that is possible without jeopardising its likely success.

Once a decision has been made that it is lawful and ethically acceptable to override a refusal of treatment, in principle there cannot be an absolute prohibition on the use of force to carry it out. However, "merely because treatment is in a competent patient's best interests does not mean the use of force is".[25] Doctors must look at the patient's overall interests, and how imposing treatment may impact on human rights. For example, the European Court has held that force feeding a patient may amount to degrading treatment,[26] although doctors must consider whether this is a proportionate interference with rights given the expected benefits. Promoting the child's welfare in the broadest sense is the overarching consideration.

Parents can have an important role to play in persuading their children to cooperate with treatment, although, if the family is dysfunctional, the views of parents may not influence the child. If attempts to persuade a young person fail, but it is judged to be in his or her best interests to proceed, rarely the only option may be to use restraint or detention.

Using restraint or detention

In addition to being difficult to achieve in practice, imposing treatment on young people when they refuse could damage the young person's current and future relationships with healthcare providers and undermine trust in the medical profession. It is important for young people to understand that restraint of any form in order to provide treatment is used only as a matter of last resort and not until other options for treatment have been explored. The child and the family must be offered continual support and information throughout the period of treatment.

Members of the health team benefit from being given an opportunity to express their views and to participate in decision making, although ultimate responsibility rests with the clinician in charge of care. All staff require support, and must not be asked to be involved in restraining a child without proper training.

If, after spending as much time as is practicable, it is impossible to persuade a child to cooperate with essential treatment, the clinician in charge of the patient's care may decide that restraint is appropriate. The following points are relevant to any action taken.

- Restraint should be used only when it is necessary to give essential treatment or to prevent a child from significantly injuring himself or herself or others.
- The effect should be to provide an overall benefit to the child and in some cases the harms associated with the use of restraint may outweigh the benefits expected from treatment.
- Restraint is an act of care and control, not punishment.
- Unless life prolonging or other crucial treatment is immediately necessary, legal advice should be sought when treatment involves restraint or detention to override the views of a competent young person, even if the law allows doctors to proceed on the basis of parental consent.
- All steps should be taken to anticipate the need for restraint and to prepare the child, his or her family, and staff.
- Wherever possible, the members of the health care team involved should have an established relationship with the child and should explain what is being done and why.
- Treatment plans should include safeguards to ensure that restraint is the minimum necessary, that it is for the minimum period necessary to achieve the clinical aim, and that both the child and the parents have been informed what will happen and why restraint is necessary.
- Restraint should usually be used only in the presence of other staff, who can act as assistants and witnesses.
- Any use of detention or restraint should be recorded in the medical records. These issues are an appropriate subject for clinical audit.

Detaining children for the purpose of providing medical treatment raises serious legal issues. Legal advice is essential before children are detained outwith the provisions of mental health legislation, and court approval will be necessary. A court asked to rule on such an issue is required to have regard to the young person's rights under the Human Rights Act 1998, and whether, in the circumstances, detention is compatible with these.

Cultural practices

Circumcision

The circumcision of male babies and children, when there is no clinical indication, is a controversial area. Parents ask for their children to be circumcised for a range of reasons, including their religion, to incorporate a child into a community, or so that sons are like their fathers. There is a spectrum of views within the BMA's membership about whether non-therapeutic male circumcision is a beneficial, neutral, or harmful procedure or whether it is superfluous, and whether it should ever be carried out on a child who is not capable of deciding for himself. The medical harms or benefits have not been unequivocally proven except to the extent that there are clear risks of harm if the procedure is done inexpertly. The BMA has no policy on whether circumcision is acceptable or not. Indeed, it would be difficult to formulate a policy in the absence of unambiguously clear and consistent medical data on the implications of the intervention. In keeping with the advice in this chapter, however, the BMA believes that parents should be entitled to make choices about how best to promote their children's interests, and it is for society to decide what limits should be imposed on parental choices. Detailed advice is available in a BMA guidance note.[27]

General advice about assessment of best interests is given on pages 136–7. In relation to non-therapeutic male circumcision, the BMA identifies the following factors as being relevant:

- the patient's own ascertainable wishes, feelings and values
- the patient's ability to understand what is proposed and weigh up the alternatives
- the patient's potential to participate in the decision, if provided with additional support or explanations
- the patient's physical and emotional needs
- the risk of harm or suffering for the patient
- the views of parents and family
- the implications for the family of performing, or not performing, the procedure
- relevant information about the patient's religious or cultural background
- the prioritising of options that maximise the patient's future opportunities and choices.

Circumcision – best interests

J was a 5-year-old boy who lived with his mother, a non-practising Christian. His father, a non-practising Muslim, wanted him to be circumcised. Asked to decide whether J should be circumcised, the Court of Appeal considered all the factors relevant to J's upbringing and concluded that J should not be circumcised because of three key facts.

(Continued)

- He was not, and was not likely to be, brought up in the Muslim religion.
- He was not likely to have such a degree of involvement with Muslims as to justify circumcising him for social reasons.
- As a result of these factors, the "small but definite medical and psychological risks" of circumcision outweighed the benefits of the procedure.

Re J (a minor) (prohibited steps order: circumcision)[28]

It is essential that doctors should perform male circumcision only where this is demonstrably in the best interests of the child. The responsibility to demonstrate that non-therapeutic circumcision is in a particular child's best interests falls to his parents. The BMA is generally very supportive of allowing parents to make choices on behalf of their children, and believes that neither society nor doctors should interfere unjustifiably in the relationship between parents and their children. It is clear from the list of factors that are relevant to a child's best interests, however, that parental preference alone is not sufficient justification for performing a surgical procedure on a child.

When there is agreement that non-therapeutic circumcision is in a child's best interests, consent may come from competent children or people with parental responsibility.

The BMA and the General Medical Council (GMC)[29] have long recommended that consent for non-therapeutic circumcision should be sought from both parents. Although parents who have parental responsibility are usually allowed to take decisions for their children alone, non-therapeutic circumcision has been described by the courts as an important and irreversible decision that should not be taken against the wishes of a parent.[30] It follows that, when a child has two parents with parental responsibility, doctors considering circumcising the child must satisfy themselves that both have given valid consent. If a child presents with only one parent, the doctor must make every effort to contact the other parent in order to seek consent. If parents disagree about having their child circumcised, the parent seeking circumcision could seek a court order authorising the procedure, which would make it lawful, although doctors are advised to consider carefully whether circumcising against the wishes of one parent would be in the child's best interests. When a child has only one parent, obviously that person can decide.

All children who are capable of expressing a view should be involved in decisions about their care and have their wishes taken into account. The BMA cannot envisage a situation in which it is ethically acceptable to circumcise a competent, informed young person who refuses the procedure. When children cannot decide for themselves, their parents usually choose for them. Although they usually coincide, this chapter explains that the interests of the child and those of the parents are not always synonymous. There are, therefore, limits on parents' rights to choose and parents are not entitled to demand medical procedures contrary to their child's best interests.

Male circumcision in cases where there is a clear clinical need is not normally controversial.[31]

Summary – male circumcision

- The welfare of child patients is paramount and doctors must act in the child's best interests.
- Children who are able to express views about circumcision should be involved in the decision making process.
- Consent for circumcision is valid only where the people (or person) giving consent have the authority to do so and understand the implications and risks.
- Both parents must give consent for non-therapeutic circumcision.
- When people with parental responsibility for a child disagree about whether he should be circumcised, doctors should not circumcise the child without the leave of a court.
- As with all medical procedures, doctors must act in accordance with good clinical practice and provide adequate pain control and aftercare.
- Doctors must make accurate, contemporaneous notes of discussions, consent, the procedure, and its aftercare.

Female genital mutilation

Female genital mutilation is a collective term used for a range of practices involving the removal or alteration of parts of healthy female genitalia. It is carried out by communities in Africa, Southeast Asia, and the Middle East, and by immigrants from those areas, for reasons ranging from hygiene to enhancement of male sexual pleasure. It involves suffering and mutilation and can give rise to very serious health risks. Female genital mutilation was made illegal in the UK by the Prohibition of Female Circumcision Act 1985, although there have, to date, been no prosecutions under the Act.

There is a pressing need to raise awareness about the health and legal issues, and about the services and sources of information that are available among communities that practise female genital mutilation. There are a small number of specialist clinics offering reversal procedures, and doctors should encourage women who have been mutilated to consider this option before they become pregnant. Doctors must also be alert to the possibility that girls may be at risk of genital mutilation.

If it becomes apparent that a girl is at risk of female genital mutilation, the GP or other doctor caring for her, for example, the community paediatrician, must ensure that there is discussion with the family about the health and legal issues. This may also involve counsellors, supportive local community groups or other clinicians with experience of working with communities that have a tradition of female genital mutilation. Doctors must ensure that their approach is sensitive to the beliefs and culture of the family, while remembering that female genital mutilation is illegal in the UK and that participation by any person, including a doctor, is a criminal offence. The aim is to find effective mechanisms for ensuring the protection of the child in a way that promotes her overall welfare. Doctors are unlikely to be able to initiate all of this work as individuals and should consider seeking help from social services, counsellors, and other health professionals. In initial enquiries to seek general help, advice, and information, it is unlikely to be necessary to identify the child or family.

Female genital mutilation is perceived in the UK as a form of child abuse; it is illegal, performed on a child who is unable to resist, medically unnecessary, extremely painful, and poses severe health risks. Members of communities that practise female genital mutilation do so, however, with the best intentions for the future welfare of their child and do not intend it as an act of abuse. When parents cannot be persuaded that their daughter should not be subjected to female genital mutilation, doctors will have to find sensitive ways to explain that steps may be taken to prevent the child from being mutilated. It is usually appropriate for doctors to contact social services when they believe a girl is at risk of female genital mutilation, for example, when a mother becomes pregnant again in a family whose existing daughters have been mutilated in infancy.

Parents' rights to control information about their young children may be overridden when this is necessary to protect the child from serious harm, although whenever possible, their permission for disclosure of information to social services or another appropriate agency should be sought. In judging how to broach the issue with parents, doctors must bear in mind the likely attitude of the parents in such circumstances and the risk that the child may simply disappear by being concealed within the community or sent to relatives abroad. This can be extremely difficult and doctors must take great care to ensure that their reactions are supportive of the child's overall welfare wherever possible.

When there are fears that a girl may be taken abroad for genital mutilation, doctors should counsel the parents, explain the health and legal[32] issues, and try to persuade them not to do it. Involving community paediatricians may be helpful. Ultimately, a doctor may have to consider initiating child protection proceedings if there is no other feasible way of protecting the child (see pages 156–62).

A guideline offering advice for doctors caring for women who have undergone female genital mutilation, and how to protect girls at risk of the procedure, is published by the BMA.[33]

Withdrawing or withholding life prolonging treatment

From birth, all people have the right to expect care and treatment appropriate to their needs. Some, however, believe that a willingness for late termination of pregnancy because of serious handicap means that more leeway should be allowed regarding withholding or withdrawing life prolonging treatment from handicapped newborns than from similarly impaired older babies, children, or adults. Legally and ethically, however, the considerations are the same. Any decision not to treat, or to stop providing a particular treatment, must be based on whether treatment is able to provide any benefit to the child. The parents of an infant born severely malformed must never be left with the feeling that they are having to exercise their responsibility to make decisions regarding consent to the management of their child without help and understanding. They should be encouraged to seek advice and support. The doctor in charge is responsible for the initiation or the withholding of treatment in the best interests of the child. Doctors must attend primarily to the needs and rights of the child, but they must also have concern for the family as a whole. If doubt persists in the minds either of the parents or the doctor in charge as to the best interests of the infant, another independent opinion should be sought.

There is no legal or ethical obligation for health professionals to provide medical treatment that cannot achieve its clinical aim, or which does not provide an overall benefit to the child. In deciding whether treatment should be started or whether it should be stopped, health professionals should assess the relevant clinical aspects and other vital factors, including the wishes of the patient and the family. Support for the child and family is essential throughout the process of deciding about the provision of life prolonging treatment, and during and following its implementation. Constant review of the child's condition is essential, and all decisions and changes to the child's circumstances should be documented in the health record. Whether the reason for not giving active treatment is because it can provide no clinical benefit to the child, or because the child, the parents, and the health team agree it is not in the child's best interests, the child must never be abandoned. Other treatment and care options should be discussed, and palliative care must be available for all children who are dying. More advice about withdrawing or withholding treatment is given in Chapter 10 and in a separate BMA publication, *Withholding and withdrawing life-prolonging medical treatment.*[34]

Conjoined twins

The previous section explains that infants born with severe disabilities have the right to expect care and treatment appropriate to their needs. Conjoined twins are one such example of children about whom difficult decisions may need to be made. Although some twins remain conjoined and survive well into adulthood, others are separated. Sometimes the separation of twins means that one will inevitably die. Conjoined twins raise complex dilemmas, involving themes of autonomy and interdependent interests. Usually, decisions about how to manage the twins' medical needs are made by the parents and medical team together. In 2000, however, parents and the medical team were faced with an exceptionally difficult case that required the court to intervene.

Conjoined twins

Jodie and Mary were conjoined twins. They were joined at the lower abdomen and each had her own brain, heart, lungs, other vital organs, and limbs. Mary was considerably weaker than Jodie, and her brain was described as having only primitive function. Her heart and lungs were not sufficiently strong to sustain her life if she was separated from Jodie. Had she been born a singleton, she would have died shortly after her birth.

Although surgery would be extremely complex, the twins' doctors were of the opinion that it would be possible to separate them, but that separation would kill the weaker twin, Mary, within minutes. If the operation did not take place, both were expected to die within 3–6 months because Jodie's heart would eventually fail. If they were separated, Jodie would still need extensive medical care and treatment, but was expected to have a good length and quality of life.

The parents, however, said that they could not consent to separation if this would result in Mary's death. The twins were equally precious to their parents, who felt that it was "not God's will" for them or anyone to choose death for one. They could not agree to kill one even to save the other.

The High Court issued a declaration that separating the twins would be lawful. Although the parents appealed, the High Court's decision was upheld by the Court of Appeal and the twins were separated.

Re A (children) (conjoined twins: surgical separation)[35]

In the case of conjoined twins Jodie and Mary, the Court of Appeal concluded that the twins' interests were best served by giving the chance of life to the stronger twin, Jodie, even if that had to be at the cost of the life of the weaker twin, Mary. The least detrimental choice was to separate the twins. It then looked to whether it was possible to achieve this in a lawful way, since Mary was a human being and separating the twins involved a positive act of killing her. The court said that the reality was that Mary was killing Jodie. That provided the legal justification for the doctors coming to Jodie's defence and removing the threat of fatal harm to her presented by Mary. In these very exceptional circumstances, "necessity" to act made intervention by the doctors lawful.

It was a case that the court found extremely difficult. Aside from being legally complex, one of the judges described it as "difficult because of the scale of the tragedy for the parents and the twins, difficult for the seemingly irreconcilable conflicts of moral and ethical values".[36]

The court noted that, although there were those who believed most sincerely that it would be an immoral act to save Jodie if this would involve ending Mary's life prematurely, there were also those who believed with equal sincerity that it would be immoral not to save Jodie if there were a good prospect that she could live a happy, fulfilled life if the operation was performed. Subsequent commentators have argued that it was wrong to deprive parents of their usual decision making authority in a case that was so finely balanced.[37]

The court went to great lengths to make clear that the case did not set a precedent for intentional killing in order to preserve the life of another. One of the judges, Lord Justice Ward, in emphasising the uniqueness of the case, said:

> Lest it be thought that this decision could become authority for wider propositions, such as that a doctor, once he has determined that a patient cannot survive, can kill the patient, it is important to restate the unique circumstances for which this case is authority. They are that it must be impossible to preserve the life of X without bringing about the death of Y, that Y by his or her very continued existence will inevitably bring about the death of X within a short period of time, and that X is capable of living an independent life but Y is incapable under any circumstances, including all forms of medical intervention, of viable independent existence.[38]

The BMA generally believes that parents are the best decision makers for their young children, but it also acknowledges that there are occasions on which the law should intervene to determine what is in children's best interests. Any doctor caring for conjoined twins and considering their separation must consider:

- the likely clinical outcome for both twins, with and without intervention
- the legal and moral rights of both twins
- the twins' best interests
- the views of the parents.

Where these factors lead to the conclusion that separating the twins would be the best course of action, and it is unlikely, or impossible, that both twins could survive the separation, legal advice is essential.

Child protection

Doctors are often the first professionals to realise that a child needs protecting. It is imperative that they are aware of their responsibilities in this area.

Victoria Climbié

Eight-year-old Victoria Climbié died as a result of "the worst case of child abuse and neglect" the paediatric consultant responsible for her care immediately before she died had ever seen.[39] This brief outline of her case focuses on Victoria's contact with professionals during her time in England.

Victoria was born in the Ivory Coast in 1991. In 1998 she was chosen from among seven siblings to go and live with her aunt in Europe. It was not uncommon for children born in the Ivory Coast to be entrusted to relatives living in Europe who could offer improved financial and educational opportunities for them. They moved to France in 1998 and settled in England in April 1999.

(Continued)

Shortly after their arrival in England, Victoria and her aunt were seen by a number of social services staff. No efforts were made either by the aunt or social services to enrol Victoria in any educational or day care activity. Victoria was registered with a GP in June 1999. She was seen by the practice nurse, who did not physically examine her because she was reported not to have any current health problems or complaints. Shortly afterwards, a neighbour noticed what may have been early signs of physical harm including a scar on her cheek. A few days later the neighbour made the first of two anonymous telephone calls to social services reporting her concerns about the way Victoria's aunt treated her.

In July 1999, Victoria and her aunt joined the aunt's new boyfriend in a one roomed flat where Victoria had no bed and spent the nights in the bathroom. The signs of physical abuse appeared to increase considerably soon after the move. Later that month, Victoria's childminder was worried and took her to hospital. The accident and emergency doctor who saw Victoria thought that there was a strong possibility that her injuries were non-accidental and referred her to a paediatric registrar. The registrar found a large number of injuries to Victoria's body and agreed that some may have been non-accidental. She was admitted overnight, and the police and social services were informed. She left the following day with her aunt.

Just over a week later, Victoria was admitted to a second hospital with a severe scald. She stayed on the paediatric ward for 13 nights, during which time a number of the clinical staff noticed signs of serious deliberate physical harm. When Victoria's aunt and her boyfriend visited, Victoria appeared frightened of them. Her discharge to the care of her aunt was agreed by a police constable and social worker who visited Victoria in hospital. After her discharge, Victoria's contact with the outside world during the remaining seven months of her life was limited and sporadic. Professionals saw her on only four occasions during this period, twice when her social worker made a prearranged visit and twice when she was taken to the social services office. The social workers visited and noticed nothing untoward. That Victoria was not attending school was commented on but not pursued. The aunt's application for rehousing was turned down since Victoria was not considered to be "at risk of serious harm". She was, however, advised to move out when she told the social worker that her boyfriend was sexually harming Victoria. They were due to move in with a friend, but this did not materialise and by the end of the day they were back in the boyfriend's flat. The following day Victoria's aunt retracted the allegations to a different social worker, who advised that they must not return to the boyfriend's flat while the matter was being investigated. They continued to live there, however, until Victoria's death four months later. She had no further contact with professionals of any kind until she was admitted to hospital on the night before her death.

A postmortem examination revealed death by hypothermia, which had arisen in the context of malnourishment, a damp environment, and restricted movement. The pathologist found 128 separate injuries on Victoria's body showing that she had been beaten by sharp and blunt instruments. Marks on her wrists and ankles showed that her arms and legs had been tied together. The pathologist said that it was the worst case of deliberate harm to a child that he had ever seen.

Lord Laming's report into the death of Victoria Climbié after extensive abuse by carers stated that protecting Victoria would have "required nothing more than basic good practice being put into operation".[40] The inquiry identified gross system failures, with individuals and agencies neglecting to take responsibility to act to protect Victoria from the horrific abuse she suffered. The inquiry sought to understand the failings that led to Victoria's death, and identify improvements at national and local level. There were failings in many areas of Victoria's care. In her contact with health professionals, it was clear from the evidence to the inquiry that information was known about Victoria but not documented in health records, or was recorded but not shared. Investigations and examinations were deferred, and sometimes erroneously assumed to have been carried out by somebody else. Necessary action was identified but not acted upon. Of the inquiry's 108 recommendations, 27 related specifically to health care. They focused on improving communication, ensuring communication flow, ensuring that concerns are acted upon, record keeping, and attributing clear responsibility for child protection to a single hospital consultant. The inquiry also recommended that no child about whom there are child protection concerns should be discharged from hospital without the permission of the consultant in charge or other suitable senior doctor. There must be a documented plan for the future care of the child and an identified GP.

Doctors need to be aware of the way the inquiry's recommendations are being implemented and ensure they are following best practice guidelines, including those from the health departments[41] and GMC.[42]

Doctors must try to work positively with families to enhance coping and parenting skills. In some cases, however, it is not possible to do this and also ensure the safety of children. A child or young person who comes to a doctor with a suspicious injury or other evidence of abuse or neglect should be the central focus of the doctor's concern, not the family, although the doctor must also bear in mind the safety of others who may be at risk, for example, the child's siblings. Some doctors say they feel a divided loyalty when they have as patients other members of the family, including the alleged abuser, but adults responsible for providing care have a duty to protect vulnerable people. Health professionals do not have statutory powers to intervene in family life, so, if intervention is necessary, the matter must be passed without delay to an agency that has the relevant statutory powers, namely social services, the National Society for the Prevention of Cruelty to Children (NSPCC), or the police. Informal advice from the local child protection team may be helpful. Detailed advice about confidentiality and disclosure of information is given in Chapter 5.

Refusal of medical or psychiatric examination under the Children Act

Children have a statutory right to refuse to submit to medical or psychiatric examination or other assessment that has been directed by the court for the purpose of an interim care, supervision, child protection, or emergency protection order, provided that the child is "of sufficient understanding to make an informed decision".[43] This provision of the Children Act and its equivalents in other UK jurisdictions is often quoted out of context, resulting in the erroneous impression that the Act gives young people a general statutory right to refuse examination for care or treatment. On the contrary, the provisions apply only in the limited cases specified in law as described above. Even in these cases, however, the English High Court has dealt with competent young people refusing examination under the Children Act in the same way as other refusals by competent young people, by overriding their statutory right to refuse.[44] This approach is controversial, and doctors faced with a competent young person refusing examination in such circumstances should seek legal advice, particularly in Scotland, where the point has not been tested and there may be less scope for overriding a competent young person's wishes.

Confidentiality and disclosure of information about abuse or neglect

Everybody is entitled to confidentiality, but when abuse or neglect occurs, other imperatives are likely to take centre stage. Abused children are entitled to have their confidentiality respected in the same way as other patients. As with all areas of caring for children and young people, the patient should be involved as much as possible in decisions, and this includes decisions about the disclosure of information. The child's rights to confidentiality should be explained, but it must also be emphasised that where there are grounds for concern, there is a professional duty to take action to prevent serious harm to patients and others. This means that doctors must consider what action best promotes the welfare of the abused child and protects others from the risk of harm. Doctors must be able to justify any decision about whether or not to refer a case to an outside agency and much depends on the evidence or reason for the suspicion that a child or young person is being neglected or abused. The same applies to the way in which doctors should respond to requests for information from outside agencies such as social services.

Decisions about disclosure in this area are complex and must be taken carefully and without delay. If a competent child cannot be persuaded to agree to voluntary disclosure, and there is an immediate need to disclose information to an outside agency, he or she should be told what action is to be taken unless to do so would expose the child or others to an increased risk of serious harm. When a child lacks the competence to make decisions about disclosure, doctors must protect that child's interests and encourage the child's cooperation. It is clearly in the public interest to identify and prevent abuse of children.

Cases in which the patient does have the capacity to take decisions about disclosure, but refuses to permit disclosure so that action against an abuser can be taken, are very difficult. Although it is essential to ensure child protection, it is also ethically important to respect the wishes of a competent patient. Disclosing against a competent patient's wishes may be unproductive. The patient may feel betrayed and lose trust in the doctor, and could refuse to cooperate with any investigation of alleged abuse. If it is possible without exposing them to danger, patients should be given time to come to a firm decision about disclosure. Counselling and support in the interim may help the patient to decide, and are essential throughout. Doctors must weigh the advantages and disadvantages of disclosure versus non-disclosure and make a decision based on the individual circumstances. Disclosure without consent will be justified in some cases and it follows that doctors should never make promises of secrecy.

Disclosure in order to prevent abuse may involve the identification of alleged abusers, and may include information that the doctor has learnt in his or her professional capacity as the abuser's doctor. The interests of the child are paramount, and in some cases this will require a doctor to breach a third party's confidentiality. While ensuring the safety and welfare of the child, however, efforts must also be made to protect the relationship of trust between the health professionals involved and others to whom they have provided health care. Published guidance in the area of child protection emphasises that although it is the child whose interests are paramount, doctors do have obligations to others who are their patients, and it is acknowledged that doctors may find it extremely difficult to take decisions about disclosure when alleged abusers are also their patients.[45] Responding to requests for information from social services is discussed in Chapter 19 (page 690).

If it is possible to involve parents and carers in the decision to disclose information concerning abuse, this may be helpful in encouraging all parties to work together towards what is in the best interests of the family. A goal of child protection is to work to keep families together and promote good parenting and family relationships. The interests of family members are often interrelated and solutions ideally involve working with all concerned. The consent or refusal of family members regarding disclosure will not always be determinative in the decision whether to disclose, and where permission is not forthcoming disclosure may still be justified. Sometimes, however, this is not only inadvisable but could proliferate the risks to victims of abuse.

Summary – action in cases of child protection[46]

- Being alert to a child's welfare

  - Everybody who works with children should be able to recognise, and know how to act upon, indicators that a child's welfare or safety may be at risk. These indicators may become apparent through contact with children and also their families.
  - Due regard must be given to the child and family's rights to confidentiality (see below).

- Help and advice

  - Doctors should know what services are available locally and how to access them, who to contact for sources of further advice and expertise and how, and when and how to make a referral to the local authority social services department.

- There should be a designated senior doctor and nurse in each area to provide help and advice.
- Although help and advice are essential, doctors should not delay if emergency action is needed to protect a child.

- Record keeping

  - All concerns about a child's welfare should be recorded in the child's health record, even if no further action is taken.
  - All discussions about the child's welfare should be recorded in the child's health record, including what has been agreed as future action, and who will take that action.

- Referral to social services

  - If doctors believe that a child may be suffering, or may be at risk of suffering, significant harm, they should refer these concerns to the local authority social services department without delay. In addition to the social services department, the police and the NSPCC have powers to intervene.
  - Doctors should aim to discuss any concerns with the family and, where possible, seek agreement to work positively with social services unless to raise the issue with carers would place the child at increased risk of serious harm.
  - Doctors should make a note of any referrals in the child's health records and ensure that it is clear who will be taking what action (or that no further action will be taken).
  - After a referral, the social services department has responsibility for clarifying the nature of the concerns, how and why they have arisen, and what the child and family need.
  - If there has been a criminal offence against a child, it is the responsibility of the social services department (or the NSPCC if relevant) to inform the police at the earliest opportunity. The police should then work in partnership with social services and/or other child welfare agencies, and should take into account the views of those agencies in considering whether it is appropriate to take action. It is recognised that cases will arise where the best interests of the child are served by an intervention led by the social services rather than a full police intervention.

- Assessment by social services

  - This must be done within seven days, and addresses the needs of the child, the parents' abilities to respond appropriately to those needs, protection from significant harm, promotion of the child's health and development, and whether action is needed to safeguard and promote the child's welfare. It is likely to involve speaking to the child and the family.
  - A course of action is decided upon based on the outcome of this assessment.

- Immediate protection

  - When there is a likelihood of serious immediate harm, the local authority, police, or NSPCC will act quickly to ensure the immediate safety of the child, usually after a strategy discussion between the police, social services, and other agencies as appropriate.
  - Emergency action may involve removing the child to a safe place.

- Enquiries and core assessment

  - Doctors may be asked to contribute to social services' core assessment of a child. If to do so would not increase the risk of the child suffering harm, consent to disclosure of information should be sought. If consent cannot be sought, or is not forthcoming, doctors may release information essential to protect a child from serious harm in accordance with the GMC's rules.[47]
  - The local authority will make all reasonable efforts to persuade parents to cooperate with these enquiries. If they refuse, a court may direct the parents to cooperate with an assessment of the child.

- Effects on the child and family

  - Enquiries must always be carried out in such a way as to minimise distress to the child and to ensure that families are treated sensitively and with respect.

- Child protection conferences

  - A conference will be convened if the agencies involved judge that a child may be at risk of suffering significant harm.
  - The purpose of the conference is to assess all relevant information and plan how to safeguard the child and promote his or her welfare. This forms the child protection plan.
  - Only information that is relevant to the purpose of the case conference and in the best interests of the child should be disclosed. Doctors will occasionally have to request that certain information is given in a limited forum or in writing to the chairman of the conference. Such measures should be used selectively for highly sensitive information and be avoided as regular practice.

- Child protection register

  - All children who are considered to be at continuing risk and for whom there is a child protection plan are included on a child protection register.
  - The purpose of the register is to make agencies and professionals aware of those children who are judged to be at continuing risk and in need of active safeguarding.

References

1 Children (Scotland) Act 1995. The Children (Northern Ireland) Order 1995.
2 United Nations High Commissioner for Human Rights. *Convention on the rights of the child*. Geneva: Office of the United Nations High Commissioner for Human Rights, 1989. (TS 44; Cm 1976.)
3 W v UK (1987) 10 EHRR 29.
4 Advice on good practice from government health departments includes: Department of Health. *Seeking consent: working with children*. London: DoH, 2001. Welsh Assembly Government. *Reference guide for consent to examination or treatment*. Cardiff: Welsh Assembly Government, 2002. Department of Health, Social Services and Public Safety. *Good practice in consent. Consent for examination, treatment or care*. Belfast: DHSSPS, 2003: part 2.
5 Young B, Dixon-Woods M, Windridge KC, Heney D. Managing communication with young people who have a potentially life threatening chronic illness: qualitative study of patients and parents. *BMJ* 2003;**326**:305–8.
6 See, for example: Law Commission. *Consultation paper 119, Mentally incapacitated adults and decision-making: an overview*. London: HMSO, 1991. This is also the approach adopted in the Adults with Incapacity (Scotland) Act 2000 (see Chapter 3).
7 For detailed advice about assessing competence see: British Medical Association. *Consent, rights and choices in health care for children and young people*. London: BMJ Books, 2001.
8 For discussion of children's abilities and willingness to participate in decisions see: Alderson P. *Children's consent to surgery*. Buckingham: Open University Press, 1993.
9 Advice for GP surgeries about promoting the notion of confidentiality to young people can be found in: British Medical Association, Brook, Medical Defence Union, Royal College of General Practitioners, Royal College of Nursing. *Confidentiality and young people. Improving teenagers' uptake of health advice. A toolkit for general practices*. London: Brook and RCGP, 2000.
10 Re M (child: refusal of medical treatment) [1999] 2 FLR 1097: 1100C-D.
11 *Ibid:* 1100G.
12 Apart from people with parental responsibility, any person who has care of a child, for example a grandparent or childminder, may do "what is reasonable in all the circumstances of the case for the purpose of safeguarding or promoting the child's welfare". Children Act 1989 s3(5). The Children (Northern Ireland) Order 1995 art 6(5). Children (Scotland) Act 1995 s5(1).
13 Houston (applicant) (1996) 32 BMLR 93. Children (Scotland) Act 1995 s15(5)(b).
14 Department of Health. *Consent forms*. London: DoH, 2001. Department of Health, Social Services and Public Safety. *Good practice in consent. Consent for examination, treatment or care. Op cit*. Trusts in Wales produce their own forms. At the time of writing, there are no standard forms for use in Scotland, although the Scottish Executive Health Department intends to produce forms in the future.
15 Family Law Reform Act 1969 s8(1). Age of Majority Act (Northern Ireland) 1969 art 4(1). Age of Legal Capacity (Scotland) Act 1991 s1(1)(b).
16 Gillick v West Norfolk and Wisbech AHA [1985] 3 All ER 402. Age of Legal Capacity (Scotland) Act 1991 s2(4).
17 Re W (a minor) (medical treatment: court's jurisdiction) [1992] 4 All ER 627.
18 Re O (a minor) (medical treatment) [1993] 2 FLR 149. Re S (a minor) (medical treatment) [1993] 1 FLR 377.
19 Thomson JM. *Family law in Scotland, 4th ed*. Edinburgh: Butterworths/Law Society of Scotland, 2002:189–90. Wilkinson AB, Norrie KMcK. *The law relating to parent and child in Scotland, 2nd ed*. Edinburgh: Green, 1999. Sutherland EE. *Child and family law*. Edinburgh: Clark, 1999: para 3·71.
20 Re C (a minor) (medical treatment), sub nom Re C (a minor) (withdrawal of lifesaving treatment) [1998] 1 FLR 384:389.
21 *Ibid.*
22 Children Act 1989 s1(1). The Children (Northern Ireland) Order 1995 art 3(1). Children (Scotland) Act 1995 s16(1).
23 Re J (a minor) (prohibited steps order: circumcision) sub noms Re J (child's religious upbringing and circumcision); Re J (specific issue orders: Muslim upbringing and circumcision) [2000] 1 FLR 571.
24 British Medical Association. *Consent, rights and choices in health care for children and young people. Op cit*.
25 Grubb A. Commentary: court's inherent jurisdiction (child): detention and treatment. *Med Law Rev* 1997;**5**:227–33:231.
26 X v Germany (1985) 7 EHRR 152.
27 British Medical Association. *The law and ethics of male circumcision – guidance for doctors*. London: BMA, 2003.

28   Re J (a minor) (prohibited steps order: circumcision), sub noms Re J (child's religious upbringing and circumcision) and Re J (specific issue orders: Muslim upbringing and circumcision) [2000]. *Op cit.*

29   General Medical Council. *Guidance for doctors who are asked to circumcise male children.* London: GMC, 1997.

30   Re J (a minor) (prohibited steps order: circumcision), sub noms Re J (child's religious upbringing and circumcision); and Re J (specific issue orders: Muslim upbringing and circumcision) [2000]. *Op cit.*

31   For advice about circumcision for medical purposes see: British Association of Paediatric Surgeons, Royal College of Nursing, Royal College of Paediatrics and Child Health, Royal College of Surgeons of England, Royal College of Anaesthetists. *Statement on male circumcision.* London: Royal College of Surgeons of England, 2001.

32   The Prohibition of Female Circumcision Act 1985 does not contain provision to stop children being taken out of the country for mutilation, although at the time of writing there are proposals before Parliament to reform the law to contain such provision. Meanwhile, other legal mechanisms may be available to social services departments to protect children at risk of being mutilated abroad.

33   British Medical Association. *Female genital mutilation. Caring for patients and child protection.* London: BMA, 2001.

34   British Medical Association. *Withholding and withdrawing life-prolonging medical treatment, 2nd ed.* London: BMJ Books, 2001.

35   Re A (children) sub nom Re A (conjoined twins: medical treatment) sub nom Re A (children) (conjoined twins: surgical separation) [2000] 4 All ER 961.

36   *Ibid:* 968j – 969a.

37   Gillon R. Imposed separation of Siamese twins – moral hubris by the English courts? *J Med Ethics* 2001;**27**:3–4.

38   Re A (children) sub nom Re A (conjoined twins: medical treatment) sub nom Re A (children) (conjoined twins: surgical separation) [2000]. *Op cit:* 1019bc.

39   The Victoria Climbié Inquiry. *Report of an inquiry by Lord Laming.* London: The Stationery Office, 2003:1.

40   *Ibid.*

41   Department of Health, Home Office, Department for Education and Employment. *Working together to safeguard children. A guide to inter-agency working to safeguard and promote the welfare of children.* London: The Stationery Office, 1999. Department of Health. *What to do if you are worried a child is being abused.* London: DoH, 2003. The National Assembly for Wales. *Working together to safeguard children. A guide to inter-agency working to safeguard and promote the welfare of children.* Cardiff: National Assembly for Wales, 2000. Scottish Executive. *Protecting children. A shared responsibility. Guidance for health professionals in Scotland.* Edinburgh, Scottish Executive Health Department, 2000. Department of Health, Social Services and Public Safety. *Co-operating to safeguard children.* Belfast: DHSSPS, 2003.

42   General Medical Council. *Confidentiality: protecting and providing information.* London: GMC, 2000.

43   Children Act 1989 s38(6). The Children (Northern Ireland) Order 1995 art 57(6). Children (Scotland) Act 1995 s90. The Scottish legislation gives competent young people the right to refuse to submit to medical or psychiatric examination or other assessment that has been directed by the court or a children's hearing for the purpose of supervision requirement, assessment, protection or place of safety order.

44   South Glamorgan CC v B sub nom South Glamorgan CC v W and B [1993] FLR 574.

45   Department of Health, British Medical Association, Conference of Medical Royal Colleges. *Child protection: medical responsibilities.* London: DoH, 1992.

46   The bullet points are based on Chapter 5 of: Department of Health, *et al. Working together to safeguard children. A guide to inter-agency working to safeguard and promote the welfare of children. Op cit.*

47   General Medical Council. *Confidentiality: protecting and providing information. Op cit.*

5: Confidentiality

The questions covered in this chapter include the following.

- Is all health information confidential?
- What does the law say about confidentiality?
- Is information about deceased patients confidential?
- Is consent always needed before information is disclosed?
- What form should consent take?
- When may confidentiality be breached "in the public interest"?

The ethos of confidentiality

Respect for privacy allows people time and space to express their thoughts and feelings without fear of being misunderstood or judged by unsympathetic third parties. It has been described as being essential for "sexual, religious, and imaginative impulses to flourish" as well as necessary for people making important life choices such as those related to medical treatment.[1] Despite this, people are often interested in the private lives of others. In medicine, others – typically relatives or employers – sometimes believe that it is important for the protection of their own interest to discover information about patients. Health professionals' duties of confidentiality prevent such access without patients' consent.

Important aspects of the right to privacy are the choice and control it gives people. The importance of confidentiality goes wider than this, however, because this encompasses respect for the privacy of people who cannot choose or exercise control. The duty of confidentiality applies to all patients. Maintaining respect for the privacy of all people (a respect that continues after their death) engenders trust that facilitates the provision of health care.

We have seen in Chapter 1 that trust in the doctor–patient relationship depends on reciprocal honesty. Frank and open exchange between health professionals and patients is the ideal, and patients need to feel that their privacy will be respected before they can enter into such an exchange.

As well as the individual interest in maintaining confidentiality, there is a strong public interest in confidential health care. Patients who do not believe that their secrets will be protected may withhold information that is important not only to their health but possibly to the wellbeing of others. Patients who, for example, conceal a condition such as epilepsy, which would make driving dangerous, put both themselves and others at risk. Good quality health information also improves epidemiological and other study outcomes that advance medical knowledge and understanding.

The right to privacy that confidentiality protects is an essential element of human rights, but it is not absolute and may be countered when the rights of others to be protected from harm are jeopardised in a serious way. When rights such as these collide, a balance must be struck between the importance of maintaining confidentiality and the harms that could be avoided if confidentiality was breached. When patients cannot be persuaded to disclose voluntarily, a judgment will often fall to doctors, who may even be considered negligent in some circumstances if they fail to breach confidentiality to the authorities or the police when there is an overwhelming public interest in doing so.

As well as expecting that carers will keep details confidential, patients also rightly expect that information about them will be shared and made available when this is necessary for their care. Information systems must reflect the right balance between protecting privacy and the trust this engenders, and making information available when it is needed.

On the whole, patients have a high level of trust in the NHS and its ability to protect information. Although acknowledging that some information is particularly sensitive and requires additional safeguards, patients surveyed in 2002 were found to be generally happy for their GP, hospital doctors, and the emergency services to have access to health information about them.[2] They thought that other people who were treating them should have access only on a "need to know" basis and that disclosures outside the health service should be either of anonymous data or only with their permission.

This chapter answers many of the questions that doctors most commonly ask the BMA. The confidentiality issues for doctors with dual obligations, when colleagues are sick or failing and in relation to public health, are covered in detail in other chapters.

General principles

"Patients have a right to expect that information about them will be held in confidence by their doctors."[3]

The following basic principles underpin the advice in this chapter.

- Information about patients must be properly protected to prevent malicious, thoughtless, or inadvertent breaches of confidentiality.
- All people who come into contact with personal health information in their work should have training in confidentiality and security issues.
- Patients must be informed properly about the way information about them is used.
- Consent should usually be sought for the use or disclosure of personal health information.
- Occasionally, when it is not possible to obtain consent, information may be disclosed with strict safeguards.
- Data should be anonymised wherever possible.
- Disclosures should be kept to the minimum necessary to achieve the purpose.
- When patients request disclosure, their wishes should be respected.
- Doctors must always be prepared to justify their decisions about the use of personal health information.

What is confidential?

Once information is anonymised effectively, it is no longer confidential and may be used with relatively few constraints. All health information that doctors have about identifiable individuals learnt in a professional capacity is subject to the duty of confidentiality.

> ## An informal discussion?
>
> A GP and a dentist were both found guilty of breaching confidentiality after discussing a mutual patient during a round of golf.
>
> The GP told the dentist that the patient had had a termination of pregnancy two years earlier. The dentist repeated this to his wife, who told a friend, who then revealed to the patient that she knew about the termination.
>
> Both the doctor and dentist were found guilty of serious professional misconduct and suspended from their professional registers for six months.[4]

Doctors often enquire about which particular pieces of patient information are classified as confidential personal health information. Common questions concern whether the fact that a patient is registered with one doctor rather than another is confidential, or whether a list of patients who have attended a surgery can be given to the police, for example, after a petty theft has taken place. In the BMA's view, these, and all information collected in the context of health care, are confidential. Examples include matters that patients tell doctors, the content of health records and appointment books, x-ray films, videos, and audio recordings of patients. The activator of their release is usually patient consent. Other interests sometimes compete with the obligation to keep information confidential and, in exceptional circumstances, an overriding public interest may be the justification for disclosure when consent cannot be obtained. Additionally, patients may choose to put information in the public domain or statutory obligations may require disclosure.

The BMA believes that all doctors have duties of confidentiality to the people they see in a professional capacity, even when those people are not "patients" in the traditional sense of the word. For example, a doctor who is employed by an insurance company to write a medical report about an insurance applicant has a duty of confidentiality and may disclose information in the report only with consent. Of course, this may cause difficulties if the subject of the report refuses consent, but rather than breaching confidentiality in such cases doctors should indicate that they are unable to write a report. Similarly, police surgeons have a duty of confidentiality to the people they examine on behalf of the police. (Dual obligations of this nature are discussed further in Chapters 16 and 17.)

On the other hand, information that doctors acquire outside the sphere of their professional practice is arguably unconstrained by confidentiality and doctors are subject to the same conventions as other citizens. However, whether or not doctors are engaging in their professional practice depends to some extent on the perception of the person giving the information. If any doubt exists, the higher (professional) standard of confidentiality should prevail.

Regulation

Professional obligations to safeguard the privacy of living and deceased patients are enunciated clearly in ethical and professional codes. In the past, doctors have been generally happy to look to these codes (from the General Medical Council (GMC), for example) to explain the scope and limits of the duty of confidentiality. In the late 1990s, however, some doctors began to feel that the GMC's advice, although entirely consistent with the law, was out of step with some of their activities, particularly in relation to disclosure to cancer and other disease registries, and for public health surveillance. At around the same time, the Data Protection Act 1998 and the Human Rights Act 1998 gave new protection to information about living patients, and demand grew for clear advice about the law. This section explains the main legal provisions that impact on information about living patients. Data protection and human rights legislation do not apply after death, and there is no common law duty of confidentiality to the deceased, although the Department of Health, the GMC, and the BMA all agree that the ethical duty endures beyond death. This position appears to have some support in law because legislation that gives access to health records after death prohibits access to information that the patient did not want disclosed (see Chapter 6, pages 220–1; Chapter 12, pages 436–9).[5]

The legal position is complex. Legal responsibilities in respect of confidential health information cannot be gleaned from common law or statutes alone, and doctors must look at the overall effect of the law, not each aspect in isolation. For example, the Data Protection Act sets out circumstances in which the use of data may be lawful. The common law generally requires consent for disclosure. Doctors must be sure that any use of data falls into the relevant Data Protection Act categories and meets the common law requirement for consent.

The common law

Much of the law affecting confidentiality is not set out in legislation but is common law. It imposes a duty on health professionals to respect the confidences of patients.[6] This duty arises where information is confidential (such as health information) and is imparted in circumstances where an obligation of confidence is implied (such as the doctor–patient relationship). The courts have suggested that this duty may arise when there is a public interest that confidentiality should be protected,[7] or when the confider would suffer from revelation of the information.[8]

The effect of the common law is that information may be disclosed with consent or where the law requires it. Legal judgments have also established that confidentiality may be breached, but only when there is a public interest that overrides the patient's right to privacy. Decisions are made on a case by case basis, and health professionals must be able to justify their decisions.

Disclosure in the public interest

W suffered from paranoid schizophrenia and shot and killed five people and injured two others in 1974. At his trial, his plea of guilty to manslaughter on the grounds of diminished responsibility was accepted and he was detained indefinitely in a secure hospital.

In 1986 the responsible medical officer recommended to the Secretary of State that W be transferred to a regional secure unit, which could eventually lead to him returning to the community. The Secretary of State refused consent. W then applied to a mental health review tribunal. To support his application for a transfer to a regional secure unit he sought a report from an independent consultant psychiatrist, Dr Egdell.

Dr Egdell's report did not support W's application. It disclosed that W had a longstanding and continuing interest in homemade bombs and did not accept the view that W was no longer a danger to the public. W withdrew his application to the tribunal and refused to consent to Dr Egdell disclosing the report to the medical officer at the secure hospital.

Dr Egdell, however, was of the view that the report should be known to those treating W, and disclosed the report to the medical officer. Copies were subsequently sent to the Secretary of State and the Department of Health and Social Security. W challenged this decision. The Court of Appeal held that it was necessary to balance the public interest in maintaining confidentiality against the public interest in protecting others against possible violence. W lost his case because Dr Egdell's disclosure had been in the public interest and in accordance with the advice of the GMC.

W v Egdell[9]

The public interest in confidentiality

X was a health authority from whom two HIV positive GPs had sought medical advice. This information was apparently sold to a newspaper reporter (Y) by an employee of the health authority. Y used the information to contact one of the doctors concerned. The newspaper Y worked for intended to publish an article identifying the doctors and describing the cause and consequences of their condition. X asked the High Court to prevent Y or his employer from revealing any confidential information about the doctors.

The court held that, although there was a public interest in the freedom of the press and in knowing about doctors with AIDS, this was substantially outweighed by the public interest in maintaining a confidential health service. A permanent injunction was issued.

X (health authority) v Y and others[10]

Data Protection Act 1998

The Data Protection Act 1998 is a complex and lengthy piece of legislation that governs the processing of data that identify living individuals. The Act is not limited to electronic data. It incorporates other areas of law on confidentiality by its blanket requirement that data processing is "lawful".

At the heart of the Act are eight data protection principles which state that data must be:

- fairly and lawfully processed
- processed for limited purposes and not in any manner incompatible with those purposes
- adequate, relevant and not excessive
- accurate
- not kept for longer than necessary
- processed in line with the data subject's rights
- secure
- not transferred to countries without adequate protection.

The Act's requirement that all data processing must be "fair and lawful" means that patients must know when and what information about them is being processed (the "fair processing requirement"), and the processing itself must meet all the legal standards that apply, including the common law duty of confidentiality.

There are additional rules for when sensitive personal data are processed. The processing must also meet at least one of the conditions in each of Schedules 2 and 3 of the Act. These include, for example, that there is consent from the data subject, that processing is necessary for the administration of justice or for the vital interests of the data subject or another person, or is undertaken by a health professional for "medical purposes", something that is defined very broadly in the Act. The scope of the conditions is so wide that almost any disclosure from patient records for NHS purposes is likely to come within their remit. Even if these conditions are met, however, the requirement for processing to be fair and lawful still stands.

Human Rights Act 1998

A right to "respect for private and family life" is guaranteed in the Human Rights Act 1998. This right is not absolute, and may be derogated from where the law permits and where "necessary in a democratic society in the interests of national security, public safety or the economic well-being of the country, for the prevention of disorder or crime, for the protection of health or morals, or for the protection of the rights and freedoms of others".[11] The effect is similar to that of the common law: privacy is an important principle that must be respected, but confidentiality may be breached where other significant interests prevail.

Health and Social Care Act 2001

In limited circumstances, the Health and Social Care Act permits the disclosure of personal health information without consent. The Act applies only in England and Wales, and was introduced as a temporary measure to permit disclosure for purposes such as disease registries where the electronic systems that gathered information could not accommodate a patient's refusal. The relevant provisions are explained on pages 182–3.

Anonymous information

A principle that underpins the BMA's views on confidentiality and access to information is that information may be used more freely if the subject of the information is not identified in any way. Although there should be safeguards to prevent inappropriate use or abuse of even anonymous information, in general the Association believes that it is not ethically necessary to seek consent for its use. It should be noted, however, that research shows conflicting evidence about whether patients see a distinction between anonymous and identifiable information.[12]

In the past, discussion about the use of anonymised information has focused on what can be considered to be truly anonymous. For example, pieces of information such as date of birth, diagnosis, or postcode may not alone identify an individual, but may do so in combination. Similarly, an NHS number may replace other identifiers, but the information cannot be said to be anonymous if NHS numbers are widely used as identifiers and many people are able to translate the number into a name and address. Indeed, it is arguable that information that is about an individual cannot be anonymised and true anonymisation can arise only with aggregation. The GMC alludes to this in its advice that information about people as individuals, for example, case histories, may be published in media to which the public has access, for example journals and text books, only when there is express consent (see Chapter 6, page 207).[13] Usually, however, data can be considered to be anonymous where clinical or administrative information is separated from details that may permit the individual to be identified. Doctors must take reasonable steps to anonymise data to this extent and take technical advice about anonymisation techniques. Anonymisation is a permanent process. Reversible anonymisation, or pseudonymisation, is discussed next.

When data are anonymised, they may be used without patient consent. This is also the position in law. The Court of Appeal, in a decision about the sale of prescribing data, clarified that there was no legal duty of confidentiality when data were anonymous.[14]

Confidentiality and anonymous data: the Source Informatics case

Source Informatics was an American company that wanted to obtain information about doctors' prescribing habits in order to sell this on to pharmaceutical companies, so that those companies could market their products more effectively. The identity of the prescribing doctors, and the products they prescribed, was of interest to Source, but the identity of patients was not. Source proposed that pharmacists should collect anonymous data by computer and pass it to Source for a fee.

In 1997 the Department of Health issued guidance that said this would involve a breach of confidentiality. Although the judge at first instance upheld this position, his decision was overturned in the Court of Appeal, which held that confidentiality was not breached when patients' identities were protected. The Department of Health's guidance was therefore withdrawn.

R v Department of Health, ex parte Source Informatics Ltd[15]

Pseudonymised data

Pseudonymisation is sometimes referred to as reversible anonymisation or key coding of data. True patient identifiers, such as name, address, or NHS number, are substituted with a pseudonym that allows the data to be reconstructed as required. Where those who are using data have no means to reverse the process, and so no way to identify an individual from the data they have (or from the data they have and any they may acquire), the data may be treated as anonymised and there is no common law requirement to seek consent for their use. Processing should still meet at least one of the requirements in each of Schedules 2 and 3 of the Data Protection Act, however, since it is possible that pseudomymised data fall within the Act's definition of "personal data". This point has not been tested in court, although the Information Commissioner advises NHS bodies and clinicians to apply the Act in these circumstances. For those who have access to both pseudonymised data and the means to reconstitute them, on the other hand, they should be treated as identifiable.

Pseudonymisation is a useful technique where the identity of individuals is not important for the day to day uses of the data, yet it is important to be able to distinguish between individuals or to link data to identity at a later stage. The use of pseudonymised data is common in research (see Chapter 14).

Disclosures required by law

In addition to the overarching legal framework of the common law, human rights, and data protection legislation, doctors are required by law to disclose certain information, regardless of patient consent. They must be aware of their obligations to disclose in these circumstances and ensure that they do not disclose more information than is necessary. The principal subjects of regulations are potential dangers to society from serious communicable diseases and the interests of order and justice.

Examples of obligatory disclosures

Under public health legislation, doctors must notify local authorities of the identity, sex, and address of any person suspected of having a notifiable disease, including food poisoning (see Chapter 20, pages 727–8).

Deaths, major injuries, accidents resulting in more than three days off work, certain diseases and dangerous occurrences must be reported under health and safety legislation.[16]

Abortion legislation requires identifying details to be passed to the Chief Medical Officer. There are standard forms that must be used. In the past, the woman's name and address were passed on, but, since 2002, in England and Wales, doctors completing the form are asked to provide a patient reference number (for example an NHS number), date of birth and full postcode wherever possible.[17] Only when these details are not available should a name and address be provided. At the time of writing, Scotland is considering making similar changes to its procedures.

Where a statutory requirement exists, the patient's consent to disclosure is not necessary, and the patient has no right to refuse, but he or she should be told of the fact and purpose of the disclosure, and reassured that disclosure is to a secure authority.

Some statutes permit, rather than require, disclosure. In the case of the Health and Social Care Act 2001, disclosure is permitted without consent. Unless the legislation is explicit about not needing consent, however, consent is still a legal and ethical requirement. An example is the Crime and Disorder Act 1998, which permits disclosure to partner organisations, such as the police, local authority, or probation service. In such cases, doctors may disclose information only when the patient has given consent or there is an overriding public interest (see pages 189–96).

If health professionals have any doubts about whether the disclosure requested by police, lawyers, or others is a statutory obligation, they should ask the person or body applying for the information to specify under which legislation it is sought. Similarly, doctors and their representative bodies will wish to question statutory requirements when these appear contrary to ethical principles.

In any situation where disclosure is made in the absence of the subject's consent, careful consideration must be given to the question of to whom it is proper to disclose the information. This varies with the circumstances of the case and the objective that is sought. Indiscriminate disclosure is never justifiable. Where there is a statutory requirement for disclosure, the recipient of the information is usually identified and in such cases the information released should be the minimum to fulfil the requirement. It should not normally involve transfer of an individual's entire record. Doctors should seek legal advice if they believe that complying with a statutory obligation to disclose information would cause serious harm to the patient or another person.

Disclosure in connection with litigation

Health records that are required in litigation proceedings are usually acquired via legal provisions for patients to access their own records (see Chapter 6, pages 216–8). Doctors releasing information to lawyers acting for their patients should ensure that they have the patient's written consent to disclosure, and that the patient understands the nature and extent of the information to be disclosed. The BMA and the Law Society in England publish a standard consent form that it is hoped will improve the process of seeking consent by ensuring that patients are well informed about these matters.[18]

Additionally, the courts, including coroner's courts, some tribunals, and persons appointed to hold inquiries, have legal powers to require disclosure, without the patient's consent, of information that may be relevant to matters within their jurisdiction. Doctors are justified in disclosing information when they believe on reasonable grounds that information falls within this category, and should disclose only as much information as is requested. Failure to comply with a court order to release records may be an offence, but doctors should object to the judge or presiding officer if they believe that the records contain information that should not be disclosed, for example, because it relates to third parties unconnected with the proceedings. Whenever possible, patients should be informed of disclosures required by a court.

Laws affecting all citizens

In addition to laws specifically requiring disclosure by health professionals, doctors may also be affected by the disclosure statutes that apply to all citizens. Examples are the obligation to inform the police of a suspicion of terrorist activity,[19] and the requirement to provide the police, on request, with information that may identify a driver alleged to have committed a traffic offence.[20] The latter does not require doctors to volunteer information about drivers, but they must respond to requests from a police officer even if the information is subject to the professional duty of confidentiality.

Need for clarity in the law

Since the early 1980s, the BMA has been deeply concerned with the effects that modernisation of the health service may have on patient confidentiality. The NHS is responding to the new challenges brought by large, and potentially readily accessible, repositories of data. There is an increasing recognition of the importance of seeking consent and of anonymising information whenever possible. The system of appointing a senior member of staff to be a Caldicott guardian who oversees confidentiality issues within an organisation emphasises the health service's corporate responsibility for confidentiality in a way that complements the duties of individual practitioners and staff.[21] There remains a lack, however, of a clear legal basis for confidentiality that covers all patients. Although the Data Protection Act and the Human Rights Act go some way to improving the situation, the fundamental duty of confidentiality is still in common law and these pieces of legislation have not clarified that. Piecemeal legal provisions, and a combination of legislative and non-legislative solutions to legal inadequacies north and south of the border, cause confusion (see page 182). Apparent willingness from Government to embrace the issues and provide comprehensive review, comment, and guidance on the issues is welcomed. The appointment of Caldicott guardians in the late 1990s was an important gesture towards recognising the importance of these increasingly complex issues, but there is still room for clear statutory protection of confidential information that permits use and disclosure in well defined circumstances. It is said that the current legal position generates "too much uncertainty about the exceptions to the obligation of confidence and insufficient protection for confidentiality within the NHS bureaucracy".[22] It is not clear at present that there are adequate penalties against non-health professionals who breach confidentiality. Individual contracts of employment may be insufficient to safeguard confidentiality because nothing can be done about misdemeanours discovered after an employee has left.

An aim of the BMA is to protect the professional ethos of respect for patient autonomy and to allow individuals to decide how information about themselves is used. In 1992 the then Data Protection Registrar said that he was "unconvinced that the common law provides as good a constraint on the use and disclosure of personal health information as could be provided were there to be appropriate statutory provisions".[23] The Collection, Use and Disclosure of Personal Health Information Bill 1996 would have satisfied this requirement. The bill was a result of work by the BMA and other bodies representing health professionals, and had an unopposed second reading in the House of Lords in March 1996. The bill did not progress, however, and the health departments have not supported the introduction of an overarching statute in this area.

Summary – what is confidential?

- The sum of the ethical and legal rules about confidentiality is that health professionals are responsible to patients for the confidentiality and security of the health information they hold.
- There should be no use or disclosure of any confidential information gained in the course of professional work for any purpose other than the clinical care of the patient to whom it relates. There are three broad exceptions to this standard:

  - where there is appropriate consent
  - where the law requires disclosure or
  - where there is an overriding public interest in disclosure.

- Anonymous information may be used for legitimate purposes without consent.
- The confidentiality of deceased persons must be respected.

Consent for disclosure of information

Consent is the most common facilitator of disclosure. Usually, identifiable information may not be used or disclosed without the consent of the individual concerned, or an appropriate proxy (see pages 177–8). Disclosure with consent by an informed adult is unproblematic, although it is generally advisable that evidence of the patient's consent to disclosure to third parties, such as insurers or employers, is kept on the patient's file.

Consent can be defined as freely given, informed agreement. In relation to decisions about disclosure, it is helpful to see consent as having three key elements: information, choice, and evidence.[24]

Information

Consent must be informed. Patients need information about the nature and purpose of the disclosure: broadly speaking, who will have access to it, for what purpose, and what they will do with it. The more significant the potential implications, the more detail patients are likely to want. Patients cannot give consent to something if they do not understand the nature and potential implications of their decision. Put another way, consent applies only to those activities of which the patient is aware at the time, not to any subsequent uses or disclosures of information. Doctors must bear in mind that they may not know or have control over what happens to data once they have been disclosed, and they should make any uncertainties clear to patients when seeking consent.

Choice

Patients must be given a genuine choice about the use and disclosure of their information, and must have the mental capacity to make a decision. It is sometimes argued that attaching conditions to consent renders it invalid. Provided that the conditions are not too onerous, however, the BMA does not share this view. There are clearly circumstances in which duress or coercion do render consent invalid,[25] but some conditions are not necessarily a bar to valid decision making. For example, when a person needs a medical report for insurance purposes, there is clear pressure to agree to disclosure, but that does not, in the BMA's view, make the choice invalid.

Evidence: express or implied consent?

Patients need to convey their decision in some way. Consent may be expressed, or made explicit,[26] when a patient actively agrees to what is proposed. It can be given orally or in writing. Occasionally, the law requires such express consent. Examples are communication between the health team at a fertility clinic,[27] or at a genitourinary medicine clinic,[28] and the patient's GP.

Consent may also be implied (or assumed) from patients' actions. In the context of care and treatment, it has been noted in Chapter 2 that consent is implied by patients who agree to requests to open their mouth for examination, position their arm for blood pressure to be taken, or attend a doctor and give information about an illness. In relation to health information, consent for its use or disclosure may be implied when a patient is referred to another health professional for care and a relevant medical history is passed on. Similarly, because patients generally understand that a medical secretary will type the referral letter, consent to information being passed on for this purpose is implied. Occasionally, however, the particular circumstances of the case mean that the general rules are not suitable. In a small community, for example, the doctor may be aware that the medical secretary is known personally to the patient and it would be helpful to confirm that the patient understands the usual procedure and is offered a choice.

Implied consent is not a lesser, or less valid, form of consent. It must still be informed and based on a real choice. The evidential aspect is different, however. Guidance from the Information Commissioner suggests that, for consent of any sort to be given, there must be some "active communication" between the parties.[29] If hospital department personnel wrote to former patients asking them to contact the department if they wished to opt out of having their records used in research, for example, it would not be sufficient to rely on their non-response as being valid consent. However, if the same department wrote to its current patients and those patients did not object and continued to attend for treatment, they could be assumed to have agreed.

The BMA shares the view of the Department of Health,[30] the Information Commissioner[31] and the GMC[32] that implied consent is acceptable for uses or disclosures of information that directly contribute to the diagnosis, care, or treatment of a patient, and to the quality assurance of that care. This includes record keeping, transfer of information within a healthcare team and between health professionals providing care, and clinical audit. When identifiable information is needed for other purposes, for example, research, teaching or financial audit, competent patients must be asked to give their express consent. Express consent is, by its very nature, less ambiguous than implied consent and so should be used where there is a risk of misunderstanding.

When the patient cannot give consent

In the BMA's view, confidentiality is owed to all patients, regardless of their age, status, or mental capacity. The fact that individuals are unable to give valid consent (be it due to immaturity, temporary or permanent lack of capacity, or an inability to communicate) neither implies that their information can be less closely guarded nor that it cannot be used or disclosed when doing so would be in their interests or satisfies some broader public interest test.

Unless unconscious, most people with some degree of mental incapacity can make valid decisions about some matters that affect them. When they cannot decide, decisions about the use and disclosure of information about incapacitated people are based on patients' best interests. Doctors have always had discretion to release information when it would clearly be in an incapacitated individual's interests to do so and the person has not expressed an objection. If a patient lacks the ability to understand, decisions must be based on an evaluation of the incapacitated person's best interests, which should reflect the individual's current or previously expressed wishes and values. Disclosure of information about mentally incapacitated patients may be essential for their protection or wellbeing, or may permit a proxy decision maker, lawyer, or advocate acting on the patient's behalf to further the person's interests. Confidential information may also be disclosed to proxies or people close to patients in order for carers to help patients to manage their condition. When the patient lacks the capacity to give consent to information being shared with carers, it is most important that respect is paid to the "need to know" principle. Obviously, doctors have to take decisions to share information in some circumstances, but they should always have clear grounds for disclosure and a good idea of what they expect the recipient to do with the information revealed. Disclosure for the purposes of research is discussed in Chapter 14.

In addition, in some circumstances the law allows a third party to authorise disclosure on behalf of a person who is unable to give consent. When a proxy decision maker has been appointed, for example to manage a patient's property and affairs or, in Scotland only, to make healthcare decisions, access may be given to information necessary to carry out the role. People with parental responsibility for an immature minor may also authorise disclosure, although young people who have the competence to understand the implications may make their own decisions.

Occasionally, young people seek medical treatment, for example contraception, but are judged to lack the capacity to give consent. In the BMA's view, even when the doctor considers the young person is too immature to consent to the treatment requested, confidentiality should still generally be maintained concerning the consultation. The BMA considers that doctors' duty of confidentiality is not dependent upon the capacity of the patient and, unless there are very convincing reasons to the contrary, for instance if abuse is suspected, the doctor should keep confidential a minor's request for treatment such as contraception. This is so even if the doctor believes the minor to be insufficiently mature for the request to be fulfilled. Further advice should be taken if there is any doubt.

In an emergency when patients are unable to make decisions, information should be made available where this is necessary to provide treatment or to avert immediate and serious harm to any person. It is likely to be extremely rare, but if the patient has previously made explicit that disclosure is not permitted, and has acknowledged the risks to himself or herself, information must not be released unless it is essential to prevent another person from suffering serious harm. Emergency care is discussed further in Chapter 15.

Deceased persons

Deceased persons are owed a duty of confidentiality. In the past, it was assumed that an executor or a close relative could authorise or prohibit disclosure of information about deceased patients. These people have rights of access to information when they are pursuing a claim arising from the patient's death (see Chapter 6, pages 220–1), but generally they do not control the use or disclosure of information. Additionally, a coroner or procurator fiscal may need information in connection with an inquest or fatal accident inquiry.

It is common for relatives to approach the doctor of a deceased person, asking for information about their loved one's last illness. Doctors should weigh the benefits to the patient's partner or family of disclosing information against the duty of confidentiality. Unless the patient had requested confidentiality, it is likely to be appropriate to discuss in general terms the deceased's last illness and medical history. Providing better access for relatives after a patient's death was one of the issues raised by the Shipman Inquiry (see Chapter 12).

Summary – consent

- Consent to disclosure has three key elements:

  - information: patients must be informed
  - choice: patients must be given a choice and be competent to make a decision
  - evidence: decisions must be conveyed to those seeking consent.

- Implied consent is generally acceptable for uses or disclosures of information that directly contribute to the diagnosis, care, or treatment of a patient, and to the quality assurance of that care.
- Express consent is needed for other uses of information.
- People with parental responsibility may give consent for the sharing of information about children who lack the capacity to decide.
- Proxy decision makers may give consent for the disclosure of information about incapacitated adults when this is necessary as part of their role as a proxy.

Disclosures necessary to provide effective health care

When patients are able to make a choice, implied consent is usually the basis for sharing information for purposes necessary to provide effective health care. When patients are unable to make decisions about disclosure, information may be shared with other health professionals for purposes necessary to provide effective health care, provided that this is in, or not contrary to, the patient's best interests (see Chapter 3, pages 108–9). Proxies may also authorise disclosure (see pages 177–8).

Implied consent for disclosure as part of the direct provision of health care

In the absence of evidence to the contrary, patients are normally considered to have given implied consent for the use of their information by health professionals for the purpose of providing the care they have come to receive. Information sharing in this context is acceptable to the extent that health professionals share what is necessary and relevant for the episode of care on a "need to know" basis. Health and social care, although often closely related, do not always fall into the same category, and disclosure of information to social services usually requires express consent from competent patients (see page 183).

In order for implied consent to be valid, it is important that patients are made aware that information about them will be shared and with whom it will be shared, and of their right to refuse. Doctors bear responsibility for the disclosures they make, so when consent is taken to be implied, they must be able to demonstrate that the assumption of consent was made in good faith and based on good information. Leaflets and posters can play a part in conveying to patients the reality and necessity of information sharing within healthcare teams.

Sometimes two competing interests come into conflict, such as an individual's informed refusal to allow disclosure and the need to provide effective treatment to that person. A patient's refusal to allow information sharing with other health professionals may compromise the patient's safety, but if this is an informed decision by a competent person it should be respected. Individuals may knowingly compromise their own safety but not that of other people. Health professionals, although not abandoning the patient, may ethically curtail the range of procedures they offer if the outcome could foreseeably be unsafe or ineffective owing to lack of information. Patients must be informed if this is an implication of their choice, and must be offered further advice about their options.

Some health information is so sensitive that legislation has been introduced to cover the sharing of it with other health professionals. NHS trusts and primary care trusts, for example, are required to take all necessary steps to ensure that any information capable of identifying an individual examined or treated for any sexually transmitted infection is not disclosed by any of their members or employees except in limited circumstances.[33] Those circumstances are where disclosure is to a doctor, or somebody working for a doctor, in connection with treating people with the disease or preventing its spread. The regulations do not prevent other healthcare staff, for example, the patient's GP, from disclosing information with appropriate consent.

Clinical audit

It is acceptable to rely on implied consent for clinical audit undertaken within the health care organisation providing care. Patients should be informed that the quality of care is reviewed through the process of clinical audit. Wherever possible, a member of the health team responsible for the patient's care should produce anonymous data for this purpose. When this is not practicable, consent should be sought before identifiable information is disclosed outside the healthcare team, for example, to a member of a hospital's audit staff for the purpose of anonymising the records. This consent may be express or implied. When this is not feasible, in England and Wales it may be possible to rely on the Health and Social Care Act and disclose without consent (see pages 182–3).

Increasingly, health professionals, and sometimes others from outside the health service body, are commissioned to carry out clinical audit. Commercial agencies are also sometimes involved in audit. Commissioners of such services must ensure that employees have firm contractual, as well as any professional, obligations to preserve confidentiality. When a third party is to be brought in to carry out audit, there must be added safeguards to ensure that confidentiality and anonymity are preserved. Ideally, information should not be released to people who do not have an enduring professional responsibility to maintain confidentiality. The BMA recognises that this may not be practical in all cases, but health professionals should aim for maximum protection for patients.

Pharmaceutical companies are also sometimes interested in sponsoring the audit of aspects such as prescribing habits in return for basic information resulting from the project. Doctors offered such services should consider whether there would be any conflict with the GMC's requirement that doctors must not accept any inducement or gift that may be seen to affect their judgment (see also Chapter 13, page 469).[34] They should also enquire about the uses to which information is likely to be put and ensure that no identifiable data leave the healthcare organisation. This requires monitoring not only that patient names and addresses are excluded but also that other identifiers are omitted to ensure anonymity (see pages 171–2).

The advice in this section applies to audit being undertaken by the healthcare body providing care. Sometimes, however, audit is undertaken across organisational boundaries, for example, medication reviews of GP records by local pharmacists. When information is disclosed to people outwith the healthcare body that provided care, express consent is needed.

Summary – disclosures necessary to provide effective care

- Patients need information about the way health information is shared between health professionals providing care.
- When patients are informed and do not object, their consent to the sharing of information for care and clinical audit is implied.
- Competent refusals to allow information to be shared must be respected.
- When patients lack capacity, information may be disclosed when this is in the patient's best interests.
- In emergencies, information necessary to provide care should be shared promptly.

Disclosure for purposes associated with providing health care

Unless there is specific legal provision to suggest otherwise, express consent is generally needed to use or disclose information for purposes associated with health care. Some such purposes are essential to the safe and effective running of the health service, although they may not fall into the previous category because they do not support the direct provision of care to individual patients. Public health surveillance, disease registries, and research are examples. Usually, doctors would be expected to have express consent from patients to use identifiable information for these purposes. It became clear in 2000, however, that this approach was not possible in some circumstances, for example, where data were needed from very large numbers of patients or where systems were in place to transfer information automatically to disease registries. In England and Wales, the Government chose to legislate to make disclosure of information for purposes such as these lawful, as a temporary measure until mechanisms could be put in place to seek and record consent, or to use anonymous information.[35]

Disclosures under Section 60 of the Health and Social Care Act 2001

Section 60 of the Health and Social Care Act 2001 gave the Secretary of State power to make regulations permitting the disclosure of identifiable information without consent in certain circumstances. Regulations may be made to support "medical purposes" that are in the interests of patients or the wider public when consent is not a practicable alternative and where anonymised information will not suffice. The Act was intended largely as a transitional measure while consent or anonymisation procedures were developed. This was reinforced by the need to review each use of the power annually.

When the Act came into force, proposals were developed by the Department of Health and by those wishing for support in law for the processing of information. All proposals for regulations are considered by the Patient Information Advisory Group, which advises the Secretary of State; many proposals have been the subject of public consultation. Regulations must be debated in Parliament by each House.

The first regulations[36] covered:

- cancer registries
- communicable disease and other risks to public health
- anonymising data
- research into locations at which disease or medical conditions occur
- contacting patients to seek consent for a further purpose (such as the use of information in research)
- bringing information from multiple sources (for example, to check for duplication)
- audit and quality assurance.

These purposes are very general, and at the time of writing it is not clear how they will be interpreted or relied upon in practice. The BMA has called on the Department of Health to issue advice to doctors who need to consider whether a particular disclosure is covered by the regulations.

The regulations permit the use of identifiable information without consent where a purpose falls within their scope, it is not possible to anonymise the information, and it is not possible to seek patients' consent. If there is any doubt about whether processing is covered by regulations, advice should be taken from the Information Policy Unit of the Department of Health.

At the time of writing, Scotland has opted not to legislate to permit disclosures of this nature, and Northern Ireland is consulting about whether to follow this legislative approach. Information about developments in this area will be made available on the BMA's website.

Social care

When patients are receiving care from, or are being referred for care to, social services, those who are competent should be asked for consent to share relevant information between agencies. When patients lack the capacity to choose, information may be shared with other people or agencies, such as social services, independent sector care providers, representatives, carers, or near relatives of the individual when:

- it is clearly necessary in the individual's interests
- the disclosure is not contrary to the individual's express request or known wishes
- information is released on a "need to know" basis.

Public health

Public health surveillance and research rely on vast quantities of data. Data come from many different sources and their appropriate handling by public health physicians is essential. Anonymised data should be used wherever possible.

In some cases, the law requires the reporting of infectious diseases (see Chapter 20, pages 727–8). Doctors must comply with such statutory requirements and tell patients what information will be disclosed and why, and reassure them that information will be used in an identifiable form only where required by law.

Where there is no statutory requirement to disclose information, and it is not possible to anonymise data, consent should be sought. Patients are generally happy for their information to be disclosed when there are good grounds and satisfactory safeguards to protect the data. Exceptionally, when it is not possible to seek consent, doctors in England and Wales may look to the Health and Social Care Act to see whether there is section 60 approval for the disclosure (see pages 182–3). In the rest of the UK, there is, at the time of writing, no support in law for disclosures of identifiable information without consent that do not meet a "public interest" justification for breach of confidentiality (see pages 189–92).

The responsibilities of doctors in relation to protecting the public's health, including how confidentiality impacts on this, is covered in detail in Chapter 20.

Research

Wherever possible, research should use anonymised data. Pseudonyms or other tracking mechanisms may be helpful for data that cannot be anonymised, as a way of ensuring accuracy and minimising the use of personal identifiers.

When it is not possible to anonymise data, consent should be sought before information can be disclosed for research. All research, both within and outside the NHS, must be subject to approval by an appropriately constituted research ethics committee, which has responsibility for considering confidentiality issues.

When doctors are asked to release information for research that has been approved by an ethics committee, but have doubts about whether the issues of confidentiality and consent to disclosure have been fully addressed, information should not be disclosed until the issue has been resolved. Ethics committee approval is not sufficient to justify a breach of confidentiality. For example, doctors may be aware of specific circumstances relating to their population of patients, or to individuals, which may not have been brought to the attention of the approving committee. The BMA advises doctors to bear these matters in mind when they are asked to disclose information and to ensure that any disclosures can be justified.

When it is not possible to anonymise data or seek consent from patients, doctors in England and Wales have the additional option of seeking approval under the Health and Social Care Act (see pages 182–3).

Chapter 14 on research and innovative treatment addresses these issues in detail, together with discussion of the particular questions that arise when the subjects of research are incapacitated adults or children who are unable to give consent.

Teaching

Teaching is an essential process but, in the BMA's view, it is contrary to the public interest to use identifiable material for teaching purposes without appropriate consent. Wherever possible, anonymous information should be used. Patient identifiable materials cannot be used without consent even in the context of teaching hospitals, although there are no necessary restrictions on anonymous information being used in teaching.

When a patient is unable to give consent, information may be used when consent is given by a proxy who is legally entitled to give it on the patient's behalf. That could be a proxy appointed under the Adults with Incapacity (Scotland) Act 2000, or somebody with parental responsibility for a young child (although consent should be sought from the young person once he or she is able to give it if identifiable materials continue to be used). In other cases, the BMA considers it acceptable to involve people who are unable to consent in teaching, provided that involvement is not contrary to the known wishes of the patient, and that the same objective could not be achieved with patients who are able to give consent. Health professionals should discuss involvement in teaching with those close to the patient. This may include a nominated representative or advocate, spouse, principal caregiver, next of kin, close relative, or other person whom, in the opinion of the health professional, it is reasonable in the circumstances to ask. The purpose of discussion is to ascertain whether involvement in teaching would be contrary to the interests of the particular patient, given his or her ascertainable preferences.

This and the issues that arise when potential medical students want to observe medical practice are covered in detail in Chapter 18 on education and training.

Financial audit

Health records are often used for purposes that may broadly be termed financial audit. Commissioning bodies frequently seek this information from GPs, for example. Wherever possible, data should be anonymised or pseudonymised before disclosure. It is often possible to separate clinical from financial information, and it is important that only relevant data are disclosed.

When the data are identifiable to the body to which they are disclosed, express consent from patients is needed. The courts have made clear that the disclosure of identifiable information at the request of a commissioning body requires consent from patients, unless a court has ordered that disclosure without consent is acceptable.[37]

Complaints

When patients initiate a complaint, they should be made aware of who will see information about them, and the safeguards that are in place to minimise any risks to confidentiality. Guidance on maintaining confidentiality in the NHS complaints procedures is available from the health departments.[38] If complaints are heard in a public forum, or a forum to which the media has access, this should be made clear. Some complaints systems, including that of the GMC, protect complainants' identities from the press. Although patients should not be discouraged from pursuing legitimate complaints, it is important that they understand, in advance, if there is any potential for media usage of health information and speculation about their condition.

Sometimes patients involve their MP or other elected representative in the complaints process. Patients may, of course, share information about themselves with whomsoever they wish. They are also entitled to authorise third parties to exercise rights of access to health records on their behalf (see Chapter 6, page 217). Doctors who are asked to disclose information in these circumstances must be satisfied that the patient has given valid consent to the disclosure.

The BMA is sometimes asked whether doctors may disclose information to their own representatives when a patient is pursuing a complaint. This should be discussed with the patient, although if the patient refuses, but the complaint is pursued, doctors must be allowed to disclose information necessary to defend themselves. The Department of Health has made clear that GPs must be entitled to copies of records they made about their former patients for this purpose.[39]

Similarly, information may be disclosed in response to an official request from a statutory regulatory body for any of the healthcare professions, where that body determines that this is necessary in the interests of justice and for the safety of other patients.[40] If records are needed by a statutory regulatory body investigating a health professional's fitness to practise, consent should be sought before disclosing information about patients. If patients withhold consent, or it is not practicable to seek consent, anonymised records should be used wherever possible. Occasionally, the statutory body may require their disclosure even if the patient objects.[41] Doctors should discuss this with patients whenever possible.

Summary – disclosure for purposes associated with providing health care

- In addition to the direct provision of care and ensuring the quality of that care, personal health information is used for purposes associated with health care such as research, teaching, and complaints.
- Wherever possible, information should be anonymised.
- Express consent is generally needed for use of identifiable information for purposes associated with health care.
- In England and Wales, it may be possible to rely on the provisions of section 60 of the Health and Social Care Act for the use of information without consent.

Uses of health information for purposes not associated with providing health care

This section covers uses of health information for purposes not associated with providing health care. Because disclosure to prevent harm is a large area, and the considerations are slightly different, it is covered separately on pages 189–92, with examples given on pages 192–6.

Spiritual care

Spiritual care is provided by a range of spiritual advisers. Hospital chaplains can provide vital support and care to people in hospital. Some patients are happy for information about their religious affiliation to be passed to the chaplain, who may then arrange spiritual care in accordance with the patient's wishes. Information about affiliation, and clinical information about the patient's health and care, should not, however, be passed on without the consent of a competent patient. When patients give consent, health professionals should share records in accordance with the patient's wishes.

When patients lack the capacity to give consent, for example because they are unconscious, doctors must make decisions about whether to pass very general information about patients and their condition to a spiritual adviser, based on the patient's best interests. Discussion with people close to the patient about his or her likely wishes is essential.

Disclosure to the media

When doctors are asked to disclose information to the media, the usual rules about confidentiality apply. Express consent is generally needed, but when this cannot be sought, or even when it is refused, there may be exceptional reasons to justify disclosure.

GMC rules about disclosure to the media[42]

- "Remember that information which a doctor has learnt in a professional capacity should be regarded as confidential, whether or not the information is also in the public domain.
- Whenever possible, obtain explicit consent from patients before discussing matters relating to their care with journalists, whether or not the patients' names or other identifying information is to be revealed. Explicit consent must be obtained if patients will be identifiable from details disclosed.
- Remember that patients can be identified from information other than names or addresses. Details which in combination may reveal patients' identities include: their condition or disease, their age, their occupation, the area where they live, their medical history, the size of their family.
- Always consider and act in accordance with the best medical interests of patients when responding to invitations to speak to the media about patients."

Doctors are asked to disclose information to the media in many different circumstances; each demands a slightly different approach. What they have in common is that any decision to disclose information must be justified on a case by case basis and should be limited to the minimum necessary in the circumstances. Hospital doctors will want to take advice from their trust's solicitors and GPs from their defence bodies.

- Comment on the condition of celebrity patients

  - When the patient has the capacity to make decisions about disclosure, consent is essential before any information is released to the media. When the patient lacks capacity, legal advice should be sought.

- After incidents involving harm to many people

  - After major disasters, for example a fire, road traffic accident, or terrorist attack, it is important that requests for information are dealt with sensitively, while not breaching the confidentiality of patients. It will not usually be necessary to give identifying or detailed clinical details of the people involved. Liaison with injured people and their families is essential.

- Discussion of individual cases in the media

  - Occasionally, patients approach the media to publicise information about their case or care. When the purpose is educational, the BMA has no objections to doctors engaging in this process if there is consent from the patient for them to do so.[43]
  - The situation is different, however, when patients use the media as a vehicle to complain. The BMA does not believe that entering into an argument about the facts of a case in the media is an appropriate way for doctors to respond to allegations made by patients.
  - Doctors should, of course, have the opportunity to defend themselves against complaints. Many doctors feel strongly that patients forfeit their rights to confidentiality by going to the media, and that they should be entitled to "set the record straight" and correct any inaccuracies, but, in practice, doctors who did this would risk criticism and breach GMC guidance on confidentiality if the patient does not give consent.
  - Where misleading information has been presented to the media, doctors who wish to respond should limit their comments to pointing out that the information is inaccurate or incomplete. Patients, and others pursuing complaints on their behalf, should be informed of any forthcoming statement. It is important to maintain the reputation of the health service as a secure and confidential service.[44]

- During fly on the wall documentaries about health care

  - Using images of competent patients in television programmes is generally not problematic provided that consent has been sought. Images of children may also be used provided that the child's parents have given informed consent, the child agrees, and it is not contrary to the child's interests either at the time or in the future.
  - Whether it would be lawful to use images of patients for whom consent is not available is not clear. Doctors approached by the media to involve incapacitated adults in such projects must take legal advice.

Employment, insurance, and other affairs

When third parties such as insurers or employers ask for information, doctors must have written consent from the patient or a person properly authorised to act on the patient's behalf. This should be provided by the third party, as either the original consent form or a copy. An electronic copy of the signed form is sufficient, provided that the third party can satisfy the doctor that there are robust mechanisms in place to ensure that the form has not been tampered with in any way. The use of medical information in insurance is covered in Chapter 16, pages 570–6.

There is reluctance from some third parties, such as insurance companies and the Benefits Agency, to provide doctors with a copy of a signed consent form. Sometimes this is because of the administrative burden of doing so, sometimes because the third party would prefer not to ask their client to sign a form, for example, during an online insurance application. If evidence of consent is not provided to doctors, however, they themselves need to confirm that consent has been given. This may involve writing to the patient, or telephoning to confirm that there is valid consent. These processes are likely to be considerably less efficient than the requesting party simply sending a copy of a form. In the case of government departments such as the Benefits Agency, however, the GMC advises doctors that they may accept written assurances from an officer of a government department (civil servant) that the patient has given written consent to disclosure.[45] In other cases information should not be provided unless evidence is produced.

GPs are sometimes asked to provide information to a patient's family or solicitor when the family is seeking to exercise power of attorney. This usually happens when the patient's capacity is in doubt and can be very difficult for doctors. Relatives may report aberrant behaviour but, if the patient refuses to cooperate with an assessment of his or her capacity, it is unclear to health professionals whether they are justified or not in providing medical information that would enable another person to act in the patient's interests. The BMA's advice in such cases is that health professionals must assess the information that is available from the patient's record and from third parties. They should attempt to discuss with patients their needs and preferences and weigh up whether they appear to be making a valid refusal regarding the assessment or the sharing of information resulting from it.[46]

Disclosures in the public interest

On occasions, the public interest may be seen to override the privacy of an individual. Disclosure that is essential to prevent or lessen a serious and imminent threat to public health or to the life or health of another individual typifies this category of justification. The facts must be subject to close scrutiny as to whether there is a genuine necessity for disclosure. Aptly, it has been said that "there is a wide difference between what is interesting to the public and what is in the public interest".[47]

Generally, public interest disclosures centre around the prevention of serious harm. Confidentiality is too important a principle to be sacrificed for vague goals or indefinable harms, but it should give way where there is some "serious" threat to people. The BMA has identified threats to living people as significant in a way in which threats to property or financial interests are not. In line with this reasoning, the risk of an assault, a traffic accident, or an infectious disease may be seen as more compelling grounds for disclosure than risk relating to fraud or theft.

In reality, such neat divisions are not entirely satisfactory and, in many cases, harm is multifaceted. Serious fraud or theft involving NHS resources, for example, may harm individuals awaiting treatment. Even comparatively minor prescription fraud may reveal a serious harm if prescriptions for controlled drugs are being forged.

In this comparatively narrow sphere there is no broad consensus of how harm to people should be evaluated or from whose perspective it should be judged. For the victim who suffers harm or loss, it may be perceived in very different terms than by a decision maker outside the situation who is trying to weigh it up. The BMA's advice is that, where feasible, health professionals should try to envisage the seriousness of the potential harm from the viewpoint of the person likely to suffer it.

Some serious crimes almost invariably justify disclosure of information to the police. Examples include murder, manslaughter, and rape. Serious harm, however, is a much wider concept than that of serious criminal activity and it encompasses omissions, such as neglect, as well as acts. It must also take account of psychological as well as physical damage. Child neglect or abuse is an example of treatment whose psychological sequelae may be considerably more profound than the physical harm suffered, and the psychological damage may be experienced not only by the actual victim but also by siblings who know of it. When considering non-consensual disclosure, health professionals rightly take into account that the degree of psychological harm for victims may be influenced by the manner in which the disclosure is handled.

Advisory bodies, such as the BMA, cannot tell doctors whether or not to disclose information in a particular case, but can provide general guidance about the categories of cases in which decisions to disclose may be justifiable. Doctors should be aware that they risk criticism, and even legal liability, if they fail to take action to avoid serious harm.

Balancing benefits and harms

A decision to disclose is often not based on the interests of the person concerned but is made to protect other people or the public at large. The decision to disclose is based partly on a balancing of several moral imperatives, including the risk and likelihood of harm if no disclosure is made, and the need to maintain the trust of the patient. Health professionals can be in an invidious position in having to weigh speculative as well as known facts, and assess whether a perceived harm can be better averted by making a disclosure or by maintaining the trust of an individual while attempting to persuade him or her to disclose voluntarily. It may be helpful to discuss situations on an anonymous basis with colleagues, and to seek advice from professional and indemnifying bodies.

In some cases, although a duty of confidentiality is owed, the need to protect other people may tip the balance. In many cases, however, clear and unambiguous information upon which to judge the scope of the potential threat is unavailable.

Scraps of information may be pieced together but, even after discussion with the patient and with experienced colleagues, it may be impossible to ascertain the degree of actual risk in order to make a fair and justifiable decision about disclosure. Time, patience, and repeated discussions with the individual may be needed to clarify the real dimensions of the threat. Non-consensual disclosure is generally considered justifiable only in cases where the threat appears serious and imminent, and disclosure is likely to limit or prevent it occurring.

The urgency of the need to disclose

In all cases, delay is inadvisable when the risks are imminent, serious, and foreseeable. Health professionals who are unable to persuade an individual to disclose voluntarily information that could prevent serious harm to other people are likely to be justified in disclosing without consent.

Involving the individual

It is desirable for individuals to be encouraged strongly to take responsibility for disclosure themselves, while being made aware that a reluctance to do so may oblige the health professional to take action. Persuasion may require time, counselling, repeated consultations, and possibly discussion of the case on an anonymous basis with colleagues or with other agencies. Health professionals must therefore weigh up the potential immediacy of the risk in relation to the likelihood of eventually persuading the individual and consider whether the objective of preventing harm is achievable by other means.

In some cases, it is clearly inadvisable to alert the individual to the fact that health professionals are considering disclosure. Such cases arise, for example, when telling the patient would exacerbate the threat, possibly also resulting in violence against the health professional, or it may give time to destroy evidence that is necessary to secure the long term protection of the other people at risk.

Making a disclosure

Decisions to disclose information in the public interest should be taken by health professionals, not by other health service staff, and may involve discussion among the whole healthcare team. Whenever possible, the clinician with overall responsibility for care must be consulted.

Disclosure without consent should reveal the minimum of information required to deal with the risk and careful thought must be given to the question of to whom the information should be released.

A doctor must be prepared to justify any decision regarding disclosure, and may be asked to do so before the GMC.

Seeking advice

Health professionals should remember that advice about these issues can always be sought from professional, regulatory, and indemnifying bodies.

Summary – public interest disclosures

When considering disclosing information to protect the public interest, doctors must:

- consider how the benefits of making the disclosure balance against the harms associated with breaching a patient's confidentiality
- assess the urgency of the need for disclosure
- consider whether the person could be persuaded to disclose voluntarily
- inform the person before making the disclosure and seek his or her consent, unless to do so would enhance the risk of harm
- reveal only the minimum information necessary to achieve the objective
- seek assurances that the information will be used only for the purpose for which it was disclosed
- be able to justify the decision.

Examples of disclosures in the public interest

Health professionals have clear moral duties to individual patients and to colleagues that may come into conflict with wider obligations to avert serious and preventable harm to others. This section takes some examples of situations where disclosure could be in the public interest, and discusses what doctors should do if patients refuse to permit this. Dangers arising from the health or performance of colleagues, and decisions to disclose information, are discussed in Chapter 21. Specific issues that arise in public health are discussed in Chapter 20.

As stated previously, the BMA does not seek to lay down "blanket" rules in such situations and recognises that there may be scope for negotiation with patients that allows them to make the disclosure at their own pace, without exposing others to risk. It is hoped there will be few such cases that cannot be resolved in this way. Doctors must bear in mind that they may have to justify the decisions they take. When there is any doubt, advice should be sought in confidence from professional bodies.

Health

When a person has a medical condition that puts others at risk, for example, a risk of infection or because of dangerous behaviour, doctors must discuss with the patient how to minimise the risk to others. In the case of HIV infection, for example, doctors should discuss with the patient the need to inform sexual partners, and the options for safer sex. Exceptionally, if patients refuse to modify their behaviour or inform others, doctors are advised by the GMC that they may breach confidentiality and inform a known sexual contact of an HIV positive patient.[48] Wherever possible, patients should always be told before this step is taken.

The same considerations apply to circumstances where the potential disclosure relates to a colleague who poses a threat to the health of his or her patients by reason of illness, incompetence, or addiction (see Chapter 21).

Public safety

A common example of what can be categorised as public safety occurs in connection with the assessment of patients with, for example, diabetes, epilepsy, defective eyesight, or serious cardiac conditions who have been advised by health professionals to discontinue driving, but who nevertheless continue. When an individual has insight into the problem, it is advisable for health professionals to attempt to persuade that person to either discontinue the risky behaviour or agree to disclosure being made to a responsible body as one step towards a change of behaviour. In some cases, the individual is unable or unwilling to follow the recommended course of action and health professionals have to weigh up the likelihood of serious harm and the need to breach confidentiality. Disclosure to the Driver and Vehicle Licensing Authority is not mandatory, but health professionals must consider whether non-disclosure in relation to a foreseeable and serious threat could leave them open to a possible charge of negligence if grave harm results from the non-disclosure.

Issues of public safety may similarly arise in circumstances where an individual who legitimately possesses firearms is thought by health professionals to be a risk because of drug or alcohol addiction or a medical condition such as depression (see Chapter 16, pages 578–9). The police should be informed if anybody is thought to be at risk.

Serious crime and national security

Disclosure necessary for the prevention, detection, investigation, or punishment of a serious offence is widely regarded as justifiable and desirable. The definition of what constitutes a "serious" crime is a matter of debate. The Police and Criminal Evidence Act 1984 contains some definitions of what it calls a "serious arrestable offence": an offence that has caused or may cause serious harm to the security of the state or to public order; serious interference with the administration of justice or with the investigation of an offence; death; serious injury; or substantial financial gain or serious loss.[49] These definitions include such crimes as murder, manslaughter, rape, treason, and kidnapping. Generally, crimes that may result in serious harm or loss of life for individuals can be regarded as very substantially more significant than crimes involving theft, fraud, or damage to property.

The BMA recommends that, in such cases, health professionals should seek advice from their professional, regulatory and indemnifying bodies. When time permits, further discussion, the provision of counselling or therapy for the person alleging the offence, and whether that person claims to be either the victim or the perpetrator, may clarify the issues.

When it is not possible to seek consent for disclosure of information about a crime, the following conditions should be satisfied before relevant information is disclosed.

- The crime must be sufficiently serious for the public interest to prevail.
- It must be established that, without the disclosure, the task of preventing or detecting the crime would be seriously prejudiced or delayed.
- The information is not available from a source that would not necessitate a breach of doctor–patient trust.

A common source of enquiry to the BMA is the situation in which many GPs find themselves, when the police are investigating a crime near the practice premises and want to know who attended the surgery in a given time period. The fact of attendance is, in itself, confidential and should not be disclosed unless disclosure can be justified according to the criteria set out above.

Similarly, doctors are often asked to speculate on the identity of the perpetrator of a minor crime, such as the theft of personal belongings from healthcare premises. It is unlikely that such crime would be considered to be of sufficient severity to warrant a breach of confidentiality. The police do not have an automatic right of access to information, and advice can always be sought from professional, regulatory, or indemnifying bodies when there is any doubt.

Crimes in the past

Although it is widely accepted that information should be disclosed to prevent or detect a serious crime, or bring to justice the suspected perpetrator before the crime can be repeated, it is sometimes argued that the obligation to disclose is weakened if there is no continuing danger. Whereas the justification for disclosing information about a serious current or future threat is clear, the public safety justification for doing so with regard to a past offence is less so if the individual is unlikely to repeat it. Such arguments have been raised with the BMA in relation to either confessions or allegations against others of past child abuse or "mercy killing". As in all other cases, doctors need to assess the particular situation, and may find it helpful to take advice. There is some additional discussion of this issue in Chapter 17, page 608.

In general, however, health professionals should be very wary of concealing any information of substance that would lead to the resolution of a past serious crime against a person. The public interest in ensuring that serious crimes are solved and innocent people are not wrongly punished is likely to require disclosure even in cases where there is no fear of future repetition.

Safety in the workplace

Disclosure is justifiable when failure to do so in regard to the health status of an employee could foreseeably result in a substantial risk to others. For example, an occupational health doctor has a responsibility to take action if he or she is aware that the health of an employee threatens the safety of others (see Chapter 16, pages 587–8). Similarly, GPs may need to take action if they become aware that a patient they consider to be a threat to vulnerable people begins working with young children, elderly people, or other vulnerable groups.

Action may be necessary if a colleague poses a threat to the health of his or her patients by reason of illness, incompetence, or addiction. This issue is addressed in Chapter 21.

Abuse and domestic violence

Knowing what to do when patients do not want confidential information to be disclosed, despite this being the best way to ensure that they do not suffer harm or abuse, is very difficult for doctors. Abuse of dependent elderly or young people may fall into this category, as may domestic violence (covered in Chapter 15 on emergency care).

Victims may be concerned that disclosure of what has occurred may lead to further maltreatment. There are no easy solutions, but doctors must bear in mind such factors as whether other people in institutions or in the family are also at risk and the possibility of continued or more severe abuse resulting in permanent damage. The mature patient may need time to come to a firm decision about disclosure. Counselling and support in the interim may help the patient to decide. In the case of a minor, doctors should not make promises to the patient about maintaining confidentiality that they may not be able to keep, but in the case of any patient, trust in the doctor is best maintained if disclosure is not made without prior discussion between doctor and patient. Doctors cannot personally protect children from further abuse, so they should ensure that statutory bodies with such powers are involved when necessary.

GMC advice: abuse or neglect of people who lack capacity

"If you believe a patient to be a victim of neglect or physical, sexual or emotional abuse and that the patient cannot give or withhold consent to disclosure, you should give information promptly to an appropriate responsible person or statutory agency, where you believe that the disclosure is in the patient's best interests. You should usually inform

(Continued)

the patient that you intend to disclose the information before doing so. Such circumstances may arise in relation to children, where concerns about possible abuse need to be shared with other agencies such as social services. Where appropriate you should inform those with parental responsibility about the disclosure. If, for any reason, you believe that disclosure of information is not in the best interests of an abused or neglected patient, you must still be prepared to justify your decision."[50]

A confidential service that shares information

There has been some struggle by the medical profession to stress the importance of confidentiality to the public. Rightly, the priority of patients in almost every case is the availability of their records and effective sharing of information between those providing care. Yet, at the same time, patients need to be able to trust doctors and the health service not to share information without sufficient justification. Confidence in a secure service is essential and this must be maintained while meeting patients' other priorities, including effective communication between carers (see Chapter 19).

References

1   Boyd KM, Higgs R, Pinching AJ, eds. *The new dictionary of medical ethics*. London: BMJ Publishing Group, 1997:197.
2   NHS Information Authority. *Share with care! People's views on consent and confidentiality of patient information*. Birmingham: NHSIA, 2002.
3   General Medical Council. *Confidentiality: protecting and providing information*. London: GMC, 2000: para 1.
4   Anonymous. GP struck off after golf club gossip *Pulse* 1997;(Mar 8):12.
5   Access to Health Records Act 1990. Access to Health Records (Northern Ireland) Order 1993.
6   Stephens v Avery [1988] 2 All ER 477.
7   Attorney-General v Guardian Newspapers (No. 2): Same v The Observer Ltd and Ors: Same v The Times Newspapers Ltd and Anor [1988] 3 All ER 545.
8   Discussed in Stephens v Avery [1988]. *Op cit*. The need for detriment is not universally accepted, see X (health authority) v Y and Ors [1987] 2 All ER 648.
9   W v Egdell and Ors [1990] 1 All ER 835.
10 X (health authority) v Y and Ors [1987]. *Op cit*.
11 Council of Europe. *European convention on human rights 1950*:article 8(2).
12 Patients were found not to distinguish between identifiable and anonymous data in: Willison DJ, Keshavjee K, Nair K, Goldsmith C, Holbrook AM. Patients' consent preferences for research uses of information in electronic medical records: interview and survey data. *BMJ* 2003;**326**:373–6. On the other hand, patients were found to be happy not to be asked for consent to share anonymised data in: NHS Information Authority. *Share with care! People's views on consent and confidentiality of patient information*. *Op cit*.
13 General Medical Council. *Confidentiality: protecting and providing information*. *Op cit*: para 32.
14 R v Department of Health (Respondent), ex parte Source Informatics Ltd (Appellant) and (1) Association Of The British Pharmaceutical Industry (2) General Medical Council (3) Medical Research Council (4) National Pharmaceutical Association Ltd (Interveners) [2000] 1 All ER 786.
15 *Ibid*.
16 Reporting of Injuries, Diseases, and Dangerous Occurrences Regulations 1985. (SI 1985 No. 2023 as amended.)

17 Department of Health. *Guidance note for completing the abortion notification form HSA4*. London: DoH, 2002.

18 British Medical Association, The Law Society. *Consent form (releasing health records under the Data Protection Act 1998)*. London: BMA, 2003.

19 Terrorism Act 2000.

20 Road Traffic Act 1988.

21 For information about the role and function of guardians, see: NHS Executive. *Protecting and using patient information: a manual for Caldicott guardians*. Leeds: NHSE, 1999.

22 Montgomery J. *Health care law, 2nd ed.* New York: Oxford University Press, 2003:288.

23 Data Protection Registrar. *Eighth report of the Data Protection Registrar*. London: HMSO, 1992:9.

24 Information Commissioner. *Use and disclosure of health data. Guidance on the application of the Data Protection Act 1998*. Wilmslow: Information Commissioner, 2002.

25 An example of this in relation to consent to treatment is seen in the case of: Re T (adult: refusal of medical treatment) [1992] 4 All ER 649, discussed in Chapter 3.

26 The GMC uses the term "express consent" in its guidance. The Department of Health uses "express" and "explicit" interchangeably.

27 Human Fertilisation and Embryology Act 1990 as amended by the Human Fertilisation and Embryology (Disclosure of Information) Act 1992.

28 National Health Service (Venereal Diseases) Regulations 1974. (SI 1974 No. 29.)

29 Information Commissioner. *Use and disclosure of health data. Guidance on the application of the Data Protection Act 1998*. Op cit: p. 15.

30 Department of Health. *Confidentiality: a code of practice for NHS staff (draft)*. London: DoH, 2002. A final document is expected in 2003.

31 Information Commissioner. *Use and disclosure of health data. Guidance on the application of the Data Protection Act 1998*. Op cit.

32 General Medical Council. *Confidentiality: protecting and providing information*. Op cit.

33 NHS Trusts and Primary Care Trusts (Sexually Transmitted Diseases) Directions 2000.

34 General Medical Council. *Good Medical Practice*. London: GMC, 2001: para 55.

35 Health and Social Care Act 2001 s60.

36 The Health Service (Control of Patient Information) Regulations 2002. (SI 2002 No. 1438.)

37 A Health Authority v X and Ors [2002] 2 All ER 780.

38 Department of Health. *NHS complaints procedures: confidentiality*. London: DoH, 1998. (HSC 1998/059.) Scottish Executive Health Department. *Guidance for NHS complaints: hospital and community health services. Guidance for NHS complaints: family health services. Guidance for NHS complaints: health boards*. Edinburgh: SEHD, 1999. Northern Ireland has not published guidance on the confidentiality aspects of complaints procedures.

39 Department of Health. *Confidentiality of medical records: procedure where a patient's former GP wishes to refer to medical records*. London: DoH, 1988. (FPCL 08/88.)

40 General Medical Council. *Confidentiality: protecting and providing information*. Op cit: para 46.

41 Medical Act 1983 (as amended); s35A gives the GMC powers to require doctors to supply any document or information that appears relevant to the discharge of the GMC's professional conduct, professional practice, or fitness to practise functions.

42 General Medical Council. *Media inquiries about patients*. London: GMC, 1996.

43 The BMJ offers advice to its contributors in: British Medical Journal. *Guidelines on publishing articles critical of doctors or other health professionals*. London: BMJ, 2003.

44 In Ashworth Hospital Authority v MGN Ltd [2002] 4 All ER 193, the House of Lords ruled that the management of a high security mental hospital still had an independent interest in keeping health records confidential even when the data subject had put the information in the public domain.

45 General Medical Council. *Confidentiality: protecting and providing information*. Op cit: para 34.

46 Further advice, including a chapter on the practical aspects of the assessment of capacity, is given in: British Medical Association, The Law Society. *Assessment of mental capacity: guidance for doctors and lawyers, 2nd ed.* London: BMJ Books, in press.

47 Lord Wilberforce in the case of British Steel Corporation v Granada Television [1981] 1 All ER 417: 455.

48 General Medical Council. *Serious communicable diseases*. London: GMC, 1997: para 22.

49 Police and Criminal Evidence Act 1984 s116.

50 General Medical Council. *Confidentiality: protecting and providing information*. Op cit: para 39.

6: Health records

The questions covered in this chapter include the following.

- What should be put in health records?
- How much control do patients have over what does and does not go into them?
- How long must records be kept?
- Are there special rules for photographs and videos?
- Are there any limits on patients' rights of access to their health records?

Records and record keeping

Health records exist to provide a record of patients' contact with healthcare providers. They act as an *aide memoire* and facilitate communication with and about patients. Their primary purpose is to support patient care, but they also contain information that is useful for clinical audit, financial planning, management, and research aimed at providing better patient care in the future. As is discussed further in other chapters, they are also increasingly used for a range of social purposes at the request of patients.

The information doctors put in health records falls into four broad categories:

- description from the patient or perhaps a relative or friend concerned about the patient's health
- observation by the health professional, including the outcome of examinations or tests
- an interpretation of these two sets of information, usually in the form of diagnosis or assessment of the problem
- documentation of the problem's management, including treatment, referral, prescription and outcome.

Records include notes made during consultations, correspondence between health professionals such as referral and discharge letters, results of tests and their interpretation, x ray films, videotapes, photographs, and other materials produced in the course of care. Tissue samples taken for diagnostic purposes may also be considered an extension of the record and subject to similar controls. The principles in this chapter apply to all identifiable patient information, however it is stored.

General principles

Many of the ethical issues that arise in relation to records are to do with confidentiality and disclosure of information. These issues are dealt with in

Chapter 5. This chapter focuses on the practical issues to do with records and record keeping. The following principles apply to all types of records, whether they are held manually, on computer, or stored in some other way, for example archived onto microfiche.

- The primary purpose of health records is to support direct care to the patient.
- Secondary purposes include audit, teaching, and research.
- Good quality records are factual, accurate, contemporaneous, and legible.
- Records must be stored and handled securely.
- Sharing the content of records with patients helps to strengthen the doctor–patient relationship and can help to improve accuracy.

Record keeping

Content of records

Doctors must keep "clear, accurate, legible, and contemporaneous patient records that report the relevant clinical findings, the decisions made, the information given to patients, and any drugs or other treatment prescribed".[1] The key information that is recorded includes:

- presenting symptoms and reasons for seeking health care
- relevant clinical findings and diagnosis
- options for care and treatment discussed with the patient
- risks and benefits of care and treatment options, as explained to the patient
- decisions about care and treatment, including evidence of the patient's agreement
- action taken and outcomes.

Some matters that are recorded in health records are speculation, or may later prove to be incorrect. Doctors should not be wary of recording their speculations when these have a bearing on decisions about care or treatment. It is not uncommon for doctors to provide treatment based on an interim diagnosis that later investigations disprove. It is important that the health records show a continuous record of all action taken and outcomes, and this type of information should remain on the records even if further investigation suggests a different approach. The records should, of course, indicate clearly such changes in approach, and put any previous diagnoses and management into context.

Personal views about the patient's behaviour or temperament should not be included in health records unless these have a potential bearing on treatment. Where behaviour or temperament are being recorded, the record should include a factual account. Recording the patient's actual words or phrases can be helpful.

Aggressive behaviour

Doctors sometimes ask whether they may record in a health record that the patient has been aggressive or threatening to staff. Patients should be aware, perhaps through the use of notices in waiting rooms, that such behaviour will not be tolerated, and any incidents will be documented in their records. Dealing with violent and aggressive patients is addressed in Chapter 1 on the doctor–patient relationship.

Records should be made promptly. A contemporaneous record is more likely to be an accurate reflection of actual events, rather than an interpretation with the benefit of hindsight. Retrospective documentation may suggest that a course of action was based on dubious reasoning, or needs extensive justification. It is also important that records show clearly the reasoning behind treatment or management. Documenting the thought-processes not only benefits health professionals using the records in the future, it also protects the health professional in cases of litigation. Even if additional, or non-contemporaneous, entries to a record are entirely accurate, the mere fact of tampering could jeopardise a legal case. If after the contemporaneous note has been made it becomes clear that more information should have been included, a fresh entry should be made, dated accordingly, with an explanation of why additional information is now considered necessary.

Tampering with records – examples from the Medical Defence Union

In one case defended by the Medical Defence Union, the original health record contained an entry by a doctor concerning a consultation with a patient. At a pre-trial conference where the records were being discussed, a photocopied set of the same records was produced that did not contain this entry. The copies had been taken when the claim was first notified and before the doctor had had the opportunity to make his later, spurious entry in the records.

In another case, a 5-year-old child with an apparently simple viral infection was seen by a GP. Five hours later, the child became moribund and was taken to hospital by the parents. The child was diagnosed with meningococcal meningitis and septicaemia. The child recovered, but was left brain damaged. The parents sued and the child's records were disclosed to their solicitors. It was clear that the records were false for three reasons.

- The note of the contact with the GP was considerably longer and more detailed than the records of other consultations.
- The form on which the notes were made was printed two years after the incident.

(Continued)

- A questioned documents forensic expert would be able to show that the notes of the event were not contemporaneous, by using microscopes, tracing infrared and ultraviolet techniques, measuring subtle handwriting changes, and dating the age of the inks.

In both these cases, even if the new entries were an accurate reflection of the events, the mere fact that records had been tampered with would jeopardise the doctors' defence.[2]

Records do not necessarily have to include every piece of paper received in connection with patients or every piece of information. Nor does everything that is added to a record necessarily become a permanent feature of that record that may never be deleted. GPs and trusts (in consultation with doctors) should determine which elements should be considered as a permanent part of the record, and which are transient and may be discarded as they cease to be of value. A common question to the BMA is whether GPs need to retain appointment books. The information in these books is duplicated in patients' records, and so there are no reasons why they cannot be destroyed once they have outlived their usefulness to the practice.

Omitting information from health records

Patients sometimes take steps to avoid information being recorded in their GP record. For example, a patient may choose to go outside his or her GP practice for HIV testing. In the past, even a negative test for HIV had adverse implications for insurance applications, with insurers assuming that anybody who had been tested was at increased risk of infection. Since 1994, however, the Association of British Insurers has instructed its members not to make such inferences. Insurers should not ask for negative HIV test results and doctors should not provide this information. Patients should be encouraged to allow their usual GP to be informed about care they are receiving elsewhere, and be reassured that all doctors are obliged to keep information about patients confidential.

Similarly, some patients ask their doctor not to make a note of some clinical fact. It has been argued that conditions for which there is no effective treatment or programme of management are sometimes irrelevant to health records. Before doctors omit such information from the record, they should be absolutely convinced that doing so could have no detrimental effect on the care of the patient, for their own protection as well as that of the patient. A doctor could be open to criticism if relevant clinical information was omitted from the record and the patient suffered harm because of it. Explaining to the patient how confidentiality will be ensured can help to allay concerns about inadvertent disclosure.

Removing information from health records

Closely linked to requests to omit information from records is when patients ask for information to be removed. Reasons for a request for removal may be very similar to requests for information to be omitted, although these can be more difficult to handle. Once relevant clinical information has been recorded in a health record there are difficulties with removing it. It may be that a doctor is faced with a request to remove information which, although factually accurate and clinical in nature, he or she might have decided not to record in the first place.

There is, of course, no ethical difficulty with removing or correcting inaccurate or misleading information, or making a clear addition to incomplete information. It is obviously important that records do not contain information that may mislead another health professional who uses them. Indeed, the Data Protection Act 1998 gives patients a right to have inaccurate records amended.

It is inadvisable, on the other hand, to remove relevant (usually considered in terms of "medically relevant") information from patient records. It is important that notes provide a contemporaneous record of consultations and information gained about patients. To remove relevant medical information may, for example, give the impression that the notes have been tampered with for an underhand reason, and may make later treatment and care decisions seem unsupported. The purpose of the health record is to record the patient's contact with healthcare providers and any interventions that took place. If it becomes obvious that interventions were inappropriate, this must be reflected clearly in the notes. The fact that a particular treatment was given may have long term implications, however. Interventions generally reflect important aspects of the patient's contact with caregivers and an accurate record is essential. It follows that doctors must take care to ensure that the records show all significant aspects of care, and clearly identify any decisions that were later found to have been inappropriate so that future carers do not misinterpret the patient's medical history.

If there is a dispute about the accuracy of information, for example, that which was recorded by a previous GP, doctors should take reasonable steps to ascertain the veracity of the records. If this is not possible, a note explaining the patients' views should be appended to the records. This allows health professionals who use the records in the future to be wary of placing undue weight on disputed information.

Transsexualism

GPs sometimes ask what to do with the records of people who are transsexual, which should reflect the gender by which these persons are commonly known. New NHS numbers are available for these patients. In Scotland and Northern Ireland, NHS numbers are not changed until the patient has undergone surgery.

(Continued)

Information about gender reassignment surgery should be kept in accordance with the usual rules about retaining medically relevant information. It would be inappropriate to remove all reference to a person's pre-surgery gender, for example.

Patients sometimes request the removal of information that is "social" or which they feel is not relevant to their health and so should not have been recorded. The BMA has no objection to the deletion of such information, provided that both parties agree, and it is done in a way that makes clear that the record has not been inappropriately changed. Doctors may consider that some social information is relevant, however, and could be used, for example, if a GP was asked to comment on suitability for clinical assistance with reproduction. Decisions must be made on a case by case basis, taking into account the particular circumstances. If a decision to remove irrelevant information is taken, a deletion should be made clearly, with an explanation that the deletion is of irrelevant information.

Adoption

What to record about the fact that a patient has been adopted raises questions about record keeping. The fact of adoption may not, in itself, be medically relevant, but the fact that a child is not genetically related to his or her parents may be. Similarly, if the true parents are known to be carriers of a genetic condition, this may have implications for the child's future care. It is worth noting, however, that many children are not the genetic child of those whom they assume to be their father and assumptions about genetic ties may not always be true.

Decisions about whether to include information on adoption must be taken on a case by case basis. Parents of adopted children are encouraged to be frank with them about the fact of adoption. It may be helpful to talk to parents about whether they are planning to tell the child about his or her adoption so that the risks of inadvertent disclosure are put within context. It could be harmful or distressing for individuals to discover inadvertently, and when unprepared, that their background is not as they had been led to believe.

If patients ask for relevant information to be removed from their records, doctors should explain why the information should be included and reassure the patient that nobody, including the patient's family, friends, employer, or insurer, can access the record without the patient's permission. Doctors should reassure patients that even though they will be assumed to have given implied consent for their information to be shared within the healthcare team, they do have the option to object if they wish, although refusal to allow information to be shared could, in some circumstances, jeopardise their care. It may also reassure patients to know that everybody who comes into contact with personal health information is obliged to keep it confidential. If the patient's primary concern is insurance or employment, doctors should point out that they could not be untruthful in a report. Even if a sensitive diagnosis is not included in the record, doctors could not omit relevant information of which they are aware from a report, because to do so could expose them to allegations of fraud.

Facilitating access to records

Doctors should ensure that their manner of keeping records facilitates access by patients. Patients are entitled to see, and have copies of, their health records, although occasionally information has to be withheld, for example, where it identifies a third party such as a family member (see page 217). Doctors should order, flag, or highlight records so that when patients seek access to their records, any information that should not be disclosed can be separated easily from the information to be disclosed.

Documenting patients' views about confidentiality

If patients express views about future disclosure to third parties, this should be documented clearly in the records. Occasionally, it may appear to doctors that disclosure of information will become an issue at a time when the patient is unable to express a view, if he or she becomes incapacitated, for example, or after his or her death. Doctors may want to counsel their patients about such future disclosures and record their wishes in the records. People receiving hospital care are often asked to nominate their next of kin, the person whom health professionals keep informed about their care (see Chapter 1, pages 34–5). This should be explained to patients on admission.

Tagging records

Occasionally, doctors consider tagging patients' records to draw immediate attention to a piece of information, which may be clinical or social. In the past this has meant that coloured stickers have been used on patients' files so that everybody who sees the file knows that the patient is, for example, diabetic, allergic to certain medication, or linked to an at risk register. The BMA has some concerns about such systems. They potentially compromise confidentiality since, as well as drawing the attention of health professionals to important information, they may incidentally alert all staff to clinical details or social facts such as child abuse. It is preferable to find an alternative that maintains confidentiality. Tagging is acceptable only when it is the sole effective system and involves less inadvertent disclosure than the available alternatives.

With electronic records, tagging may mean including a specific screen with the important information. Access to the screen should be restricted to those who need to know the information as part of their work, so maintaining confidentiality should be less problematic.

In all cases in which records are tagged, patients should be told and their consent sought. When young children's records are tagged, permission will usually come from their parents until the child is able to decide for himself or herself. Patients' wishes about tagging when it compromises their confidentiality should be respected unless there is an overriding public interest that warrants a breach of confidentiality, for example when there is a risk of future violence. Dealing with violent patients is discussed in Chapter 1 (pages 58–60).

Summary – record keeping

Records must:

- be clear, accurate, factual, legible, and contemporaneous
- include relevant clinical findings, decisions made, information given to patients, drugs, or treatment prescribed
- identify clearly information that the patient does not want revealed to third parties.

Records must not:

- contain personal views about the patient's temperament or behaviour if these have no bearing on health care
- be altered or tampered with other than to remove incorrect or misleading information (amendments must be made in a way that makes clear why they have been altered).

Recordings

The general principles about record keeping apply to all types of records. There are some additional principles that are important for photographs and audio and video recordings.

The General Medical Council (GMC) advises doctors to:

- seek permission to make the recording and obtain consent for any use or disclosure
- give patients adequate information about the purpose of the recording when seeking their permission
- ensure that patients are under no pressure to give their permission for the recording to be made
- stop the recording if the patient asks, or if it is having an adverse effect on the consultation or treatment

- not participate in any recording made against a patient's wishes
- ensure that the recording does not compromise patients' privacy and dignity
- refrain from using recordings for purposes outside the scope of the original consent for use, without obtaining further consent
- make appropriate secure arrangements for storage of recordings.[3]

Identifiable recordings

Generally, consent is needed before a recording is made. Patients should be told if they are being recorded as part of their assessment or treatment, for audit, for research, or for medicolegal purposes. They should understand the purpose of the recording, who will be allowed to access it, whether copies will be made, the arrangements for storage, and how long the recording will be kept. Clearly, some recordings are an integral part of assessment or treatment, and refusal may affect the ability to provide care. Patients need to understand the effect of any refusal. Generally, however, refusals should not affect the quality of care patients receive.

When people cannot give consent for themselves, agreement should be sought from a close relative, a carer, or, in Scotland, a proxy decision maker. Parents are usually responsible for authorising recordings of young children, while competent young people choose for themselves. In emergencies, where patients cannot give consent, recordings that would be valuable for audit or teaching may be made if this would not prejudice the patient's care or treatment, and provided that people close to the patient do not object. Consent for making recordings of anaesthetised patients should ideally be sought in advance, but if there is an unexpected development, a recording of which would be valuable, the recording may be made and consent to keep and use it sought once the patient regains consciousness. Again, it is important that the making of the recording does not prejudice the patient's care.

After a recording has been made, patients should be given the opportunity to see it and to withdraw consent for its future use. Minors must be able to withdraw consent upon attaining maturity. When the minor continues to be a patient, there should be opportunities to discuss permission as he or she becomes able to decide. Similarly, incapacitated patients should be given the opportunity to decide if they regain the capacity to make a decision. It is good practice to reaffirm consent for all continued use of identifiable recordings, and this regular contact may provide an opportunity for previously incapacitated people to decide.

Except when patients have given specific consent to other arrangements, patient identifiable recordings should remain part of the patient's confidential medical record, subject to the same safeguards as other data. No identifying material may be published in textbooks or journals, or used for teaching without express patient consent, and patients should understand that, once material is published and in the public domain, it is unlikely to be possible to withdraw it from circulation. That aside, the BMA takes the view that consent is not blanket permission but should be periodically renewed, at intervals of five years for example, when there should be the option to withdraw material from use or limit its future use. When consent is withdrawn, as far as possible all copies and the master material should be destroyed and only material that is part of the patient's health record should be kept.

Covert surveillance is discussed in Chapter 1 (pages 45–7).

Anonymised recordings

Some recordings, unless associated with other details, do not identify patients. The GMC identifies five categories that fall into this group of anonymous recordings:

- images from pathology slides (glass slides from microscopy)
- x ray films
- laparoscopic images
- images of internal organs
- ultrasound images.

The GMC advises that these recordings may be made during treatment without separate consent from patients, although it is clearly good practice to tell patients that images are being made as part of their care or treatment. When these images are not labelled in a way that identifies the patient, the GMC advises that they may be used for any purpose, for example in research, audit, or teaching, without consent.[4] The GMC also advises that it is acceptable to use these anonymous images in publications without patients' consent, since they cannot be recognised from these images alone. Of course, an image of this type, when used in connection with a case history could make a patient identifiable, and would, therefore, require permission.

The images listed above are, when presented alone, intrinsically anonymous. Other images may be anonymised by removing identifying details, after which they may be used more freely than those that remain identifiable. Anonymisation must be effective; simply printing a bar across a patient's eyes would not be sufficient, for example. The GMC draws a distinction between the use of these types of anonymised recordings for purposes such as teaching and the publication of images in media to which the public may have access, including medical journals. As a general rule, any image that is anonymised may be used for teaching without consent; but, since apparently insignificant features may be capable of identifying an individual, and it is difficult to be absolutely certain that a patient cannot be identified from an image, no recording other than those mentioned above may be published in publicly accessible media without consent.

Photographs

Photographic records are used in some specialties, especially in paediatric, and accident and emergency departments. Whenever feasible, photographs should be taken only with the patient's consent. Children's parents should also be asked for permission; this is essential if children are unable to give consent for themselves.

Even when children are not able to give valid consent, there is a clear duty to seek their cooperation and to explain the purpose of the photograph if this is feasible. Whenever possible, photography and video recording of children should be undertaken by a properly accredited medical illustrator.

Documenting suspected cases of child abuse sometimes involves photographic records. Although parental consent should be sought, if such clinical illustration is required for legal purposes, for example because it is required by a court, and alerting the parent would put the child at increased risk, photographs may be taken without consent.

When photographs are used in teaching or research, whenever possible they should be anonymised. If this is not possible, consent from the patient is essential. The consent of parents of young children who are unable to decide for themselves is needed. As with all recordings used in these ways, agreement for continued use should be reconfirmed at regular intervals. This provides an opportunity to seek consent from young people who attain sufficient maturity and understanding to give consent after the recording was made.

Stillborn babies and neonates who are on the point of death are sometimes photographed at the request of the parents, but photographs should not be used for any other purposes, unless the parents indicate that this would be acceptable. Great sensitivity is required regarding this issue.

Video recordings

Video recordings are becoming increasingly common in clinical use, especially in the field of paediatric psychiatry and as a teaching tool. These records should be subject to the same general safeguards as other confidential, patient identifiable material. Patient consent is generally required for making a recording; further consent is required for its use in an identifiable form in teaching, audit, or research, and additional consent is required for its wider dissemination to, for instance, medical video libraries. Some bodies, including the BMA, have been concerned that doctors are not able to exercise adequate control over such visual teaching material, which could be copied illegally. It is difficult, if not impossible, to police provisions that all material must be withdrawn if the patient revokes consent to its use, although all efforts should be made to destroy or anonymise these recordings.

One solution is that video recordings can be edited and anonymised by obscuring or "digitising" identifying features. Although this is not universally possible, it is recommended that this procedure be followed wherever feasible. Patients' facial expressions, however, are important for some purposes, such as teaching that involves neurological and neuropsychological conditions. Unfortunately, this often involves patients who are incapable of giving consent. In practice, relatives, or proxy decision makers in Scotland, authorise the use of such material for teaching, provided that this is not contrary to the patient's interests and a recording of a patient who is able to give consent would not suffice. Even when their authorisation has no basis in law, the BMA considers this to be good practice.

Audio recordings

In many areas, not only in health care, telephone calls are recorded for medicolegal purposes. When telephone calls to a practice or out of hours service are recorded, patients need to be told that conversations are being recorded and why. A failure to do so could mean that these recordings are unlawful. Information should also be available concerning how long recordings are kept and how patients can access them. As a general rule, the BMA encourages doctors to share information with patients whenever possible. If patients want to listen to recordings, this should be facilitated, if possible via the doctor who usually provides their care. The recording forms part of the patient's medical record, and could be accessible under the access provisions of the Data Protection Act (see pages 216–20).

A recommendation of *The report of the public inquiry into children's heart surgery at the Bristol Royal Infirmary 1984–1995* (the Bristol report) is that "tape-recording facilities should be provided by the NHS to enable patients, should they so wish, to make a tape recording of a discussion with a healthcare professional when a diagnosis, course of treatment, or prognosis is being discussed".[5] The BMA supports the concept when the aim is to assist patients to understand and recall facts. Doctors worry, however, if they feel that they are being recorded for future complaints or litigation, and may be less likely to want to express opinions freely. This issue is discussed further in Chapter 1 (pages 50–1).

Summary – recordings

- Audio and video recordings form part of health records.
- Consent should be sought before recordings are made.
- When consent is not available because the patient lacks capacity, recordings may be made when this is not contrary to the patient's interests and authorisation is given by parents or people close to the patient.
- When the patient is temporarily incapacitated, consent must be sought for the use of the recordings once the patient regains capacity.
- Images from which it is impossible to identify the patient, generally internal images and pathology slides, may be used for teaching, audit, or research without consent, but such uses of identifiable images require consent.

Databases

A database is a system that allows data to be stored and retrieved. Systems that store health records, manually or on paper, for example, are databases. Other databases hold information for specific purposes, such as for use in research, teaching, public health surveillance, or disease management. The principles in this chapter about access, data integrity, security, and retention apply equally to personal health information that is stored in databases. Similarly, the principles in Chapter 5 about the use and disclosure of information are relevant.

The World Medical Association has identified some additional ethical considerations relevant to the use and storage of health data on databases.[6] In particular, it recommends that there should be a medically qualified guardian of a database to help to focus responsibility for monitoring and ensuring compliance with the principles of confidentiality and security. It also proposes that ethical review committees should be involved in decisions about the use of data on databases.

Ownership

For most purposes, establishing who owns the information or health record is not significant. What matters is who has control of records and information. The question of who owns health records is sometimes asked, however. In law, the concept of ownership of information is very underdeveloped. Many differentiate between the information, which belongs to the patient, the opinion, which the doctor brings to that raw information, and the documentation of this process. Private doctors, or occasionally their employers, are considered to own the records they make (for discussion of what happens to records when private practitioners retire or leave their employer see page 216). NHS records are understood in law to be the property of the Secretary of State for Health. In the past, the BMA has expressed grave anxiety about this situation because, in the absence of conditions to the contrary, ownership implies control. Generally, unless there is overriding statutory authority, conditions set by the owner of records must be observed. Prior to 1998, there was no such statutory authority and, arguably therefore, nothing to prevent the Secretary of State from imposing inappropriate conditions on record holders. In 1998, however, the Data Protection Act made it a statutory requirement for data processing to meet common law standards for confidentiality. The Act applies to all manual and computerised health records, and clearly prohibits inappropriate conditions being imposed by data "owners".

Security

All health professionals, and everybody else employed by or working under contract to a healthcare establishment, have obligations of confidentiality. They should be asked to sign a confidentiality agreement stating that they understand the obligation of confidentiality and will not breach it. In addition doctors have particular obligations relating to the storage and use of health information, and may be held responsible for any breaches of confidentiality resulting from insecure handling. Doctors could face criminal charges as well as private actions by patients if they fail to provide adequate protection for health information. Protection is needed against both external threats such as burglary and internal threats such as inappropriate access by staff. Even the simplest security measures can be effective.

- Lock doors, offices and filing cabinets.
- Avoid leaving paper or computer files open where they may be seen by others.
- Do not leave files unattended.
- Password protect computer systems and do not share passwords with other people.

When records are stored remotely, for example on a centralised server, doctors must ensure that the remote facility has in place adequate safeguards to protect the information.[7] The Information Commissioner has said that while he does not necessarily expect each GP practice, for example, to develop its own IT system capable of concealing the identities of patients from those who do not need to know them, he does expect those who are developing IT systems for use by GPs to build in such a capability and would certainly consider action against a GP (or any other data controller) who did not make use of the features available on a system for maximising the privacy of patients.[8]

Practice staff

Staff in GP practices may know people who are patients of the practice. The BMA is aware of cases in which GP reception staff have inappropriately accessed the records of family members or acquaintances. There should be security measures in place to prevent inappropriate "browsing" of records. Having more than one member of staff on duty at all times can help, for example. Electronic systems should make use of the ability to restrict individuals' access to a level that is suitable for their job.

GPs are also advised to take only necessary information with them when they leave the surgery to visit patients, because occasionally records have been stolen from doctors' cars. In many cases, the danger of possible loss or theft is outweighed by the improved quality of care that can be provided when the health records are available, but all reasonable precautions must be taken to ensure that identifiable information is not left unattended in risky situations. The level of protection for electronic data being taken home on laptops or other portable electronic equipment is exactly the same as would be expected in the surgery.

For the record

In 1995 the Audit Commission published the results of its study of hospital medical records. It found poor standards of record keeping, missing case notes and untidy and overcrowded libraries. Its report said that:

> In nearly two thirds of the hospitals visited casenotes were taken out of the hospital by clinical staff for research and other purposes. They had been known to be left under the doormat in doctors' residences and in the boots of cars. In one instance a doctor sold his car with patients' casenotes still in the boot.[9]

Health records should be stored in a secure way, with proper environmental control and adequate protection against fire and flood. Where records that are not in regular use are held only in electronic form, extra care may be needed to prevent corruption or deterioration of the data. Re-recording or migration of data may also need to be considered as equipment and software become obsolete.

Transmission

Frequently, doctors ask about the implications of using technology to communicate patient details electronically, by fax or email, for example. The Association recognises that these are common and convenient media, but reminds doctors that they are responsible for ensuring that identifiable information does not arrive in the wrong hands. The GMC states that doctors "must be satisfied that there are appropriate arrangements for the security of personal information when it is stored, sent or received by fax, computer, e-mail or other electronic means".[10] Whenever possible, clinical details must be separated from demographic data so that, should information fall into the wrong hands, it cannot readily be linked to an individual. Obvious measures, such as using a unique identifying number rather than the patient's name and address, may be useful. In addition, all data transmitted by email must be encrypted.[11] This is necessary both to protect confidentiality and to ensure that doctors do not breach their obligation under the Data Protection Act to take adequate precautions to protect the confidential nature of information being transmitted. Doctors should also make sure that, when data are being sent by email, messages will be received and dealt with, including if the intended recipient is absent, for example on holiday.

When information is being transmitted by fax, it is sensible to enquire whether the receiving machine is in a publicly accessible area, such as a waiting room, or in a private office. The BMA recommends that patient-identifiable information should be faxed only when the receiving machine is known to be secure both during and out of working hours. These and other mechanisms for ensuring that patient information is received only by the intended recipient are described as "safe-haven" procedures. All health service organisations should have such procedures in place. The Department of Health gives detailed advice about safe haven procedures that includes the following key points.[12]

- All information exchanged should be between safe haven contact points.
- Audit procedures should track the movement of all confidential information.
- Photocopying of confidential information should be avoided as far as possible.
- When not in use, paper-based information should be kept within folders, envelopes or other containers that prevent sight of the paper, and be kept locked securely away.
- Information being transferred between safe haven points should be in a locked briefcase or other secure device.
- Physical access to the safe haven area should be restricted to those with the appropriate authority.

- Safe haven areas should have only one "normal" entry point.
- Archived material should be kept locked and access to it restricted.
- Offices in safe haven areas should be locked when not in use.
- Access should be on a need to know basis only.
- Measures must be in place to prevent casual scanning of information, including by password control on computer systems.
- The identity of telephone callers must be confirmed.

All members of staff should be aware of the procedures for the safe handling of confidential information.

Transfer of GP records

The health records of a patient who leaves a GP practice are transferred to the patient's new GP via the primary care trust (PCT) or, in Northern Ireland, the Central Services Agency (CSA). If a patient leaves a computerised practice, a hard copy of his or her medical record at that date should be sent to the PCT or CSA inside the manual record envelope, for onward transmission to the patient's new GP. Electronic transfer of records should also be encouraged, and systems are being established to allow this to be done successfully. Advice should be sought from the PCT or CSA about electronic transfer.

Strictly speaking, it may be a breach of the Data Protection Act for GPs to retain information about patients who are no longer under their care. The Act's fifth principle prohibits doctors from keeping data for longer than is necessary. The BMA is, however, concerned about the potential for records to be corrupted or lost in transfer. Until such a time as electronic records (and their associated audit trail) can be transferred reliably between practices, the BMA advises doctors not to delete the electronic records of patients who have left their practice. It is essential that a complete and uncorrupted version of the record exists at all times, in the interests of both patients and doctors. This position has been agreed with the Office of the Information Commissioner, the independent supervisory authority that enforces and oversees the Data Protection Act. During this interim period, when a patient is no longer receiving services from a practice, his or her record should be archived and accessed only when there is a valid reason to do so.[13] The BMA has received complaints about doctors who continue to use information, for example to send unsolicited letters to people who are no longer their patients.

Retention of records

The primary purpose of making and maintaining health records is the provision of health care to the patient. Records serve many other useful purposes, however, and, with appropriate authorisation, may be useful for research, teaching, and litigation, virtually without limit of time, although there are legal rules governing the time limits within which actions for personal injuries or death may be brought.

The health departments give detailed advice about the retention of NHS records. A summary of the main points for GP and hospital records is given in the tables below. The recommendations apply to electronic and manual records, and the BMA advises private practitioners to follow the same rules. The retention of pathology records is covered in Chapter 12 (page 439).

After the appropriate minimum period has expired, the need to retain records further should be carefully, and if necessary periodically, reviewed. Records retained after these minimum periods remain confidential and should be stored and handled appropriately. In some cases, for example, it may be appropriate to anonymise records that are being maintained for historical research purposes. It may be a breach of data protection legislation to retain identifiable information about living patients for longer than is necessary, although special considerations apply for computerised records that cannot be transferred successfully (see page 213).

Records could be required in litigation virtually without limit of time, so it is inevitable that some may be destroyed that might otherwise subsequently have been required for litigation. The Department of Health has taken the view that the cost of indefinite retention of records would greatly exceed the liabilities likely to be incurred in the occasional case where defence to an action for damages may be handicapped by the absence of records. However, doctors must be careful to ensure that, if it is known that records may be needed in litigation, they are not destroyed.[14] Private practitioners are unlikely to be criticised if they retain records for the minimum period recommended by the NHS.

Recommended minimum lengths of retention of GP records (England, Wales, and Northern Ireland)[15]

Type	Retention period
Maternity records	25 years
Records relating to children and young people (including paediatric, vaccination and community child health service records)	Until the patient's 25th birthday, or 26th if an entry was made when the young person was 17; or 10 years after death of a patient if sooner
Records relating to persons receiving treatment for a mental disorder within the meaning of mental health legislation	20 years after no further treatment considered necessary; or 10 years after patient's death if sooner
Records relating to those serving in HM Armed Forces	Not to be destroyed
Records relating to those serving a prison sentence	Not to be destroyed
All other personal health records	10 years after conclusion of treatment, the patient's death or after the patient has permanently left the country

Recommended minimum lengths of retention of hospital records (England, Wales, and Northern Ireland)[16]

Type	Retention period
Maternity records (including all obstetric and midwifery records, including those of episodes of maternity care that end in stillbirth or where the child later dies)	25 years
Children and young people	Until the patient's 25th birthday, or 26th if young person was aged 17 at conclusion of treatment; or 8 years after patient's death if death occurred before 18th birthday
Mentally disordered persons within the meaning of mental health legislation	20 years after no further treatment considered necessary, or 8 years after the patient's death if the patient died while still receiving treatment
Donor records	11 years post-transplantation
Oncology	8 years after conclusion of treatment
Patients involved in clinical trials	15 years after conclusion of treatment
All other records	8 years after conclusion of treatment

Summary of minimum retention periods for personal health records (Scotland)[17]

Type	Retention period
Maternity records	25 years
Records relating to children and young people (under 16 years on admission)	Until the patient's 25th birthday, or 3 years after death of the patient if sooner
Psychiatric records	3 years after the patient's death, unless containing entries made on or before 31 December 1960, in which case, not to be destroyed
Oncology	3 years after the patient's death
All other personal health records	6 years after conclusion of treatment, or 3 years after the patient's death
GP records	3 years after the patient's death

Disposal

When doctors are responsible for destroying records, they must ensure that the method of destruction is effective and does not compromise confidentiality. Incineration, pulping, and shredding are appropriate methods of destroying paper records. Doctors must similarly ensure that electronic data are deleted effectively. Again, this may involve incineration or other methods of physical destruction.

Private records

When private practitioners retire and there is a successor for their practice, the records should be passed to the new doctor. If there is no successor, records should be stored securely for the appropriate period (see pages 213–5) or, with the patient's consent, passed to another doctor who is providing care. Patients should be informed of any changes in arrangements for their records.[18]

Private doctors should make a will with instructions for how their records should be handled after their death. Ideally, the records should be transferred to another doctor to take responsibility for their care. If there is no arrangement for succession to a private practice, the person administering the estate distributes the deceased's property. If no doctor can be found to take the records, one option is for the records to be given to the patients to take with them to their next doctor. Alternatively, and if there is no other reason to retain records, those falling outwith the recommended minimum retention periods may be destroyed. Those administering a deceased doctor's estate should bear in mind that the patients to whom the records relate are entitled to expect that their confidentiality will be maintained. Patients may have a right to sue the holder of the records if information about them is wrongly disclosed. To minimise risks to confidentiality, therefore, ideally a registered health professional should sort through records to establish which ones may be destroyed. Those with custody of records should bear in mind that patients also retain their rights of access to their records (see below).

For information about occupational health records see pages 590–2.

Access to health records

Access by patients

In the past, the concept of confidentiality meant that health records were kept secret from patients themselves. Nowadays, there is broad support for openness and frankness between doctors and patients. Although patients have long had the opportunity to apply for access to their health records, few exercise this right and many do not know why they are being referred to another practitioner, or what is being said about them. The Government has promised to give all patients a clear explanation of what is happening to them in the course of their care, and why. For example, from 2004 patients in England and Wales can expect to receive copies of letters between clinicians about their care and, provided that they are found to be effective, smart cards to improve access to health records.[19] The idea is to give patients their own personal record of their contact with the health service. Unfettered access to information also gives the opportunity for patients to check its accuracy, and so can improve the quality of information that is held in records.

Doctors have long had the discretion to show patients the contents of records and the BMA encourages doctors to give patients informal access to their records. Only when releasing information would cause serious harm to the patient or another person, or compromise the confidentiality of a third party, may it be appropriate to withhold information. Withholding access solely because disclosure would be embarrassing for doctors or may give rise to legal claims against them is not acceptable.

Patients also have a statutory right of access to information about themselves, as enshrined in the Data Protection Act 1998. This covers all health records, including reports written to satisfy the requirements of mental health legislation and, in the BMA's view, medical reports written by independent doctors who have no other professional relationship with the patient. The Access to Medical Reports Act 1988 and Access to Medical Reports (Northern Ireland) Order 1991 relate specifically to medical reports for insurance or employment purposes that are written by the patient's own doctor (see page 221) and give rights of access to them. There are limited rights of access to information about deceased patients in the Access to Health Records Act 1990 and Access to Health Records (Northern Ireland) Order 1993.[20]

The law gives patients the right to see and receive copies of their health records. Competent patients, including young people, may apply for access to their own records, or may authorise a third party, such as their solicitor, to do so on their behalf. There is a schedule of fees that may be charged, which vary according to whether the records are held manually or on computer, and whether a copy is requested.[21] Requests for access are made to the person in charge of keeping the records. This is usually the health professional responsible for the patient's care but, when it is not, decisions about disclosure must still be made by an "appropriate health professional".

The law also exempts certain categories of data from its subject access provisions. The category most likely to arise is confidential information that identifies or relates to someone else. No information that identifies any other person can be revealed to the patient without the consent of the person so identified (unless that person is a health professional who has been involved in the patient's care, or it is reasonable to release the information without consent). This may be an area where doctors would have to consider the interests of other parties in allowing the patient access. Information may also be withheld if the doctor believes it would be harmful to the patient or another person, although this should be extremely rare. Doctors may find it helpful to consult others who have contributed to the record for help in assessing the nature and extent of any risk. Detailed advice about access under the Data Protection Act is available from the BMA.[22]

At the time of writing there is considerable debate about whether the exemptions in the legislation are appropriate. Some groups, typically those representing the interests of patients, argue that people should be entitled to see all records held by health professionals about them and their care. Others argue that giving completely open access could, albeit in very rare circumstances, lead to avoidable serious harm to the patient or another person. It could also inhibit the candour with which relatives and people close to patients speak to doctors about their concerns for their loved one. It is not uncommon, for example, for a spouse to approach the family GP to express concerns about a partner's health that he or she does not feel able to address directly. Similarly, GPs in particular may hold information about possible genetic conditions in close relatives, of which they may be aware because of their professional relationship with the relative. The BMA considers that the use of information in this way can benefit patients, but would not want to see family members' confidentiality eroded by requiring doctors to disclose this information to others. If there are any changes to these or other aspects of access rights, information will be made available on the BMA's website.

Older entries in health records were often not written in the expectation that patients would see the records or receive copies of them, and the BMA is aware of some concern about how to deal with giving access to records written in a way that patients could find upsetting. Doctors may not withhold this type of information if patients exercise their right of access, but they should offer to delete any inappropriate comments. It may be helpful to discuss any potentially distressing entries with patients in advance of access. Attempting to amend entries before giving patients access could give the impression that the records were tampered with for an underhand reason; this could be more damaging than an explanation of, and an apology for, the original comment.

Inappropriate comments

The Medical Defence Union found a strange entry in a medical record during preparations for trial.[23] The entry read: "Still holds bottle".

It turned out that a few additions and deletions had produced this odd comment from the defamatory one of: "Silly old bat".

Needless to say, the patient found out about the original comment and did not appreciate the sentiment expressed.

As a matter of courtesy, doctors sometimes feel that they should inform other doctors about a request for access to records when it is known that litigation is contemplated. There is no obligation to do so, but doctors may wish to inform a colleague when the patient does not object.

Access to the records of children and young people

All competent young people, whatever their age, may exercise a statutory right of access to their own health records. Additionally, people with parental responsibility have a statutory right to apply for access to their child's health records, unless a court has imposed specific conditions to the contrary. This is an area where the tension between parents' rights and young people's developing maturity can come into conflict. It can also highlight tension between parents if unmarried fathers who do not have parental responsibility for their child (see Chapter 4, pages 114–5) believe they have the same rights as their child's mother.

If patients are minors (under 16 in Scotland, under 18 in the rest of the UK) but capable of giving consent, parents can apply to have access to their records only with the young person's consent. As discussed in Chapter 4, parents should ideally help young people to make medical decisions and should be aware of information about their child's care. In some cases, however, young people may wish to keep confidential from their parents some of the matters they have raised with their doctor. Contraceptive advice, examination for sexually transmitted infections, assistance in stopping smoking or drug abuse are examples of matters that young people may wish to conceal from their parents, although doctors should encourage them to involve them whenever possible.

In cases in which a child cannot understand the nature of the application, but parental access would be in his or her interests, the law allows such access. Parental access to a minor's medical record should not be allowed when it conflicts with the child's interests. Any information that the child previously gave in the expectation that it would not be revealed should not be released, although it must be noted that, exceptionally, doctors can breach the confidentiality of any patient if they consider that there are sufficiently serious grounds to justify it (see Chapter 5 on confidentiality).

Parents may exercise this aspect of their parental responsibility separately. If one parent applies for access, there is no requirement to inform the other, although if this would be in the child's best interests, it may be appropriate in some cases. GPs in particular can find themselves in a difficult position when separated parents, independently of each other, want information about their young child's health care. Some parents who do not live with their child ask the GP to contact them each time the child is brought to the surgery. There is no requirement on GPs to agree to such requests, which could entail much time and many resources if the child presents frequently. It is clearly better if parents are able to communicate with each other about their child's health, although doctors may agree to contact a parent under certain circumstances, for example if something serious arises. In any case, both parents may apply for access to the health records at reasonable intervals of time. Doctors are also usually prepared to discuss the child's health informally without requiring that the procedures in the legislation are followed. The aim is to ensure that both parents are involved in the child's health care without imposing a disproportionate burden on the doctor. Only if disclosure to either parent would be contrary to the child's interests, or contrary to a competent child's wishes, should information be withheld.

A problem may arise if a young person who has been prescribed contraception refuses to allow her doctor to grant parental access to her medical record in order to conceal this fact, even though the doctor believes it would be in her best interests for her parents to be informed. The decision to prescribe in such cases turns on the competence and understanding of the patient, so it would follow that a patient capable of making up her mind about contraception should also be able to control access to her health record. More difficult perhaps is the case of a young person who requested contraception that the doctor declined to prescribe on grounds of a lack of comprehension of what was involved. Such decisions are subject to the doctor's clinical judgment in each case, but, unless there are very convincing reasons to the contrary, the doctor should keep this type of request secret even if he or she believes the patient is insufficiently mature for the request to be granted. If, however, the doctor considers the child to be at risk of exploitation or abuse, the limits of confidentiality should be discussed and the young person told that information may exceptionally need to be disclosed.

Access to the records of incapacitated adults

In addition to sharing information with people who are close to an incapacitated patient when this is in his or her interests, in some circumstances a third party may exercise rights of access to the patient's records. When the patient is incapable of managing his or her own affairs, a person appointed by a court to manage those affairs may seek access to the records under the Data Protection Act. Access should be restricted to the information necessary for the appointee to carry out his or her functions. Disclosure is acceptable insofar as it is commensurate with the best interests and previous wishes of the patient. Information given by patients at a time when they were competent and believed it would be kept confidential cannot be disclosed subsequently to other people. Confidentiality and general issues around sharing information with people close to incapacitated adults are discussed in Chapter 5.

Access to the records of deceased persons

The Access to Health Records Act 1990 and Access to Health Records (Northern Ireland) Order 1993 permit limited access to the records of deceased patients. Access may be sought by any person who may have a claim arising from the death of a patient, and rights of access are limited to information directly relevant to that claim. For example, a personal representative or executor can access information to benefit the deceased's estate, as can an individual who was a dependent of the deceased and who has a claim relating to that dependency that has arisen from the death.

Information may be withheld if:

- it identifies a third party who has not given consent for disclosure, unless that person is a health professional who has cared for the patient
- in the opinion of the relevant health professional, it is likely to cause serious harm to somebody's physical or mental health, or
- the patient gave it in the past on the understanding that it would be kept confidential.

It follows that doctors should counsel their patients about the possibility of disclosure after death and solicit views about eventual disclosure where it is obvious in the circumstances that there may be some sensitivity. Such discussions should be documented in the records. In addition to the legal provisions, people who were close to a deceased patient often ask to see the records in order to learn more about the illness of their loved one. Confidentiality and handling requests of this nature are covered in Chapter 12 (pages 436–8).

Access to medical reports

The Access to Medical Reports Act 1988 and Access to Medical Reports (Northern Ireland) Order 1991 give patients rights in respect of reports written about them for employment or insurance purposes. They cover reports written by the applicant's GP or a specialist who has provided care, including an occupational health doctor. Reports written by an independent medical examiner are not covered but, in the BMA's view, patients are entitled to access these reports under the data protection legislation (see pages 216–8).

The administrative requirements of the legislation fall mainly upon the body that requests the report (the applicant). Applicants must inform patients of their rights, including:

- to withhold permission for the company to seek a medical report (that is, to refuse consent to the release of information)
- to have access to the medical report after completion by the doctor either before it is sent to the company or up to 6 months after it is sent
- if seeing the report before it is sent, to instruct the doctor not to send the report
- to request the amendment of inaccuracies in the report.

Patients must be informed when a report is sought and notified in writing of their rights. From the time that the doctor is notified that the patient wants to see the report, the patient has 21 days in which to do so and the doctor should not dispatch the report during this period. If the patient does not contact the doctor within that 21 days, the doctor may send the completed report to the applicant. If the patient sees the report and withdraws consent for it to be released, it must not be dispatched and the doctor should inform the applicant.

Patients are entitled to have any factual inaccuracies in the report corrected. If the doctor does not agree that there is an error, he or she must append a note to the report regarding the disputed information. Doctors must not comply with patients' requests to leave out relevant information from reports. If a patient refuses to give permission for certain relevant information to be included, the doctor should indicate to the applicant that he or she cannot write a report, taking care not to reveal any information the patient did not want revealed.

Summary – access to health records and reports

- Patients and their representatives are entitled to have access to their records and to have copies of them.
- Competent patients may authorise a third party, such as a lawyer, to access records on their behalf.

- Parents may have access to their child's records if this is in the child's best interests and, when the child is competent, if he or she gives consent.
- People appointed to manage the affairs of mentally incapacitated patients may have access to information necessary to fulfil their function.
- Information may be withheld if revealing it may cause serious physical or mental harm to the patient or, in certain circumstances, it relates to a third party who is not a health professional who has cared for the patient.
- Doctors should facilitate information access by patients, and be willing to show them the contents of their records.
- There are fees that may be charged for providing access and copies.
- The records of deceased patients may be accessed by anybody with a claim arising from the patient's death, although information may be withheld if the patient had not wanted it revealed.
- Separate legislation gives additional rights in respect of insurance and employment reports written by the patient's usual doctor.

References

1 General Medical Council. *Good medical practice*. London: GMC, 2001: para 3.
2 Schütte P, Gilberthorpe J. Altering records – beware of the pitfalls. *J Med Defence Union* 1994;**1**:6–7.
3 General Medical Council. *Making and using visual and audio recordings of patients*. London: GMC, 2002: para 1.
4 General Medical Council. *Making and using visual and audio recordings of patients*. Op cit: para 5.
5 The Bristol Royal Infirmary Inquiry. *Learning from Bristol: the report of the public inquiry into children's heart surgery at the Bristol Royal Infirmary 1984–1995*. London: The Stationery Office, 2001: recommendation 10. (Cm 5207(II).)
6 World Medical Association. *Declaration on ethical considerations regarding health databases*. Geneva: WMA, 2002.
7 For discussion of the issues raised by the remote storage of records see: General Practitioners Committee. *Remotely held records and centralised servers*. London: British Medical Association, 2002.
8 Information Commissioner. *Use and disclosure of health data. Guidance on the application of the Data Protection Act 1998*. Wilmslow: Office of the Information Commissioner, 2002.
9 Audit Commission. *Setting the record straight: a study of hospital medical records*. London: HMSO, 1995:31.
10 General Medical Council. *Confidentiality: protecting and providing information*. London: GMC, 2000:21.
11 General Practitioners Committee. *Consulting in the modern world*. London: British Medical Association, 2001.
12 Department of Health. *Handling confidential patient information in contracting: a code of practice*. London: DoH, 1992.
13 General Practitioners Committee. *The Data Protection Act 1998: an updated code of practice for GPs*. London: British Medical Association, 2000.
14 An Appeal Court judge expressed his dissatisfaction with a health authority's destruction of x ray films after 3 years when it was known that legal proceedings were being contemplated, having received initial requests from solicitors for a patient's notes. Hammond v West Lancashire Health Authority [1998] Lloyd's Rep Med 146.
15 Department of Health. *Preservation, retention, and destruction of GP general medical services records relating to patients*. London: DoH, 1998. (HSC 1998/217.) Welsh Office. *Preservation, retention and destruction of GP general medical services records relating to patients*. Cardiff: Welsh Office, 1999. (WHC (99) 7.) Department of Health, Social Services and Public Safety. *Preservation, retention, and destruction of GP medical records*. Belfast: DHSSPS, 2000. (HSS (PCCD) 1/2000.)
16 Department of Health. *For the record – managing records in NHS trusts and health authorities*. London: DoH, 1999. (HSC 1999/053.) National Assembly for Wales. *For the record – managing records in NHS trusts and health authorities*. Cardiff: National Assembly for Wales, 2000. (WHC (2000) 71.) Department

of Health, Social Services and Public Safety. *Communication from information and analysis unit, regional information branch 27 February 2002*. Belfast: DHSSPS, 2002.

17 The Scottish Office. *Guidance for the retention and destruction of health records*. Edinburgh: The Scottish Office, 1993. (NHS MEL (1993) 152.)

18 Under the Data Protection Act 1998, patients must be informed when there is a change of data controller.

19 Department of Health. *The NHS plan*. London: The Stationery Office, 2000. NHS Wales. *Improving health in Wales. A plan for the NHS with its partners*. Cardiff: National Assembly for Wales, 2001.

20 The parts of these pieces of legislation that dealt with access to the records of living patients were repealed by the Data Protection Act 1998.

21 For detailed advice about the Act and the fees, see: British Medical Association. *Access to health records by patients*. London: BMA, 2002.

22 *Ibid.*

23 Schütte P, *et al*. Altering records – beware of the pitfalls. *Op cit.*

7: Contraception, abortion, and birth

> The questions covered in this chapter include the following.
>
> - What factors should be considered when a person aged under 16 requests contraception?
> - Can a woman with severe learning disabilities be sterilised?
> - In what circumstances is abortion lawful?
> - Should prenatal genetic testing be offered for adult onset disorders?
> - Is it acceptable to continue to provide life support for a permanently unconscious pregnant woman in order to give her fetus the greatest chance of survival?
> - Should women be able to choose to deliver by caesarean section?
> - Can a woman refuse a caesarean section if that refusal would result in the death of a viable fetus?

The nature of reproductive ethics

The increasing ability of people to exercise control over fertility and reproduction has led to major changes in the way people live their lives. Women are now able to exercise choice over whether and when to have children to a greater extent than ever before. This and the next chapter discuss the issues raised concerning reproduction in the broad sense of the range of issues that arise throughout an individual's "reproductive career". They cover the decision of whether to have children (issues around contraception, sterilisation and abortion), dilemmas raised by pregnancy and birth, and the increased ability to help people to have children through assisted reproduction. The issues discussed concern not only individuals but, in some cases, their families and society at large. Although inevitably much of the discussion focuses on the rights and duties of women, as those who physically bear children, this is in no way intended to dismiss or undermine the important role of men in reproduction. Although emphasis is often placed on the provision of contraception to young women, boys and men also need advice about contraception and sexual health. Similarly, although decisions about the progress of a pregnancy ultimately rest with the woman carrying the fetus, fathers also have a role to play in decision making, particularly when they intend to take an active part in bringing up the child.

Reproduction differs from many other areas of medical practice because of its complexity and because tension can sometimes arise between the rights of women to make decisions about their own bodies and the moral duties owed to unborn children. It is this aspect of reproduction that is at the root of many of the ethical, legal, social, and psychological questions that continue to trouble society. Control over one's body, abortion, reproduction, and parenthood are matters about which most people hold strong views. For many, such views are based on moral, religious, or cultural convictions. Given the existence of such diversity of opinion, it is clear that some of these questions can never be resolved to the satisfaction of all sections of society, but will be the subject of continuing ethical debate. Broad areas of moral consensus can, however, be sketched out after wideranging consultation and public debate, and these form the basis of legislation, guidance, and practice in this area.

General principles

When considering questions about contraception, abortion, and birth, the following general principles should apply.

- The confidentiality of all patients, including those aged under 16, should be respected except in exceptional cases.
- Young people who are sufficiently mature to understand the nature and implications of the treatment requested are able to give valid consent, but parental involvement should be encouraged.
- No treatment may be provided to a competent adult without valid consent.
- Adults are presumed to be competent unless there is clear evidence to the contrary. (Being in labour does not, in itself, render a woman incompetent to make decisions.)
- Women should be encouraged to participate to the greatest possible extent in decisions about their pregnancy.
- A woman who plans to carry her fetus to term has special moral responsibilities towards the unborn child, but neither health professionals nor society can force her to fulfil those duties.
- Discussion about reproduction inevitably focuses primarily on women, but the role of men should not be undermined. Contraception and sexual health are the responsibility of both sexes.

Autonomy, rights, and duties

The autonomy of pregnant women

It is an accepted principle of medical law and ethics that competent adults have the right to refuse any treatment or medical intervention, even if that refusal results in their avoidable death. The courts have held that this rule applies equally to a woman who is pregnant even if she is carrying a viable fetus capable of being born alive. The fetus, up to the moment of birth, does not have any separate legal interests capable of being taken into account by a court, and therefore the legal position is that the woman's right to refuse treatment overrides all other legal considerations.

Refusal of caesarean section

MB was 40 weeks pregnant and the fetus was in breech position. She signed a consent form for a caesarean section delivery, but refused to consent to a venepuncture because of her fear of needles. She subsequently gave and then withdrew her consent to the anaesthetic. The health authority sought and obtained a declaration that it would be lawful to perform a caesarean section, with the necessary anaesthetic, to deliver the fetus. MB appealed against this decision. The Appeal Court heard the case immediately and rejected it on the grounds that, because of her needle phobia, MB was temporarily incompetent and unable to give a valid refusal. On the following day she agreed to the anaesthesia and a healthy male infant was delivered by caesarean section.

Despite rejecting MB's appeal, Lady Justice Butler-Sloss restated the legal position that a competent pregnant woman has an absolute right to refuse treatment, even if that refusal would result in the death or serious handicap of the child she is carrying. It was made clear that, in such cases, the courts do not have the jurisdiction to declare medical intervention lawful and the question of best interests does not arise. If a competent pregnant woman refuses medical intervention, the doctors may not lawfully do more than attempt to persuade her to accept the treatment. If that persuasion fails, there are no further steps that can be taken.

Re MB (medical treatment)[1]

Although refusals of treatment that would save an unborn child are uncommon, official statistics on maternal deaths do occasionally report cases in which women have died after not seeking or declining various treatments.[2] Such cases are deeply tragic for the individuals and families concerned and the health professionals who offer treatment, but they have been seen as a risk that society must allow in order to protect the integrity and autonomy of all competent patients. Some fear that usurping the decision making rights of a competent pregnant woman demeans women in general and sets a precedent for invading the bodies of some patients in order to benefit others. The idea that a woman should be forced to undergo surgery for another's benefit has been widely rejected.

Is there a right to reproduce?

A woman's right to refuse life prolonging treatment is one of a number of "rights" that are frequently appealed to in relation to reproduction. A distinction is often made between negative and positive rights or between a liberty and a right. Negative rights simply involve being free from interference and are based on the notion that the state should not interfere with essentially private decisions. In terms of reproduction, this confers the right not to be prevented from procreation, for example by non-consensual sterilisation. Positive rights, however, would include the right to demand appropriate health care. In terms of reproduction, this would include a positive obligation on the state and health professionals to support the individual's reproductive choices, including providing reproductive technology for every person who requires it. Claims to positive rights are often seen as problematic in that they suppose that there is a corresponding obligation on other people to supply what the right holder claims. The courts have made clear that, in the UK, there is not a positive right to assistance to reproduce (see Chapter 8, pages 270–1).

Does the fetus have any legal rights?

Although in the case of MB it was confirmed that the fetus does not have any separate interests capable of being taken into account in considering a woman's refusal of caesarean section, it is not the case that the embryo or fetus is totally without legal protection. There are, for example, restrictions in law on the use of human embryos for research (see Chapter 14, page 517) and there are limits applied to the availability of abortion. Lady Justice Butler-Sloss referred to this inconsistency saying:

> Although it might seem illogical that a child capable of being born alive is protected by the criminal law from intentional destruction, and by the Abortion Act from termination otherwise than as permitted by the Act, but is not protected from the (irrational) decision of a competent mother not to allow medical intervention to avert the risk of death, this appears to be the present state of the law.[3]

It has been suggested that the right of everyone to have their life protected by law, under Article 2 of the Human Rights Act 1998, could extend to the unborn. The European Court has, so far, avoided making a decision as to the scope of the term "everyone" in this context. Given, however, that individual states are allowed broader scope for interpretation on matters of a moral nature, discussion on the subject within the European Commission[4] and the way in which UK law has developed in this area, it is unlikely that a fetus would be considered, by UK courts, to have such rights.

Do we have duties towards unborn babies?

The fact that there is a straightforward legal precedent for the situation in which a woman refuses treatment that could save the life of her fetus, does not mean that the situation is unproblematic or straightforward from an ethical perspective. Most of those who accept that embryos and fetuses do not have rights nevertheless believe they are deserving of respect by virtue of their potential for development and for becoming the holder of rights after birth. As a society we do not regard human embryos and fetuses as having the same status as children or adults, but neither do we consider them to be merely cells or tissues. This "special status" is reflected in the law, which gives them some, but not absolute, protection. The extent of the duties owed to embryos and fetuses depends upon gestational age because the nearer they come to developing individual rights, after birth, the stronger their claim to protection. This approach of increasing duties owed according to age can be seen to underpin the legal limits for permissible interference. In the UK, human embryos, up to 14 days after fertilisation, may be used for carefully controlled and licensed research (see Chapter 14, pages 517–8); abortion is permitted in some circumstances up to the 24th week of gestation and, in more restricted cases, up to term (see pages 242–4).

Although all members of society have certain duties and responsibilities, a pregnant woman who plans to carry a fetus to term can be seen to have particular moral obligations towards that unborn child. This means that she has a responsibility not to harm the unborn child deliberately and also to take positive steps to protect it. The BMA's general view is that some duties are owed to the fetus even though its claims may not override the mother's claim to autonomy over her body. The fact that a woman is perceived to have moral responsibilities towards the fetus, however, does not mean that she can or should be forced, legally or ethically, to fulfil those duties.

Contraception

The continuing high number of unwanted or unintended pregnancies demonstrates a clear need for better access to, and uptake of, family planning information and services. The Government has for many years been encouraging cooperation between various agencies, including health and education services, the voluntary sector, and service users to try to improve family planning services. This includes recognition of the need for specific training to enable providers to assess, and explain to patients, the range of contraceptive methods available and to provide general advice about sexual health to accompany the provision of contraceptives. Most women who seek contraceptive advice and services do so from their GP or, increasingly, from their practice nurse, although many younger women tend to prefer the anonymity of specialist clinics. (In 1999 about a fifth of women aged 16–49 who required family planning services in England went to family planning clinics; most of the remainder went to their GPs.[5]) Patients are sometimes unaware that they can register with a second GP for contraceptive services only. It is important to maintain a diversity of provision of advice and services, including specialist sexual and reproductive health clinics in parallel with GP services, in order to offer patient choice.

Contraception and those aged under 16

Public policy

Young people in particular need access to contraceptive advice because studies show that one of the main reasons for the high number of teenage pregnancies in England is a lack of accurate knowledge about contraception.[6] A report by the

Social Exclusion Unit found another important explanation to be young people's low expectations about their future. Young women did not see any prospect of obtaining a job and expected to end up on some form of state benefit; essentially, they saw no reason not to get pregnant. Many of those questioned also felt that society was giving mixed messages about young people and contraception. Although young people are bombarded by images of sexuality in the media, and sexual activity amongst young people is seen as the norm, there is still a reluctance to talk to young people about sex and contraception. One teenager told the Unit that it seems, sometimes, as if sex is compulsory but contraception is illegal.[7] Evidence shows that ignoring the issue does not lead to less sexual activity among young people, but to more unwanted pregnancies. In 2001 in England and Wales almost 96 000 teenagers became pregnant, around 7900 of whom were aged under 16 and nearly 2300 were aged 14 or under.[8]

In 1999 the Government launched a cross-government teenage pregnancy strategy with a target of halving the under-18 conception rate in England by 2010, with an interim target, set out in 2000 in the NHS plan,[9] of a 15% reduction by 2004. Each top tier local authority area has its own teenage pregnancy strategy, developed with local health partners, to reach locally agreed reduction targets. These strategies are managed by teenage pregnancy partnership boards, involving representation from the relevant commissioning body and led by a local teenage pregnancy coordinator. As part of its strategy, the Teenage Pregnancy Unit carried out research to establish the most appropriate and effective methods for reaching young people, and for providing information about sexual health and contraception.[10] The research showed clearly that "just say no" messages are not effective, but what can work is a campaign that does not lecture but tells young people to take control, be prepared, be responsible, and not to feel pressurised into having sex before they are ready. Health professionals, particularly GPs, have an important role in reinforcing these messages because many young people are likely to turn to their family doctor if they have confidence that their requests for contraceptive advice or treatment are kept confidential.[11] From a survey undertaken in 1999 by Brook,[12] however, it is clear that, in spite of attempts to reassure young people about confidentiality, this still represents one of the main areas of concern. Teenagers were most concerned about:

- deliberate breaches of confidentiality: for example, if an under 16-year-old revealed she was pregnant, teenagers thought the doctor would have to tell her parents
- informal, inadvertent breaches of confidentiality by staff: for example, mentioning a teenager's recent visit to the surgery in the course of a conversation with a parent
- "gossipy" receptionists
- confidential information being sent in the post and intercepted by parents.

Every opportunity should be taken to offer reassurance to young people that the duty of confidentiality owed to them is the same as the duty to an adult.

Consent and confidentiality

Controversy about the issue of "underage" contraception is a recurring phenomenon, particularly in relation to the provision of oral contraceptives to those under the age of 16.

Provision of contraception to people aged under 16

Mrs Gillick took her local health authority to court because it refused to assure her that her five daughters, all aged under 16, would not be given contraceptive advice and treatment without her knowledge and consent. The case followed the publication of a Department of Health and Social Security circular advising that doctors consulted at a family planning clinic by a girl under 16 would not be acting unlawfully if they prescribed contraceptives, provided that they acted in good faith and to protect the young woman from the harmful effects of sexual intercourse. In seeking a declaration that this advice was unlawful, Mrs Gillick argued that a young girl's consent was legally ineffective and inconsistent with parental rights. She said that it was therefore necessary to involve parents.

This argument was rejected by the House of Lords, where the majority opinion was that the relevant test was whether the girl had reached an age where she had sufficient understanding and intelligence to enable her to understand fully what was proposed. If she had, a doctor would not be acting unlawfully in giving advice and treatment.

Gillick v West Norfolk and Wisbech AHA[13]

The BMA has a clear policy, based on the Gillick judgment, that the patient's maturity and understanding of the nature of the consultation and of the treatment proposed should be the guiding factors. It is sometimes argued that very young patients may not understand either the concept of confidentiality or the implications of the treatment they request. They may have an erroneous impression of the purpose of contraceptives. An example would be that of a 9-year-old seeking contraceptives because she knows older friends have them. Kennedy[14] raises this hypothetical case, but such cases are likely to be exceptional. Minors who seek contraception are usually either sexually active or intending to be so. In such cases, when patients understand the treatment, their autonomy and confidentiality should be respected. The BMA emphasises the importance of the doctor trying to persuade the patient to agree to parental involvement but, if the patient refuses, there is a duty to maintain the confidentiality of the consultation.

Before providing contraception to young people, health professionals must:

- consider whether the patient understands the potential risks and benefits of the treatment
- consider whether the patient understands the advice given
- discuss with the patient the value of parental support (Doctors must encourage young people to inform parents of the consultation and explore the reasons if

the patient is unwilling to do so. It is important for persons aged under 16 who are seeking contraceptive advice to be aware that, although the doctor is obliged to discuss the value of parental support, he or she will respect their confidentiality (see Chapter 5).)

- take into account whether the patient is likely to have sexual intercourse without contraception
- assess whether the patient's physical or mental health or both are likely to suffer if the patient does not receive contraceptive advice or treatment
- consider whether the patient's best interests would require the provision of contraceptive advice or treatment or both without parental consent.

These are known as the "Fraser Guidelines". They were issued after the judgment in the Gillick case.

Even if the doctor is unwilling to supply contraception on the grounds of the patient's immaturity, he or she still maintains a general duty of confidentiality unless there are exceptional reasons for disclosing information without consent. Such reasons could occur when, for example, the request for contraception arises in the context of sexual exploitation, incest, or other sexual abuse. In such exceptional cases the doctor has a duty to protect the patient and this may eventually involve a breach of confidentiality, although with counselling and support the patient may feel able to agree to disclosure. Nevertheless, it is important that doctors avoid making completely unconditional promises about secrecy to individual young people, while at the same time making it clear that confidentiality as a general principle extends to all consultations. The BMA has worked with other organisations, including the Royal College of General Practitioners and Brook, to produce a toolkit on confidentiality and young people, which is specifically designed for those working in primary care.[15] Guidance on the provision of effective contraception and advice services for young people has been issued by the Teenage Pregnancy Unit.[16] This includes confidentiality as a key issue in the criteria against which services should be commissioned and provided.

Young people with learning difficulties

It is generally accepted that, if they wish to do so, young people with learning difficulties should be able to experience aspects of life from which they may have been protected in the past, including sexual relationships. It may be, however, that these are something that they explore at a later stage than many of their peers because most young people with significant learning difficulties have a highly supervised life. Clearly, there is no justification for providing contraception – particularly using invasive methods – if there is no evidence that the young person is interested in an intimate relationship and there is no identifiable risk of pregnancy. Doctors consulted in relation to a request for contraception for a young person with learning difficulties need to bear in mind the points made previously concerning contraception for any minor. Also, as with other patients, they need to ensure that any product supplied is the most appropriate for that patient's needs. Some young women with a learning disability can be reliable pill takers, although they may require help from their carers. Implants or other long term contraceptive methods, such as a hormonally loaded intrauterine system, are appropriate for some patients. It is lawful to provide contraception to a young person who is incapable of giving consent if a person with parental responsibility consents to the treatment, or if it is in the best interests of the patient. Obviously, however, lack of capacity to consent to the treatment would raise concerns about the individual's capacity to consent to sex, if that is the purpose of providing contraception. In cases of doubt or difficulty, doctors should consult their lawyers.

Emergency hormonal contraception

The development of drugs that prevent the establishment of pregnancy after intercourse has provided another option for women when a regular contraceptive method has not been used or has failed. The General Household Survey for 1998 found that 10% of women aged 16–49 had used emergency contraception at least once in the two years prior to interview.[17] The main barriers to its use are confusion about the timescale within which it must be taken (up to 72 hours after intercourse, although it is most effective when taken within the first 24 hours) and access, particularly outside normal practice opening hours. Fears that making access to emergency contraception easier would encourage promiscuity and discourage the use of more reliable contraception appear to be unfounded. Research evidence shows that women with ready access to emergency hormonal contraception use it neither irresponsibly nor as an alternative to other methods.[18]

Changes introduced throughout the UK in January 2001 enabled emergency hormonal contraception to be sold by pharmacists to women aged 16 or over, without a doctor's prescription.[19] The BMA strongly supported this change, while recognising that pharmacists would need specific training in giving advice about contraception and sexual health, and would require facilities for private discussions in order to protect confidentiality. The BMA has also called for emergency contraception to be available free of charge from pharmacists.[20] Whether provided by doctors or by pharmacists, it should usually be accompanied by advice and counselling on sexual activity, future contraception, and related matters such as sexually transmitted infections.[21]

The principles involved in the provision of contraception to people aged under 16 apply equally to emergency hormonal contraception. The BMA believes that a range of measures are needed to bring down the number of teenage pregnancies and that access to emergency hormonal contraception through pharmacies could have been extended to those under 16. The BMA hopes that this issue will be kept under review.

Emergency "contraception" or early abortion?

There has, in the past, been some uncertainty about whether certain types of contraceptives that prevent implantation, such as emergency hormonal contraception and intrauterine devices, should be classed as abortifacients, which could be issued only under the terms of the Abortion Act 1967. This question was addressed in a parliamentary answer in May 1983, in which the Attorney General stated that the provision of postcoital contraception designed to prevent implantation does not constitute "procuring a miscarriage".[22] This view was tested and confirmed in the case of R v HS Dhingra[23] in 1991 and by a judicial review in 2002.

Judicial review on emergency hormonal contraception

The Society for the Protection of the Unborn Child applied for a judicial review of the decision of the Secretary of State for Health, made in 2000, to make emergency contraception available from pharmacists without a prescription. The claimant contended that the "morning after pill" was not a contraceptive but an abortifacient because it procured a miscarriage within the meaning of the 1861 Offences Against the Persons Act. Its use, therefore, would be lawful only if prescribed by two doctors, as required by the Abortion Act 1967. The Secretary of State argued, however, that the meaning of "miscarriage" was the loss of a fertilised egg that had become implanted in the endometrium of the uterus. Emergency hormonal contraception causes the loss of an egg before implantation, so there is no miscarriage and therefore no criminal offence.

The judge, in the High Court, held that the decision had to turn on the meaning of "miscarriage" now and not its meaning in 1861. Today, miscarriage is taken to mean the termination of an established pregnancy and therefore the application was dismissed.

R (on the application of Smeaton) v Secretary of State for Health[24]

Conscientious objection to the provision of contraceptive services

Although GPs are not obliged by their terms of service to provide contraceptive services, most do so. When a practice does not offer contraceptive advice it is important that patients are aware of this fact and are appraised of alternative practitioners or family planning services.

Although, legally, the use of contraceptives that are capable of preventing implantation does not constitute an abortion, the BMA recognises that some doctors, believing that life begins at fertilisation, may have an ethical objection to their use. Those who take this view may choose not to provide such services. In the BMA's view, however, doctors with a conscientious objection to providing contraceptive advice or treatment have an ethical duty to refer their patients promptly to another practitioner or family planning service.

Summary – contraception

- Health professionals have an important role to play in reducing the number of unwanted pregnancies, particularly among young people.
- The provision of contraception should be accompanied by advice and information about sexual health.

- Young people who are sufficiently mature to understand the implications are able to give valid consent to treatment, but parental involvement should be encouraged.
- Confidentiality of all patients, including those aged under 16, should be respected except in exceptional circumstances where there is serious concern about exploitation or abuse.
- Emergency hormonal contraception is an important step in the drive to reduce unwanted pregnancies and should be made available to those who need it.
- Health professionals with a conscientious objection to some or all forms of contraception are not obliged to provide them, but they have an ethical duty to refer their patients promptly to another practitioner.

Sterilisation

Male or female sterilisation is usually expected to produce permanent sterility (although this is not necessarily the outcome). Although some people have conscientious objections to sterilisation for contraceptive purposes, within society as a whole it appears to be viewed as an acceptable form of family planning, as long as individuals are adequately informed of the implications of the procedure and no pressure is exerted upon them. Non-consensual sterilisation of those who are unable to give valid consent has, however, been the subject of intense debate.

Consent

As discussed in Chapter 2 on consent, the patient's agreement to treatment is valid only when adequate information about the procedure and its implications has been provided. This should include information about the likelihood of success and the possibility that the procedure could fail. The degree of patient understanding should be commensurate with the gravity of the treatment; in other words, where the procedure is irreversible, a high level of understanding is needed. Some men enquire about storing their semen prior to sterilisation in case their circumstances change in the future. This is generally discouraged because it demonstrates ambivalence about a procedure designed to render permanent sterility. Some clinics, however, agree to semen storage; a limited number of treatment centres are also able to store oocytes prior to treatment likely to affect a woman's future fertility. Information about centres licensed to store gametes is available from the Human Fertilisation and Embryology Authority (see Chapter 8, page 273).

The same considerations about information and consent apply whether the intention is to sterilise the patient or, as with hysterectomy, permanent sterility is an inevitable side effect of a procedure undertaken for medical reasons. As part of the consent process, discussion should take place about the likelihood of the patient already being pregnant and how to proceed if that is found to be the case.

Inadequate consent for hysterectomy

In 2002 a consultant obstetrician and gynaecologist was found guilty of serious professional misconduct by the GMC for his management of a patient's total abdominal hysterectomy and bilateral salpingo-oophorectomy. The patient had been referred to the consultant by her GP because of symptoms of abdominal pain and vaginal discharge. Part of the case against the doctor was that he had failed to ensure that the patient understood the nature and purpose of the operation and that she had given her informed consent. The GMC's Professional Conduct Committee found that, during the course of the operation, the doctor had cause to suspect that the patient may have been pregnant but nonetheless continued with the operation, without her consent, thereby terminating the pregnancy. This action was held to be inappropriate because the doctor knew, or should have known, that the patient had not given her consent for termination of pregnancy and yet he made no effort to consult her about it, despite the fact that the operation would prevent her from ever having any children. The consultant was severely reprimanded.[25]

Any treatment affecting an individual's reproductive capacity also has potential implications for that person's partner or future partners. In the past, consent to treatments such as sterilisation was sought routinely from the patient's partner. This is now acknowledged to be inappropriate because it is for the individual patient to decide whether to be sterilised. In addition, with limited exceptions in Scotland, nobody can consent to treatment on behalf of another adult. Partners should be consulted only if the patient has given specific consent, although it is good practice to encourage patients to discuss such procedures with their partners.

Sterilisation of people with learning disabilities

Individuals with learning disabilities have varying degrees of difficulty in making decisions that influence the course of their lives. Like all patients, they should be encouraged to make for themselves all those decisions whose implications they broadly understand and with which they feel comfortable. The rights of people with learning disabilities to enjoy sexual relationships in private has been an issue of historical debate, and sterilisation of those who lack the capacity to give valid consent has been controversial. Debate on this issue has focused primarily on proposals to sterilise women – where the consideration must include the risks of harm arising from the pregnancy as well as the difficulties of bringing up a child – but sterilisation of men with learning disabilities has also been proposed. Proposals to sterilise those who are not able to give consent present a number of difficulties. The harm against which it seeks to protect may not be sufficient to justify the intervention or it may be proposed more for the benefit of carers than the individual. There are also concerns that it may more easily expose the patient to sexual abuse and misdirect attention towards preventing pregnancy rather than protecting vulnerable people from abuse. It has also been argued that non-consensual sterilisation can be seen as contravening a fundamental freedom to reproduce. Article 12 of the European Convention on Human Rights (the right to marry and found a family) is frequently referred to in this context.

As a matter of principle, contraceptive services for people with learning difficulties should not impede the exercise of autonomy more drastically than is essential to protect against an unwanted pregnancy. Advances in the development of contraceptive devices mean that, for many patients, other less drastic methods of contraception are available and these should always be considered before sterilisation. In the past hysterectomies, or sterilisation, may have been carried out prematurely on young women who could have coped successfully with other forms of contraception and who might have been capable of making their own decisions about motherhood at a later stage. This point was implicit in a 1976 case where the judge refused to authorise the sterilisation of an 11-year-old girl, pointing to the frustration and resentment the patient would be likely to experience in later life, arising from her inability to have children.[26] To perform a sterilisation on a woman for non-therapeutic reasons and without her consent, the judge said, would be a violation of the individual's basic human rights to have the opportunity to reproduce.

A similar point was made in the 1989 case of Re F (see below). Although heard some time ago, this case is important because it set the legal parameters for the medical treatment of adults who are unable to consent for themselves. It confirmed that the courts cannot give consent on behalf of an adult and that, in all cases involving the treatment of an incompetent adult, the treatment must be in the patient's best interest (see Chapter 3, pages 108–9), which was defined as:

- necessary to save life or prevent deterioration or ensure an improvement in the patient's physical or mental health and
- in accordance with a practice accepted at the time by a responsible body of medical opinion skilled in the particular form of treatment in question.

Sterilisation of a woman with severe mental disorder

F was 36 years old and suffered from severe mental disorder. She was described in court as having the verbal capacity of a 2-year-old and the general mental capacity of a 4- or 5-year-old. F had been a hospital inpatient for more than 20 years and over that period had made great progress such that she was given increased freedom within the confines of the hospital. Her mental capacity was not, however, expected to improve. Over time, F had developed a sexual relationship with another patient. It was said that the psychiatric consequences for F of becoming pregnant would be "catastrophic". Consideration had been given to the option of preventing F from forming sexual relationships, but the view was taken that this could be achieved only by seriously restricting her already limited freedom. Less invasive methods of contraception had been considered, but none was suitable, so an application was made for a declaration that it would not be unlawful to sterilise F despite her being unable to give consent. All parties were agreed that sterilisation would be in F's best interests, but a number of legal and procedural issues needed to be resolved.

(Continued)

The House of Lords ruled that the common law allowed doctors to give medical or surgical treatment to an adult patient who is incapable of consenting when it is in the best interests of the patient to do so. Where the treatment proposed was sterilisation for non-therapeutic purposes, however, it was recommended that an application should be made to the court for a declaration that the operation was not unlawful and was in the patient's best interests.

Re F (mental patient: sterilisation)[27]

Sterilisation (unless for therapeutic reasons) is one of a small number of procedures that must not be carried out without applying for a court declaration (see pages 118–20). This is because of its intended irreversible nature, which deprives the individual of what is, according to one judge, "widely and rightly regarded as one of the fundamental rights of a woman, the right to bear a child".[28]

This "right to reproduce" has also been raised, in the specific context of Article 12 of the European Convention on Human Rights, in a more recent case about male sterilisation.

Sterilisation of a man with Down syndrome

In Re A, an application for the sterilisation of a 28-year-old man with Down syndrome was rejected. A was cared for by his mother, who supervised him, but who was concerned that when, given her ill health, he moved into local authority care he may have a sexual relationship and be unable to understand the possible consequences. The judge at the High Court found that, although A was sexually aware and active, he did not understand the link between intercourse and pregnancy. Nevertheless, the judge refused the declaration on the basis that the effect on A would be minimal.

A's mother took her case to the Appeal Court but it was dismissed. Although decided shortly before the Human Rights Act 1998 came into force, in dismissing the appeal Lady Justice Butler-Sloss warned that the courts should be slow to take any step that could infringe the rights of those who are unable to speak for themselves. The case was decided on the basis that sterilisation would not be in A's best interests, taking account of medical, emotional, and all other welfare issues. It was made clear in the judgment that the concept of best interests in such cases relates to the mentally incapacitated person, not to carers or other third parties.

Re A (male sterilisation)[29]

Sterilisation and young people

Sterilisation is occasionally requested for young people with serious learning difficulties. Of course, every case requires assessment and balancing of the relevant factors, but sterilisation for contraceptive purposes should not normally be proposed for young people aged under 18. Even when there are exceptional circumstances in which there is agreement that sterilisation is the best option for a young person, court authorisation is essential.[30]

Sterilisation for contraceptive purposes in young women usually involves tubal ligation. Before authorising such a procedure, the court will scrutinise the reasons for the request and require evidence concerning the inappropriateness of other options (see below). Health professionals must be able to demonstrate to the court that less invasive alternatives, such as oral, injectable, or intrauterine contraception would still be unsuitable even if the patient were given help and support. Whenever possible, the young woman's own views need to be heard. Efforts should be made to make the patient as much at ease as possible. A gynaecological examination is likely to be needed to assess or eliminate the possibility of organic disease. Health professionals should make every effort to ensure that the patient understands what the examination involves and gives consent for it. Concern is sometimes expressed that the treatment may be sought primarily for the benefit of carers rather than in the interests of the patient herself. Although attention is often drawn to the difficulty of separating out the "interests" of individuals in the family context, the court will need to be convinced that sterilisation is the best option for the young woman.

Hysterectomy may, in the past, have seemed appropriate treatment for a young person who is approaching adulthood and who will never achieve the capacity to make a valid choice about treatment to manage heavy menstrual bleeding. In most cases, however, the objective of menstrual management can be achieved by lesser means than surgery. Given that evidence-based clinical guidelines examining these issues have been published by the Royal College of Obstetricians and Gynaecologists,[31] it is hard to see how doctors could be satisfied that no less intrusive means of treatment is available. Oral or injectable contraception or a hormonally loaded intrauterine device may regularise and lighten menstrual bleeding. It must also be borne in mind that most women with a learning disability can manage their own menstruation with appropriate education and support. Some may need assistance from their carers. In many cases, referral to special learning disability services rather than to gynaecological services is most appropriate. In all cases where surgery is being considered, doctors must take legal advice and it is likely that a court ruling will be needed.[32]

Court authorisation for sterilisation

Sterilisation of those who are unable to consent should be carried out without judicial review only when there are unambiguous therapeutic grounds.

England and Wales

The Official Solicitor for England and Wales has issued a practice note providing legal guidance on this matter.[33] This states that the sterilisation of a minor or a mentally incompetent adult will, in virtually all cases, require the prior sanction of a

High Court judge. The judge needs to be satisfied that the patient is incapable of making his or her own decision about sterilisation and is unlikely to develop sufficiently to make an informed judgment in the foreseeable future. Those proposing sterilisation must be seeking it in good faith and their paramount concern must be for the best interests of the patient rather than their own or the public's convenience. In considering whether sterilisation would be in the patient's best interests the following factors must be considered.

- It must be shown that the patient is capable of conception and is having or is likely to have full sexual intercourse. In relation to a young woman who has no interest in human relationships with any sexual ingredient, a high level of supervision is an appropriate protection. Any risk of pregnancy should be identifiable, not speculative.
- The physical and psychological consequences of pregnancy and childbirth for the patient should be analysed by obstetric and psychiatric experts. In the case of a male patient, these considerations will be different. Psychiatric evidence concerning the patient's likely ability to care for and/or have a fulfilling relationship with a child should be adduced. Evidence that any child born would have a disability is likely to be irrelevant. If the proposed procedure is intended to affect the patient's menstruation, then evidence about any detriment caused by her current menstrual cycle must also be adduced.
- The court requires a detailed analysis of all available and relevant methods of addressing any problems found to be substantiated under the above two points. This analysis should be performed by a doctor with expertise in the full range of available methods. The expert should explain the nature of each relevant method and then list its advantages and disadvantages for the individual patient, taking into account any pertinent aspects of the patient's physical and psychological health.

The question of whether sterilisation of incompetent adults should continue to require court approval in England and Wales was discussed in the Lord Chancellor's department's 1997 consultation on decision making for mentally incapacitated adults.[34] However, in 1999 the Government announced that it did not intend to proceed with any changes to the existing position.[35]

Northern Ireland

There have been no reported cases of sterilisation of incapacitated adults in Northern Ireland, but the procedure recommended in Re F and the criteria set out in the practice note for England and Wales would apply (see above).[33]

Scotland

It is a requirement of the Adults with Incapacity (Scotland) Act 2000 that non-therapeutic sterilisations of those who are unable to consent for themselves must have prior court approval.[36] Detailed guidance has not been issued, but doctors should ensure that the criteria set out above for assessing best interests are met.

Summary – sterilisation

- As with other irreversible procedures, those seeking sterilisation should be given sufficient information about the procedure and its implications in order to make an informed decision.
- Patients should be encouraged to discuss sterilisation with their partners, but the decision of whether to involve the partner rests with the patient.
- Sterilisation of those who are unable to consent, except where there are unambiguous therapeutic grounds, will in virtually all cases require a court declaration.

Abortion

BMA policy and background to the abortion debate

The BMA represents doctors who hold widely diverse moral views about abortion. In the 1970s and 1980s, the Association approved policy statements supporting the 1967 Abortion Act as "a practical and humane piece of legislation".[37] The BMA does not consider that abortion is necessarily unethical but, as with any act having profound moral implications, the justifications must be commensurate with the consequences. The BMA's advice to its members is to act within the boundaries of the law and of their own conscience. Patients are, however, entitled to receive objective medical advice and referral as appropriate to another practitioner, regardless of their doctor's personal views for or against abortion.

In order to understand the very contentious background to the abortion debate, it may be helpful to mention briefly the main strands of the argument. People generally give one of three common types of response to abortion: prochoice, anti-abortion, and the middle ground that abortion is acceptable in some circumstances. The main arguments in support of each of these positions is set out below.

Arguments in support of abortion being made widely available

Those who support the wide availability of abortion consider the matter to be primarily one of a woman's right to choose and to exercise control over her own body. These arguments tend not to consider the fetus to be a person, deserving of any rights, or owed any duties. Moralists who judge actions by their consequences alone could argue that abortion is equivalent to a deliberate failure to conceive a child and, since contraception is widely available, abortion should be too. Others take a slightly different approach, believing that, even if the fetus has rights and entitlements, these are very limited and do not weigh significantly against the interests of people who have already been born, such as parents or existing children of the family. Most people believe it is right for couples to be able to plan their families and for women to have control over when they become pregnant. Although contraception is understood to be the appropriate means to avoid unwanted pregnancy, all methods have a failure rate. When contraception fails, or when couples fail to use it effectively, many people accept that abortion is preferable to forcing a woman to continue with an unwanted pregnancy.

Arguments against abortion

Some people consider that abortion is wrong in any circumstances because it fails to recognise the rights of the fetus or because it challenges the notion of the sanctity of all human life. They argue that permitting abortion diminishes the respect society feels for other vulnerable humans, possibly leading to their involuntary euthanasia. Those who consider that an embryo is a human being with full moral status from the moment of conception see abortion as intentional killing in the same sense as the murder of any other person. Those who take this view cannot accept that women should be allowed to obtain abortion, however difficult the lives of those women or their existing families are made as a result. Such views may be based on religious or moral convictions that each human life has unassailable intrinsic value, which is not diminished by any impairment or suffering that may be involved for the individual living that life. Many worry that the availability of abortion on grounds of fetal abnormality encourages prejudice towards any person with a handicap and insidiously creates the impression that the only valuable people are those who conform to some ill defined stereotype of "normality".

Some of those who oppose abortion in general nevertheless concede that it may be justifiable in very exceptional cases when termination is seen as the lesser moral offence. This could include cases such as where the pregnancy is the result of rape, or the consequence of the exploitation of a young girl or a mentally incompetent woman. Risk to the mother's life may be another justifiable exception, but only when abortion is the only option. It would thus not be seen as justifiable to abort a fetus if the life of both fetus and mother could be saved by implementing any other solution.

Arguments used to support abortion in some circumstances

Many people argue that abortion may be justified in a greater number of circumstances than those conceded by antiabortionists, but that it would be undesirable to allow "abortion on demand". To do so could incur undesirable effects, such as encouraging irresponsible attitudes to contraception. It could also lead to a devaluation of the lives of viable fetuses and trivialise the potential psychological effects of abortion on women and on health professionals. These types of argument are based on the premise that the embryo starts off without rights, although having a special status from conception in view of its potential for development, and that it acquires rights and status throughout its development. The notion of evolving fetal rights and practical factors, such as the increasing medical risks and possible distress to the pregnant woman, nurses, doctors, or other children in the family, gives rise to the view that early abortion is more acceptable than late abortion.

Some people support this position on pragmatic grounds, believing that abortions will always be sought by women who are desperate and that it is better for society to provide abortion services that are safe and can be monitored and regulated, rather than to allow "back street" practices.

The law on abortion

England, Scotland and Wales

In England, Scotland, and Wales, a registered medical practitioner may lawfully terminate a pregnancy, in an NHS hospital or on premises approved for this purpose, if two registered medical practitioners are of the opinion, formed in good faith:

(a) that the pregnancy has not exceeded its twenty-fourth week and that the continuance of the pregnancy would involve risk, greater than if the pregnancy were terminated, of injury to the physical or mental health of the pregnant woman or any existing children of her family; or

(b) that the termination is necessary to prevent grave permanent injury to the physical or mental health of the pregnant woman; or

(c) that the continuance of the pregnancy would involve risk to the life of the pregnant woman, greater than if the pregnancy were terminated; or

(d) that there is a substantial risk that if the child were born it would suffer from such physical or mental abnormalities as to be seriously handicapped.[38]

(The above conditions are lettered and ordered as set out in the Act, which differs from the form completed by doctors authorising, or referring a patient for, termination of pregnancy.)

In addition, when a doctor "is of the opinion, formed in good faith, that the termination is immediately necessary to save the life or to prevent grave permanent injury to the physical or mental health of the pregnant woman"[39] the opinion of a second registered medical practitioner is not required. Nor, in these limited circumstances, are there restrictions on where the procedure may be carried out.

The Abortion Act was amended in 1990 to remove the pre-existing links with the Infant Life Preservation Act 1929, which had made it illegal to destroy the life of a child that is capable of being born alive, with an assumption that this would be so after 28 weeks gestation. Thus, terminations carried out under sections 1(1)(b) – 1(1)(d) of the Abortion Act may be performed at any gestational age.

The question of what constitutes a "serious handicap" under section 1(1)(d) is not addressed in the legislation. It is a matter of clinical judgment and accepted practice. Practical guidance for health professionals involved with terminations for fetal abnormality is available from the Royal College of Obstetricians and Gynaecologists.[40] The types of factor that may be taken into account in assessing the seriousness of a handicap include the following:

- the probability of effective treatment, either *in utero* or after birth
- the child's probable potential for self awareness and potential ability to communicate with others
- the suffering that would be experienced by the child when born or by the people caring for the child.

Northern Ireland

The Abortion Act does not extend to Northern Ireland, where the law on abortion is different and is based on the Offences Against the Person Act 1861, which makes it an offence to procure a miscarriage unlawfully. The Bourne judgment of 1939,[41] in which a London gynaecologist was found not guilty of an offence under this Act for performing an abortion on a 14-year-old girl who was pregnant as a result of rape, was based on an interpretation of the word *unlawfully* in this Act. The defence argued, and the judge accepted, that in the particular circumstances of the case, the operation was not unlawful because continuation of the pregnancy would severely affect the young woman's mental health. In reaching this decision, the judge turned to the wording of the Infant Life (Preservation) Act 1929, which gave protection from prosecution if the act was carried out in good faith for the purpose only of preserving the life of the mother. This formed the basis of the judgment and extended the grounds for a lawful abortion to include the mental and physical wellbeing of the woman.

It is known that abortions are carried out in Northern Ireland and abortion is lawful in some circumstances.[42] However, without specific legislation, doctors are left with the task of interpreting the word "unlawfully" as discussed in the Bourne judgment.

Abortion in Northern Ireland

K became pregnant at the age of 13 while in the care of a children's home. By the time of the court hearing in October 1993, K was 14 years old and 14 weeks pregnant. K wanted an abortion and had threatened to kill herself and the baby and had cut her wrists with broken glass, declined food, and punched herself in the stomach. The judge declared that abortion would be lawful in Northern Ireland in these circumstances and that an abortion would be in K's best interests. Although it had been declared lawful in Northern Ireland, no doctor could be found to carry out the termination, not because of any moral qualms but because of the fear of litigation. K was taken to Liverpool, where the abortion was performed.

Re K (a minor), Northern Health and Social Service Board v F and G[43]

In the subsequent case of Re A the judge clarified the circumstances in which abortion would be lawful, stating that:

The doctor's act is lawful where the continuance of the pregnancy would adversely affect the mental or physical health of the mother. The adverse effect must, however, be a real and serious one and it will always be a question of fact and degree whether the perceived effect of non-termination is sufficiently grave to warrant terminating the unborn child.[44]

Although case law has provided some clarification of the law in Northern Ireland, these cases also indicate the continuing legal uncertainty concerning the precise circumstances in which abortion is lawful. The BMA recognises the difficulties caused by this lack of legal certainty and supports the extension of the 1967 Abortion Act to Northern Ireland.[45] In 2001 the Family Planning Association sought a judicial review of the situation regarding termination of pregnancy in Northern Ireland, arguing that the Health Minister had acted unlawfully in failing to issue advice and guidance to women and doctors on the availability and provision of services to terminate pregnancy. In July 2003 the court rejected the FPA's claim. The judge, however, invited the Department of Health, Social Security and Public Safety to consider issuing guidance even though it was not legally required to do so.[46]

Women from Northern Ireland frequently travel to England or Scotland for termination of pregnancy. Adequate provision should be made for the aftercare of these patients.

Early medical abortion

Since 1991 mifepristone (formerly known as RU486) has been available in England, Scotland, and Wales for early medical abortions. These can be performed at up to 9 weeks gestation and must comply with the terms of the 1967 Act (as amended). A 1990 amendment to the Abortion Act specifies that the power to approve premises for termination of pregnancy includes the power to approve premises for the administration of medicinal terminations. Without this amendment, the administration of mifepristone would have been lawful only if carried out on premises approved for surgical terminations. Those considering administering mifepristone should discuss with the woman the advantages and disadvantages of this technique compared with surgical abortion.

The additional ethical issue raised by its use is that, it is said that mifepristone makes abortion too "easy", the implication being that women may undertake the procedure too lightly.[47] Some have predicted that the availability of such early abortion may result in a diminished sense of moral responsibility to avoid unwanted pregnancy, leading couples to neglect to take contraceptive measures. Others, however, have argued that the decision to terminate an unplanned pregnancy is unlikely to be trivialised in this way and have criticised the attitude that appears to claim that abortion requires punitive aspects for the woman in order to be taken seriously.[48] The Royal College of Obstetricians and Gynaecologists emphasises the benefit of being able to offer a choice of methods in its guidance, *The care of women requesting induced abortion.*[49]

Abortion and young people

As with other medical interventions, a person who has sufficient understanding of the issues, and is acting free from pressure, may give valid consent to the termination of pregnancy, regardless of age. Some competent young women requesting abortion insist that parents must not be informed. Patients may fear, for example, that their parents will disown them or threaten them if they find out. Awareness of the potential emotional and psychological sequelae of abortion, however, makes doctors anxious about the lack of family support mechanisms for such patients. Counselling may help the patient to identify supportive adults within or outside the immediate family. Ultimately, however, a patient's request for confidentiality should not be overridden except in very exceptional cases (see Chapter 5). The courts have confirmed that a parent's refusal to give consent for a termination cannot override the consent of a competent young person.[50]

The case of P and the limits of parents' power to refuse abortion

P was aged 15 and in local authority care after a conviction for theft when she gave birth to a baby boy. Soon after the baby's birth, she became pregnant again and, as with her first pregnancy, her parents refused to consent to an abortion. Part of their objection was on religious grounds since P's father was a Seventh Day Adventist. P herself wanted to terminate her second pregnancy. The local authority made P a ward of court and asked the High Court to authorise a termination. P's father opposed this, suggesting that P should give birth and take care of the second child while he and his wife raised the first. The judge, however, concluded that the second pregnancy endangered P's mental health, impeded her schooling, and endangered the future of P's existing child. She had no doubt that continuance of the pregnancy involved greater risk for P and her existing child than the risks of the termination. P's welfare, as a ward of court, had to be the judge's paramount consideration and the court also had to consider the welfare of P's existing son. The judge concluded that the parents' objections did not outweigh the risks to P's mental health if the pregnancy continued. Termination was ruled to be in P's best interests.

Re P (a minor)[51]

If a young pregnant person is assessed as lacking competence, somebody with parental responsibility can legally give consent for her to have a termination of pregnancy, provided the legal requirements of abortion legislation are met (see pages 242–4). In all cases, the patient's views must be heard and considered. If an incompetent minor refuses to permit parental involvement, expert legal advice should be sought. This should clarify whether the parents should be informed against the girl's wishes. A termination cannot proceed without valid consent, except in an emergency. This may require an application to the courts. If doctors believe that the patient is insufficiently mature to consent validly to termination of pregnancy, this raises the question of whether she was also unable to consent to sexual intercourse.

The first duty of health professionals concerns the welfare of the patient, who may need to be referred for specialist counselling. For more information about consent for termination of pregnancy see the BMA's separate guidance.[52]

Involvement of fathers

Although women should generally be encouraged to discuss their decision to terminate a pregnancy with the father, male partners have no legal rights to involvement in the decision.

Male partner opposing abortion

Mr Paton applied for an injunction to prevent the British Pregnancy Advisory Service and his wife from causing or permitting an abortion to be carried out. He originally argued that his wife had no proper legal grounds for seeking the termination of pregnancy and that she was being spiteful, vindictive, and utterly unreasonable in doing so. He later accepted that the provisions of the Abortion Act had been correctly complied with, but contended that he had the right to have a say in the destiny of the child he had conceived. The judge referred to the highly emotional nature of such cases but confirmed that his task was to apply the law free of emotion or predilection. He considered the terms of the Abortion Act and concluded that the husband had "no legal right enforceable in law or in equity to stop his wife having this abortion or to stop the doctors from carrying out the abortion."[53]

Mr Paton took his case to the European Commission of Human Rights, claiming that his Article 8 right to respect for family life had been breached. The Commission found that the decision insofar as it interfered with the applicant's right to respect for his family life was justified under paragraph (2) of Article 8 as being necessary for the protection of the rights of another person.

Paton v United Kingdom[54]

Selective reduction of multiple pregnancy

The increased use of fertility treatment has led to higher numbers of multiple pregnancies. Careful monitoring of ovulation induction and a reduction in the maximum number of embryos replaced in *in vitro* fertilisation treatment can help to reduce the number of multiple pregnancies, but this cannot be avoided in all cases. High order multiple pregnancies are known to carry an increased risk of the death or serious handicap of one or more of the fetuses. This risk may be reduced by "selective reduction", which involves killing one or more of the fetuses *in utero* in order to give the others a greater chance of a successful outcome. The procedure itself is not without hazard and the risk of obstetric complications is far from negligible. Delayed spontaneous abortion of all fetuses is one risk, which varies according to the technique used. Other risks include maternal infection and some possible risk of fetal malformation. Some also see the procedure as posing medical, ethical, and psychosocial problems, not least because of the paucity of information about how women and their partners cope with the experience and its after effects. It is said, for example, that women are insufficiently informed about selective reduction, including the subsequent sense of loss and grief that many parents experience.[55]

Until 1990 the legality of selective reduction of multiple pregnancy was unclear because the Abortion Act referred to the termination of a "pregnancy" and, in selective reduction, the pregnancy itself is not terminated. This was clarified by section 37(5) of the Human Fertilisation and Embryology Act 1990, which amended the Abortion Act explicitly to include "in the case of a woman carrying more than one fetus, her miscarriage of any fetus". Thus, selective reduction of pregnancy would be lawful provided the circumstances matched the criteria for termination of pregnancy set out in the 1967 Act and the procedure was carried out in an NHS hospital or premises approved for terminations. The same ethical and legal considerations apply to termination of all or part of a multiple pregnancy as to the termination of a singleton pregnancy. Under the new section 5(2) of the Abortion Act, selective reduction of a multiple pregnancy may lawfully be performed if:

(a)   the ground for termination of the pregnancy specified in subsection (1)(d) of [section 1] applies in relation to any fetus and the thing is done for the purpose of procuring the miscarriage of that fetus; or

(b)   any of the other grounds for termination of the pregnancy specified in that section applies.

It has been suggested that a general risk of serious handicap to the fetuses, if the multiple pregnancy is not reduced, would not be covered by the Act and the risk must be to a specific fetus. Where, however, there is an increased risk to the mother, as a result of the multiple pregnancy, the selective reduction may be lawful under section 1(1)(a), (b) or (c).[56]

Like gender selection (see Chapter 8, pages 296–8), selective reduction is a procedure that has arisen from medical necessity, but which could arguably be offered as a consumer choice to parents who are not prepared to accept a natural multiple pregnancy.

Abortion of a healthy twin

In August 1996, it was reported in the media that a 28-year-old woman had aborted a healthy twin at 16 week's gestation on the grounds that she would be unable to cope with two babies.[57] The woman, Miss B, was reported to have one child already and to be in "socially straitened circumstances". She allegedly told her consultant that she would keep one baby but could not keep two, and if she could not have selective reduction, she would terminate the pregnancy. This case caused considerable disquiet, not only amongst those who were fundamentally opposed to abortion or those who objected in principle to selective reduction. Some believed that it was wrong to use selective reduction for "social" reasons, while others thought that aborting any fetus at 16 weeks for purely social reasons was unacceptable.[58]

The BMA considers selective termination to be justifiable when the procedure is recommended for medical reasons (both physical and psychological). Women who have a multiple pregnancy should be carefully counselled when medical opinion is that continuation, without selective reduction, will result in the loss of all the fetuses, but they cannot be compelled or pressured to accept selective abortion. The Association does not, however, consider it acceptable to choose which fetuses to abort on anything other than medical grounds. When there are no medical indications for aborting a particular fetus, the choice should be a random one. The Association would not consider it acceptable, when making this decision, to accede to the parents' desire for a male or a female child. For further discussion of sex selection, see Chapter 8 (pages 296–8).

Abortion on grounds of fetal sex

Fetal sex is not one of the criteria for abortion listed in the Abortion Act and therefore termination on this ground alone has been challenged as outwith the law. There may be circumstances, however, in which termination of pregnancy on grounds of fetal sex would be lawful. It has been suggested that, if two doctors, acting in good faith, formed the opinion that the pregnant woman's health or that of her existing children would be put at greater risk than if she terminated the pregnancy, the abortion would be arguably lawful under section 1(1)(a) of the Abortion Act.[59] The Association believes that it is normally unethical to terminate a pregnancy on the grounds of fetal sex alone, except in cases of severe sex linked disorders. The pregnant woman's views about the effect of the sex of the fetus on her situation and on her existing children should nevertheless be carefully considered. In some circumstances doctors may come to the conclusion that the effects are so severe as to provide legal and ethical justification for a termination. They should be prepared to justify the decision if it were challenged.

Conscientious objection to abortion

The Abortion Act has a conscientious objection clause that permits doctors to refuse to participate in terminations, but which obliges them to provide necessary treatment in an emergency when the woman's life may be at risk. The BMA supports the right of doctors to have a conscientious objection to termination of pregnancy and believes that such doctors should not be marginalised. Some have complained of being harassed and discriminated against because of their conscientious objection to termination of pregnancy. There have also been reports of doctors who carry out abortions being subjected to harassment and abuse. The Association abhors all such behaviour and any BMA members who feel they are being pressured, abused, or harassed because of their views about termination of pregnancy should contact their regional office for advice and support.

Legal scope

The scope of the conscientious objection clause in the 1967 Act was clarified by the House of Lords in 1988.[60] In that case, a doctor's secretary (Janaway) refused to type the referral letter for an abortion and claimed a conscientious objection under the Act. The House of Lords, in interpreting the word "participate" in this context, decided to give the word its ordinary and natural meaning; that is, in order to claim conscientious exemption under section 4 of the Act, the objector had to be required to actually take part in administering treatment in a hospital or approved centre. The same view emerged in a parliamentary answer in December 1991.[61] This made it clear that conscientious objection was intended to be applied only to participation in treatment, although hospital managers were asked to apply the principle, at their discretion, to those ancillary staff who were involved in the handling of fetuses and fetal tissue.

In the Janaway case the judge said that the signing of the certificate would not form part of the treatment for the termination of pregnancy. This would seem to support the view that GPs cannot claim exemption from giving advice or performing the preparatory steps to arranging an abortion if the request meets the legal requirements. Such steps include referral to another doctor as appropriate. Doctors with a conscientious objection to abortion should make their views known to the patient and enable the patient to see another doctor without delay if that is her wish. Although they may not impose their views on others who do not share them, doctors with a conscientious objection may explain their views to the patient if invited to do so. General practitioners with a conscientious objection who are working in a group practice may ask a partner to see patients who seek termination. The restrictions imposed by GPs' terms of service, however, may prevent single handed GPs from referring patients to another GP and oblige them to refer directly to a specialist. The position of medical students was clarified in a personal communication with the Department of Health that has been passed to the BMA for information. This made clear that the conscientious objection clause may be used by students to opt out of witnessing abortions.

The BMA's advice is that those who have a conscientious objection should disclose that fact to supervisors, managers or GP partners (whichever is appropriate) at as early a stage as possible so that this fact can be taken into account when planning provisions for patient care.

Distinction between legal and moral duties

In some cases a distinction can be made between the legal and ethical obligations. Although noting the legal view, the BMA considers that some things that arguably fall outside the legal scope of the conscience clause, such as completion of the form for abortion, are arguably an integral part of the abortion procedure and thus fall morally within its scope. Other preliminary procedures, such as clerking in the patient, are incidental to the termination and are considered outwith the scope of the conscience clause, both legally and morally. Nevertheless, where such tasks are unavoidable, health professionals and other staff must pursue a non-judgmental approach to the women concerned.

Delays in referral

Much concern has been expressed about avoidable delays in referral. Unreasonable delay with the intention, or the result, of compromising the possibility of a termination being carried out is unethical and may possibly leave the practitioner open to litigation. Referral need not be a formal procedure. In some cases, it may simply consist of arranging for the patient to see a partner in the practice. In other cases, it involves arranging a specific appointment with a colleague. It is not sufficient simply to tell the patient to seek a view elsewhere because other doctors may not agree to see her without an appropriate referral. The Royal College of Obstetricians and Gynaecologists has issued guidance on recommended referral times.[62]

Questions about abortion in job applications

The BMA is frequently asked what enquiries may be made about a doctor's views on abortion in job advertisements and at interview. The Department of Health published guidance on this issue in 1994,[63] which states that, for training grade posts, no reference to abortion should be included in the job advertisement or the job description, and applicants should not be questioned about their attitude to termination of pregnancy prior to the appointment. For most career grade posts, no information should be included in the advertisement but, if certain conditions have been satisfied, reference may be included in job descriptions and some questions may be asked at interview. At interview, however, enquiries about duties that relate to termination of pregnancy should be confined to matters of professional intention and not extend to questions about the applicant's personal beliefs. The Department of Health has confirmed that this guidance is not intended to cover the advertising of career posts that have little content other than termination of pregnancy duties.[64] Trusts can therefore advertise explicitly when the duties of career posts are entirely for the termination of pregnancy. At the time of writing Scottish guidance on this subject is in preparation.

Summary – abortion

- In England, Scotland, and Wales abortion is lawful in the circumstances set out in the Abortion Act 1967. Abortion is also lawful in more limited circumstances in Northern Ireland.
- A young person aged under 16, who has sufficient understanding and competence, may consent to termination of pregnancy, but parental involvement should be encouraged.
- Although women should generally be encouraged to discuss their decision to terminate a pregnancy with the father of the fetus, male partners do not have the legal right to decide.

- Doctors with a conscientious objection to abortion are not obliged to participate, except in an emergency situation where the woman's life may be at risk. Patients should, however, be referred to another health professional without delay.

Prenatal diagnosis

Some form of screening or testing is offered routinely to every pregnant woman in the UK. It is often presented as a standard part of antenatal care but, in fact, it raises significant ethical dilemmas that need to be addressed. These issues are discussed in some detail in the BMA's publication on genetics.[65] The main issues are summarised below.

Objectives of prenatal diagnosis

In the past, some health professionals restricted access to prenatal diagnosis to those individuals who planned to terminate an affected pregnancy,[66] but this approach is now widely regarded as paternalistic and unacceptable. The BMA believes that parents should be given as much information as necessary to enable them to make an informed decision about whether to opt for testing and, if so, how to respond to an unfavourable result.

The termination of an affected pregnancy is one possible outcome of prenatal diagnosis, but there are a number of reasons why parents may wish to know the health of their fetus. For many people, prenatal diagnosis brings reassurance, but for those who receive an unfavourable result there can be practical benefits in having advance warning. In some cases, for example, knowledge of a disorder prior to the birth allows arrangements to be made for delivery at a specialised unit with facilities and expertise available to provide for the immediate medical needs of the child. Advance knowledge of disability can also prevent misdiagnosis and lead to earlier treatment or management of the condition. With a very small number of conditions, such as congenital adrenal hyperplasia, there is also the option of *in utero* treatment. When treatment is not a possibility, parents may still find it helpful to know in advance, to give them and their family time to come to terms with the child's disability, to find out more information about the condition, to access support networks, and to plan for the child's future. Even with fatal conditions, some people prefer to "let nature take its course", allowing time for the parents and their family to come to terms with the inevitability of the child's death.

The Royal College of Physicians set out the objectives of prenatal diagnosis as:

- to allow the widest possible range of informed choice to women and couples at risk of having children with an abnormality;
- to provide reassurance and reduce the level of anxiety associated with reproduction;

- to allow couples at risk to embark on having a family knowing that they may avoid the birth of seriously affected children through selective abortion;
- to ensure optimal treatment of affected infants through early diagnosis.[67]

Prenatal screening

Prenatal screening is frequently used as a means of identifying those at higher than average risk of having a child with a disability, who are then offered more specialised testing. Prenatal screening may be by family history, serum screening, molecular tests, or ultrasound. Ultrasound scanning is currently offered routinely to all pregnant women in the UK. Although undertaken to monitor the development of the fetus, it is also able to detect both major and minor defects. Often it is offered as "routine" and some women have reported difficulties in refusing it. Concerns have also been expressed that women may accept screening unquestioningly without giving due consideration to the implications of an unfavourable result. Health professionals have a general ethical and legal duty to ensure that patients are given sufficient information to understand what is proposed and are given the opportunity to give or withhold consent. The BMA believes that, when giving information to patients, health professionals should present the possibility of refusing all prenatal screening as a reasonable and acceptable option.

Prenatal genetic testing

Prenatal genetic testing is offered to those who are known to be at risk of carrying an affected child. This may be because of previous affected pregnancies, a family history of a particular disorder, or because they have been identified, from screening, as being at higher than average risk of having an affected child. The majority of prenatal genetic testing is carried out during pregnancy using either amniocentesis or chorionic villus sampling. (Some success has also been achieved with testing embryos for particular conditions before implantation; this is discussed in Chapter 8 (pages 291–2).) It has been suggested that those who are at high risk of passing on a severe genetic disability have a duty to future generations and to their partner either not to reproduce[68] or to seek appropriate testing and termination of an affected pregnancy. Harris, for example, argues that an individual's moral obligation to future generations is both positive and negative. Not only must we not deliberately act to cause harm to our offspring, but we also have an obligation to remove dangers that would cause harm.[69] Depending upon the notion of harm in this context, this could be interpreted as a moral obligation for women to avail themselves of prenatal diagnosis and, where the child would be affected, to terminate the pregnancy. The BMA does not support this position, believing that it would be unacceptable to prevent people from reproducing or to force women to have testing and terminate affected pregnancies. Neither is it reasonable to impose on those who suffer from genetic disorders moral responsibilities over and above those that apply to the rest of the population. Information should be provided and women and couples should be supported in whatever decision they make. When the parents disagree with each other about whether to seek testing, or about whether to terminate an affected pregnancy, they should each be given the opportunity to discuss their views and wishes. In some cases it may also be appropriate to offer expert counselling. If agreement cannot be reached, the woman's view about the progress of her pregnancy should hold sway within the constraints imposed by the law.

Social implications

Some people see prenatal diagnosis, not as part of a duty of care to the potential child, but as a personal and societal drive to eliminate non-standard individuals and to what has been termed the "tyranny of normality", leading to an ever narrowing definition of normality and tolerance. This, in turn, leads to higher expectations among parents and makes them less able to accept disability when it happens. This can manifest itself in anger when a child is born with a disability and can result in the parents grieving for the loss of the normal, healthy baby that, they considered, was almost guaranteed. Although disability is a fact of life, it is suggested that people are less able to cope because, with the emphasis on prenatal diagnosis, "normality" within a narrow range of variation is expected.

There are also concerns that, as prenatal diagnosis becomes more widespread, those who decide not to have testing when they are known to be at risk of a genetic disorder, or who decide to continue with an affected pregnancy, may come to be seen as irresponsible. When the child will be severely disabled and require long term and expensive treatment it is possible that society will become increasingly unwilling to pay for the necessary care, seeing the parents as "to blame" for the birth and therefore individually responsible for the cost of treatment. In the USA there have been reports of private insurance companies attempting, unsuccessfully, to withhold reimbursement for the medical care of children whose disability was detected before birth.[70] Any such moves in this country must be vigorously opposed. The availability of resources for the care and treatment of a disabled child must not be contingent on whether the parents knew of the disability before the child was born.

Little research has been undertaken into the effect of prenatal diagnosis on public attitudes towards disability, either to confirm or refute these predictions. It is important that the potential for increased discrimination is recognised and that public attitudes towards disability are carefully monitored.

Setting boundaries

A frequent question in relation to prenatal diagnosis is where the boundaries should be set. Is it acceptable, for example, to terminate a pregnancy because the child, if born, will develop a serious disorder in middle age? Could, and should, the technology be used to meet parental desires for children with particular characteristics or looks? The BMA has considered these questions in some detail and has reached the following conclusions.

- The criteria for prenatal diagnosis should be sufficiently flexible to allow for consideration of individual cases, when the following factors should usually be taken into account:

  - the sensitivity and specificity of the test and the level of predictability obtained from the results
  - the pregnant woman's own perception of the situation and her existing family circumstances
  - the severity of the disorder
  - the age of onset of the condition
  - the options available, including the possibility of effective treatment, either *in utero* or after birth.

- The BMA has concerns about the routine use of prenatal diagnosis for adult onset disorders, but accepts that, in some circumstances, after careful counselling and consideration, such testing could be appropriate.
- Genetic information and technology should be used primarily to reduce suffering and impairment. Their use for trivial reasons or as a means of satisfying parental desires for certain physical or enhancing characteristics in healthy children is inappropriate.

Summary – prenatal diagnosis

- When giving information to patients about prenatal diagnosis, health professionals should present the possibility of refusing all prenatal screening and testing as a reasonable and acceptable option.
- When the parents disagree with each other about whether to seek testing, or about whether to terminate an affected pregnancy, they should each be encouraged to discuss their views and wishes. If agreement cannot be reached, the woman's view should hold sway within the constraints imposed by the law.
- Parents should not be seen as "to blame" for the birth of a disabled child, irrespective of whether they refused testing or knew of the disability before the child was born.
- Medical technology should be used to reduce suffering and impairment and its use for trivial reasons or for satisfying parental desires for certain physical or enhancing characteristics is inappropriate.

Pregnancy

Protecting the fetus from harm during pregnancy

There has been considerable debate, both in the UK and elsewhere, about ways of protecting a fetus from harm caused by its mother's actions during pregnancy by, for example smoking, or the abuse of alcohol or drugs. In Re F (see below) the Appeal Court rejected an application to make a fetus a ward of court in order to protect it from harm from its mother, who suffered from severe mental illness, abused drugs, and had a nomadic lifestyle. It was held in that case that the court did not have the power to make an unborn child a ward of court and that any such action would necessarily involve controlling the mother.

Attempt to make a fetus a ward of court

F was 36 years old and since her early 20s had suffered from severe mental disturbance, accompanied by drug abuse, and she suffered from delusions and hallucinations. She lived a nomadic existence, travelling through a number of European countries. F had a son, G, who had been taken into the care of long term foster parents and adoption proceedings had commenced; F's access to her son had been terminated after repeated unsuccessful attempts at rehabilitation. F became pregnant again and, shortly before the anticipated date of delivery, the local authority applied to make the fetus a ward of court in order to protect it from possible harm arising from its mother's actions. The application was dismissed on the grounds that the court did not have the jurisdiction to make a fetus a ward of court.

This decision was upheld by the Court of Appeal.

Re F (in utero)[71]

Although a child may sue a third party for damages caused by negligent acts in the antenatal period, in England, Wales, and Northern Ireland a child cannot sue its mother for harm caused by her actions during pregnancy (with the exception of harm resulting from a road traffic accident).[72] This followed a Law Commission report published in 1974.[73] Influential in its decision were the arguments that: the relationship between a disabled child and its mother would inevitably be difficult and the situation would be exacerbated if she was liable to pay compensation for the child's disabilities; it was not clear where the mother would find the funds to pay any compensation to the child without causing hardship to the rest of the family; and such a course of action could easily become a weapon in cases of matrimonial conflict. Concern was also expressed about the problem of setting limits to the type of maternal conduct that would render the woman liable for any subsequent disability. Although women should be alerted to the likely risks to the fetus caused by their behaviour, and should be encouraged to refrain from risky activities for the duration of the pregnancy, there is no way of compelling them to do so. In Scotland this issue remains open because there is no law excluding a claim by the child against its mother in relation to prenatal injuries, although it has been suggested that a Scottish court would be unsympathetic to such claims, on policy grounds.[74]

Routine screening of pregnant women

In addition to prenatal screening and testing of the fetus (see page 252), pregnant women themselves are offered screening for disorders for which treatment or appropriate management during pregnancy and birth can prevent the disorder being passed to the baby. A good example of this is screening for HIV infection. Guidance from the health departments states that all maternity units should offer and recommend HIV testing as a routine part of antenatal care.[75] This is consistent with BMA policy dating back to 1991 that all pregnant women should be offered routine screening for HIV antibodies. If a woman tests positive, the risk of vertical transmission to her baby can be reduced from 25% to less than 5% by the avoidance of breastfeeding, the use of antiretroviral drugs, and delivery by elective caesarean section. Clearly, the greater the ability to intervene effectively to prevent harm, the greater the argument for offering screening. The aim is to reduce by 80% the number of babies with HIV acquired from an infected mother during pregnancy and birth, or through breastfeeding.

Providing life support to a pregnant woman for the benefit of a fetus

Decisions to withhold or withdraw life prolonging treatment are difficult and controversial, but they are even more so when the patient is a pregnant woman and withdrawing treatment would result in the death of an otherwise healthy fetus. Thankfully, such situations are rare, but when they occur they raise difficult legal and ethical questions about the acceptability of continuing to provide life support for the benefit of the fetus. These questions have yet to be properly resolved. This section explores some of the legal and ethical factors that would need to be taken into account. When there is no benefit to the pregnant woman of providing treatment, it is likely that a court declaration would need to be sought.

As discussed in Chapter 3, when adults do not have the capacity to give consent to medical treatment, the doctor in charge of the patient's care must assess, and act in, that individual's best interests. A proxy decision maker may also have a role (see Chapter 3, pages 110–2). When starting or continuing treatment is not in the patient's best interests, it may be withdrawn, even if this results in the patient's death. If the woman has a valid advance directive refusing all life prolonging treatment in the circumstances that have arisen and which specifically states that the directive should apply while she is pregnant, the directive should be followed. If the advance directive does not state that it should apply when the woman is pregnant, and the life of the fetus could be saved by continuing to provide life support to the mother, legal advice should be sought and it may be necessary to seek a court declaration. The Law Commission, in its report on mental incapacity, recommended that women making an advance directive should be explicit about whether the directive should apply during pregnancy.[76] In the absence of such a statement, it is likely that the courts will assume that the woman had not intended the directive to apply during pregnancy and rule it invalid.

In the absence of any clear expression of the patient's previous wishes, the primary duty of the doctor is to provide necessary and appropriate treatment for the mother. So, when life support is likely to provide clinical benefit to the patient, this should be provided. This is true even if the treatment will jeopardise the health or life of the fetus, since the mother's interests prevail over those of her fetus in such cases.[77] When, however, an alternative treatment could be provided that does not jeopardise the fetus, this would be the preferred option. If the fact of pregnancy itself jeopardised the chances of survival for the woman, the legal grounds for terminating the pregnancy would be met. A more difficult situation arises when clinical assessment reveals that there is no hope of survival for the woman and, although continuing to provide life support would increase the chance of a successful live birth, it will involve prolonging the dying process for the mother. The question then arises as to whether treatment may be provided for the benefit of the unborn child or whether saving the child could be seen to be in the woman's emotional or psychological best interests.

Providing life support for a pregnant woman

Ms Karen Battenbough was 24 years old and 4½ months pregnant when a car accident in 1995 left her in a coma with virtually no chance of survival. She could breathe unaided and was given artificial nutrition and hydration to prolong her life. On 3 May 1995 she delivered a daughter by caesarean section; according to her family this was a baby she desperately wanted. She never regained consciousness and died in December 1996.[78] This case did not go to court and it is unclear from the media reports whether, had she not been pregnant, her doctors would have judged the provision of life prolonging treatment to be in her best interests. The fact that treatment was continued after the delivery, however, implies that her doctors considered that she was deriving benefit from it. Even if there had been no clinical benefit, it is likely that the woman's previously expressed views about her pregnancy would have been influential in assessing that her best interests would be met by providing treatment to give the child the best chance of survival.

The case described above would have been more complex if the woman had not known she was pregnant before the accident, she had not planned the pregnancy, and she had never discussed her views about pregnancy. In that situation, it would be difficult to argue that it would be in the woman's best interests to continue life support in order to increase the chance of a healthy child. Then, the only grounds for continuing to provide the treatment would be for the benefit of the fetus, but, in considering cases of enforced caesarean section, the courts have made clear that they do not have the jurisdiction to take the interests of the fetus into account.[79] Similarly, in a review of the common law on consent, McLean highlighted the fact that "the best interests test requires evidence that the intended intervention is for the benefit of the individual concerned. Thus, no attention should be paid to possible benefits to third parties".[80] Peart *et al.* point out that, using the reasoning in Bland[81] (see Chapter 10, page 359), "it would be unlawful to keep a pregnant woman in such circumstances on life support solely for the benefit of her unborn child, because it would not be in her best interests. Life support should be withdrawn and she should be allowed to die, regardless of the effect that this has on her unborn child".[82] They go on to say, however, that it seems improbable that a court would sanction the withdrawal of treatment, if continuing it was not *contrary* to the woman's interests (or if she was perceived to have no interests) and it would be possible to save the life of the unborn child. They take the view that

> a pregnant woman in [persistent vegetative state (PVS) or similar irreversible condition] ... has no interest in being alive, nor does she have an interest in being dead. Prolonging her existence until after the birth of her child therefore does not conflict with her interests, because she no longer has interests in any meaningful sense. ... We would therefore conclude that decisions about treatment of a pregnant PVS patient should be made in the interests of her unborn child, because the patient's condition and prognosis have effectively deprived her of the sort of interests which normally underpin treatment decisions.[83]

Although, intuitively, it would appear appropriate to save the life of a child, when this is possible without causing harm to the mother, this is not straightforward either legally or morally. Legally, treatment may be provided to incompetent adults only if it is in their best interests, or in Scotland under the general authority to treat if it is considered to be of benefit, or with the consent of any appointed healthcare proxy (see Chapter 3, pages 110–2). To provide treatment in other circumstances would constitute battery. Given that under the current law the best interests test cannot include the interests of any third party, including a fetus, treatment cannot lawfully be provided to an incompetent woman for the benefit of her unborn child. Arguments about "not being contrary to interests", which have been proposed in the academic literature, have not been tested in the courts. From an ethical perspective, unless it is assumed that all women have moral obligations to their unborn children that can be enforced, such action could be seen as assault on the woman's autonomy, bodily integrity, and dignity. It has been argued, for example, that keeping a woman on a ventilator after her death to permit the safe delivery of her child would, in the absence of any indication of her wishes, involve a violation of her autonomy, be an act of disrespect, and would amount to treating her as a "human incubator" or "fetal container".[84]

The UK courts have not considered a case where treatment is not in the best interests of a pregnant woman (or where she is perceived to have no interests) and where her own wishes are not known. The question of whether the presumption should be in favour of providing life support or withholding it, in such circumstances, remains unresolved. Should such a case arise, legal advice should be sought and a declaration from the courts may be needed.

Summary – pregnancy

- Women should be alerted to any risks to their fetus arising from their behaviour during pregnancy, but they cannot be compelled to refrain from such activities.
- Even where there are concerns that a mother's actions are putting her fetus at risk, the fetus cannot be made a ward of court.
- It is unclear whether, legally, life support could continue to be provided to a pregnant woman solely for the benefit of the fetus. If such a situation arises, legal advice should be sought.

Childbirth

During the 1990s there was a shift towards greater patient choice in where and how to give birth, articulated in the Department of Health's report *Changing childbirth*.[85] Some women have exercised this choice to opt for more medical intervention, by requesting elective caesarean section as their chosen mode of delivery. Others have sought to reduce medical intervention by requesting natural, water, or home births, or by refusing a medically indicated caesarean section. Wherever and however a woman wishes to give birth, she must be given adequate, accurate information to enable her to make an informed choice. There should be clear agreement among the health professionals involved about who takes responsibility for different elements of the woman's care. In most cases, a midwife assumes sole responsibility for normal deliveries, calling upon a doctor for assistance only if complications arise.

Home births and the role of GPs

Changing childbirth emphasised that every effort should be made to accommodate the wishes of women and their partners about how and where they give birth. This specifically included the option of having a midwife as the lead professional responsible for their care and presenting home birth as a realistic option.

When a woman is considering a home birth, with the support of her midwife, she should be given sufficient information to enable her to make an informed decision, based on both the actual and perceived risks and benefits of giving birth outside a medical environment. With home births, as in hospital, the lead role is usually taken by the midwife, with medical assistance called upon or hospital admission arranged only if complications arise. In an emergency situation, the patient is likely to be admitted to hospital but, if called, the GP would be required to attend and to give such assistance as is reasonable, judged by the standards of an ordinary GP. In some cases, the patient's GP attends during the labour, in order to give personal support to the woman or to provide additional backup to the midwife who is managing the birth. However, the majority of GPs do not have obstetric skills and they are not expected to provide specialist intervention. GPs who are asked to support a woman's choice of a home birth should ensure that their patient is aware of what, if any, additional training in obstetrics they have received, and the role they will take in the delivery. It is important that a woman is aware of the limitations of the support her GP is able to provide.[86]

When, in a particular case, GPs have concerns about the safety of a home birth, this should be discussed with the patient, midwife, and obstetrician. Every effort should be made to reach a mutually acceptable position through discussion, negotiation, and the offer of seeking another expert opinion. When agreement cannot be reached, it is important that the patient does not feel abandoned by any of the healthcare providers. Nor should GPs be excluded from their patient's care, since they have a continuing duty of care to the woman and, possibly, other members of her family. Even if GPs make clear their concerns about the choice of a home birth, they are still obliged to attend if called in an emergency situation. Although women cannot be obliged to attend hospital or a maternity unit for delivery, they do not have a legal right to demand medical assistance in support of their choice of a home birth. The Nursing and Midwifery Council position statement on home births, however, advises that "if mutually acceptable alternative arrangements cannot be agreed [after providing an explanation of the risks of a home birth and the alternatives available], the midwife should not withdraw care, thereby potentially placing the woman at risk of delivering unattended".[87]

Many women who have wanted to give birth at home when there were no medical contraindications have been unable to do so because of a shortage of midwives. As part of a concerted effort to improve maternity services, in May 2001 the Government announced the recruitment of 2000 more midwives by 2005. It also announced a National Service Framework for children and maternity services to ensure that:

- women will have access to a midwife dedicated to them when in established labour 100% of the time
- all women will have access to care delivered by midwives they know and trust and
- there is an end to the lottery in childbirth choices, so that women in all parts of the country, not just some, have greater choice, including that of a safe home birth.[88]

Requests for caesarean section

The number of women giving birth by caesarean section has increased dramatically, such that one in five women in England and Scotland now gives birth in this way.[89] Part of the explanation for this increase is that women are delaying childbirth until later in life and it is known that older mothers are more likely to deliver by caesarean section. However, research has found that, despite this correlation, the higher number of caesarean deliveries is not explained by higher rates of complications, as could be expected.[90] Instead, as the authors of the study suggest, the results may support existing speculation that physician and maternal preference has played a significant role in the increase. Evidence of patient demand for caesarean section in affluent parts of London[91] appears to mirror the media portrayal of caesarean delivery as a new "designer" lifestyle choice. This follows publicity surrounding the birth choices of a number of high profile celebrities who, it has been suggested, are unwilling to endure the pain and long term sequelae of vaginal delivery and favour the convenience of a planned delivery date. Others see the increase in caesarean sections as evidence of defensive medicine by obstetricians and "a process in which women are finally given less information and less choice and in which obstetricians appropriate the central role of childbirth at the expense of women".[92] It has been suggested that maternal preference is, in fact, strongly influenced by the views of medical practitioners, many of whom have vested interests in making "the well worried".[93] Doctors should ensure that information is provided objectively and is, wherever possible, evidence based, acknowledging uncertainty where it exists. All requests for elective caesarean section should be assessed individually, taking account of the most recent guidance available, including that from the National Institute for Clinical Excellence.

Why women choose caesarean section

A study, carried out in 1999 by Graham *et al.*, found that, out of 166 women who delivered by caesarean section, maternal preference was a direct factor in 7% of cases.[94] The reasons why women choose to deliver by elective caesarean section, rather than by a vaginal birth, has been the subject of much debate. Some have speculated that "health has become secondary to a sexually attractive body"[95] and that the fear of genital damage represents another aspect of society's popular obsession with body image. A genuine fear of vaginal delivery, as well as concerns about the long term sequelae and fear of harm to the baby, were reported in interviews carried out by Weaver *et al.* with women who said that the issue of caesarean section arose during their pregnancy.[96] An expert advisory group that considered the increased rate of caesarean sections in Scotland, reported a variety of reasons why women choose this option, including bad experiences at previous vaginal delivery, fear of intimate examinations, and previous sexual abuse.[97]

Views are mixed about whether women should be given the right to choose a caesarean section when this is not required for medical reasons. In Scotland, an expert advisory group appeared to support giving women that option. Its report concluded that "women's views and preferences should be acknowledged as a major factor in the joint decision between clinicians and women to deliver by caesarean section".[98] The recommendations went on to say that, when a decision is made for a caesarean delivery, in the absence of obstetric indications, clinicians must ensure that the woman has the necessary information to reach a truly informed choice.

261

Those who oppose giving women this choice stress that caesarean section is a major operation, carrying risks for both mother and child, and that to expose women and their unborn babies to those risks when there is no medical need to do so would be wrong and contrary to the doctor's duty of care. Those who support giving women the choice of caesarean section argue that, provided they are properly informed of the risks, women themselves are the best judge of what is right for them. In a society that is increasingly intolerant of risk, where antenatal screening and care is positively encouraged, it has been argued that women should be given the option of a caesarean section if they find that more acceptable.

Central to this debate is the balance of risks between vaginal and caesarean delivery. Caesarean section has traditionally been seen as exposing both mother and baby to higher risk than vaginal delivery. It has been argued, however, that much of the data on mortality and morbidity rates after caesarean section are taken from emergency caesareans, where there are existing complications, and that the risks of vaginal delivery are frequently underestimated.[99] More research and clinical guidance is needed to provide objective, comparative data about risk in order to assist those facing such requests. Some argue that, until there is evidence that elective caesarean section is at least as safe as vaginal delivery, it should not be offered when there are no medical indications. Others take the view that, in the absence of clear and undisputed evidence, the woman's own assessment of the risks and benefits to her should provide the crucial deciding factor. This is an area that needs to be explored further because the closer the balance of risks between the two modes of delivery, the stronger the argument for allowing women to choose. Inevitably, however, the resource implications of giving all women the option of elective caesarean section, at far greater cost than vaginal delivery, cannot be ignored.

When presented with a request for a caesarean section on grounds of maternal preference rather than medical necessity, the doctor should ensure that the patient is provided with up to date information about the relative advantages and disadvantages. The woman should be encouraged to discuss any fears or concerns, and steps should be taken to address these before deciding on the most appropriate course of action. An obstetrician who is concerned about the risks of carrying out an elective caesarean in these circumstances would not be obliged to comply with the request. The courts have frequently stated that they would not force doctors to act contrary to their clinical judgment. The doctor should discuss the concerns with the patient and explain the reasons for not wishing to proceed. If the patient still wishes to have a caesarean section, she should be offered the option of transferring to the care of another doctor. Where elective caesarean section is not provided on the NHS, the patient should be informed of this and offered a referral for private treatment if that is her wish.

Refusal of caesarean section

Health professionals who provide care for women during their pregnancy and labour aim to promote the greatest benefit to both mother and fetus with the least risk. In a small number of cases, problems arise because the pregnant woman and her doctors fundamentally disagree about the action believed to be in the best interest of the mother or fetus or because medical advice conflicts with the woman's beliefs, religious or otherwise. Pregnancy and labour are particularly recognised as processes in which women's wishes should be supported and health professionals normally try to accommodate patients' wishes when this can be done without incurring grave risks.

Questions inevitably arise, however, about the validity of the patient's decision when it conflicts with her known desire to have a healthy baby or when she is subject to involuntary compulsion. Such is the case where a woman wishes to deliver a healthy child, but refuses a caesarean section or other medical intervention that is considered necessary to achieve that aim. The courts have made clear that whether treatment may be provided without consent in such cases depends upon if the woman is competent to make the decision. Assessing competence in this situation is not always easy and in some cases specialist psychiatric examination may be required. Despite the pain and distress that can be associated with childbirth, being in labour is not incompatible with being competent to make decisions. For women over the age of 16, there should be a presumption that they are capable of giving or withholding consent, and that their decisions will be respected. The fact that the healthcare team disagrees with the decision a woman has made does not mean that she is not competent to make the decision. There are, however, some cases in which a woman becomes temporarily incapacitated during labour, for example if her refusal of treatment is caused by a needle phobia as in the case of Re MB (see page 226). In these situations, attempts should be made to alleviate the reasons for the incompetence, wherever possible, in order to obtain a competent decision.

If the woman is competent, her refusal must be respected. If she is not competent, the doctor in charge of her care must act in the woman's best interests, taking account of any previously expressed wishes. If there is genuine doubt about the woman's competence, an application may be made to the courts to decide if treatment may be provided lawfully.

Refusal of caesarean section

Ms S was 36 weeks pregnant and had not previously sought antenatal care. She was diagnosed with pre-eclampsia and was advised that she needed urgent attention, bed rest, and admission to hospital for an induced delivery. Although she understood that without this treatment both her life and that of the fetus were in danger, she rejected the advice, wanting her baby to be born naturally. S was seen by an approved social worker and two doctors, and was admitted against her will for assessment under the Mental Health Act 1983. She was then transferred to St George's Hospital where she continued to refuse treatment. An application was made to the court, and was granted, to dispense with the need for her consent and a caesarean section was carried out, delivering a baby girl. Shortly afterwards her detention under the Mental Health Act was terminated.

Ms S appealed against the original judgment. Upholding the appeal, the decision from the Appeal Court was:

(Continued)

> while pregnancy increases the personal responsibilities of a woman it does not diminish her entitlement to decide whether or not to undergo medical treatment. Although human, and protected by the law in a number of different ways ... an unborn child is not a separate person from its mother. Its need for medical assistance does not prevail over her rights. She is entitled not to be forced to submit to an invasion of her body against her will, whether her own life or that of her unborn child depends on it. Her right is not reduced or diminished merely because her decision to exercise it may appear morally repugnant.[100]
>
> It was further held that the Mental Health Act could not be used to detain an individual against her will merely because her "thinking process is unusual, even apparently bizarre and irrational, and contrary to the views of the overwhelming majority of the community at large".[101]
>
> *St George's Healthcare NHS Trust v S*[102]

The BMA considers that health professionals should encourage pregnant women to consider carefully the options available to them and the implications of a refusal to accept a caesarean section in such cases. Usually, once women realise that acceding to the medical intervention recommended is the best, or perhaps only, way of saving the life of the fetus, they agree to the treatment. In the minority of cases in which women continue to oppose a caesarean section, and they are competent to make that decision, the refusal must be respected. Health professionals must tread a delicate line between advising women honestly of the implications of their decisions and unreasonably pressurising them to consent to the intervention. The refusal of treatment is discussed further in Chapter 2.

Pain relief

Sometimes questions are raised with the BMA about whether a "birth plan" that refuses any pain relief would be binding if the woman subsequently changed her mind during labour. A birth plan is one form of advance directive and, as such, becomes active only when competence is lost. Women in labour generally retain competence to give consent and so their contemporaneous decisions should be respected. Some women make birth plans that include a stipulation that any request for drugs during childbirth should be ignored. Doctors who become aware of such plans should discuss them in advance with the women concerned and explain that any contemporaneous requests for drugs will be taken to override the birth plan. It should be made unambiguously clear that a birth plan refusing particular interventions becomes active only if the patient is not competent to express any views. General discussion about advance statements can be found in Chapter 3 (pages 113–6).

Summary – childbirth

- In home births, as in hospital, the lead role is usually taken by the midwife.
- A GP who is approached about a woman's choice of a home birth should ensure that the patient is aware of the limitations of the support the GP is able to provide.
- Even if a GP makes clear his or her concerns about the choice of a home birth, the GP is still obliged to attend if called in an emergency situation.
- An obstetrician with serious concerns about the risks of carrying out a caesarean section requested for maternal preference rather than medical necessity, would not be obliged to comply with such requests.
- A competent adult's refusal of medical intervention must be respected even if both she and her fetus may die as a result. When there is genuine doubt about the patient's competence, an application may be made to the courts.
- Women in labour generally retain competence to give consent. A birth plan refusing any pain relief during pregnancy would be overridden by a contemporaneous request for drugs.

Reproductive ethics: a continuing dilemma

Reproduction is an area that covers a number of different strands, all of which raise complex legal and ethical questions. This chapter's focus on contraception, abortion, and birth seeks to provide guidance on the type of practical questions raised with the BMA, while also discussing some of the more unusual and perhaps more theoretical scenarios. These are issues that will continue to challenge doctors and society. The next chapter focuses more specifically on the issues raised by assisted reproduction, including some of the major policy decisions that require debate within society.

References

1   Re MB (medical treatment) [1997] 2 FLR 426.
2   Department of Health, Welsh Office, Scottish Office Department of Health, Department of Health and Social Services, Northern Ireland. *Why mothers die. Report on confidential enquiries into maternal deaths in the United Kingdom 1994–1996*. London: The Stationery Office, 1998.
3   Re MB (medical treatment). *Op cit:* p. 441.
4   Paton v United Kingdom (1980) 3 EHRR 408. See also H v Norway (1990) (Case No C-17004/90, unreported).
5   Department of Health. *NHS contraceptive services, England: 1999–2000. Statistical Bulletin 2000/27.* London: DoH, 2000.
6   Social Exclusion Unit. *Teenage pregnancy.* London: The Stationery Office, 1999. (Cm 4342.)
7   *Ibid:* p. 7.
8   Office for National Statistics. Conceptions in England and Wales, 2001. In: *Health statistics quarterly 17.* London: The Stationery Office, 2003.
9   Department of Health. *The NHS plan. A plan for investment. A plan for reform.* London: The Stationery Office, 2000. (Cm 4818-1.)
10 Teenage Pregnancy Unit. *Teenage pregnancy national campaign. Findings of research conducted prior to campaign development.* London: Department of Health, 2000.

11 British Medical Association, Royal College of General Practitioners, Family Planning Association, Brook Advisory Centres. *Confidentiality and people under 16*. London: BMA, 1994.

12 Brook Advisory Centres. *You think they won't tell anyone. Well you hope they won't*. London: Brook Advisory Centres, 1999.

13 Gillick v Wisbech and West Norfolk AHA [1985] 3 All ER 402.

14 Kennedy I. *Treat me right*. Oxford: Oxford University Press, 1988:112.

15 British Medical Association, Brook, General Practitioners Committee, Medical Defence Union, Royal College of General Practitioners, Royal College of Nursing. *Confidentiality and young people. Improving teenagers' uptake of health advice. A toolkit for general practice, primary care groups and trusts*. London: RCGP and Brook, 2000.

16 Teenage Pregnancy Unit. *Best practice advice on the provision of effective contraception and advice services for young people*. London: Department of Health, 2000.

17 Office for National Statistics. *Living in Britain 1998 general household survey*. London: The Stationery Office, 2000.

18 Glasier A, Baird D. The effects of self-administering emergency contraception. *N Engl J Med* 1998;**399**:1–4.

19 The Prescription Only Medicines (Human Use) Amendment (No. 3) Order 2000. (SI 2000 No. 3231.)

20 British Medical Association Annual Representative Meeting, 2001.

21 For further information on sexually transmitted infections see: British Medical Association. *Sexually transmitted infections*. London: BMA, 2002.

22 The Attorney General. *House of Commons official report (Hansard)*. 1983 May 10; col 236.

23 R v HS Dhingra – Birmingham Crown Court Judgment 24 January 1991. *Daily Telegraph* 1991 Jan 25.

24 R (on the application of Smeaton) v Secretary of State for Health [2002] 2 FLR 146.

25 GMC Professional Conduct Committee hearing, 27–30 May 2002.

26 Re D (a minor) [1976] 1 All ER 326.

27 Re F (mental patient: sterilisation) sub nom F v West Berkshire Health Authority [1989] 2 All ER 545: 566.

28 *Ibid:* p. 552.

29 Re A (male sterilisation) [2000] 1 FLR 549.

30 Re B (a minor) (wardship: sterilisation) [1987] 2 All ER 206. In Scotland, contraceptive sterilisation of people aged over 16 is regulated by the Adults with Incapacity (Scotland) Act (see Chapter 3).

31 Royal College of Obstetricians and Gynaecologists. *The management of menorrhagia in secondary care*. London: RCOG, 2000.

32 Re S (sterilisation: patient's best interests) sub noms Re SL (adult patient: medical treatment), SL v SL [2000] 1 FLR 465.

33 The Office of the Official Solicitor. *Practice note (official solicitor: declaratory proceedings: medical and welfare decisions for adults who lack capacity)*. London: Office of the Official Solicitor, 2001.

34 Lord Chancellor's Department. *Who decides? Making decisions on behalf of mentally incapacitated adults*. London: The Stationery Office, 1997. (Cm 3803.)

35 Lord Chancellor's Department. *Making decisions. The government's proposals for making decisions on behalf of mentally incapacitated adults*. London: The Stationery Office, 1999. (Cm 4465.)

36 Adults with Incapacity (Specified Medical Treatments) (Scotland) Regulations, 2002. (SSI 2002/275.)

37 British Medical Association Annual Representative Meeting, 1978.

38 Abortion Act 1967 s1.

39 *Ibid:* s1(4).

40 Royal College of Obstetricians and Gynaecologists. *Termination of pregnancy for fetal abnormality in England, Wales and Scotland*. London: RCOG, 1996.

41 R v Bourne [1939] 1 KB 687.

42 Lee S. An A to K to Z of abortion law in Northern Ireland: abortion on remand. In: Furedi A, ed. *The abortion law in Northern Ireland. Human rights and reproductive choice*. Northern Ireland: Family Planning Association Northern Ireland, 1995.

43 Grubb A. Abortion and children. Re K (a minor), Northern Health and Social Service Board v F and G (1993). *Med Law Rev* 1994;**2**:371–4. Lee S. An A to K to Z of abortion law in Northern Ireland: abortion on remand. *Op cit*.

44 Grubb A. Treatment without consent (abortion): adult. Re A (Northern Health and Social Services Board v AMNH) (1994). *Med Law Rev* 1994;**2**:374–5.

45 British Medical Association Annual Representative Meeting, 1985.

46 Anonymous. Abortion clarity request denied. *BBC Online*, 2003. http://news.bbc.co.uk (accessed 7 July 2003).

47 Henshaw RC, Templeton AA. Mifepristone: separating fact from fiction. *Drugs* 1992;**44**:531–6.
48 *Ibid.*
49 Royal College of Obstetricians and Gynaecologists. *The care of women requesting induced abortion.* London: RCOG, 2000.
50 Re P (a minor) [1986] 1 FLR 272. Re B (wardship: abortion) [1991] 2 FLR 426.
51 Re P (a minor) [1986]. *Op cit.*
52 British Medical Association. *The law and ethics of abortion: BMA views.* London: BMA, 1999.
53 Paton v British Pregnancy Advisory Service Trustees [1978] 2 All ER 987: 991.
54 Paton v United Kingdom (1981). *Op cit.*
55 Price F. Tailoring multi-parity: the dilemmas surrounding death by selective reduction of pregnancy. In: Morgan D, Lee R, eds. *Death rites: law and ethics at the end of life.* London: Routledge, 1994.
56 Lee RG, Morgan D. *Human fertilisation and embryology. Regulating the reproductive revolution.* London: Blackstone Press, 2001:254–6.
57 Phillips C, Hadfield G. A mother wanted me to abort one of her healthy twins. It may sound unethical but it was either that or for both babies to die. *Sunday Express* 1996 Aug 4;12–13.
58 John Habgood, Lord. Moral implications of aborting a twin and of destroying human embryos [letter]. *The Times.* 1996 Aug 7;15.
59 Morgan D. *Issues in medical law and ethics.* London: Cavendish Publishing, 2001:147–9.
60 Janaway v Salford HA [1988] 3 All ER 1079.
61 Bottomley V. *House of Commons official report (Hansard).* 1991 Dec 20; col 355.
62 Royal College of Obstetricians and Gynaecologists. *The care of women requesting induced abortion. Op cit.*
63 NHS Executive. *Appointment of doctors to hospital posts: termination of pregnancy.* London: Department of Health, 1994. (HSG (94) 39.)
64 Department of Health, personal communication, 2003 Feb 19.
65 British Medical Association. *Human genetics: choice and responsibility.* Oxford: Oxford University Press, 1998.
66 Green JM. Obstetricians' views on prenatal diagnosis and termination of pregnancy: 1980 compared with 1993. *Br J Obstet Gynaecol* 1995;**102**:228–32.
67 Royal College of Physicians. *Prenatal diagnosis and genetic screening. Community and service implications.* London: RCP, 1989:1.
68 Dickenson D. Carriers of genetic disorder and the right to have children. *Acta Genet Med Gemellol* 1995;**44**:75–80.
69 Harris J. *Wonderwoman and superman.* Oxford: Oxford University Press, 1992:178.
70 Wertz DC. Ethical and legal implications of the new genetics: issues for discussion. *Soc Sci Med* 1992;**35**:495–505.
71 Re F (in utero) [1988] 2 All ER 193.
72 Congenital Disability (Civil Liability) Act 1976.
73 The Law Commission. *Report on injuries to unborn children. (Law Com No. 60.)* London: HMSO, 1974: paras 54–64.
74 Mason JK, McCall Smith RA, Laurie GT. *Law and medical ethics, 6th ed.* Edinburgh: Butterworths, 2002: para 5·53.
75 NHS Executive. *Reducing mother to baby transmission of HIV.* London: Department of Health, 1999. (HSC 1999/183.) Scottish Executive Health Department. *Offering HIV testing to women receiving antenatal care.* Edinburgh: SEHD, 2002. (NHS HDL (2002) 52.) Department of Health, Social Services and Public Safety, Northern Ireland. *Infection screening for pregnant women and reduction of mother to baby transmission.* Belfast: DHSSPS, 2002. (HSS (MD) 11/02.)
76 Law Commission. *Mental incapacity – Report 231.* London: HMSO, 1995: paras 5·25–5·26.
77 Peart NS, Campbell AV, Manara AR, Renowden SA, Stirrat GM. Maintaining a pregnancy following loss of capacity. *Med Law Rev* 2000;**8**:275–99.
78 Anon. Mother who gave birth in coma dies. *The Daily Telegraph* 1996 Dec 5.
79 Re MB (medical treatment). *Op cit.*
80 McLean SAM. *Review of the common law provisions relating to the removal of gametes and of the consent provisions in the Human Fertilisation and Embryology Act 1990.* London: Department of Health, 1998: para 1·7.
81 Airedale NHS Trust v Bland [1993] 1 All ER 821.
82 Peart NS, *et al.* Maintaining a pregnancy following loss of capacity. *Op cit:* p. 290.
83 *Ibid:* pp. 292–3.
84 See, for example: Jones DG. *Speaking for the dead.* Aldershot: Ashgate Dartmouth, 2000:96–9. Purdy LM. Are pregnant women fetal containers? *Bioethics* 1990;**4**:273–91.
85 Department of Health. *Changing childbirth.* London: HMSO, 1993.

86 General Practitioners Committee. *General practitioners and maternity medical services. Guidance for GPs in England and Wales.* London: British Medical Association, 1999.

87 United Kingdom Central Council for Nursing, Midwifery and Health Visiting (now Nursing and Midwifery Council). *Position statement. Supporting women who wish to have a home birth.* London: UKCC, 2000: para 17.

88 Department of Health press release. *Milburn announces £100 million boost for maternity units; 2000 extra midwives by 2005.* 2001 May 2. (2001/0212.)

89 Royal College of Obstetricians and Gynaecologists Clinical Effectiveness Support Unit. *The national sentinel caesarean section audit report.* London: RCOG, 2001:2.

90 Bell JS, Campbell DM, Graham WJ, Penney GC, Ryan M, Hall MH. Do obstetric complications explain high caesarean section rates among women over 30? A retrospective analysis. *BMJ* 2001;**322**:894–5.

91 Eftekhar K, Steer P. Women choose caesarean section. *BMJ* 2000;**320**:1073.

92 Castro A. Commentary: increase in caesarean sections may reflect medical control not women's choice. *BMJ* 1999;**319**:1401–2.

93 Bewley S, Cockburn J. The unfacts of "request" caesarean section. *Br J Obstet Gynaecol* 2002;**109**:597–605.

94 Graham WJ, Hundley V, McCheyne AL, Hall MH, Gurney E, Milne J. An investigation of women's involvement in the decision to deliver by caesarean section. *Br J Obstet Gynaecol* 1999;**106**:213–20.

95 Bastian H. Health has become secondary to a sexually attractive body [commentary]. *BMJ* 1997;**319**:1402.

96 Statham H, Weaver J, Richards M. Why choose caesarean section? *Lancet* 2001;**357**:635. Weaver J, Statham H, Richards M. High rates may be due to perceived potential for complications [letter]. *BMJ* 2001;**323**:284.

97 Expert Advisory Group on Caesarean Section in Scotland. *Report and recommendations to the chief medical officer of the Scottish Executive Health Department.* Edinburgh: Scottish Executive Health Department, 2001.

98 *Ibid:* p. 5.

99 Paterson-Brown S. Should doctors perform an elective caesarean section on request? Yes, as long as the woman is fully informed. *BMJ* 1998;**317**:462.

100 St George's Healthcare NHS Trust v S, R v Collins and others, ex parte S [1998] 3 All ER 673: 692.

101 *Ibid:* p. 693.

102 *Ibid.*

8: Assisted reproduction

The questions covered in this chapter include the following.

- What responsibility do those providing fertility treatment have towards the resulting children?
- Should there be limits on who should have access to fertility treatment?
- To what extent should parents be able to express preferences about the characteristics of their children?
- Should children born from donated gametes be able to find out the identity of the donor?
- What is the role of health professionals in surrogacy arrangements?

New reproductive technologies, new dilemmas?

Developments in assisted reproduction represent one of the success stories of the late twentieth century. The inability to procreate is a common and distressing problem. Although statistics can be only an approximate guide, one in ten couples are said to be infertile and one in six experience some difficulty in conceiving. Assisted reproduction allows some of these people to have children when nature has failed them. Although initially viewed as an experimental procedure, in vitro fertilisation (IVF) is now a well established, routine, and increasingly popular method of treatment for those who suffer infertility. Although still relatively low, success rates have improved. Between 1978 and 1999 over 50 000 babies were born after IVF treatment in the UK, over 50% of whom were born since 1995.[1] An unintended and generally unwelcome effect of the more frequent use of assisted reproduction was a large increase in the number of multiple births, including in some cases high order multiple births, which have serious consequences for both the individual families and NHS services. Real efforts have been made to overcome this problem, most notably by reducing the number of embryos that may be replaced in a single cycle of IVF, but this continues to be an issue that requires attention. Reports that some forms of assisted reproduction, such as intracytoplasmic sperm injection,[2] may be associated with a higher rate of birth defects has also been a matter of concern. In response, the Medical Research Council and the Human Fertilisation and Embryology Authority (HFEA) set up a working group in 2002 to consider the current knowledge of IVF and its possible health effects, and to advise what further research and follow up may be needed.[3]

In addition to the practical benefits and risks of this treatment, it is also acknowledged that assisted reproduction raises moral and social issues of profound importance. The creation and use of human embryos outside the body promotes complex debate about fundamental questions such as when life and "personhood" begin and at what stage people begin to matter morally. When donated gametes or surrogacy are used, our basic concepts of family relationships, personal identity, and the definitions of "mother" and "father" are challenged. Reproductive technology enables women to have children long after their natural reproductive ability has ceased and to an extent frees women from the restrictions imposed by their natural biological clock, although, often, public expectations exceed what can be delivered, in terms of both the technical possibilities and the level of success achievable. Techniques that were originally developed to help people to overcome some pathology that meant they were unable to reproduce, are increasingly being used to allow people greater choice in their reproductive decisions. For many, this continual pushing back of the barriers is regarded as a very positive and exciting step, allowing women to take greater control over their bodies and reproduction, but, for others, this excitement is tinged with fear and anxiety about where it may lead and about the need for society to set some moral barriers that it will not cross.

Is there a positive right to assistance to reproduce?

People are now able to exercise more choice over their reproductive decisions and are less governed by biological constraints, so some have increasingly perceived control over reproduction as a "right". This tendency to focus on reproductive rights has gained added impetus since the Human Rights Act 1998 came into force, with appeals not only to natural rights but also to enforceable legal rights. It is not surprising, therefore, that one of the first cases to be considered as a challenge under the Human Rights Act was a claim relating to Article 12 (the right to marry and found a family). The case of Gavin Mellor, however, gave an early and clear statement that the Human Rights Act does not give a positive right to assistance to conceive.

The right to found a family

Gavin Mellor was serving a life sentence for murder when he met and married his wife. In 1997 he applied for permission to be allowed to inseminate his wife artificially, arguing that Article 12 of the European Convention gave him the right to found a family. The Secretary of State refused the request on the grounds that artificial insemination was not needed for medical reasons but was sought in order to circumvent the normal consequences of imprisonment. Furthermore, the Home Secretary argued that there were serious concerns about the stability of the relationship, which had not been tested under normal circumstances.

Mr Justice Forbes held that the Secretary of State's decision did not contravene Mr Mellor's Article 12 rights. It had been clearly established that the Article 12 right to found a family did not mean that a person must be given, at all times, the actual possibility of procreating his descendants. In reality, what Mr Mellor was seeking was to be granted the privilege or benefit of being afforded access to artificial insemination services because an inevitable consequence of his lawful detention in custody was that it was impossible for his wife to conceive a child by natural means. The Secretary of State was therefore entitled to formulate a policy for dealing with such requests by prisoners and to decide whether the privilege should be made

(Continued)

available in a particular case. The application was dismissed. In upholding this decision, at the Court of Appeal, Lord Philips emphasised that it will not always be justifiable to prevent a prisoner from inseminating his wife. In this case, however, there were no exceptional circumstances, for example to demonstrate that a refusal would not merely delay the founding of a family but would prevent it altogether.

R v Secretary of State for the Home Department, ex parte Mellor[4]

Duties to the different parties

As in other areas of medicine, focus on rights without any discussion of duties and responsibilities is both incomplete and unreflective of existing practice. In many circumstances, however, doctors' duties are primarily focused on the patient before them, whereas in assisted reproduction there is another party to be considered, that is, the child born as a result of medical intervention. Disputes continue about the ethical obligations, if any, owed to the unborn child. The BMA's general view is that the fetus deserves respect but does not have absolute claims that can override those of an autonomous person, usually the mother (see Chapter 7, pages 227–8). In the case of any form of assisted reproduction, however, the "person" to whom a duty is owed is not only unborn, but also not yet conceived. There has been considerable debate about whether duties can be owed to a "potential person" and whether any life is invariably better than no life. Whereas many individuals experiencing pain, abuse, neglect, or other substantial disadvantages are nevertheless glad to have been born, most people regard it as axiomatic that it would be wrong to generate a pregnancy knowing that the future child would be harmed.

In the BMA's view, as well as in the view of the law, doctors who are asked to intervene to help to generate a pregnancy have particular duties to consider the welfare of any resulting children. The child is the most vulnerable party and doctors' obligations are held to be significantly greater than in any case in which the doctor assumes management of an already existing pregnancy. The extent of these duties is discussed in more detail on pages 274–8.

General principles

When considering the types of dilemma that arise with assisted reproduction, the following general principles should be kept in mind.

- Doctors who help to initiate a pregnancy have particular duties to address the welfare of any future child.
- All people are entitled to a fair and unprejudiced consideration of their request for treatment, so individual cases should be considered and blanket restrictions should not be applied to certain groups.

- Many of the dilemmas that arise have far reaching implications for society as a whole, so public debate should be encouraged and facilitated.

Public debate and regulation

Over recent decades there has been an almost constant barrage of news, information, and debate about developments in assisted reproduction, resulting in the UK having one of the most comprehensive and hitherto effective regulatory mechanisms in the world. The starting point for this period of public debate was the Warnock Committee, which reported[5] in July 1984 and laid the foundations for the enactment of the Human Fertilisation and Embryology Act in 1990.

The Warnock Committee

A committee of inquiry was appointed in 1982 under the chairmanship of Mary Warnock (now Baroness Warnock) to consider "recent and potential developments in medicine and science related to human fertilisation and embryology; to consider what policies and safeguards should be applied, including consideration of the social, ethical and legal implications of these developments; and to make recommendations".[6] The fact that the Warnock report is still referred to some 20 years on shows the way in which the report, and the wide ranging debate that stemmed from it, helped to shape public opinion on these matters. This is not to say that its recommendations were uncontroversial, but they represented the beginning of a long process of education and debate that helped to shape the current regulatory mechanism.

The Human Fertilisation and Embryology Act 1990

The Human Fertilisation and Embryology Act put in place in the UK a statutory regulatory mechanism for assisted reproduction as recommended by the Warnock Committee. The Act established the HFEA and made it a criminal offence to undertake licensable activities without a licence from the statutory body. The activities that are licensable are:

- the creation and use of human embryos *in vitro*
- the storage of gametes and embryos
- the use of donated sperm, eggs, or embryos.

Several duties are imposed on clinics by the Act, such as an obligation to take account of the welfare of any child born or affected by the treatment, the duty to use gametes and embryos in accordance with the consent obtained, and the requirement to offer counselling to anyone seeking licensed treatment. The Act also permits research to be undertaken using human embryos within certain limits (see Chapter 14, pages 517–20).

The Human Fertilisation and Embryology Authority

The HFEA issues a code of practice that gives detailed guidance to clinics about their responsibilities under the legislation and the requirements of the Authority.[7] Every clinic is inspected annually by a team of inspectors from the HFEA to assess the protocols, facilities, and staffing, and to ensure compliance with the Act and the code of practice. The HFEA is also required to maintain a confidential register of information (see pages 285–6) containing details of every cycle of IVF and donor insemination (DI) carried out in the UK, and of all donors and all children born as a result of licensed treatment.

One of the responsibilities of the HFEA is to provide information to the public about the services available. It does this primarily through the annual publication of patients' guides to IVF clinics and DI, each of which gives a list of licensed clinics, the services they provide, and their individual success rates. An annual report presents composite data and a review of activities during the previous 12 months.

Access to treatment

Despite the massive increase in the amount of fertility treatment carried out in the UK, it is not freely available to all. Access to treatment is restricted both on financial grounds and, sometimes, because of concerns about the welfare of future children.

NHS funding

For many years there has been debate about whether involuntary childlessness is a medical issue deserving of a publicly funded medical remedy. Although the Warnock Committee concluded that it was, others disagreed, arguing that those affected by infertility are not "ill" and most infertile people lead normal, healthy lives. Although it is recognised that considerable psychological morbidity and depression stems from involuntary childlessness, it is often seen as a social rather than a medical problem. This argument is sometimes put forward to justify the relative scarcity of NHS funded treatment centres.

In order to assess the extent of variation in provision around the country, the Department of Health undertook a survey of NHS funded infertility services in England and Wales during the financial year 1997/98.[8] The results confirmed anecdotal evidence of widespread variation in the policies of health authorities towards infertility services (16 of the 100 health authorities approached had no policy at all on the purchase of infertility treatment). The amount of money spent on infertility ranged from zero to more than £400 000, but by far the greatest number of health authorities fell into the £0–£100 000 range. There was a similar pattern with the number of infertility treatments carried out: although the range was from zero to over 400, more than half of the health authorities questioned either provided no treatment or fell into the 0–50 range. Virtually all of the health authorities that did provide IVF used eligibility criteria for funding based on factors such as age, number of previous children, minimum length of relationship, and number of previous cycles. In November 2000, the Government announced its intention to tackle the "postcode lottery of infertility treatment" by asking the National Institute for Clinical Excellence to consider and update existing clinical guidelines so that best practice could be available in all parts of the NHS.[9]

It has been suggested that the lack of NHS provision of fertility treatment, and its sporadic provision around the country, leading to "postcode rationing", was an area where there could be a challenge under the Human Rights Act. Article 14 (which is not a freestanding right) gives a right not to be discriminated against in the enjoyment of a substantive right under the Convention. Thus, it has been argued that the inconsistent funding of fertility treatment by the NHS discriminates against people (on grounds of their place of residence and ability to pay) in their enjoyment of their Article 12 right (the right to found a family).[10] Given the clear statement from the court in the Mellor case (see pages 270–1) that there is no positive right to receive fertility treatment, the success of any such claim may be in doubt.

Welfare of the child

Clinics offering licensable treatments are required, by law, to take account of "the welfare of any child who may be born as a result of the treatment (including the need of that child for a father), and of any other child who may be affected by the birth".[11] Although some see this as discriminatory against infertile people, since society does not generally attempt to prevent unsuitable parents from conceiving naturally,[12] others consider that by intervening with treatment to help people to have children, doctors have special responsibilities to ensure that these children will not be greatly disadvantaged. As stated above, the BMA supports this latter view.

The question of eligibility for treatment is a difficult one that demands social judgments that go beyond the purely medical and require multidisciplinary and non-clinical assessments. If, however, it is known that a couple's existing children have been physically and psychologically abused and taken into care, and it is considered very likely that future children too would be abused, it would in our view be inappropriate to help that couple to have more children. However, what about someone who has a history of violence, but has not offended for many years, or someone who has a history of alcoholism or of mild psychiatric problems? What about those who have an unusual lifestyle, who live in a caravan or in a commune, or whose existing children "look unkempt"? There is clearly a risk that individual opinions and prejudices about appropriate and inappropriate lifestyles and family makeup could unfairly influence judgment. Although health professionals must take account of the welfare of the resulting child before offering fertility treatment, such assessments should be carried out fairly and to avoid prejudice. The vast majority of those seeking assisted reproduction are ordinary people who are simply unable to conceive without assistance, rather than those who may legitimately raise concerns. Such assessments should, in the BMA's view, seek to identify those few cases in which a future child is at clear risk of serious harm, rather than seeking to restrict treatment to the minority of the population who fulfil some idealised image of a "happy family".

Although assisted reproduction was originally developed to help couples suffering from infertility, it also allows people to have children outside biological constraints. By using donated gametes, women who are past their normal reproductive age can have children and single women and members of lesbian couples can reproduce without the need for a male partner. The increasing use of assisted reproduction in these types of case reflects growing societal acceptance of a broad range of family relationships, including single parents, and formal recognition of homosexual relationships. The Human Fertilisation and Embryology Act does not exclude any category of patient from treatment but focuses on the clinic's assessment of the prospective patient's ability to meet the needs of a child. The HFEA's code of practice states that "people seeking treatment are entitled to a fair and unprejudiced assessment of their situation and needs, which should be conducted with the skill and sensitivity appropriate to the delicacy of the case and the wishes and feelings of those involved".[13] The BMA also supports this view and has consistently rejected the idea of applying inflexible rules on access to fertility treatment, believing instead that each application should be considered on its merits. Although aspects such as age or stability of the relationship may be relevant items to take into account, assessments should be made on the individual factors in each case rather than according to blanket restrictions applied to certain categories of people.

Although, in practical terms, treatment is likely to be denied only very rarely on the grounds of the welfare of the child, fertility treatment has been refused to people whose lifestyle doctors considered to be unsuitable. When challenged, a court did not find it unreasonable to refuse to provide IVF treatment because of concerns about the welfare of any future child, provided there was not a blanket policy of refusal to treat members of particular religious or ethnic groups (see below).

Welfare of the child

A woman who was having difficulty with conceiving a child applied to adopt or foster a child. Her applications were refused on the grounds that her criminal record, which included allowing premises to be used as a brothel and soliciting for prostitution, made her unsuitable as a foster parent. She then sought IVF treatment but was turned down. She sought a judicial review to quash the decision of the hospital's ethical committee on the grounds that she had not been given the opportunity to make representations before the decision not to treat her was made.

(Continued)

> The court held that, as an advisory committee, the ethical committee was not required to receive representations before reaching a decision. The decision made, that the consultant should make up her own mind as to whether the treatment should be given, was not objectionable as would have been the case had the decision been to refuse treatment to anyone of particular religious or ethnic groups.
>
> *R v Ethical Committee of St Mary's Hospital, ex parte Harriott*[14]

Although it may be easy to identify some forms of discrimination as unlawful, the correct procedure in individual cases, which can involve a variety of complex factors, may be much harder to define objectively and advice may be needed. Despite having some initial reservations about the use of clinical ethics committees, the HFEA now positively encourages clinics to establish such committees and to seek their advice whenever necessary.[15] The HFEA has also produced guidelines for treatment ethics committees, explaining their role in the decision making process, giving guidance about the code of practice, and providing recommendations as to their constitution.[16] The BMA welcomes this shift of opinion and would encourage all clinics to have access to such independent scrutiny of difficult cases.

The need for a father

Although the Human Fertilisation and Embryology Act does not exclude any category of woman from being considered for treatment, clinics are required to take account of "the need of ... [the] child for a father".[17] This statement is rather ambiguous because it has not been interpreted as preventing single women or lesbian couples from having treatment. Rather, the HFEA advises that, where the child will have no legal father, the centre must "have regard to the child's need for a father"[18] and give particular consideration to the mother's ability to meet the child's needs throughout his or her childhood. This could be achieved by considering whether there is anyone else in the mother's family or social circle who is willing and able to share the responsibility for bringing up, maintaining, and caring for the child.

Postmenopausal women

The use of donor oocytes was originally used as a treatment to help those of normal reproductive age who had suffered a premature menopause. Reports, however, have focused on a small number of cases of this treatment being provided for women in their mid to late 50s. The HFEA has resisted calls to set an upper age limit for treatment, arguing that clinics have a responsibility to consider every case on its individual merits. The HFEA has given reassurances that it will continue to monitor the use of oocyte donation for older women and will require clinics to justify the decision to proceed in individual cases, using the general criteria set out in the code of practice. The BMA supports this approach believing that, although age may be one relevant factor to consider, it is the ability of the parents to provide a safe and supportive environment to a child throughout his or her childhood that is the most relevant factor.

Assessments

The HFEA code of practice gives guidance on the types of factors that should be taken into account when clinics are assessing whether people should be accepted for licensed treatment. These include:

- their commitment to having and bringing up a child or children
- their ability to provide a stable and supportive environment for any child produced as a result of treatment
- their medical histories and the medical histories of their families
- their health and consequent future ability to look after or provide for a child's needs
- their ages and likely future ability to look after or provide for a child's needs
- their future ability to meet the needs of any child or children who may be born as a result of treatment, including the implications of a possible multiple birth
- any risk of harm to the child or children who may be born, including the risk of inherited disorders or transmissible diseases, problems during pregnancy and of neglect or abuse
- the effect of a new baby or babies upon any existing child of the family.

The code of practice requires centres to satisfy themselves that the GP of each prospective patient (including the woman's partner if she has one) knows of no reason why they may not be suitable for the treatment to be offered, including any factors that could adversely affect the welfare of any resulting child. Some GPs have expressed concern about such enquiries, believing that they are being asked to speculate about the suitability of their patients for treatment. In fact, the responsibility, as stated above, rests very clearly with the clinic offering treatment. The GP's role is limited to providing factual information that may be important for the clinic to take into account in reaching its decision. The HFEA has issued guidance for GPs about such requests, which states very clearly that

you are not being asked to speculate on lifestyles or on the probability that a patient of yours might behave in certain ways. We are not asking you to assess your patient's suitability to act as parent. You are being asked for relevant factual information, medical or otherwise, within the scope of the information available to you, which you think the clinic needs to know before they consider providing fertility treatment.[19]

If a clinic requests information that appears to be asking the doctor to speculate or to go beyond the information available to him or her, the question should not be answered and the reason for this should be passed on to the clinic.

As in other cases, GPs should ensure that they have their patient's written consent before providing information to a third party. The clinic requesting information should enclose a copy of the patient's signed consent with any request for information but, if this is not enclosed, the information should not be provided without checking with the patient directly or asking the clinic to forward a copy of the consent form. Some GPs are concerned about their continuing relationship with the patient if they disclose information that may harm the patient's chances of being accepted for treatment. Clearly, however, the doctor must not knowingly provide false information or withhold relevant information at the patient's request. When sensitive information is to be disclosed, it is important that this is discussed with the patient. If the patient subsequently withdraws consent to the release of the information, this fact should be relayed to the clinic concerned. A failure to give consent or the subsequent withdrawal of consent to the provision of information is likely to raise concern in the clinic. The HFEA code of practice advises that failure to give consent should be taken into account in considering whether to offer treatment.

Summary – access to treatment

- Doctors who help people to conceive have particular responsibilities to take account of the welfare of the future child.
- Assessments should be carried out fairly and avoid prejudice. They should seek to identify those cases where there is a clear risk of serious harm, rather than to restrict treatment to those who meet some idealised image of a "happy family".
- Assessments should be made on the individual factors in each case rather than according to blanket restrictions applied to certain categories of people.
- GPs who are asked to provide information to a fertility clinic should do so only with their patients' consent. They should not speculate, but provide only factual information.

Consent to the storage and use of gametes and embryos

The Human Fertilisation and Embryology Act requires that consent for the storage or use of gametes or embryos must be in writing and that, before giving consent, the person must have been given information and the opportunity to receive counselling. Consent to storage must specify the maximum period of storage (if less than the statutory limits of 10 years for gametes and 5 years for embryos) and what should be done with the gametes or embryos if the person who gave the consent dies or is unable, because of incapacity, to vary or withdraw the terms of the consent. Consent to the use of gametes or embryos must specify whether they may be used for treatment with a specified person, for the treatment of others, or for use in licensed research. Individuals may withdraw or vary their consent at any time up to the point at which the gametes or embryos are used in treatment or research.

The consent provisions of the legislation were subject to review by Professor Sheila McLean and subsequent consultation[20] in 1997, after the highly publicised case of Diane Blood (see box below).

Posthumous use of gametes

In 1995 Mr Blood contracted meningitis and died. Prior to her husband's death, Mrs Blood asked the doctors to remove sperm samples from him; two samples were taken and stored. Mrs Blood's subsequent request to use the samples in treatment was denied on the grounds that her husband had not given written consent, or received information or the opportunity for counselling, as required by the Human Fertilisation and Embryology Act, and therefore the stored sample could not lawfully be used. In her evidence, Mrs Blood claimed that she and her husband had a genuine commitment to having a family together and that they had even discussed what should happen if he should die before conception occurred.

The HFEA's refusal to permit either the use of the sperm in the UK or its export to another European country for treatment was challenged by Mrs Blood. The Appeal Court held that the HFEA was correct that the sample could not lawfully be used in the UK. In considering its decision on export, however, the court held that the HFEA had taken insufficient account of Mrs Blood's right, under European law, to seek treatment in another country. The matter was referred back to the HFEA, which subsequently withdrew its objection, leaving Mrs Blood free to seek treatment in another country. She has since had two children after treatment with the exported sample.

R v Human Fertilisation and Embryology Authority, ex parte Blood[21]

This case led to considerable debate in the media, the medical profession, and among the public. There was tremendous support and sympathy for Mrs Blood and many people argued vociferously for her right to fulfil her husband's previously expressed wish to have a child. Others, including the BMA, although understanding Mrs Blood's desire to have her late husband's child, were concerned about the broader implications of subjecting incompetent adults to medical procedures from which they would not benefit personally, but which were essentially for the benefit of a third party. It is interesting that both groups used "best interests" arguments to support their case. McLean's review clarified that, legally, the best interests test required evidence that the intended intervention was for the direct benefit of the individual concerned and that no attention could be paid to possible benefits for third parties. It therefore confirmed that the taking, storage, and use of sperm in this type of situation was unlawful under UK law; the consultation that followed sought views on whether the law in this respect should be amended.

In its response to the consultation, the BMA took the view that it should be lawful to permit the collection of gametes without consent, but *only* when the patient is likely to regain competence in the future. The removal of gametes in such cases could be in the patient's best interests, in that it would preserve the option of having children in the future. In these limited circumstances, the BMA believes the HFEA should be able to waive the requirement for consent to storage until the individual can decide, on regaining competence, whether the gametes should continue to be stored, be used in treatment or research, or destroyed. If the patient does not regain competence, the gametes should be allowed to perish. The BMA does not believe that gametes should be removed if, as in the case of Mr Blood, the patient is not expected to recover. In fact, the BMA goes further by rejecting all posthumous use of gametes or embryos even when consent has been given in advance. (An exception to this general rule would be required for donated gametes so that clinics would not be required to verify that the donor was still alive before using stored donated material.)

The report issued after the consultation made a number of recommendations, including the following.[22]

- No change should be made to the existing common law position that gametes can lawfully be removed if to do so would be in the best interests of a patient who is expected to regain competence.
- The Human Fertilisation and Embryology Act should be amended so that where an individual is incompetent and is undergoing treatment, after which the patient is expected to recover but will be rendered infertile, the HFEA may authorise the storage of gametes until the patient is able to make a decision personally.
- The discretionary powers of the HFEA should be limited to preclude the exercise of discretion to permit export of gametes that have been unlawfully obtained.
- Consideration should be given to amending section 28(6) of the Human Fertilisation and Embryology Act (which renders children born from the posthumous use of sperm legally fatherless) to allow men whose sperm is used posthumously to be recorded as the legal father of the resulting child.

In 2001 Tony Clarke MP introduced a private members' bill, the Human Fertilisation and Embryology (Deceased Fathers) Bill, to implement the last of these recommendations and to make its provisions retrospective. Despite Government support for the bill, there was insufficient parliamentary time for it to progress. A similar private members' bill was introduced by Stephen McCabe MP in December 2002, which was given added impetus by a declaration from the High Court, in February 2003, that section 28(6) of the Human Fertilisation and Embryology Act was incompatible with the Human Rights Act.[23] This became the Human Fertilisation and Embryology (Deceased Fathers) Act 2003.

During 2002, another attempt was made to use the courts to overcome a lack of the valid consent required by the Human Fertilisation and Embryology Act. Two women who had embryos stored with the consent of their former partners wished to use the embryos for treatment despite both men having withdrawn their consent. In one of the cases, the embryos offered the only possibility of the woman having her own genetic children. Although the Act is clear that there must be valid consent for storage and use of gametes and embryos, both women argued that the consent requirements, which essentially give one party a veto over the use of stored embryos, are inconsistent with Articles 8 and 12 of the Human Rights Act. They also used the analogy that if they became pregnant naturally and the embryos were in their bodies, then their partners would have no say at all over the future of the pregnancy. There are, however, clear differences between an embryo that is implanted and is therefore inextricably linked to the mother and one that is in storage. In the former case any attempt to end the pregnancy would involve carrying out an invasive procedure on the mother, which she is entitled, both legally and ethically, to refuse. Where the embryo is not implanted, then both partners' views about whether they wish to be parents should be considered. The women's claims were rejected by the High Court.

Summary – consent to the storage and use of gametes and embryos

- Consent for the storage or use of gametes or embryos must be in writing and, before giving consent, the person must have been given information and the opportunity to receive counselling.
- Individuals may withdraw or vary their consent at any time until the gametes or embryos are used.
- Although the collection of gametes from an unconscious patient who is expected to recover may, in some circumstances, be lawful, it is unlawful to store or use the gametes without consent.
- The BMA believes that the law should be changed to allow the HFEA to waive the requirement for consent to storage but only when the patient is expected to recover. Consent should continue to be required for the use of gametes.
- The BMA does not support the posthumous use of gametes or embryos in any circumstances, including when the individual had given his or her prior consent.

Use of donated gametes or embryos

For many people who are infertile, the use of donated sperm, oocytes, or embryos may provide the opportunity to have a much wanted child. All types of treatment involving donated genetic material must be licensed by the HFEA and may be undertaken only in licensed clinics. The "welfare of the child" assessment undertaken by the clinics, before offering treatment, is supplemented in these cases by specific consideration of:

- a child's potential need to know about his or her origins and whether or not the prospective parents are prepared for the questions that may arise while the child is growing up
- the possible attitudes of other members of the family towards the child, and towards his or her status in the family
- the implications for the welfare of the child if the donor is personally known within the child's family and social circle
- any possibility known to the centre of a dispute about the legal fatherhood of the child.[24]

There are two aspects of the use of donated gametes and embryos that have raised most concern and debate: payment of donors and the anonymity of donors.

Payment of donors

The question of whether sperm and oocyte "donors" should be paid, in money or in kind, has been a matter of considerable debate for over a decade and still remains a contentious issue. Section 12(e) of the Human Fertilisation and Embryology Act states that: "no money or other benefit shall be given or received in respect of any supply of gametes or embryos unless authorised by directions". In July 1991 the HFEA issued a direction allowing payment to donors of up to £15 plus reasonable expenses or "other benefits" (defined as treatment services and sterilisation) for each donation. This maintained the *status quo* at that time, but in its second annual report, in 1993, the HFEA stated that its intention was that payment should be phased out in the longer term. Striving towards this aim, a conference was held in June 1995 and, in its 1996 annual report, the HFEA announced its decision that "a donation should be a gift, freely and voluntarily given".[25]

Wary of the risk of seeing a serious drop in the number of donors, the HFEA decided to take time to consider the best way to implement this broad policy decision. In February 1998 the HFEA issued a consultation document on how to implement the policy and to consider how payment could be withdrawn without adversely affecting the supply of donors. In December 1998, while still stressing its commitment to altruistic donation, the HFEA reversed its policy and decided, for pragmatic reasons, to continue to allow payment, in both money and other benefits. A new direction was issued on 7 December 1998 allowing all clinics to offer payment of up to £15 per donation, the reimbursement of expenses (including loss of earnings and child minding expenses), and treatment services or sterilisation in return for donation.[26] The difficulty the HFEA encountered with implementing its policy demonstrates the tension that can arise between principle and pragmatism. Purely altruistic, voluntary donations are considered preferable, but many people are unwilling to accept the likely consequence of adopting such a policy. Research into the motivation of gamete donors (see below) gives a strong indication that, if payment were withdrawn, the number of donors would decrease below levels of demand. This would mean that some people who need or want treatment using donated gametes would be unable to receive it and must remain childless. (The same dilemma arises in the debate on donor anonymity; see pages 285–91)

Motivations of donors

Researchers, on behalf of the HFEA, interviewed 144 potential sperm donors attending 14 UK clinics for screening and a control group of 136 male students who had never donated.[27] They found that all of the potential sperm donors interviewed believed that they should be paid and 62% said that they would not have donated if they had not been paid. Of the control group, a third had considered donating sperm, 71% of whom had been motivated by the payment. The attitudes of 135 women students towards egg donation were also examined and, although 90% were aware of the possibility of donating eggs, only 10% had considered doing so, almost all of whom were motivated by a wish to help others.

As part of this research, enquiries were also made concerning the number of donors approaching centres, in order to consider the accuracy of anecdotal evidence that the number of sperm donors had fallen. It was found that the number of donors approaching clinics had not reduced, but fewer were passing the rigorous screening standards. The main reasons for rejecting potential donors were associated with poor sperm quality and poor motility after thawing. A significant minority were rejected because of past and present psychiatric or genetic disorders. The study confirmed that there was a shortage of donors to meet the increasing demand. Almost all centres (97%) reported that they paid sperm donors and the large majority of respondents believed that they would lose at least 80% of their donors if they did not pay them.

Arguments for and against payment

The BMA contributed to the debate on the payment of donors and, in its consideration of the issue, took account of the following arguments.

- In support of payment

  - Without payment it is impossible to ensure that the supply of donors is maintained and fewer people will be able to have a child using DI.
  - Prohibiting payment could lead to people paying for sperm in private arrangements and thus bypassing the clinics and the screening and counselling they provide.
  - Individuals should be free to do whatever they wish with their own gametes, including selling them, provided they have given informed consent and are not harming anyone else.
  - Payment that induces individuals to donate does not necessarily constitute exploitation. Donors are exploited only if, under different financial circumstances or with full information, they would have refused to donate. Removing payment for donation will not improve their financial situation and may remove one of the few options open to them to make money.
  - Payment can be seen as compensating the donor, rather than as payment, and also as a way of symbolically ending the donor's involvement and rights in relation to any child born.

- Against payment

  - Paying donors for sperm and eggs can be seen as degrading for the individual.
  - Payment for gamete donors can be seen as treating people as commodities and, arguably, undermining the moral obligation to show respect for persons.
  - Some people are reluctant to see an act as morally acceptable if the motive is self interest rather than altruism.

- People may begin to expect payment and this will change the nature of the act, leading to an overall reduction in altruism in society and a demand for payment for other acts currently based on altruism, such as blood donation.
- Paid donors would be likely to transmit more diseases than voluntary donors because of the type of person the payment would attract, and the possibility that they would lie about any illnesses or risk factors in order to obtain the money.
- Payment in money or in kind constitutes exploitation.

The BMA's Medical Ethics Committee debated all of these issues and concluded that, as with other forms of donation (blood, organs, etc.) gamete and embryo donation should be a gift, freely and voluntarily given. Any payment that could act as an inducement to donate should, therefore, be phased out. Donors should not, however, lose out financially as a result of their altruistic act and therefore genuine expenses should be paid. As discussed above, the HFEA reached the same conclusion from an ethical perspective, but decided not to implement it because of concerns about the number of people willing to donate without payment.

Egg sharing

In practice, although sperm donors are given monetary payment, egg donors are not. Many women donate oocytes purely altruistically, while others may receive a benefit in kind, usually free IVF treatment in a scheme that has become known as "egg sharing". For many people, payment in kind is no different, morally, from payment in money. If this is the case, most of the arguments set out above apply to egg donors as well as to sperm donors. Unlike sperm donation, however, egg donation is not without risks. The biggest risk is ovarian hyperstimulation syndrome developing as a result of the drugs given to stimulate the ovaries. Usually the symptoms are very mild, but in around 1% of cases the complications can require hospital treatment, and in a very small number this condition has been fatal. Many people find the procedure of egg collection painful, although there is no evidence of any long term problems. The fact that egg donation includes risks has been used both to justify and to exclude payment and other inducement for egg donors. Some argue that women should not be given any incentive for taking a risk, whereas others argue that the payment should be higher than for sperm donors to compensate for the increased risk. It has also been argued that egg sharing is, in fact, morally preferable to purely altruistic donation since, with egg sharing, the woman is not exposed to any additional risk for the sake of another person.[28]

The main concerns that have been expressed about egg sharing are about consent and, in particular, the risk of coercion or exploitation. The monetary equivalent of a free IVF treatment cycle is likely to be many thousands of pounds and can therefore be seen as a major incentive to donate. Those seen as most vulnerable to exploitation are women who could not otherwise afford to pay for IVF and so agree to participate in an egg sharing scheme as their only way of receiving treatment. Concerns have been expressed about the risk of psychological harm to the donor if she does not become pregnant, but is aware that the recipient may have been successful. However, if these women are fully informed of the procedures, risks, and possible outcomes, does this necessarily constitute exploitation? Some would argue that it does because they were vulnerable and their weak position was used as a means to the ends of others. Others would argue that this constitutes helping two women with different problems, one wanting IVF treatment, the other donated eggs; prohibiting such schemes could be seen as detrimental to both.

When the BMA considered egg sharing, it expressed serious concerns about the validity of the consent, given the very strong incentive provided, and did not support the use of such schemes. The HFEA, however, reported in its 2000 annual report that it had been persuaded that, if properly regulated and monitored, egg sharing could, in some cases, be beneficial to participants.[29] The HFEA therefore decided to allow egg sharing subject to strict guidelines designed to protect all those involved in the arrangements. These guidelines set out the requirements around the provision of information and counselling, consent, and confidentiality. All centres participating in such schemes are required to have a written policy that should include the centre's procedures for determining how the eggs will be shared between the provider and the recipient. The guidelines state that "the egg sharing agreement should make it clear that where there are fewer eggs collected than the minimum needed for sharing, the egg provider should be given the option of using all the eggs at no additional cost to her and with no further commitment".[30]

Anonymity of donors

Since 1991 the HFEA has been required to collect, and hold on a register, information about gamete and embryo donors, those receiving licensed fertility treatment, and any children born as a result of the treatment.

The Human Fertilisation and Embryology Act 1990 states the following at section 31.

- When people reach the age of 16, they can ask the HFEA whether they may be related to someone they intend to marry.
- When people reach the age of 18, they may ask the HFEA whether they were born as a result of fertility treatment using donated gametes or embryos.
- If people aged 18 or above are told that they were born after the use of donor gametes or embryos, they can receive as much information as is stated in regulations about their genetic parents.

The Department of Health issued a consultation document in December 2001 to consider whether regulations should be made and, if so, what information should be provided to those making enquiries.[31] In the UK the vast majority of sperm, oocyte, and embryo donation is carried out on an anonymous basis (the few exceptions are when a known donor, such as a sibling or a friend, is used). A provision was inserted in the Human Fertilisation and Embryology Act that regulations could not require the HFEA to release identifiable information about donors who donated before the regulations came into force; thus, any decision to allow the release of identifying information would not be retrospective. Although some concerns have been expressed that the Government may renege on this agreement, the consultation document confirmed that "there is no question whatsoever of making any changes in the law which would allow the identification of people who have already donated sperm, eggs, or embryos".[32]

Psychological studies of people born after donor insemination

Although it is often suggested that people are likely to suffer psychological harm from not being able to trace their genetic parents, there is no definitive research that assesses the impact of this on individuals. One of the difficulties of assessing the impact on people born after donation is that the majority of parents still do not tell their children the circumstances of their conception. The social father is named on the birth certificate, so people usually have no reason to question their genetic parentage.

A European study of assisted reproduction families was set up in the mid-1990s to compare family relationships and the social and emotional development of children in families created as a result of IVF and DI compared with control groups of families with naturally conceived and adopted children. The first phase of the study was undertaken when the children were aged between 4 and 8 years old,[33] and the second phase took place when each child reached the age of 11–12 years.[34] Both studies found that all groups were similar for many aspects of the quality of parent–child relationships. In the later study, to the extent that differences were found, these reflected mainly more positive functioning among the assisted reproduction families. There were no differences between the groups of children on any of the measures of psychological adjustment and no differences were identified between the IVF and DI families for any of the variables relating to parenting or the psychological wellbeing of the children. It was noted in the article, however, that only 8.6% of DI children had been told about their genetic origins and so the ability of this study to assess whether people are harmed by being unable to access information about donors is very limited. Research on this specific question is further hampered by the traditionally high dropout rate among donor families taking part in longitudinal studies.

Research has also been undertaken involving adults who know they were born as a result of donation. This found some evidence of mistrust within families, feelings of loss caused by the lack of knowledge about their genetic background, and frustration in being thwarted in the search for their biological fathers.[35] Many individuals reported feelings of anguish, resentment, and anger as well as a loss of a sense of self and of identity.[36] In a number of cases, those interviewed had found out about the DI at a late stage and in an unplanned and sometimes confrontational way. For many of these it was not clear whether their feelings were caused by when and how they found out, or by being unable to obtain information about the donor, or by a combination of both.

Telling children about donor insemination

Studies from around the world show remarkable consistency in the number of parents who do not tell their children they were born after DI and who have no intention of doing so. Overall, in the 2002 European study referred to above, 69·9% had definitely decided not to tell and 78·4% of the British parents had reached that decision (a similar figure has also been found in the USA). The reasons the parents in the European study gave for opting for secrecy include:

- the wish to protect the child from distressing information
- concern about the impact on family relationships, particularly the father–child relationship
- fear about the possible negative reactions of other people
- the wish to protect the father
- the belief that there was no need to tell the child.[37]

The first of these reasons is at odds with the strong emphasis placed on disclosure in other areas of medicine. Although, generally, non-disclosure of distressing news to very young children by their parents is accepted, as they develop understanding and reach maturity, their own interests and needs take precedence. The non-disclosure of information about DI, even to adults, can be seen to reflect closely the type of paternalism that is now considered inappropriate in medical treatment because of the patients' right to autonomy in terms of making decisions about their own values, beliefs, and preferences. The BMA would not suggest that it is the role of doctors to disclose this information to people born as a result of DI, but believes parents should be encouraged to be open with their children about their origins. Baroness Warnock has gone further and argued that "all such deception is an evil".[38]

In Sweden, where children have had a right since 1985 to find out the identity of the donor, a study found that 89% of parents had not informed their children about the DI.[39] The number of parents who expressed an intention to tell the child, however, was higher in Sweden (at 41%) than that found in other countries. Even so, the authors conclude that compliance with the law must be considered low because only 52% of the parents had either told (11%) or intended to tell (41%). It is interesting that none of the countries that have removed anonymity have formalised a system for telling these children about the nature of their conception; this is still left to the parents to decide. Frith makes the argument that "if it is felt that knowledge of one's genetic inheritance is indeed a fundamental right then it might seem unsatisfactory to leave such a decision solely to the parent's discretion".[40]

Effect on the number of donors

One of the major arguments against a switch to identifiable donors has been that it is likely to lead to a reduction in the number of donors available, so that some people in the future may be unable to obtain treatment. As a result, it is feared that some will make private arrangements that will potentially put women at risk because of the absence of screening for HIV and other infectious diseases. Those who support a shift to identifiable donors have questioned whether the likely effect on the number of donors has, in fact, been overstated. They go on to argue, however, that, even if there is likely to be a large drop in donations, the interests of those born after DI should not be sacrificed for the sake of maintaining the DI programme at its current level.[41] In fact, the number of DI treatment cycles carried out has been dropping over the last decade, from 16 299 in 1991/92 to 5586 in 2001/02.[42] This is likely to be, at least in part, because developments such as intracytoplasmic sperm injection have opened up other treatment options for male infertility.

Studies in the UK have, however, added support to concerns about a drop in the number of donors if anonymity were to be removed. A survey of 144 potential donors in the UK was carried out in 1993, seeking information about their motivation and their views on payment and anonymity. Only 8% believed that identifying information about the donor should be given to the child and 63% of donors stated that they would not donate sperm if the law allowed identifying information to be given to the offspring.[43] In a more recent survey of licensed clinics, fear of being traced by offspring, should the law change, was given as the most likely deterrent to men donating sperm. According to the clinic staff, this was of less concern to older men with children than to younger students.[44]

The experience in other countries appears to show that the removal of anonymity led to an initial drop in the number of donors, but that over a period of time the numbers increased, with a shift in the type of donors away from young students to older, married men.[45] The UK has traditionally tended to recruit mainly student donors[46] and, if anonymity is removed, there may need to be a shift in recruitment strategies. Reports from those who have already made this shift indicate that recruitment of older donors is possible, but requires considerably more effort and resources.[47]

The arguments for and against anonymity

The arguments for and against anonymity for gamete and embryo donors are finely balanced. This is illustrated by the fact that the BMA's Medical Ethics Committee and its Representative Body (the main policymaking body) reached different conclusions on this point. The Medical Ethics Committee had advised that the interests of those born after donation should take precedence, but this was overruled by the Representative Body, which was very concerned about the likely impact on the number of available donors. BMA policy therefore supports continued anonymity.

The main points that were raised during the discussions that took place within the BMA are summarised below.

- Those who argue for identifying information to be available usually do so on the basis of the "right" of the individuals born as a result of treatment to know their genetic parents. Many people who were conceived naturally, however, are not the children of those they believe to be their parents and, unless paternity tests are to be available to everyone (irrespective of the views of the "parents"), it cannot be argued as a principle that there is a general entitlement to know one's parents. The BMA accepts, however, that people born after donation have a strong interest in knowing the identity of the donor and that this can be very important for some individuals.

- The situation of people born subsequent to DI is different from those conceived naturally because information about the donor is available and is held by a public body (the HFEA). Generally, medical ethics argues for openness and transparency and, unless there are good reasons for withholding information, it is usually considered appropriate to share information with those for whom it has personal relevance.
- It is generally considered to be in the interests of those who are adopted to have access to identifying information about their birth parents, an interest that since 1975 has been enshrined in law. Although there are differences between adoption and DI, it is not self evident that those differences justify dissimilar treatment in terms of access to identifying information about genetic parents.
- It is very likely that, if anonymity were removed, the number of donors would drop, at least initially, and some people may be unable to receive treatment. A particular concern was the likely effect on the number of ethnic minority donors, of whom there was already a shortage. Because masturbation is taboo or prohibited in some religious groups, there was real concern that the risk of being identified as a donor could further deter donors from ethnic minorities.
- Studies from around the world show consistently that around 70–75% of parents decide not to tell their children that they were born after DI. Although anybody can make inquiries to the HFEA about whether they were born subsequent to a donation, it is difficult to envisage people doing so unless they have some reason to doubt their genetic parentage. The impact of removing anonymity is therefore likely to be limited.
- There is no definitive research showing the impact of the availability of identifiable information on parents' decisions about whether to tell their children about their origins. It could make it easier for parents because they have more information available to give to these children, or it could make it more difficult because the fact the children may want to trace the donors could be perceived as threatening to the parents. If the latter is the case and more families opt not to tell their children they were born after DI, there is a risk that the search for more openness could, in fact, lead to more secrecy. It is currently not possible to determine whether removing anonymity would lead generally to more or less openness.

As with payment to donors, this is an area where principles and pragmatism can be seen to conflict. In deciding public policy, the harm that may be caused by people being unable to receive treatment with donated gametes or embryos needs to be balanced against the interests of those born after donation in receiving identifying information about the donors. (The donors themselves would not be harmed because they could decide whether or not to donate in the knowledge that identifying information would be available to any children born.) Information on changes resulting from the consultation exercise can be obtained from the Department of Health or the HFEA.

Is there a right to information?

The Department of Health's policy on anonymity of donors was challenged during 2002 as being a breach of Article 8 of the Human Rights Act (the right to respect for private and family life) and Article 14 (discrimination in the enjoyment of that right). The argument that Article 14 was engaged centred on the discrimination that existed between DI offspring and adopted children and also between DI children born before the 1990 Act came into force and those born after.

A "right" to information about donors?

Ms Joanna Rose was born in Reading in 1972 and, when she was 7 years old, discovered that she was born as a result of DI. The circumstances of the discovery were distressing and she was sworn to secrecy; she felt grief, confusion, and guilt. As an adult Ms Rose tried to find information about the donor. Although she discovered that all records of her conception had been destroyed, she decided to pursue her challenge on behalf of other people in the same situation. In describing the importance of the information to her she told the judge:

> I feel that these genetic connections are very important to me, socially, emotionally, medically, and even spiritually. I believe it to be no exaggeration that non-identifying information will assist me in forming a fuller sense of self or identify and answer questions that I have been asking for a long time.[48]

The second claimant was EM, who was born in 1996 as a result of DI. Her parents had always been open with her about the DI and were unhappy at not having the information needed to answer her questions about the donor.

Neither claimant was seeking the provision of identifiable information against the wishes of the donor. They were, however, seeking access to non-identifying information about donors and the establishment of a "voluntary contact register" (to allow contact to be made if the donor was willing). They claimed that the Secretary of State's failure to take this action breached his duties under Articles 8 and 14 of the Human Rights Act. In assessing the scope of respect for private and family life the court held that it required that "everyone should be able to establish details of their identity as individual human beings. This includes their origins and the opportunity to understand them. It also embraces their physical and social identity and psychological integrity".[49] In May 2002 Mr Justice Scott Baker held that Article 8 was engaged in this case. Whether there had been a breach of Articles 8 and 14 in these cases would be considered at a later date.

Rose v Secretary of State for Health and Human Fertilisation and Embryology Authority[48]

Summary – use of donated gametes or embryos

- Regulations issued by the HFEA permit payment of up to £15 per donation, the reimbursement of expenses, and treatment services or sterilisation in return for donation.
- "Egg sharing", whereby a woman receives free IVF treatment in return for donating some of her eggs, is permitted subject to strict guidelines.
- The BMA does not support the payment of donors or egg sharing, believing that gamete or embryo donation should be a gift, freely and voluntarily given without inducement.
- Any change to the rules on gamete donor anonymity should not be retrospective.
- The arguments for and against anonymity for future gamete donors are very finely balanced, but BMA policy supports continued anonymity.
- Information about the outcome of the Department of Health's consultation exercise on donor anonymity can be obtained from the Department of Health or the HFEA.

Preimplantation genetic diagnosis

Preimplantation genetic diagnosis (PGD) is one form of prenatal testing and, as such, the ethical considerations discussed in the previous chapter also apply to preimplantation diagnosis. PGD involves the creation of embryos *in vitro* and the removal of one or two cells for analysis prior to implantation. For those who know that they are at risk of passing on a serious genetic disorder, this procedure offers the opportunity of selecting and replacing only those embryos that are free of the disease. This allows a woman to begin her pregnancy knowing that the child is not affected by the disorder for which there is known risk. The number of conditions for which this type of testing is available is limited, and only a small number of centres have the necessary expertise to undertake the biopsy and testing procedures. Although it has been suggested that increasing numbers of people may wish to seek PGD for "frivolous" reasons, the BMA considers this to be unlikely. The invasive nature of the technique combined with the relatively low success rates for IVF treatment and the costs of the procedure are likely to deter its widespread adoption. It is possible, however, that its use for aneuploidy screening (screening embryos *in vitro* for numerical chromosomal abnormalities) among those patients requiring IVF for medical reasons could increase. In November 2001 the HFEA agreed, in principle, to allow the use of aneuploidy screening for older women and those with a history of miscarriage or IVF failure,[50] but its broader use could be considered in the future as a way of increasing the success rates for IVF.

As PGD involves the creation and use of human embryos *in vitro*, it is a criminal offence for a clinic to carry it out without a licence from the HFEA. Recognising the public interest in this area and the range of unresolved questions about the way in which such new technology should be regulated, the HFEA and the Advisory Committee on Genetic Testing (subsequently replaced by the Human Genetics

Commission) published a consultation document in November 1999. Two years later the HFEA and the Human Genetics Commission published their findings and conclusions.[51] In addition to a number of recommendations about improving the way in which applications were assessed, it was agreed that, when deciding about the appropriateness of PGD, the following factors should be taken into account:

- the view of those seeking treatment of the condition
- their previous reproductive experience
- the likely degree of suffering associated with the condition
- the availability of effective therapy or management now and in the future
- the speed of degeneration in progressive disorders
- the extent of intellectual impairment
- the extent of social support available
- the family circumstances of the people seeking treatment.

Selecting embryos on the basis of tissue type compatibility

Between the consultation document on PGD being issued and the final report being published, the HFEA was faced with an issue that had not been specifically addressed in its consultation exercise. An application was made for PGD to be used in conjunction with human leucocyte antigen typing, not only to avoid the birth of a child with a severe genetic disorder, but also to select for replacement those embryos that were most likely to produce a child who would be a good tissue match for a very sick sibling. It was proposed that stem cells would be taken from the umbilical cord blood and so the child himself or herself would not be subjected to any intrusive or painful procedures. In December 2001 the HFEA gave approval in principle to the use of this procedure, subject to a number of conditions, including a requirement that individual requests must be considered by the HFEA on a case by case basis. In the first few months after this decision, the HFEA considered two applications (see below), one of which it approved, but the other (for a non-inherited condition) it turned down. The HFEA was criticised for both of these decisions including, for the first decision, by the House of Commons Select Committee on Science and Technology, which said "the HFEA's decision to allow tissue typing in conjunction with preimplantation genetic diagnosis went beyond the scope of its own public consultation. It is vital that the public are taken along with decisions of such ethical importance".[52]

The Pro-life Alliance sought a judicial review of the decision, arguing that the HFEA had exceeded its legal powers. Under the Human Fertilisation and Embryology Act, the HFEA can issue treatment licences only for the provision of "treatment services", defined as "assisting women to carry children". The Pro-life Alliance argued that the purpose of tissue typing was not to assist a woman to carry a child and could therefore not be licensed. In upholding the challenge, Mr Justice Maurice Kay held that, since the reason for requesting tissue typing did not arise from an impaired ability to conceive or to carry a child through pregnancy to full term and birth, it could not be argued that it was "necessary or desirable" for the purpose of assisting a woman to carry a child.[53] This decision was overturned by the Court of Appeal, which rejected this narrow interpretation. Lord Phillips said that "when concern as to the characteristics of any child that she may bear may inhibit a woman from bearing a child, IVF treatment coupled with PGD that will eliminate that concern can properly be said to be '... for the purpose of assisting women to carry children'".[54] He went on to say that decisions about what choices should be allowed raise difficult ethical questions, responsibility for which Parliament has placed in the hands of the HFEA. The appeal court's decision in this case was formally welcomed by the BMA at its Annual Representative Meeting in July 2003.

PGD with tissue typing for the benefit of a very sick sibling

Three-year-old Zain Hashmi suffered from beta thalassaemia. His parents wanted to use PGD to avoid the birth of another child with the same condition and also to select for replacement those embryos most likely to produce a child who would be a compatible donor. The intention was to use stem cells from the umbilical cord blood to produce bone marrow for the transplant, thus the child himself or herself would not be subjected to any invasive, painful, or risky procedures. Approval was given by the HFEA for this case.[55]

Three-year-old Charlie Whitaker suffered from Diamond–Blackfan anaemia, a rare life threatening blood disorder. Although some children with Diamond–Blackfan anaemia inherit this condition from carrier parents, most cases arise as a result of a sporadic mutation. In this case, the parents were found not to be carriers and so the future child was at no greater risk of developing the condition than any other child. The couple wished to use PGD solely to provide a compatible donor for Charlie. As with the Hashmi case, stem cells would be taken from the umbilical cord blood and so the child himself or herself would not be used as a donor. The HFEA turned down this application on the basis that the PGD was not being carried out to avoid a serious disorder in the future child and so it did not meet the criteria set out by the HFEA.[56]

Welfare of the child

A key concern in both of these cases was the possibility of psychological harm resulting to the child who would be selected and born to be a donor. Although likely to be as loved as any other child, would he or she resent being "selected" and feel less wanted or less respected as an individual? Alternatively, would the child feel proud of being uniquely able to save the life of his or her sibling? If treatment with cord blood were unsuccessful, would the child feel obliged to donate bone marrow? What would be the effect on the child's relationship with the parents if, despite treatment, the sibling died? Would the child feel guilty for being unable to achieve the task he or she was born to do? The response to all of these questions is that we simply do not know. Yet these hypothetical risks of harm have to be balanced against other harms, primarily the real harm to the sibling who would suffer or die without this treatment. If permission for PGD and tissue typing is refused, parents may continue to have children naturally in the hope of obtaining a match; the harm to those children, particularly if they are unsuitable as donors, needs also to be considered. The requirement in the Human Fertilisation and Embryology Act to take account of the welfare of the child usually focuses on the child who may be born as a result of the treatment, but the requirement specifically extends to taking account of the welfare of "any other child who may be affected by the birth".[57] Under the terms of the Act, therefore, it is entirely reasonable to consider the welfare of other children in the family who may be affected, in a positive or a negative way, by the birth of the new child.

It is sometimes argued that, if selection by tissue typing were permitted, children would be born as a means to someone else's ends rather than for their own sake. In reality, however, parents have children for many reasons that are often more to do with their own wishes and desires than the interests of the future child. As Gillon points out in another context,[58] it is not unusual for individuals to use each other as a means to an end. In helping each other, we do not become *merely* a tool for achieving objectives. If donor children were abandoned after the treatment, they would have been merely tools. In practice, however, the child is most unlikely to be abandoned or rejected. Nevertheless, such concerns need to be taken seriously in the debate. For those who believe that the risks to the selected child are sufficiently serious to override all other considerations, neither of the cases described above would be acceptable. The BMA does not, however, believe that selection by tissue typing is necessarily incompatible with the welfare of the child and supports the HFEA's decision in the Hashmi case, but are there reasonable grounds for differentiating between the two cases as did the HFEA?

The use of embryos

The HFEA judged there to be a fundamental difference between cases where the invasive procedure (PGD) was undertaken for the benefit of the embryos themselves and where it was being carried out solely for the benefit of others. This statement in itself, however, is controversial because it is not self evident that PGD is being undertaken for the benefit of the embryos tested, certainly not for all of them, because as a result some (those found to be affected by the disorder) are destroyed. In some ways, however, it can be seen as easier to justify this type of case. During the process of PGD carried out to help a couple to avoid the birth of a child with a serious, life threatening condition, a number of embryos are created. Given that some form of selection is required and not all of the unaffected embryos are replaced (assuming one accepts the notion of tissue typing in principle), there are good arguments for selecting, from among those that are free of the disease, the ones that can help to save a life, rather than selecting at random. The BMA has opposed the selection of embryos for trivial reasons or for meeting the desire of parents for some particular characteristics, but saving or improving the life of a very sick child is not a trivial matter.

In the second scenario, as with the Whitaker case, the embryos are not being created and tested in order to avoid a disorder but simply to select those that would provide the best possible tissue match. The HFEA's objection appears to be that an invasive procedure is being carried out on an *in vitro* embryo for the benefit of another person, but this needs to be considered in the context of the status accorded to the embryo and what interference and invasive procedures are permissible. In the UK, human embryos may be used for research to pursue questions that are important to the public good. If they are used to improve fertility treatment and contraceptive measures, is it appropriate to prohibit their use to save a child's life?

It could be that there is perceived to be a difference between embryos that are to be replaced and may become a child and surplus embryos that are otherwise destroyed, but it is not clear on what grounds such a distinction would apply. There is no evidence, and the HFEA has not argued, that the child himself or herself would be at risk of physical harm caused by the PGD procedure. Even if there was perceived to be some increased risk to the child as a result of the procedure, this does not necessarily mean that it should not be permitted. We allow parents to expose their children to some other risks for the benefit of other people, provided those risks are below a certain threshold. Young children are sometimes involved in research projects, for example, where the risk of harm is minimal and there are potential benefits for others. Similarly, society does not object to the use of a child as a bone marrow donor when there is no benefit to that child but the benefits to a sibling are great. There are also considered to be psychological benefits to the donor, and the family unit as a whole, from saving the life of a dying child. Concerns have been expressed, however, that, if a child is selected to be a donor and treatment with stem cells from umbilical cord blood is not successful, there will be tremendous pressure for the child to donate bone marrow. In the BMA's view, parents should be counselled in advance and informed that, if umbilical cord blood is not effective, then the child should not automatically be considered as a donor, but a careful analysis of the risks and benefits will be needed. The same safeguards should apply to these children as to other children who donate bone marrow to siblings.

It is not clear that any risk of psychological harm to the child, as a result of being "selected" in this way, would be greater where the procedure was undertaken primarily for selection purposes rather than to avoid a serious disorder. If there are serious concerns about the psychological harm to the child born, this must apply to all cases of selection by tissue typing rather than simply where PGD is used for tissue type selection only. The BMA does not believe that there is any morally relevant difference between the two cases, and supports, in principle, the use of PGD combined with tissue typing in all cases where this is the only possibility of treatment for a sibling whose condition is life threatening or sufficiently serious to justify the use of PGD.

Summary – preimplantation genetic diagnosis

- It is a criminal offence for a clinic to carry out PGD without a licence from the HFEA.
- The BMA believes that the invasive nature and cost of the technique combined with the relatively low success rate for IVF treatment is likely to restrict the use of PGD to serious conditions.

- The BMA supports, in principle, the use of PGD combined with tissue typing in all cases where this is the only possibility of treatment for a sibling whose condition is life threatening or sufficiently serious to justify the use of PGD.

Gender selection

One of the choices that developments in reproductive technology has made possible is that of selecting the gender of future children. The most accurate means of selection is using PGD and selecting for replacement only those embryos of the desired gender (this is known as "secondary selection" as selection takes place after fertilisation). It is also possible, with increasing accuracy, to make the selection before fertilisation takes place (primary selection) by separating out the X- and Y-bearing sperm and using the preferred sample for insemination. Gender selection is a widely accepted practice for medical reasons, such as where it is used to avoid the birth of a child with a severe disorder that affects only one sex, for example, Duchenne muscular dystrophy, which affects only boys. More controversial, however, is its use for social or cultural reasons.

Arguments for and against gender selection for social reasons

In both 1993 and 2002 the HFEA undertook public consultation exercises to seek views on whether people should be permitted to select the sex of their children in the absence of any medical imperative. In the later consultation, a distinction was made between "family balancing" (where the family already had children of one sex) and other social reasons. The arguments in this debate are set out in detail in the HFEA's 2002 consultation document.[59] The main points considered by the BMA are summarised below.

- In support of sex selection for social reasons
  - Freedom of choice should be encouraged if there is no evidence of foreseeable harm from allowing people to choose. Concerns that boys would be favoured if selection was permitted in the UK (which could affect the balance of the sexes or reinforce gender stereotypes) is not borne out by the evidence. In fact, in European societies, research has found a preference for girls among those wishing to choose.[60] Any perceived problems of this nature could be avoided by allowing sex selection only for family balancing.
  - People would be able to exercise greater control over the size of their family. Some people continue to have children until they have a child of the desired sex and there is a risk that those of the undesired sex may be abused or neglected. Allowing choice would therefore make more families happy.

- Primary and secondary sex selection is preferable to people seeking abortion based on the sex of the fetus. It is argued that this is practised, although reasons other than gender choice are given in justification. (For a discussion of abortion on grounds of fetal sex see Chapter 7, page 248).

- Against sex selection for social reasons

  - It is wrong to base the acceptance of a child on its particular characteristics. Children should be accepted and loved unconditionally. If a child of the "wrong" sex is born through a failure of the technology, then this could result in psychological harm to the child.
  - Once a decision is made to allow people to choose one characteristic it will be more difficult to prevent other choices, resulting in "designer children".
  - Although the balance of the sexes is unlikely to be upset in the UK, allowing selection here would send the wrong message to other countries where this is potentially a serious problem.

Having considered the issues, the BMA reached the conclusion that sex selection techniques should be used only for the avoidance of sex linked disorders and not for social reasons.[61]

Regulation of sex selection

After its 1993 consultation exercise, the HFEA also concluded that sex selection techniques should not be used for social reasons. Its code of practice included a rule that "centres should not select the sex of embryos for social reasons".[62] The use of secondary methods of sex selection for social reasons is therefore illegal in the UK because the HFEA licenses clinics for sex selection for medical reasons only. The HFEA's code of practice also says, in paragraph 9.10, that "centres should not use sperm sorting techniques in sex selection". So, centres that are licensed by the HFEA are not permitted to use sperm sorting techniques in sex selection, but there is nothing to stop clinics being set up solely for this purpose. Clinics not using or storing embryos or donated eggs or sperm, for example, would not require a licence and would not be bound by the HFEA's code of practice. In its 2002 consultation the HFEA considered the question of whether sperm sorting should also be subject to regulation or whether regulation should continue to be restricted to those methods of sex selection that involve the creation or use of human embryos. Further information about the outcome of the consultation exercise can be obtained from the HFEA.

Request for sex selection

In 2001 Alan and Louise Masterton appealed to the HFEA to make an exception to its prohibition of sex selection for social reasons to allow them to have a daughter. The Mastertons had four sons and their only daughter

(Continued)

(born after 15 years of trying for a girl) died in a bonfire accident at her home in 1999 at the age of 3. Mrs Masterton had been sterilised after the birth of her daughter and therefore required IVF to have another child. Mr Masterton argued that there was a pressing medical need for the procedure because of the effect on the couple, confirmed by a psychologist and their GP, of their strong desire for a daughter.

The HFEA said it could consider an application only from one of its licensed clinics in order to make an exception to its general rule, but the Mastertons were unable to find a clinic with the relevant expertise that was willing to take the case to the HFEA. The couple considered challenging this decision, using the Human Rights Act and claiming that the HFEA's refusal to consider their case was a breach of their right to a fair hearing and to respect for private and family life, but did not pursue this. They subsequently went to Italy, where IVF treatment produced only one male embryo. The embryo was not replaced, but was donated to another couple.[63]

Summary – gender selection

- It is unlawful to use PGD to select the sex of an embryo for social reasons.
- Centres licensed by the HFEA are not permitted to undertake sperm sorting procedures for social reasons.
- The HFEA has considered whether selection for "family balancing" should be permitted and whether sperm sorting should be subject to some form of regulation; information on these points is available from the HFEA.
- The BMA is opposed to sex selection for social reasons.

Surrogacy

The number of people using surrogacy is small in comparison with those using other forms of assisted reproduction, but for some it offers the only practical way of addressing the consequences of involuntary childlessness. It raises profound questions and challenges some of our most deeply held beliefs. In addition, the separation of maternity from social motherhood raises complex moral and legal issues.

Distinction can be made between "partial" surrogacy (also known as traditional or straight surrogacy) and "full" surrogacy (also known as host or IVF surrogacy). In partial surrogacy the surrogate mother provides an egg, which is fertilised with sperm from the intended father or a donor, by insemination, IVF, or another form of assisted reproduction. In full surrogacy, the woman who carries the fetus makes no genetic contribution to an embryo that she receives to gestate. The eggs and sperm used to create the embryos are usually those of the intended parents, although in some cases donated gametes may be used.

The BMA's views on surrogacy have changed over time. From advice to doctors to have no involvement with surrogacy, came a growing recognition that surrogacy is as much a social issue as a medical one. This recognition led to the BMA's acceptance, in 1990, of surrogacy as a treatment of last resort.[64] The BMA's 1996 report saw surrogacy as an acceptable option of last resort when "it is impossible or highly undesirable for medical reasons for the intended mother to carry a child herself".[65] The apparent growing public acceptance of surrogacy has led to a reduction in the amount of secrecy surrounding the practice and to a corresponding increase in the number of people requesting advice and support from the medical profession about surrogacy arrangements. The BMA's report offers health professionals advice and guidance on the legal, ethical, practical, medical, and psychological aspects of surrogacy. A brief summary of that information, and subsequent developments, is provided below. The BMA has also produced an information leaflet, jointly with the HFEA, providing basic information for those considering surrogacy.[66]

The regulatory framework

The law on surrogacy is set out in the Surrogacy Arrangements Act 1985 and the Human Fertilisation and Embryology Act 1990. The main points are summarised below.

- Agencies or individuals (other than the potential surrogate mother or intended parents) are prohibited from acting on a commercial basis to initiate, negotiate, or compile information towards the making of a surrogacy arrangement. The legislation does not, however, prohibit non-commercial agencies, or the activities of someone who may arrange surrogacy non-commercially, nor does it prohibit payment to a surrogate mother.
- All advertising (including by the potential surrogate mother or intended parents) that indicates that a person is willing to be a surrogate mother, that someone is looking for a surrogate mother, or that a person or organisation will help to initiate a surrogacy arrangement, is prohibited.
- Surrogacy contracts are unenforceable in law. This means that, if the surrogate mother wishes to keep the child, and any money she has been paid, she is entitled to do so. Equally, if the intended parents decide they do not want the child, the surrogate mother is responsible in law for its welfare because she is the child's mother, under section 27 of the Human Fertilisation and Embryology Act, regardless of its genetic makeup. In practice, a child rejected by its birth mother and the intended parents is likely to be placed for fostering or adoption.
- Any centre offering IVF or DI services (including those carried out as part of a surrogacy arrangement) must be licensed by the HFEA.
- A competent court may make a "parental order" making the intended parents in a surrogacy arrangement the legal parents of the child. A number of criteria must be met before a parental order can be made, including that the intended parents must be married to each other and at least one of them must be genetically related to the child.

The Brazier Committee

In June 1997 the Government set up a review group, chaired by Professor Margaret Brazier, to review certain aspects of surrogacy arrangements; after wide ranging consultation, the group reported in October 1998.[67] The report made the following recommendations.

- There should be a new Surrogacy Act to replace the Surrogacy Arrangements Act 1985 and section 30 of the Human Fertilisation and Embryology Act. Under the new Act:
  - surrogacy arrangements would continue to be unenforceable
  - the existing prohibition on commercial agencies and advertising would remain
  - there would be statutory provisions defining and limiting lawful payments to surrogate mothers
  - non-profit making agencies would be required to register with the Department of Health and comply with a surrogacy code of practice issued by the Department of Health
  - unregistered agencies would be prohibited
  - the existing provision for parental orders would be amended to make it a requirement that the surrogacy code of practice and the restrictions on payments had been respected.

- Payments to surrogate mothers should cover only genuine expenses associated with the pregnancy. The nature and level of expenses should be agreed before there is any attempt to initiate a pregnancy and documentary evidence should be provided of the expenses incurred. The new Surrogacy Act should define expenses in broad terms of principle, but what constitutes "reasonable expenses", and the evidence required, should be set out in directions.

- The Department of Health should consider establishing requirements for full record keeping and reporting of specified statistics.

The BMA supports these recommendations, which reflect very closely the Association's own views set out in its 1996 publication and in its evidence to the review team.

The doctor's duties in the surrogacy arrangement

Doctors have different responsibilities depending on the level of their involvement with the surrogacy arrangement. Once a surrogate pregnancy has been established, the practitioner's ethical obligations to the surrogate mother and child are no different from those owed to any other pregnant woman, although additional emotional support may be required. The duty of the healthcare team is to provide the appropriate level of support and guidance, both during and after the pregnancy.

Practitioners approached for advice by people considering self insemination should encourage those concerned to consider the issues and implications very carefully and should ensure that they are aware of how to obtain accurate information about the medical, psychological, emotional, and legal issues involved with surrogacy. They should also actively encourage those considering surrogacy to seek counselling and testing for infectious diseases. The responsibilities are greatest for those who are providing licensed treatment services aimed at establishing a surrogate pregnancy through IVF or DI. In such cases, the healthcare team must take all reasonable steps to ensure that all relevant issues have been carefully considered. Such treatment services can be provided only in clinics licensed by the HFEA and in compliance with the HFEA's code of practice. This includes storing sperm and embryos for a six month quarantine period, as well as taking account of the range of factors associated with the welfare of the child (see pages 274–8) for both the intended parents and the surrogate mother and her partner because either couple could eventually be caring for the child.

Surrogacy arrangements made in other countries

Although surrogacy arrangements are unenforceable in the UK, this is not the case in other countries. In the USA, for example, commercial agencies are permitted and surrogacy arrangements are legally enforceable. Those considering entering into a surrogacy arrangement in another country should be advised to seek specialist advice about their legal position and that of any children resulting from the arrangement. There are complicated legal questions about which jurisdiction should apply, who should be considered the legal parents of the resulting child, and, when the intended parents are from the UK, whether the child is entitled to become a UK citizen.[68]

Surrogacy arrangement in the USA

H, an English woman, entered into a surrogacy arrangement with W and B in California, where surrogacy arrangements are enforceable in law. The relationship became acrimonious during the pregnancy and H subsequently decided she wanted to keep the twins she was expecting. She returned to England, where the children were born in November 2001. W and B applied to the High Court in the UK for a declaration that H's retention of the twins was unlawful under the Hague Convention on Civil Aspects of International Child Abduction.[69] The application was rejected, but the question of who should have custody of the children was left unresolved.

W and B subsequently applied for an order for the return of the twins to California for the courts there to determine who should have their custody.[70] H argued that this would be seriously disadvantageous to her because the

(Continued)

Californian court would seek to enforce the terms of the contract, which was considered, in England, to be contrary to public policy. Mr Justice Hedley held that the future of the twins should be a matter for the family court in California because all the realistic links in the case were in California. H had entered into a contract in accordance with the law of California and she should continue to submit to the Californian courts until the matter had been resolved.

W v H (child abduction: surrogacy)[69,70]

Summary – surrogacy

- The BMA considers surrogacy to be an acceptable option of last resort in cases where it is impossible or highly undesirable for medical reasons for the intended mother to carry a child herself.
- Doctors have different responsibilities depending on the level of their involvement with the surrogacy arrangement.
- Once a surrogate pregnancy has been established, the doctor's ethical obligations to the surrogate mother and the child are no different from those owed to any other pregnant woman, although more support may be required.
- Practitioners approached for advice by those planning self insemination should encourage those concerned to consider the issues and implications carefully, ensure they know how to obtain accurate information, and encourage them to seek counselling and testing for infectious diseases.
- Doctors providing IVF or DI as part of a surrogacy arrangement must have a licence from the HFEA and follow the HFEA's code of practice.
- Those considering entering into a surrogacy arrangement in another country should be recommended to seek specialist legal advice.

Seeking treatment in other countries

It has always been possible for people to travel to other countries to receive treatment that is either not available or is more expensive in their home country. As a result of the strict regulatory mechanism in the UK, reproduction is one area where this has been a particular issue. Common reasons for what has been referred to as "fertility tourism" include older women seeking treatment with donor oocytes, couples seeking sex selection for social reasons, and those wishing to use the services of a commercial surrogacy agency, either as intended parents or as a surrogate mother. It is not unlawful for patients from the UK to go abroad for procedures that are unavailable or unlawful here (although there may be legal consequences[71]), but whether doctors should promote or facilitate such moves is another question.

The Diane Blood case (see page 279) made it clear that it is not only legally acceptable to seek treatment in another European Union country, but there may also be a legally enforceable right to export the means to effect that. In refusing to issue a direction allowing export of the stored sperm, the HFEA had argued that, in the absence of compliance with the requirements of the Act, in particular that of written consent, the applicant should not be permitted to avoid those specific requirements by exporting the sperm to a country with which she had no connections. The Court of Appeal held, however, that in making this decision, the HFEA had failed to give sufficient attention to Mrs Blood's rights to receive medical treatment in another member state. Lord Woolf said in his judgment that, although he was not required to consider whether the refusal was reasonable, he thought it unlikely that the arguments given by the HFEA for refusing the application would withstand scrutiny. Commenting on this aspect of the case, it has been stated "not only does the Court use the trump of EU law to sweep aside the hand dealt by the UK Parliament, it deals the cards with which the HFEA must now play, and apparently leaves the applicant holding all the aces".[72] In her review of the law subsequent to this case, McLean recommended that the Human Fertilisation and Embryology Act should be amended to make it clear that the HFEA's discretion to permit the export of gametes cannot extend to authorising the export of gametes that were unlawfully obtained.[73]

Arguably, if individuals are aware of the possible legal complexities and, where appropriate, any additional risks of seeking treatment elsewhere, it is a matter for them alone to decide whether to seek procedures that are not permitted in the UK. When health professionals are involved, however, either by encouraging or helping to facilitate those decisions, questions begin to arise about whether doctors have a responsibility not only to comply with the wording of the national law but also with its spirit. There have been cases reported of doctors working in clinics licensed by the HFEA setting up clinics in other countries to offer patients procedures that are not permitted in the UK, thus evading the regulatory system in the UK.[74] In contrast, it is unlawful for a person in the UK to initiate or negotiate any arrangement involving the making or offer of payment for the supply of an organ for transplantation, whether the transplant takes place in the UK or elsewhere.[75] This applies irrespective of whether payment for organs is lawful in the country in which the transplant takes place. If the regulatory mechanism in the UK, and those practising in the field of fertility, are to retain public confidence, making a similar provision for uses of reproductive technology that are unlawful in the UK may be something the HFEA needs to consider recommending to the Secretary of State, who may then seek to amend the Human Fertilisation and Embryology Act to effect this.

Time to review the law?

At the time of writing, the Human Fertilisation and Embryology Act has been in force for more than a decade. Throughout this time, the HFEA has continued to carry out the tasks delegated to it by Parliament, by applying the legislation to new and increasingly complex technological developments. As the boundaries continue to be pushed back, however, legitimate questions have been raised about whether it is for the HFEA or Parliament to decide on some of the new and ethically sensitive potential uses of reproductive technology. This, combined with the increasing number of challenges to the Act, has led to calls for the Government to take urgent action "to reconnect the Act with modern science".[76]

References

1 Human Fertilisation and Embryology Authority press release. *Over 50,000 babies born following IVF treatment in the UK since first success in 1978.* 2000 Dec 13.
2 The possible risks with intracytoplasmic sperm injection are summarised in: Human Fertilisation and Embryology Authority. *Intra-cytoplasmic sperm injection.* London: HFEA, 2002.
3 Human Fertilisation and Embryology Authority press release. *HFEA dismisses claims that IVF children need health checks as "ludicrous".* 2002 Oct 23.
4 R v Secretary of State for the Home Department, ex parte Mellor [2001] 2 FLR 1158.
5 Committee of Inquiry into Human Fertilisation and Embryology. *Report of the committee of inquiry into human fertilisation and embryology.* London: HMSO, 1984. (Cmnd 9314.)
6 *Ibid:* p. 4.
7 Human Fertilisation and Embryology Authority. *Code of practice, 5th ed.* London: HFEA, 2001.
8 Department of Health. *Survey of NHS infertility services 1997–98.* London: DoH, 2000.
9 Department of Health press release. *Working towards ending the postcode lottery of infertility treatment. NICE to update existing guidelines, announces Milburn.* 2000 Nov 30. (2000/0701.)
10 Havers P. The impact of the European Convention on Human Rights on medical law. *Med Leg J* 2002;**70**(2):57–70.
11 Human Fertilisation and Embryology Act 1990 s13(5).
12 See, for example: Harris J. *Clones, genes, and immortality.* Oxford: Oxford University Press, 1998:92–7.
13 Human Fertilisation and Embryology Authority. *Code of practice, 5th ed. Op cit:* para 3·12.
14 R v Ethical Committee of St Mary's Hospital, ex parte Harriott [1988] 1 FLR 512.
15 Human Fertilisation and Embryology Authority. *Ninth annual report and accounts 2000.* London: HFEA, 2000.
16 Human Fertilisation and Embryology Authority. *HFEA information for treatment ethics committees.* London: HFEA, 2000.
17 Human Fertilisation and Embryology Act 1990 s13(5).
18 Human Fertilisation and Embryology Authority. *Code of practice, 5th ed. Op cit:* para 3·15.
19 Human Fertilisation and Embryology Authority. *Welfare of the child: information for general practitioners.* London: HFEA, 1999.
20 McLean S. *Consent and the law: review of the current provisions in the Human Fertilisation and Embryology Act 1990 for the UK health ministers.* London: Department of Health, 1997.
21 R v Human Fertilisation and Embryology Authority, ex parte Blood [1997] 2 All ER 687.
22 McLean SAM. *Review of the common law provisions relating to the removal of gametes and of the consent provisions in the Human Fertilisation and Embryology Act 1990.* London: Department of Health, 1998.
23 Tait N. Court backs IVF paternity claim. *Financial Times* 2003 Mar 1:4.
24 Human Fertilisation and Embryology Authority. *Code of practice, 5th ed. Op cit:* para 3·14.
25 Human Fertilisation and Embryology Authority. *Fifth annual report 1996.* London: HFEA, 1996:23.
26 Human Fertilisation and Embryology Authority. *Directions given under the Human Fertilisation and Embryology Act 1990. Giving and receiving money or other benefits in respect of any supply of gametes or embryos.* London: HFEA, 1998. (D.1998/1.)
27 Human Fertilisation and Embryology Authority. *Third annual report 1994.* London: HFEA, 1994:26.
28 Lockwood G. Donating life: practical and ethical issues in gamete donation. In: Shenfield F, Sureau C, eds. *Ethical dilemmas in assisted reproduction.* Carnforth: Parthenon, 1997.
29 Human Fertilisation and Embryology Authority. *Ninth annual report and accounts 2000. Op cit.*
30 Human Fertilisation and Embryology Authority. *Guidance for egg sharing arrangements.* London: HFEA, 2000.

31 Department of Health. *Donor information consultation. Providing information about sperm, egg and embryo donors.* London: DoH, 2001.
32 *Ibid:* p. 1.
33 Golombok S, Brewaeys A, Cook R, *et al.* The European study of assisted reproduction families. *Hum Reprod* 1996;**11**:2324–31.
34 Golombok S, Brewaeys A, Giavazzi MT, Guerra D, MacCallum F, Rust J. The European study of assisted reproduction families: the transition to adolescence. *Hum Reprod* 2002;**17**:830–40.
35 Turner AJ, Coyle A. What does it mean to be a donor offspring? The identity experiences of adults conceived by donor insemination and the implications for counselling and therapy. *Hum Reprod* 2000;**15**:2041–51.
36 McWhinnie A. Gamete donation and anonymity. Should offspring from donated gametes continue to be denied knowledge of their origins and antecedents? *Hum Reprod* 2001;**16**:807–17.
37 Golombok S, *et al.* The European study of assisted reproduction families: the transition to adolescence. *Op cit.*
38 Warnock M. *Making babies. Is there a right to have children?* Oxford: Oxford University Press, 2002:66.
39 Gottlieb C, Lalos O, Lindblad F. Disclosure of donor insemination to the child: the impact of the Swedish legislation on couples' attitudes. *Hum Reprod* 2000;**15**:2052–6.
40 Frith L. Gamete donation and anonymity; the ethical and legal debate. *Hum Reprod* 2001;**16**:818–24.
41 Blyth E. A child's right to know. *New Scientist* 2002;(Jul 6):28.
42 Human Fertilisation and Embryology Authority. *Ninth annual report and accounts 2000. Op cit:* p. 12. Human Fertilisation and Embryology Authority. *Eleventh annual report and accounts 2002.* London: HFEA, 2002:13.
43 Human Fertilisation and Embryology Authority. *Third annual report 1994. Op cit:* p. 26.
44 Murray C, Golombok S. Oocyte and semen donation: a survey of UK licensed centres. *Hum Reprod* 2000;**15**:2133–9.
45 Daniels K, Lalos O. The Swedish insemination act and the availability of donors. *Hum Reprod* 1995;**10**:1871–4.
46 Murray C, *et al.* Oocyte and semen donation: a survey of UK licensed centres. *Op cit.*
47 Daniels KR, Curson R, Lewis GM. Semen donor recruitment: a study of donors in two clinics. *Hum Reprod* 1996;**11**:746–51.
48 Rose v Secretary of State for Health and Human Fertilisation and Embryology Authority [2002] 2 FLR 962: 964–5.
49 *Ibid:* p. 976.
50 Human Fertilisation and Embryology Authority. *Eleventh annual report and accounts 2002. Op cit:* p. 16.
51 Human Fertilisation and Embryology Authority, Human Genetics Commission. *Outcome of the public consultation on preimplantation genetic diagnosis.* London: HGC, 2001.
52 House of Commons Science and Technology Committee. *Developments in human genetics and embryology. Fourth report of session 2001–02.* London: The Stationery Office, 2002: para 25. (HC 791.)
53 R (on the application of Quintavalle) v Human Fertilisation and Embryology Authority [2003] 2 All ER 105.
54 R (on the application of Quintavalle) v Human Fertilisation and Embryology Authority CA [2003]: 3 All ER 257: Lord Phillips at 270.
55 Dyer C. Watchdog approves embryo selection to treat 3 year old child. *BMJ* 2002;**324**:503.
56 Human Fertilisation and Embryology Authority press release. *HFEA confirms that HLA tissue typing may only take place when preimplantation genetic diagnosis is required to avoid a serious genetic disorder.* 2002 Aug 1.
57 Human Fertilisation and Embryology Act 1990 s13(5).
58 Gillon R. Human reproductive cloning – a look at the arguments against it and a rejection of most of them. *J R Soc Med* 1999;**92**:3–12.
59 Human Fertilisation and Embryology Authority. *Sex selection: choice and responsibility in human reproduction.* London: HFEA, 2002.
60 *Ibid:* p. 26.
61 British Medical Association Annual Representative Meeting 1994; reaffirmed in 2001.
62 Human Fertilisation and Embryology Authority. *Code of practice, 5th ed. Op cit:* para 9·9.
63 Seenan G. "Designer baby" parents give away male embryo. *The Guardian* 2001 Mar 5.
64 British Medical Association. *Surrogacy: ethical considerations.* London: BMA, 1990.
65 British Medical Association. *Changing conceptions of motherhood. The practice of surrogacy in Britain.* London: BMA, 1996:2.
66 British Medical Association, Human Fertilisation and Embryology Authority. *Considering surrogacy? Your questions answered.* London: BMA, 1996.

67   Brazier M, Campbell A, Golombok S. *Surrogacy. Review for health ministers of current arrangements for payments and regulation. Report of the review team.* London: The Stationery Office, 1998.

68   Tony Barlow and Barry Drewitt had twins after a surrogacy arrangement in the USA. Although the children were granted permission to stay in Britain indefinitely they were denied UK citizenship: Anonymous. Gay fathers' twins to stay in UK. *BBC Online*, 2000 Jan 25. http://news.bbc.co.uk (accessed 28 April 2003).

69   W v H (child abduction: surrogacy) (No. 1) [2002] 1 FLR 1008.

70   W v H (child abduction: surrogacy) (No. 2) [2002] 2 FLR 252.

71   See, for example: U v W [1998] Fam 29.

72   Morgan D, Lee RG. In the name of the father? ex parte Blood: dealing with novelty and anomaly. *Mod Law Rev* 1997;**60**:840–56: 847.

73   McLean SAM. *Review of the common law provisions relating to the removal of gametes and of the consent provisions in the Human Fertilisation and Embryology Act 1990. Op cit.*

74   Cooper G. Plans for selecting babies' sex attacked. *The Independent* 1997 Feb 27.

75   Human Organ Transplants Act 1989 s1. Human Organ Transplants (Northern Ireland) Order 1989 art 3.

76   House of Commons Science and Technology Committee. *Developments in human genetics and embryology. Fourth report of session 2001–02. Op cit:* para 28.

9: Genetics

The questions covered in this chapter include the following.

- Does genetics raise different ethical issues?
- To what extent can genetic information be shared with relatives for whom it has personal relevance?
- Should children be tested for carrier status at the request of their parents?
- Should incidental findings be disclosed?
- What is the role of health professionals when patients request paternity testing?

Responding to the "genetic revolution"

The field of human genetics has been characterised by rapid and spectacular advances in knowledge. For some it represents the panacea that will revolutionise medicine, with gene chip technology, individualised treatment regimens, and the ability not only to predict but also to avoid or cure most diseases. For others, optimism about the inevitable health benefits is counterbalanced by fears about the potential for genetic knowledge to be abused or moderated by an appreciation of the limits to what is feasible. Concerns have been voiced that genetics will give an unwelcome boost to our almost obsessive striving for perfection and that it signals a rejection of disability (and, some people argue, by implication, those with disabilities). A major concern is that, with increasing genetic information becoming available and the potential uses of that information by employers and insurance companies, new areas of discrimination will develop.

Although the medical profession has an important role to play in shaping public policy in this area, the task of promoting the benefits and preventing the harms that could flow from developments in genetics falls not just to doctors but to society as a whole. In June 2003 the Government published a white paper, *Our inheritance, our future*, to focus attention on ways of ensuring that the NHS can realise the benefits that genetics has to offer. It is hoped that this will stimulate informed public debate as well as continuing discussions within the profession. Inevitably, however, health professionals begin to feel the impact of such developments at an early stage and need to have the knowledge and understanding to respond appropriately. Genetics is no longer the sphere of a limited number of experts; it is increasingly an issue for doctors from all specialties, particularly general practice, oncology, and obstetrics. That is not to say that all health professionals are expected to provide specialist genetic advice and, in most cases, referral to a specialist genetics unit continues to be the most appropriate course of action. An understanding of the basic science of genetics, however, together with knowledge of the conflicts and dilemmas that can arise and where to go for help, forms part of the core knowledge base required for all doctors.[1]

This chapter focuses primarily on the issues raised by highly penetrant genes of large effect – Mendelian single gene disorders – because these are the most likely to raise practical and ethical dilemmas. It needs to be recognised, however, that these disorders are neither typical nor common and non-geneticists are likely to come across these types of dilemmas infrequently. GPs are more likely to encounter issues of genetics in the context of predisposition to (rather than prediction of) disorders (see pages 327–8), prenatal testing (see pages 251–4) and pharmacogenetics (see pages 484–6). Although this chapter focuses on information obtained from genetic testing, it needs to be recognised that this is not the only way in which genetic information may be obtained. It may be identified, for example, in the construction of a family history or from a conversation with a patient (e.g. if a woman says that her mother and her daughter have both tested positive for the same BRCA1 mutation, then it is obvious, without the need for a test, that she too has the mutation). Genetic information may also be obtained from non-genetic tests.

General principles

When considering the types of dilemma that arise with genetic technology, the following general principles should be kept in mind.

- It should not automatically be assumed that different rules should apply to genetics. There are some ways in which genetic information is different from other types of medical information, but the extent and inevitable implications of those differences are often overstated. Individual situations need to be assessed to decide whether additional safeguards or protection are needed.
- The same rules of consent and confidentiality apply to genetics as to other areas of medical practice.
- Genetics usually affects families, so individuals should be encouraged to consider the impact of their decisions on others who may be affected by them.
- Patients should be encouraged to share genetic information with others for whom it has personal relevance but, except in very exceptional circumstances, confidentiality should be respected.
- Genetic testing should generally be restricted to patients who are able to give valid consent or where the test is needed in order to provide appropriate information or care to the individual.
- In most circumstances, a general framework for decision making is more helpful than firm rules.

Does genetics raise different ethical issues?

Emphasis on the need for doctors to understand the dilemmas raised by genetics has led to a general tendency to assume that genetics is somehow "different" from other areas of medicine and so inevitably requires special rules and added protection.

Arguments to justify these differences, however, are frequently not articulated and, in fact, many of the ethical dilemmas that arise in the genetic sphere are the same as those that arise in other areas of medicine. They centre on the traditional duties of health professionals to act in the patient's interests and to avoid harm. Facets of those duties are embodied in the accepted obligations to respect patient confidentiality, to provide information in order to obtain valid consent, to evaluate the risks and benefits of treatment, and to aim for justice and equity in decision making. In some ways, however, genetics is different, primarily because of its familial nature, which requires that these general principles are supplemented by other considerations such as the inevitable interdependence of interests and the duties owed to other family members. Although these considerations are not exclusive to genetics, it is here that the idea of a truly autonomous decision meets perhaps its greatest challenge. This does not mean that specific provision should always be made for genetics but that there are some areas in which the standard response is inappropriate or inadequate.

When considering whether, and, if so, what, additional protection is needed, the primary question that arises is whether genetic information is fundamentally different from all other medical information. One difficulty in answering this question is that "genetic knowledge" is not a homogeneous concept – it is not all predictive, or relevant to families, or medically significant – and different kinds of information have different implications. Nevertheless, the Human Genetics Commission has suggested that the following factors could be seen to distinguish genetic from other forms of information:

- the almost uniquely identifying nature of some genetic information, including its capacity to confirm, deny, or reveal family relationships
- the fact that genetic information could be obtained from a very small amount of material (such as skin, saliva, blood, or hair), possibly secured without the consent of the person
- the predictive power of some genetic information, especially across generations of certain rare genetic diseases
- the fact that genetic information may be used for purposes other than those for which it was originally collected
- the interest that some genetic information has for others, including relatives who may be affected by it themselves, insurers, and employers
- the importance that genetic information may have for establishing susceptibility both to rare inherited disease and the effectiveness of some treatments
- the stability of DNA that can be recovered from stored specimens or even archaeological material after many years.[2]

Although there are certainly some ways in which genetic information is different from other types of medical information, the extent and inevitable implications of those differences are often overstated. Many of the factors listed above are also true of other types of information. For example, a broad range of medical information could be used for purposes other than those for which it was collected, and may be of interest to third parties such as insurance companies. Genetic information is also not unique in being predictive: HIV is predictive of AIDS. There are some ways in which it is different, however, such as the ability of information about one person to reveal information about another, perhaps without that person's knowledge or consent. Genetic information could also have social implications and affect how we perceive ourselves by revealing definitive and perhaps previously unknown knowledge about our parentage. Even where genetic information is clearly different, however, that does not necessarily mean that it requires special safeguards or justifies different treatment. Individual scenarios and uses need to be considered to determine whether the situation is "different" and, if so, if it is sufficiently different to warrant special rules or treatment. The implications of this are explored throughout this chapter.

Choice and responsibility

Discussion about genetics focuses on both choice and responsibility.[3] Developments in genetics give individuals greater choice, but also impose on them certain responsibilities. Patients have a responsibility to take account of the effect of their decisions on others who may be affected; doctors have a responsibility to use the technology wisely; and society as a whole has a responsibility to ensure that the technology is used appropriately and fairly.

The chequered history of genetics and the understandable concerns and sensitivities about past eugenic practices have led to a degree of reticence about talking in terms of the "responsibilities" of those with genetic disorders. This is because the most common "responsibility" assigned historically to these people was to remain childless. In this form, the BMA rejects the notion of assigning duties to those with genetic abnormalities. Genetic decisions are not alone in having an impact on people other than the decision maker, and the BMA believes that all individuals – with or without genetic disorders – have a general moral duty to take account of the impact of their decisions on others. The fact that individuals are seen to have certain moral obligations does not, however, imply that they necessarily can or should be forced to meet those obligations.

An ethical framework

As with the rest of this book, the aim of this chapter is not to provide ready-made answers to specific questions but to provide a framework and some indicators about how to think about the types of dilemmas that arise in genetics, in order to reach balanced solutions. Where the BMA has taken a view on a particular issue, this is stated, but, as in other areas, the Association is conscious of the need for flexibility and to be responsive to exceptional circumstances. In most situations, case by case decision making is likely to be more useful than firm and inflexible rules.

In the BMA's view, any framework for decision making in the genetic sphere should take into account and attempt to integrate three themes.

- **Rights and their limits:** Showing respect for patients' decisions and rights is seen as central to good practice. Placing emphasis on rights alone, however, without any mention of corresponding responsibilities and concern for others, cannot provide complete or convincing solutions; nor does it reflect the reality of how most people make decisions. In genetics, one person's moral claim to privacy or to refuse to know information can conflict with another's claim to be forewarned of matters affecting his or her life. If one person has a right to information, then another person has a responsibility to provide that information.
- **Concern for others:** Genetics necessarily deals with the relatedness of people based on shared DNA. Although the BMA stresses that concern for others can only very rarely justify disregarding an individual's informed decision, we believe that patients should at least take into account the needs of others as well as their own. Doctors should therefore ensure that patients are aware of the implications that their decisions may have for other people and encourage them to take these factors into account in the decision making process. This concept, of a shared interest in genetic information and research, has been referred to by the Human Genetics Commission as "genetic solidarity and altruism".[4]
- **Interdependence of interests:** Whereas a concern for others implies acting altruistically in circumstances where there is no direct benefit for the individual, the concept of interdependence recognises that in helping others the individual may also accrue indirect benefits such as improved family relationships and emotional support. From a very practical perspective, with genetics there is frequently an interdependence of interests within families because people's ability to access genetic testing and counselling depends upon other family members being willing to share information about familial risk.

Genetic testing of those with a family history of genetic disease

A key aspect of developments in genetics – and a central issue for health professionals – is the increasing ability to identify and test for particular gene mutations associated with disease. There are various forms of testing, each with different outcomes and implications. The main distinctions are:

- **diagnostic testing:** where the symptoms are already manifest
- **carrier testing:** where individuals may be at risk of passing on a genetic disease to their children but will usually be unaffected themselves and
- **predictive testing:** which may be either:
    - presymptomatic testing, which is able to predict future illness with varying degrees of accuracy or
    - predisposition testing, which is able to identify those at increased genetic risk of developing a particular disorder.

In addition to general concerns around consent and confidentiality, which apply to all genetic testing, there are some specific issues that are particular to the type of testing carried out. These are discussed in the following sections.

Consent for genetic testing

As with any other medical assessment, genetic tests should be carried out only with the valid consent of someone eligible to give it. (For general information on consent see Chapters 2 and 4.) This could be a competent adult or someone with parental responsibility for a young child, provided the test is in the child's best interests. It could also be a young person who is considered sufficiently mature to make the decision, although with most genetic testing the young person should be strongly advised to involve his or her parents in the decision. The consent must be given voluntarily and free from pressure, and whoever is giving consent must be provided with sufficient information to enable him or her to make an informed decision. Because of the nature of genetic testing, this should include information about the implications for other family members, the importance of sharing information with those for whom it has personal relevance, and the implications of withholding information from family members. In some cases definitive diagnostic or predictive information can be obtained from genetic tests, but more frequently the outcome is knowledge of an increased, but often unquantifiable, likelihood of developing the condition or probability of having an affected child. An important role of health professionals is to help people to understand "risk" both as a concept and what it means for their lives. Those who specialise in genetics are well aware of the complexities of probability and the difficulties many people have in understanding risk; they adopt particular strategies to achieve the best possible understanding.[5] Special care is needed to explain this information in a way that patients can understand.

When the implications of testing are profound, particularly with presymptomatic testing, counselling may also be required before the consent is considered to be valid. Genetic counselling includes not only the provision of detailed information and discussion of the implications and options of testing, but also the offer of psychosocial support. The process involves an attempt by specially trained professionals to help the individual or family to:

- comprehend the medical facts, including the diagnosis, the probable course of the disorder, and the available management
- appreciate the way that heredity contributes to the disorder, and the risk of recurrence in specified relatives
- understand the options for dealing with the risk of recurrence
- choose the course of action that seems appropriate to them in view of their risk and their family goals, and to act in accordance with that decision
- make the best possible adjustment to the disorder in an affected family member and/or to the risk of recurrence of that disorder.[6]

The goal of genetic counselling is not to achieve a particular outcome such as reducing the number of babies born with disabilities or to increase the number of people who seek predictive testing, but to help individuals or families to reach the outcome that is right for them.

Testing of incompetent adults

It may sometimes be desirable to carry out a genetic test on an adult who is not competent to give valid consent. When the test is for that individual's direct benefit (e.g. by facilitating treatment) this may be undertaken in England, Wales, and Northern Ireland under the common law principle of best interests. In Scotland, an appointed proxy may authorise genetic testing when this would be of benefit to the incapacitated adult or, when there is no proxy, a doctor may choose to do a genetic test under the "general authority to treat", provided that testing would benefit the patient (see Chapter 3, pages 110–2).

In some circumstances, genetic testing of an incompetent adult may be suggested, not for the benefit of the individual himself or herself, but for the benefit of other family members by contributing to family linkage or a mutation search. Sometimes, when patients are aware of pending incapacity, they make specific provision for this, in the form of advance consent for the future testing of a sample for the benefit of other family members. When this has not occurred, however, it can cause considerable distress to the relatives that the assumption is that the relative would not give consent if able to do so. If the individual has been competent in the past, and has had a close relationship with other family members, there are good grounds for assuming that he or she would wish to help them in this way. It could be argued, therefore, that allowing an individual to help his or her family in a way that most people would want to do falls within the definition of "best interests", providing there is no or minimal risk or distress. Although the BMA believes these arguments are persuasive from an ethical perspective, it is not clear that taking a sample from an incompetent adult for this purpose would be lawful in any part of the UK. This will be determined by a legal interpretation of "best interests" (in England, Wales, and Northern Ireland) and "benefit" (in Scotland), which has not, so far, been forthcoming. In a comprehensive review of the common law on consent, McLean clearly stated that: "the application of the best interests test requires evidence that the intended intervention is for the benefit of the individual concerned. Thus, no attention should be paid to possible benefits for third parties".[7] This suggests that benefit to third parties, or indirect benefit to the individual by complying with that individual's likely wishes, would not fulfil the legal requirements and therefore genetic testing for the benefit of other family members would be unlawful. This is also likely to be true in Scotland.

The Human Genetics Commission, however, although acknowledging that it remains open to doubt whether such testing is lawful, concludes that "benefit to a relative, and hence indirect benefit to the interests of the tested person, should be factors to be taken into account in deciding whether genetic testing should be carried out on a person who is unable to consent to it". It goes on to say "we consider that if the intervention is in the best interests of the person concerned taking into account all the circumstances, it would be lawful".[8] This contradiction in views serves to emphasise the need for clarification on this point of law and for legal advice to be sought if such a case arises.

Future law reform in England and Wales may clarify this point by explicitly making it lawful to carry out procedures that "although not carried out for the benefit of that person, will not cause him or her significant harm and will be of significant benefit to others".[9] In its report, *Making decisions*, however, the Government announced that this aspect of its proposals would not be taken forward at this time.[10] This provision was also not incorporated into the Scottish legislation that made provision for decision making on behalf of incapacitated adults (see Chapter 3, pages 110–2). There are general plans to reform this area of law in Northern Ireland. It therefore appears that changes to this aspect of the law are not imminent, but up to date information can be obtained from the BMA's website. Another area of legal uncertainty is whether testing of an existing sample would be lawful. Until clear advice has been given by the courts, doctors who consider such testing to be ethically acceptable in a particular case should seek legal advice before proceeding. In considering the ethical acceptability of testing an incompetent adult for the benefit of others, the following factors should be taken into account:

- any previously expressed wishes of the incompetent individual
- whether the information can be obtained by other means such as testing another relative who is competent to consent or by direct testing of the individual at risk
- the potential harm to the individual being tested, including the level of invasiveness or risk of the test and the implications for that person of the information being available
- the degree of harm or benefit to others
- whether there are grounds to believe that most competent adults would wish to help others in this way.

Summary – consent for genetic testing

- Genetic tests should be carried out only with the valid consent of someone eligible to give it: a competent person, an authorised proxy in Scotland, or someone with parental responsibility for a young child when the testing would be in the child's best interests.
- Testing may be provided if it is in the best interests of an incompetent adult, for example, because it would facilitate treatment.
- Mature minors may give consent for genetic testing, but they should be encouraged to involve their parents.
- The information to be provided should include details of the implications of the result for other family members.
- Ethically it may be acceptable to test an incompetent adult for the benefit of another person if it is considered to be in that person's best interests, but such action may be unlawful and specific legal advice must be sought.

Confidentiality within families

The general principles of confidentiality apply equally to genetic information as to other information about health. With the results of genetic testing, however, there is the added dimension that the testing of one individual frequently has relevance for other family members. This can lead to a conflict between health professionals' duties to maintain patient confidentiality and their duty to protect others from avoidable harm.[11] It has been suggested that, with genetics, the real patient is the family rather than the individual and therefore confidentiality would not be breached by disclosing information to other family members. The BMA does not accept this view and believes that, as with other areas of health care, the doctor's duty of confidentiality to the individual patient is of fundamental importance and should be breached only when there is a legal requirement or overriding public interest. The General Medical Council states that information may be disclosed when "disclosure is essential to protect the patient, or someone else, from risk of death or serious harm".[12] Individuals should always, however, be encouraged to consider the implications of their decisions for other people.

There are two main ways in which genetic information about one individual directly affects another. First, testing for a dominant disorder inevitably reveals information about the genetic status of certain other people and, in some cases, it may reveal information that the other person does not know.

The impact of genetic testing on others

If a woman whose maternal grandfather has Huntington's disease sought presymptomatic testing, a positive result would reveal that her mother also carried the gene mutation. The daughter's test has given her information about her mother's genetic status that her mother does not have and may not want to know. The added complication is that whenever the daughter informs people of her genetic status, her mother's status can be inferred. Informing the mother of her daughter's genetic status without the daughter's consent would be a breach of confidentiality. This scenario raises not only issues of confidentiality, but also of consent because, essentially, the mother is receiving information about her health as though she herself had been tested without her consent. For this reason, it is important to encourage the patient to involve other family members in discussions about the decision to seek testing and to try to reach agreement about how to proceed. If agreement cannot be reached, however, testing should generally not be withheld solely on the grounds that it would reveal information about the mother.

Two studies, from the Netherlands and the UK, found that this sort of situation arises only rarely. They showed that this type of testing makes up less than 10% of all predictive testing. In most of these cases, the intervening parent was either dead or agreed to be tested, or the person seeking testing withdrew the request when agreement could not be reached. In both studies the number of cases where testing was carried out despite the intervening parent disagreeing or being unaware of the test was around 1 in 500 of the total predictive tests.[13] Similar problems can arise when one identical twin wishes to seek presymptomatic testing, but the other does not.

Another way in which genetic information can have personal relevance for others is when an individual discovers that other family members may be at risk of passing on a disorder to their children. The mother of a son with Duchenne muscular dystrophy, for example, who has tested positive for carrier status would have information that would be important for any sisters or daughters who were planning to have children, because they too could be carriers.

Experience has shown that in the vast majority of cases people are willing to share information with relatives for whom it has personal relevance. If, however, after counselling and persuasion, the individual refuses to share the information, this should be respected unless the limited criteria set out by the General Medical Council for disclosure in the public interest are met (see Chapter 5, pages 189–92). Such situations are likely to be rare but may include a scenario in which an individual refuses consent to share information with a family member who is at risk of a severe life threatening disorder for which medical intervention could delay or prevent the condition developing. In such circumstances there may be grounds for breaching confidentiality. Such decisions are not easy, but the types of factors that should be taken into account in deciding whether the risks are sufficiently serious to breach confidentiality are:

- the severity of the disorder
- the level of predictability of the information provided by testing
- what, if any, action the relatives could take to protect themselves or make informed reproductive decisions if they were told of the risk
- the level of harm or benefit of giving and withholding the information
- the reasons given for refusing to share the information, for example, mistaken beliefs about the nature of inheritance
- whether it is possible to identify the relatives without the assistance of the patient.

As with other situations, views should be sought from other members of the healthcare team and, where it is decided that a breach of confidentiality is justified, this should be discussed in advance with the patient whenever possible.

In most cases, discussion within the family is likely to occur before testing takes place, but there are likely to be some where other family members are unaware of their at risk status. Giving them this information allows them to make their own decisions about whether to seek testing but also denies them a so-called "right not to know". Withholding the information, however, involves the doctor, or family, making decisions about what is best for that individual without consulting him or her, which goes against traditional notions of autonomy. Husted takes the view that the disclosure of information about genetic risk to unsuspecting individuals is "a clear cut case of strong medical paternalism" because the decision to know or not to know has been taken out of the hands of the individual for his or her own good.[14] He says that making people aware of the information may at first appear to be an enhancement of autonomy, since it is only by having such information that individuals can make informed choices, but it is in fact a denial of autonomy, because it prevents them from making decisions without the interference of genetic information. Laurie rejects this view, pointing out that it is simply inaccurate to argue that choices made in the light of unsought knowledge are not autonomous decisions.[15] The difficulty, however, is that it is impossible to find out whether an individual wishes to know the information without revealing that there is information available that he or she may want to know. Laurie argues that those who wish to disclose information to unsuspecting individuals should be able to justify that decision by demonstrating that the benefits of disclosure outweigh the benefits, for the individual, of remaining in ignorance. This judgment will depend on a number of factors, including the type of disease, the risks, the availability of a therapy or cure, and any evidence of prior expressions indicating a desire not to receive information.[16] Careful consideration needs to be given to the likelihood of harm arising from both disclosure and non-disclosure, and a decision needs to be reached by weighing up the arguments in each case. In practice, the BMA believes that, when consent has been obtained to share information, or when, exceptionally, it is considered that a breach of confidentiality is justified, information should usually be passed to family members about their own risk, to allow them to decide whether to seek testing. When information is to be shared, people are likely to prefer to learn it in a controlled and supportive environment.

The BMA is sometimes asked whether health professionals are under a legal "duty" to disclose information about genetic risk to relatives who may be affected by it. There is no clear answer to this question because it is not an issue that has been specifically addressed by the courts in the UK. Legal commentators have argued, however, that in some limited circumstances it is feasible that a doctor could be considered negligent for not disclosing relevant information, but only when that doctor has an existing duty of care to the relatives.[17] In reality, the types of circumstances in which such a duty may arise are likely to be so exceptional that most doctors would consider themselves to be under a moral duty to disclose the information.

Summary – confidentiality within families

- Disclosure of genetic information about one person may also reveal information about another family member.
- Individuals should be encouraged to share information with others for whom it has personal relevance. However, if they refuse, confidentiality should be breached only when there is a legal requirement or if disclosure is necessary to avoid death or serious harm.
- Although some people may prefer not to know that they are at risk of a serious genetic disorder, it is impossible to find out their wishes without revealing that there is information they may want to know.

- The possible harms of disclosure and non-disclosure need to be considered, but the BMA believes that information should usually be passed to family members about their own risk, to allow them to decide whether to seek testing.
- When information is to be shared, it is preferable for people to learn it in a controlled and supportive environment.

Diagnostic testing

Genetic tests are frequently used, in the same way as other diagnostic tests, to confirm a diagnosis once symptoms have begun to appear. Consent should be sought in the usual way, but should include information about the implications for other family members. In some circumstances the tests themselves may not be genetic tests *per se*, but still reveal information about a genetic condition. In these cases there should be close liaison with the regional genetics unit, and support and advice should be obtained before carrying out the test. It would be inappropriate, for example, for a patient to be informed by a neurologist about a diagnosis of Huntington's disease without there being some prior discussion, with the patient if possible and/or his or her relatives, about the genetic nature of the condition and the consequent implications for other family members.

Carrier testing

When individuals are known to be at risk of carrying the gene for an autosomal recessive disorder, or an X linked disorder, they may seek carrier testing in order to inform future reproductive decisions. If it is found that future children would be at risk, the couple may decide to remain childless, opt for preimplantation or prenatal diagnosis, or accept the risk and proceed in the knowledge that the child may be affected by the disorder. These options are discussed in more detail in Chapter 7 (pages 251–4). When the patient is a competent adult or a mature minor, before consent is sought, information should be provided about the reliability of the test, the nature of the disorder, and the implications of carrier status. Young people should be strongly encouraged to involve their parents in the decision to seek carrier testing. When, however, they are sufficiently mature to give valid consent, they understand the implications of carrier status, and there is no suggestion that the consent is given under pressure, there are strong arguments for respecting the young person's wishes and carrying out the test. In some cases the suggestion for carrier testing may come from other family members, with the support of the appropriate health professionals. When an "active programme" is initiated, affected individuals are invited to inform their relatives of their potential risk of being a carrier and invite them to seek genetic testing. When carriers are identified through this mechanism, they are encouraged to inform their relatives of the risk and so the testing continues. This proactive strategy is called cascade testing.

Carrier testing of an incompetent adult is unlikely to be of direct benefit to the individual but there may be circumstances in which it would be of benefit to other family members. Testing in such cases may be considered ethically acceptable, but it is unclear whether it would be lawful (see pages 313–4). In such cases legal advice should be sought.

Carrier testing of children

The most ethically problematic aspect of carrier testing is dealing with parental requests for testing of young children who are not able to give consent for themselves. Given that, for most conditions, the children themselves are not affected by or do not have any symptoms of the disorder, the only benefit of knowing their carrier status is to make plans for reproduction when they are older. It has been argued that testing in childhood restricts the child's future options without any immediate benefit and that the child, and later the adult, would be denied the option of not knowing his or her genetic status. It has also been suggested that testing at the request of a child's parents and giving the parents the results denies the child, and later the adult, the confidentiality he or she would expect if tested as an adult. Despite these concerns, many parents strongly believe they have a right to know this information and requests for such testing are fairly common. A study on parents' attitudes to testing the siblings of patients with cystic fibrosis, for example, found that 90% would like to know the carrier status of their unaffected children and 91% believed they had a right to the information.[18]

Together with health professionals, parents are responsible for the health care of their children until they themselves are sufficiently mature to take over this task. It is generally accepted that parents can, and indeed should, have access to information that is necessary for them to fulfil this role. Thus a fundamental question is whether carrier testing should be seen as materially different in nature to other health information that parents would expect to be able to find out about their children. There is a difference in that the information is of no immediate benefit to the child and is not already available, but is being generated after a specific request from the parents. If information about carrier status were to be discovered inadvertently, for example while undertaking diagnostic testing, the BMA believes it would be inappropriate to withhold this from the parents unless disclosing it would clearly be contrary to the child's interests. This does not mean, however, that the parents should necessarily be able to authorise testing. Those with parental responsibility may consent to any testing of a young child if having the test is in the child's best interests. Given that the information derived from carrier testing is only of any practical benefit once he or she begins to think about having children, could it ever be in the best interests of a young child actively to seek this information?

It was suggested above that one of the factors to be taken into account in considering genetics is the interdependence of interests. This is an important factor when considering the genetic testing of children because, in reality, the interests of the child cannot be considered in total isolation from the interests of the parents and other family members. The parents' educational and caring role may be considered to put them in the best position to decide when to tell the child, as well as to help the child to understand the implications of the test. They may feel, for example, that early knowledge of carrier status gives the child a period of time to adapt and to come to terms with the information, compared with being presented with this knowledge during adolescence, which is often a difficult and emotional time. They may also feel that their own anxiety, caused by the continuing uncertainty about the child's carrier status, may affect their relationship with the child. The request may also come as a result of unresolved grief in parents who have lost a brother, sister, or child from a distressing disease and have a strong desire to know whether their children are carriers of the same condition.[19]

Carrier testing of children in Finland

A study was carried out in Finland to consider long term psychological consequences, experience, satisfaction, and recall of the test results of 25 healthy siblings of patients with aspartylglucosaminuria.[20] The age at testing ranged from 1 to 17 years (12 were 10 years or under and 6 were aged 15 or over at the time of testing). Of the 25 tested individuals, 21 reported that carrier testing had not had any influence on their lives, two reported that it had had a positive influence by ensuring the information was available for family planning, one reported both positive and negative influences, and no information was given about the remaining person. Overall, the emotional, social, and physical wellbeing of the young people tested was at least as good as those in the control group. All of those tested were satisfied with the carrier testing and had no concerns about their parents having made the decision on their behalf. In terms of accuracy of recollection, 23 of the 25 (92%) remembered and understood their test result correctly. The authors point out, however, that there was also no evidence that testing in childhood had any benefits over testing in adulthood. They concluded that, despite their findings, they did not recommend testing in childhood because the result is not needed prior to the time for reproductive decisions to be made.

The few studies that have been undertaken on the impact of carrier testing in childhood do not provide conclusive evidence about the benefit or harm of testing children.[21] In the BMA's view, the arguments are not sufficiently clear cut to justify a prohibition on carrier testing of young children, but there are good arguments for delaying testing until the child is old enough to make an informed decision. Although there should be a presumption against carrier testing of young children, it needs to be recognised that there may be some cases in which the benefits outweigh the harms and it is in the child's interests to test at a young age. In practice, most parents agree, after discussion, to delay testing, but there is a need for a flexible approach to deal with the exceptional cases where such agreement is not achieved and when testing would be appropriate in the circumstances.

Summary – carrier testing

- Before consent is sought, competent adults and mature minors should be given information about the reliability of the test, the nature of the disorder, and the implications of carrier status.
- Young people should be encouraged to involve their parents in a decision to seek carrier testing.
- If carrier testing of an incompetent adult is suggested for the benefit of other people, legal advice should be sought before proceeding.
- There is insufficient evidence of harm to recommend a prohibition on carrier testing of children, but there are good arguments for delaying testing until they are old enough to make a personal decision.
- There should be a presumption against carrier testing of young children, but flexibility is needed to deal with exceptional cases.
- Most parents, after discussion, agree to delay testing their young children.

Predictive testing

The type of genetic testing that is most frequently debated, and which has the potential for the most problems, is testing that can predict, before any symptoms have appeared, whether an individual will or may go on to develop a particular condition in the future. Within this category of testing there are two distinct groups:

- **presymptomatic tests:** for genetic mutations associated with dominantly inherited conditions with complete penetrance, such as Huntington's disease; having the gene mutation means the individual will go on to develop the disease at some stage unless he or she dies of another cause before the disease manifests itself
- **predisposition tests:** for genes that identify risk factors for particular diseases where having the gene mutation indicates an increased risk of developing the disorder, but not certainty. The likelihood of developing the condition varies, from very high with hereditary breast cancer to much lower with conditions such as Alzheimer's disease and heart disease.

Each of these types of test raises specific issues, which are discussed in the sections that follow.

Presymptomatic testing

When it is possible to treat the condition for which the individual is at risk or when some intervention, such as screening for early evidence of the disease, can facilitate treatment, early diagnosis would clearly be beneficial and so predictive testing, with valid consent and counselling, is relatively unproblematic. More debatable is testing for those conditions for which there is no useful medical intervention. This means, in practice, that individuals know they will go on to develop a very serious, and perhaps life-threatening, disorder in the future but they do not know when. Despite having this knowledge, there is nothing they can do to prevent or cure the disease. Most people who are at risk of such conditions do not want to know what is in store for them and the takeup rate of presymptomatic testing for Huntington's disease, for example, is only about 18% of those who are at risk.[22]

For some people, however, living with uncertainty is one of the most difficult aspects of being part of an at risk family and to know for certain that they will develop the disease is better than not knowing. Having access to information about future disability enables them to plan their careers, families, and lives to take account of their potential limitations. There can also be practical benefits, such as making arrangements for suitable care and support to be available, or moving to a house that can accommodate a wheelchair for example. It is important to keep these benefits in perspective, however, since in some respects uncertainty about whether an individual will develop the disease is replaced with uncertainty about when the disease will manifest itself and how severe it will be. The implications of testing need to be explored fully by the patient before consent is sought. Genetic counselling forms an integral part of the service offered in regional genetics centres.

Initial fears that for healthy people to learn they are destined to develop a serious and incurable genetic disorder would inevitably cause severe distress, stigmatisation, and suicide have not materialised. A worldwide assessment of people who have had a predictive test for Huntington's disease found that the vast majority did not subsequently experience any catastrophic events (defined as: suicide, assisted suicide, or psychiatric problems resulting in hospitalisation). However, 44 people out of 4527 in the study (0·97%) experienced such an event within two years of receiving the result (some – including all those who committed suicide – being symptomatic at the time of the event).[23] Although significantly higher than in the general population, the suicide rate in this group is not out of proportion when compared with that occurring in those with Huntington's disease or other serious progressive diseases.[24] This shows that predictive genetic testing can be carried out without harmful effects in the context of a carefully designed clinical programme that includes genetic counselling as part of the process, but that care and long term support are required to minimise the risks associated with such testing. Not surprisingly, research shows that people who receive an unfavourable result tend to be more distressed than those whose tests show they are not carriers of the gene mutation, but the distress is usually within the range of normal behaviour. In fact, people who are found to carry a gene mutation frequently experience some decrease in psychological distress as their uncertainty over their genetic status decreases.[25] Psychological research has also found some evidence among those who receive a favourable result of some initial difficulty in coming to terms with their new genetic status.[26]

Personal experience of presymptomatic testing

Sue Wright was 14 years old when, after her father's diagnosis, she found out that she had a 50% chance of developing Huntington's disease. She described her experience as "a yoyo type of existence", sometimes convinced she had the gene and at other times feeling guilty about worrying. In practical terms, it added complications with relationships, insurance, and applying for a nursing job in New Zealand. In her experience, being "at risk" meant that she was treated in the same way as if she definitely had the gene.

In January 1993 she and her long term partner went for genetic counselling to discuss the options available before deciding whether to have children. In March 1993 the gene was cloned and the option of testing became a reality. Miss Wright described her feelings about this:

> I had been waiting for years for the gene to be identified and now it was ... it was a strange feeling. We had to seriously consider whether we were better off living 'at risk' or living knowing I had the gene. There would be no going back. In the past I had considered this option but never imagined I would actually be offered it.

After further counselling she decided to have the test, which showed that she was carrying the gene. She was shocked and described her feelings as being similar to a form of bereavement. Nevertheless, she said that both she and her partner

> felt more at peace now we knew I had the gene. I'm sure fear can build up around something that might or might not happen and sometimes it's better to know the truth. In the months since this time neither of us has regretted the decision at all.[27]

Given the profound implications of predictive testing, it is essential that the individual gives the matter full and careful consideration and makes the decision that is appropriate for him or her. It is clear from experience that patients sometimes seek testing as a result of pressure from a spouse or other family member.[28] Although it is important for the patient to consider the effect of his or her decision on other people, it is the individual's decision, and testing should proceed only if the patient has given valid and unpressured consent. Partners may have a legitimate interest in knowing the genetic status of the patient, particularly if they are making decisions about whether to have children. This does not, however, give them the right to pressurise the patient into seeking testing or to receive the result of the test, unless that is the patient's own wish. Despite having no right to make the decision, it is important that the relatives and partners of those seeking testing also receive support. In one study, the partners of those who tested positive experienced more post-test distress and poorer quality of life than did the patient.[29]

The report issued by the Advisory Committee on Genetic Testing (whose role was subsequently taken over by the Human Genetics Commission) on testing for late onset disorders[30] offers the advice below on the information needed by those who are seeking testing.

- Information on the disorder being tested for should be full and accurate, and should be presented in a clear and simple manner that is readily understandable.
- Full information should be provided on the test, its consequences and limitations, and its scientific and clinical validity.
- Individuals should be fully informed of potential adverse consequences, such as for insurance, employment, and effects on other family members.
- Although written details are important, complex information should be provided face to face by an appropriately trained and experienced person.
- Voluntary organisations involved with genetic disorders can also be a valuable source of information for those considering genetic testing.
- Individuals should be given adequate time to absorb the information provided before a decision is taken to be tested or a result is given.

Health professionals caring for patients who have received an unfavourable presymptomatic test should be wary of relying too heavily on the test result and should remain open minded to other explanations for reported symptoms. There have been cases in which other conditions have been missed because the doctor wrongly attributed the clinical signs to the underlying predisposition.

Incompetent adults

Presymptomatic testing of an incompetent adult for a severe genetic disorder for which no treatment is available is unlikely to be demonstrably in the interests of the individual unless it would allow carers to take practical steps to improve the care of the patient. In very limited circumstances, such testing may be of benefit to other family members. Testing incompetent adults for the benefit of others is discussed on pages 313–4.

Young people

With presymptomatic testing where there is no medical benefit, a very high level of capacity would be required in order for a person aged under 16 to be able to consent to testing. Any health professional providing presymptomatic testing to a person under 16 years of age must be prepared to justify that decision on grounds of the individual's competence. The doctor would also have a responsibility to ensure that sufficient information had been given and understood, and that the patient had received extensive counselling and considered the implications of a positive test for himself or herself and for other family members. The young person should also be strongly encouraged to involve his or her parents or another adult in this important decision. Before proceeding with testing, health professionals should satisfy themselves that an appropriate support mechanism is available for the young person. Those over 16 years of age are presumed to be competent to consent to testing, but parental involvement should still be encouraged.

Children

The majority of predictive genetic testing that has been carried out in young children is for conditions that usually manifest in early childhood or where some medical intervention can usefully be applied. The benefits that accrue from presymptomatic testing for childhood onset disorders include appropriate diagnosis and management as well as options for preventive action or treatment. Testing for Duchenne muscular dystrophy, for example, can allow parents to meet at an early stage with specialist health professionals in order to plan for the future health needs of the child. Arguments about undermining the child's right to make decisions for himself or herself in the future and problems of confidentiality, which arise in relation to testing for adult onset disorders, do not arise when the condition usually becomes manifest in very young children. Where, however, parents request testing of a young child for a disorder that usually develops around the teens, these factors need to be taken into account. Some people take the view that it is harmful to the child to know from an early age that he or she will go on to develop a severe genetic condition, whereas others argue that young children are better able to cope with such information and will grow up in the knowledge of and accepting their impending disability. In fact, both the benefits and harms of testing in these circumstances are largely unproven and decisions need to be made on the basis of the facts of individual cases, making an assessment of the child's best interests, based on the following factors:

- the age and maturity of the child
- the length of time between the request and the estimated age of onset of symptoms
- the views of the child regarding testing, if sufficiently mature to make a judgment
- the type of disorder and the potential medical and psychological benefits of knowing the child's genetic status prior to the onset of symptoms
- why, and by whom, testing is being sought
- the potential benefits or harms for the child.

Occasionally, requests are received from parents who wish to have their children tested presymptomatically for adult onset disorders. In some cases, early treatment or regular surveillance could bring some medical benefit to the child and in these cases a careful balance needs to be reached between the amount of benefit and the potential for harm. When there is no treatment or useful medical intervention, there is general agreement that testing should be delayed until the child is old enough to make an informed, personal decision. The primary reason for this is that testing a child would deny that person, as an adult, the right to make that decision for himself or herself. Given the lack of benefit of testing in childhood, and the potential for arising harm, removing the option for a child not to know his or her genetic status cannot be justified. The privacy of the child would also be lost because the parents, or other adult requesting the test, would be informed of the results.

Another major area of concern is that the burden for children of knowing that in adult life they will develop a severe, incurable genetic disorder may be too great and rob them of a carefree childhood. It is feared that learning such news in childhood or adolescence could have a very negative effect on individuals' self esteem and ability to function properly in society. Because such testing is not generally undertaken, however, there is no evidence either to support or refute these suggestions. Some research has been carried out on the psychological effects of predictive testing for familial adenomatous polyposis (FAP), for which there are medical benefits to testing. This found that children did not show clinically significant distress over a period of one year after predictive testing.[31] Although this is not precisely the same as testing for an incurable disease, it provides some objective evidence about the psychological effects of predictive testing of children.

Predictive testing of children for FAP

One study compared the emotional state of children (aged 10–16 years) and adults (aged 17–67 years) after predictive genetic testing for FAP. It found that children receiving positive or negative results did not experience greater anxiety or depression than adults having the same tests. In fact, the only difference between children and adults was that, among those with positive results, the children were less anxious and a smaller proportion of them had anxiety scores in the clinical range. The study also found that the children, as a group, did not show clinically significant distress over a period of one year after predictive testing. This latter finding is consistent with the results of an earlier study conducted on 41 children aged between 6 and 16 years before and three months after predictive testing for FAP. This study, carried out in the USA, reported that anxiety and behavioural problems remained in the normal range for the three months after testing.[32]

Parents sometimes seek predictive testing for their children because they believe that, for them, knowing for certain that the child has or has not inherited the gene mutation will enable them to provide more appropriate care for the child. For some parents this may indeed be a benefit, but this needs to be weighed against the risk of harm resulting to the child. There are concerns, for example, that those who find their children to be affected by a late onset disorder may reflect this in the way they behave towards them. They may treat them as ill before the disorder becomes manifest, or fail to give them encouragement to do well at school or to train for a career. An unfavourable result may also harm the future life opportunities of the child through disadvantages in insurance and employment (see pages 335–7). Although these disadvantages apply equally to adults, who are in a position to make the decision for themselves about whether those risks are worth taking, for children, this irreversible decision would be taken on their behalf. Given that, as mentioned above, most adults decide that the disadvantages outweigh the advantages of testing for conditions like Huntington's disease, there are good arguments for not complying with parental requests. Those asking for the test should be given a detailed explanation about why it will not be undertaken. The fact that a child is not tested does not mean that he or she should not be informed of the risk of carrying the gene mutation and the possibility of testing in the future.

Predisposition testing

A large number of common disorders are known sometimes to have a genetic component, including some forms of cancer, coronary heart disease, and diabetes. With those forms of breast cancer that are caused by mutations in the breast cancer susceptibility genes, testing has a high predictive value with estimates of up to an 80% lifetime risk of developing the condition.[33] It has been suggested, however, that, with the exception of high risk families, the lifetime risk may be lower than this.[34] Many more disorders, such as heart disease, have a lower genetic component and the level of risk is more dependent upon the interaction between genetic and environmental factors. Thus, genetic testing for these disorders can identify only an increased susceptibility to a particular disorder, with varying degrees of predictability. With some conditions that give a very high level of predictability, there can be clear advantages to testing. For example, some people who know from information provided by an affected family member that they are at increased risk of being carriers of a BRCA1 mutation, consider having a prophylactic double mastectomy. A genetic test to determine whether the gene mutation has been inherited can inform this decision. If the gene is not present, the risk becomes slightly less than that in the general population and the mastectomy can be avoided. When testing gives a much lower indication of risk, however, the benefits are far less straightforward.

Many of the advantages of presymptomatic testing for conditions like Huntington's disease (discussed above) focus on the benefit of relief from uncertainty and of being able to plan for the future in the knowledge of impending disability. When the test result indicates only an increased risk of developing the disorder, particularly when this is low, the strength of these arguments is reduced. There may be other advantages, however, to knowing about increased susceptibility. The role played by environmental factors in these common disorders, for example, makes it possible, in some people, to alter their lifestyle to reduce the risk. In some ways, this type of testing is an extension of existing practice, rather than something totally new. Doctors have for many years identified those who are at high risk of cancer or heart disease and tried to encourage them to make changes to their lifestyle to minimise that risk. It remains to be seen whether such advice, based on genetic testing, will be any more successful than previous attempts to encourage people to live healthier lives. There is some evidence to support the concern that many people associate genetic tests with conditions that are not preventable and not treatable, which is likely to make it more difficult to encourage behavioural changes.[35] This can lead not only to a reluctance to take action to reduce the risk, because it is seen as inevitable, but also to increased levels of anxiety. A review of the available research evidence carried out by Marteau and Lerman found that providing people with DNA derived information about risks to their health did not increase motivation to change behaviour beyond that achieved with non-genetic information.[36] There was also some indication that people may adopt a fatalistic approach and, for some, genetic information may reduce motivation to change their behaviour.

If predisposition testing is to be of any benefit in common diseases like heart disease, attention needs to be paid to methods of presenting information in such a way that it motivates and encourages people to make the necessary lifestyle changes. The future use and availability of testing that gives only a relatively low predictive value depends upon there being some clear benefits to its use. It has been suggested that, without testing for common disorders, the ultimate impact of the new genetics will be limited because only a small proportion of the population are affected by Mendelian disorders.[37]

Summary – predictive testing

- When there is no useful medical intervention or treatment, most people choose not to have predictive genetic testing. However, for some, certainty that they will develop the disease is better than living with the uncertainty of their at risk status.
- Given the profound implications of predictive testing for severe life threatening disorders, it is essential that the individual gives the matter full and careful consideration and makes the decision that is appropriate for him or her.
- A very high level of capacity would be required in order for a person aged under 16 to be able to consent to presymptomatic genetic testing.
- The majority of predictive genetic testing in young children is for conditions that usually manifest in early childhood or where some medical intervention can usefully be applied.
- When there is no medical benefit to predictive testing in childhood for adult onset disorders, removing the option for the child not to know his or her genetic status cannot be justified.
- When the test result indicates only an increased risk of developing the disorder, the benefits – in terms of relief from uncertainty – are less clear cut.
- It is not clear whether people at increased genetic risk of developing a common condition will be more likely to change their lifestyle to reduce the overall risk or take a fatalistic approach and see such changes as futile.

Incidental findings

Sometimes, additional information is obtained during genetic testing. This could concern a condition other than the one being tested for or be about non-paternity.[38] If there is a reasonable chance of other information being inadvertently discovered from a particular test, this should be discussed with the patient or the parent of a young child during the consent process, in order to ascertain the individual's wishes about disclosure. The discussion should give examples of the type of information that could be discovered and the procedures that will be followed in that event.

When information is discovered unexpectedly, and this discussion has not taken place, there should be a general presumption that information will be shared because it would be wrong deliberately to withhold it on the assumption that it would not be in the individual's interests to know. There may, however, be exceptions to this rule, such as where it is judged that revealing the information could cause severe psychological harm to the patient or would be contrary to the interests of a young child. When such information is to be given, this must be done sensitively and taking a cue from the individual about how much information he or she is ready and willing to accept at that particular time.

Population genetic screening

Population screening involves testing members of a particular population for a disorder or condition for which there is no family history or other prior evidence of its presence. The population to be screened may be chosen for a number of reasons. It may be those who, because of their circumstances, would find screening useful. This could include screening those who are planning to have children for carrier status for common autosomal recessive conditions such as cystic fibrosis to enable them to make informed reproductive decisions, or the well established programme of screening the Ashkenazi Jewish population for Tay Sachs carrier status (see page 723). They may be chosen simply because of their age (e.g. some genetic screening is routinely carried out on neonates), or the population may be the self selecting group who choose to avail themselves of screening, possibly through one of the services that offers screening direct to the public (see pages 332–5). It has also been suggested that, in the future, screening may be offered routinely to the whole population to assess the genetic risk of predisposition to certain types of cancer. For further information about population screening see Chapter 20 on public health.

Screening for carrier status for autosomal recessive disorders

The introduction of population screening for carrier status for cystic fibrosis has been under discussion by the UK National Screening Committee for a number of years, but no guidance has yet been issued. As a result, availability and methods of screening vary between areas, although such programmes as exist are mainly based in antenatal units. Some studies of past practice found that the male partner was tested only if the pregnant woman was found to be a carrier, resulting in many women experiencing significant symptoms of anxiety and depression. As expected, this anxiety dissipated if the partner subsequently received a negative result. This model has now been modified so that samples are usually taken from both partners at the same time, although the father's sample will be tested only if the mother is found to be a carrier. In the past, results were given for the couple, rather than for individual persons but, in most areas, this has also changed and the mother is informed of her carrier status even if her partner is not a carrier of any of the standard mutations. This alerts her to the risk in any future pregnancy with a different partner. It also alerts the couple to the fact that, since one of them is known to be a carrier, the risk of having an affected child is slightly higher than in non-carriers (because a screen negative test does not exclude carrier status, but merely reduces the likelihood of it). If both partners are found to be carriers, they are advised of the risk to the child. Some parents opt for prenatal diagnosis in order to establish the health of the fetus before deciding how to proceed, while others proceed without further tests, knowing that the baby has a one in four chance of developing the condition.

Screening *during* pregnancy, however, precludes some of the reproductive options available, such as preimplantation genetic diagnosis (see Chapter 8, pages 291–2) or the use of donated gametes. The ideal situation is for information about carrier status to be available when people are planning a pregnancy. Despite the clear advantages to preconception carrier screening, its uptake in the UK has been minimal. One difficulty is identifying the population who would be most likely to want to use the service (i.e. those who are planning a pregnancy). Some people discuss their plans with their family planning clinic or GP, but many more do not. Another alternative is to offer screening to all people of reproductive age, although, where this has been offered, the uptake has been low, which appears to indicate a lack of interest in such screening.[39] Some people who are planning pregnancy may opt to seek carrier screening independently by using one of the services offered direct to the public. This is discussed on pages 332–5. Another option would be to offer carrier screening in the final year of secondary school, when young people are sufficiently mature to give valid consent and can be offered testing in conjunction with a formal educational component. A pilot study of this method of screening was undertaken in Montreal in 1993 with encouraging results.[40] Although there are benefits to carrier screening in schools, a number of safeguards would need to be put in place before this could be contemplated. These include difficulties around pressures on consent, confidentiality, the risk of stigmatisation, and the need to provide appropriate support mechanisms.

Neonatal screening

Neonatal screening has, historically, been less controversial than other types, since its main aim has been to identify affected neonates in order to instigate treatment at the earliest opportunity. Since the early 1960s, for example, virtually all newborn babies have been screened to ascertain whether they have inherited the genetic defect for phenylketonuria (PKU). The benefits to such screening are clear cut because early diagnosis and a special diet can avoid the worst effects of this disorder. Most parents are very happy to give consent when they appreciate the benefits of the test; when they refuse, there may be grounds for arguing that the refusal is not in the best interests of the child and therefore is not a decision the parents are able to make on their child's behalf. It is interesting, however, that the Supreme Court of Ireland upheld parents' right to refuse PKU testing, despite the very obvious benefits to children and the minimally invasive nature of the heel prick test.[41] No such cases have been considered by courts in the UK.

In some areas, all newborns are screened for cystic fibrosis because, although the evidence is less clear cut than with PKU, it is suggested that early diagnosis prevents lung damage and improves the long term prognosis. However, a complication with neonatal screening for cystic fibrosis (and other disorders such as sickle cell disease, which is offered to certain populations) is that, in addition to identifying affected babies, some carriers may also be detected. This raises a dilemma, given that there are generally good reasons for delaying carrier testing until the child is old enough to make a personal decision (see pages 319–20). When it is impossible to conduct the diagnostic test without also revealing carrier status, this should be explained to the parents in the process of seeking consent. Information that is available should not be deliberately withheld from the parents, particularly since knowledge of the child's carrier status may have implications for their own future reproductive decisions. When babies are found to be carriers, the parents should be given help and support to decide when and how to inform the child of the carrier status. This incidental information is an important factor that needs to be taken into account when considering the introduction of neonatal screening for cystic fibrosis. In view of this possible disadvantage to neonatal screening, the advantages for the child of having an early diagnosis need to be carefully examined and articulated to reach an appropriate balance. The possibility of introducing neonatal screening for cystic fibrosis is under consideration by the UK National Screening Committee.

There have also been proposals for neonatal screening for Duchenne muscular dystrophy, with pilot studies being undertaken in Wales, Germany, France, and Canada. Although there is no available treatment, there may be advantages to having an early, confirmed diagnosis of this condition, such as the ability to meet specialist health professionals, to seek genetic counselling, and to plan for the future, and also for the parents to be able to make informed decisions about future reproduction. The advantages of early diagnosis need to be balanced against the disadvantage of knowing of impending disability, perhaps a few years before the onset of symptoms. The House of Commons Science and Technology Committee considered this issue in its inquiry in 1995 and recommended that there should be no mass screening in childhood unless a treatment for the disorder exists.[42] The Government accepted this recommendation.[43]

Screening for predisposition to common disorders

As more information becomes available about the genetic contribution to complex, common disorders, the spectre of screening the full population for predisposition to particular disorders becomes an option. It has been argued, for example, that society will, at some time in the future, embrace large scale screening for susceptibility to diseases such as cancer.[44] The purpose would be to identify those who are at increased genetic risk, so that they can take steps to reduce those environmental aspects of risk that are amenable to change: such as diet and exercise, or possibly to take prophylactic medication to reduce the likelihood of the condition developing.[45] Many of the issues that arise with such screening are similar to testing those at risk because of a family history (see pages 327–8), but on a much larger scale and with the added inherent problems of population screening (see Chapter 20, pages 709–13). Unless evidence shows that such information has clear benefits, for example that people understand the result and are motivated to change their lifestyle or take other steps to reduce the risk, the disadvantages of full population screening are likely to outweigh the benefits for the foreseeable future. Eventually, however, the population is likely to be better informed about genetics and may find it far less threatening and accept genetic predisposition as simply one among many risk factors for common disorders.

Summary – population genetic screening

- Population screening involves testing members of a particular population for a disorder or condition for which there is no family history or other prior evidence of its presence.
- Screening for carrier status for autosomal recessive disorders should ideally be offered to those planning to have children, but this population group is difficult to identify. Many such screening programmes are based in antenatal units, which restricts the options for couples who are found to be carriers.
- Some forms of neonatal screening (such as for cystic fibrosis) also identify carriers of the disorder. When obtaining this incidental information is unavoidable, parents should be informed of this as part of the consent process and should be told of the results.
- In the future it may be possible to undertake population screening to detect an increased predisposition to common disorders. Unless evidence shows that such information has clear benefits, however, such as that people are motivated to change their lifestyle or take other steps to reduce the risk, the disadvantages of full population screening are likely to outweigh the benefits for the foreseeable future.

Genetic tests supplied direct to the public

Growing public interest and knowledge about genetics has led to a range of genetic tests being provided in shops, by mail, or over the internet, without the need to discuss the test or the results with a medical practitioner. Demand for such services has been lower than initially expected, however, and it is not clear whether this is an area that will continue to grow. Initially, such services were restricted to carrier testing for autosomal recessive disorders, but this expanded to, among other things, paternity testing and testing aimed at providing dietary and lifestyle advice. It is possible that other forms of testing could become available in the future, including, in theory presymptomatic tests for serious, life threatening disorders. The Human Genetics Commission issued a report on direct testing in 2003 recommending that:

- there should be stricter controls on direct genetic testing, but there should not be a statutory ban
- there should be a well funded NHS genetics service that can properly manage and allow access to predictive genetic tests
- most genetic tests that provide predictive health information should not be offered as direct genetic tests
- predictive genetic tests that rely on home testing or home sampling should be discouraged.[46]

The BMA broadly supports these recommendations. In the BMA's view, it is not self evident that all genetic tests, simply by being DNA tests, require additional protection. Arguably, individuals should be free to find out as much information as they wish to know about their own health, without interference from the state. There may be circumstances, however, in which serious harm could result from an individual receiving a genetic test result without the necessary information and support to both understand and come to terms with it. For example, research evidence has shown that, in carefully controlled situations, presymptomatic testing for Huntington's disease can be undertaken without harmful results. Given the very serious implications of the information revealed, however, both for the individual being tested and other family members, there are good grounds for believing that predictive testing without the involvement of any health professionals or specialist support could result in serious harm. In such cases, the duty of the state to protect its citizens from harm is likely to override the individual's wish to seek testing without the involvement of health professionals. Any restrictions on the availability of such testing would not prevent the individual from undergoing tests, but would simply require them to arrange these through a health professional. Although a range of non-genetic testing kits are available direct to the public, there is a precedent for restricting the availability of such tests when it is considered that serious harm could result. In 1992, for example, it was made an offence to sell HIV testing kits directly to the public.[47] The implications of HIV testing were considered to be sufficiently serious to merit restricting its availability to services provided by specialists who are able to give advice before and after testing.

A predictive test for Huntington's disease is, of course, at one end of a spectrum of tests that could in theory become available. The implications of other genetic tests are less problematic. For example, carrier testing for an autosomal recessive disorder in a couple who are planning a pregnancy, and in whom there is no family history, raises far fewer concerns, provided adequate and appropriate information is available. Carrier testing does not usually provide information about the individual's own health, or predict future disease, although an unfavourable result would have implications for other siblings or existing children, who may find out that they are also at risk of being a carrier of the disorder.

A fundamental question in relation to the need for regulation is whether a genetic test that identifies an increased susceptibility to heart disease, for example, is fundamentally different from any one of the non-genetic tests that could give the same information, such as tests for cholesterol levels or blood pressure. In the light of the research quoted on page 327, about people's understanding of genetic tests, there may be more of a risk of a genetic test being misunderstood and taken to imply that the individual will definitely develop heart disease, rather than that he or she is at increased risk. As already mentioned, this could not only lead to considerable anxiety but may also make behavioural changes appear futile. Careful attention would need to be given to the information provided in order to avoid this outcome. The identification of an increased genetic susceptibility in one individual could also have direct implications for other family members and, in this respect, it is also different from other forms of testing. The BMA believes that testing with the involvement and support of health professionals should continue to be the norm for most patients, but does not believe there is sufficient risk of harm to justify a general prohibition on "direct to the public" tests. When there is a high risk of clear and serious harm, such as with predictive testing for very serious, incurable, conditions, there are good arguments for limiting the availability of testing but, when the risk is lower, these arguments are not persuasive. Provided the services are easily accessible, most people are likely to prefer to use those within the NHS.

Although it would be feasible to restrict the advertising or sale of genetic testing kits in the UK, it is not currently possible to prevent people from using services in other countries, such as those accessed via the internet. Where services are restricted in the UK, however, it is important that the reasons for this are made clear to those who enquire about the availability of such tests. When health professionals become aware of an individual's plan to seek testing in another country, they should ensure that the patient is aware of the importance of receiving detailed information, of having the opportunity to ask questions, and of the availability of professional support. They should also be informed that, unless there is effective, local regulation, there can be no guarantees about the standards in the laboratories undertaking the test. Information provided to people seeking testing in this country should encourage individuals to discuss their wish for testing with their GP or other relevant health professional.

The Human Genetics Commission has expressed concern about the risk of DNA samples being sent for testing without the knowledge or consent of the individuals they came from.[48] There is far more risk of this happening with direct to the public testing than when there is personal contact between the individual being tested and a health professional or other specialist. With direct to the public testing, a sample of hair or saliva, for example, is sent off, usually by mail, together with a copy of a signed consent form. No checks are made that the consent form is signed by the person from whom the sample was taken. If testing kits are developed that do not need to be sent to a laboratory for testing, such as with home pregnancy testing kits, there is no requirement for a consent form to be signed at all. Owing to the ease with which such samples could be obtained and tested surreptitiously, the Human Genetics Commission has recommended the introduction of a new offence of the non-consensual or deceitful obtaining and/or analysis of genetic material for non-medical purposes.[49] The BMA supports this recommendation in principle which has also been supported by the Government.[50]

Summary – genetic tests supplied direct to the public

- It is not self evident that all genetic tests, simply by being DNA tests, require additional protection.
- The sale direct to the public of tests that have serious implications for the person being tested and/or his or her family should be restricted.
- Although testing without the involvement of a health professional may not be ideal, it would be overly paternalistic to assume that people are unable to understand the information or to make a decision for themselves on this matter.
- When health professionals become aware of an individual's plan to seek testing in another country, they should ensure that the patient is aware of the importance of detailed information, the opportunity to ask questions, and the availability of support.
- The BMA supports the introduction of a new offence of the non-consensual or deceitful obtaining and/or analysis of genetic material for non-medical purposes.

Controversial uses of genetic information

Genetic information may be used for a variety of purposes, both medical and social. It is the non-medical uses that have been most controversial and for some time there have been calls for additional protection to be afforded to genetic information. Some of the more controversial uses are discussed below.

Genetics and insurance

Insurance companies have always requested medical information in order to assess premiums, but their use of the results of predictive genetic tests has been one of the most controversial and frequently debated aspects of developments in genetics. From the patient's perspective, the main problem is perceived to be that those who have an unfavourable genetic test may be refused insurance cover or may be charged such a high premium that, in effect, they are unable to purchase the insurance they want. It is feared that this could deter people from having genetic tests that would be in their broader interests and which could, in some cases, help to delay or prevent the onset of a disorder. Insurance companies, however, are concerned about pressure to change the existing basis of the relationship whereby both the insurer and the insured have access to the same information in making decisions. They are concerned that, if clients have information that they do not reveal to the insurer, they could take out high value policies knowing that they have a great chance of making a claim. Without that relevant information, the insurance company cannot set the premiums at higher rates and so the company or other policyholders lose out financially.

The short term solution to this problem has been an agreed moratorium until November 2006 on the use of predictive genetic test results by insurance companies (see Chapter 16, pages 574–5) to allow more time for informed discussion about the most appropriate approach for the longer term. Although the agreement between the Government and the Association of British Insurers refers to a moratorium on the use of "predictive genetic test results" it does not, in fact, apply to all such tests, but only to "unfavourable" test results. The impact of the moratorium has been to restrict insurance companies' use of results that would be detrimental to the person buying the policy, while still allowing individuals to use favourable results that increase their likelihood of obtaining policies at the standard rates. In some ways this is a logical distinction, because it would appear unreasonable for a company to load an insurance policy on the basis of a family history when it is clear that the individual has not inherited the gene mutation involved, and therefore is not at increased risk. On the other hand, it seems contrary to principles of natural justice to prevent insurance companies from using information when it would help them, but to allow them to use the same information when it would help the consumer.

Although the moratorium was widely welcomed and received considerable positive media attention, its benefit to those at risk of genetic disorders should not be overstated. Those who have undergone predictive genetic testing have done so because of a family history of the disease. Although under the terms of the moratorium they are not required to disclose the result of the test, they are still required to disclose their family history. With a small number of tests, such as that for Huntington's disease, the loading of policies owing to a family history is very similar to that which would be applied as a result of an unfavourable test result. (The Human Genetics Commission has announced that it will be considering the use of family history information by insurance companies, but believes that "at present" the moratorium should not be extended to its use.[51]) The moratorium also applies only to predictive tests, not to diagnostic tests carried out once symptoms have begun to appear.

Continuing the moratorium indefinitely is not a reasonable option because people who are seeking testing need to know whether they will be required to divulge their test results to insurance companies at any time in the future. One way around this problem would be for special provision to be made for those who have tests carried out while the moratorium is in force. The period in which the moratorium is in force needs to be used to consider the range of options available in the longer term. The discussion should look more broadly at the use of medical information by insurance companies, rather than focusing solely on genetic information. In the BMA's view the review should also consider whether there are logical, objective reasons or sound political reasons for treating genetic information differently from other medical information in the context of insurance. The BMA has explored these issues in more detail elsewhere[52] and will continue to contribute to this debate. Practical advice for doctors who are asked to complete medical reports for insurance companies can be found in Chapter 16 (pages 570–6).

Genetics and employment

The use of genetic information by employers has been the subject of less public debate and this reflects the fact that, when enquiries were made during 2001, very few employers were seeking access to such information.[53] This may change in the future and it is important that this issue is addressed before such requests become commonplace, to assess whether, and, if so, what, safeguards are required. A thorough review of the use of genetic information in employment is scheduled for 2005.[54]

A report on the implications of genetic testing for employment, published in 1999 by the Human Genetics Advisory Commission (which preceded the Human Genetics Commission), recommended that "an individual should not be required to disclose the result of a previous genetic test unless there is clear evidence that the information it provides is needed to assess either their current ability to perform a job safely or their susceptibility to harm from doing a certain job".[55] The Government accepted this recommendation.[56] The BMA also supports the principle that pre-employment medical reports should focus on the individual's current ability safely to carry out the work in question and genetic information should be used only by employers for that purpose. Practical advice for doctors who are asked to provide pre-employment medical reports or to undertake genetic testing on behalf of employers can be found in Chapter 16 (pages 581–6).

Paternity testing

Another common use of genetic information is to establish family relationships, usually but not exclusively paternity. In the past this involved the taking of blood samples, so health professionals were invariably involved in the process, but developments in technology have led to tests being carried out on other material such as a few hair follicles or a mouth swab, and also to the provision of paternity testing direct to the public, using testing kits that are sent off for analysis. This raises the possibility of samples being tested without individuals' consent. Although samples from the putative father and the child are always required, it is no longer necessary for the mother to provide a sample in order to obtain a meaningful result. This raises the possibility of testing without the knowledge or consent of the mother. In 2001 the UK health departments published a *Code of practice and guidance on genetic paternity testing services,* which sought to address some of these issues.[57]

The legal position

As with other invasive procedures, consent is required before a sample of blood, saliva, or hair is taken for analysis. People with parental responsibility may give consent on behalf of children or young people, but when they are capable of understanding the issues, the young people's own views should be sought and taken into account in deciding whether testing would be in their best interests. Each case must be considered on its merits. If, after discussion, a mature minor decides to withhold consent to paternity testing it may not be in that person's best interest to proceed, regardless of the views of the adults involved.

When one of the adults does not consent to paternity testing, it is possible for a direction to be sought from the court.[58] When the court issues a direction for the test to be carried out on a blood sample, this does not authorise the taking of blood without consent but "inferences" can be drawn from an adult's refusal to provide blood for testing. If the person with parental responsibility refuses to consent to the testing of a child under the age of 16, this may proceed in England, Wales, and Northern Ireland with an order from the court, which allows blood to be taken from a person under the age of 16 "if the court considers that it would be in his best interests for the sample to be taken".[59] (At the time of writing there are no plans to make similar provision in Scotland.) The courts have taken the view that in the vast majority of cases the child's best interests are served by learning the truth.

Paternity testing

Mrs R gave birth to twins in 1997. At the time of conception Mrs R was having sexual relationships with both her husband (Mr R) and Mr B. Both Mr R and Mr B believed themselves to be the father of the twins. Mr R was unaware of his wife's relationship with Mr B and became the twins' primary carer. The relationship between Mrs R and Mr B ended acrimoniously in 1999 and Mr B applied to the court for contact and parental responsibility. The result was a consent order for DNA testing, with which Mrs R did not comply. At the subsequent hearing, Mr B applied for a ruling that testing could be undertaken on the children without Mrs R's consent on the grounds that it would be in their best interests.

Mr R submitted a statement to the court in which he asserted his inability to continue as the primary carer of the twins, should the court order a test that established Mr B's paternity and that, in that event, he would forsake them. In weighing "the advantage of scientific truth against uncertainty" the judge said he must "consider the interest that the community has in establishing such certitude on the one hand and on the other hand the possible, and I believe, ... probably disastrous disintegrative effects of a finding that Mr B in fact is the father".[60] The judge also took account of the fact that he thought it unlikely that the matter would become the subject of local gossip and that it was therefore also unlikely that the children themselves would ever get to know about the uncertainty concerning their paternity. He therefore dismissed the application, arguing that the tests would not be in the children's best interests.

In allowing an appeal against this decision, Lady Justice Butler-Sloss held that the judge had given insufficient weight to the importance of certainty. She referred to the leading case from the 1970s, in which Lord Hodson said: "the interests of justice in the abstract are best served by the ascertainment of the truth and there must be few cases where the interests of children can be shown to be best served by the suppression of the truth".[61] The application was submitted for retrial in order that all of the facts could be carefully considered.

H and A (children) (paternity: blood tests)[62]

Ethical obligations

Although, legally, paternity testing may be undertaken without further investigation when the necessary consents have been obtained, from an ethical perspective, the BMA considers that health professionals should agree to provide assistance with testing only when this is considered to be in the best interests of the child. In some cases, the certainty of knowing may be better for the child than a persistent unresolved suspicion. However, there are likely to be cases in which, because of the ease with which such testing can be obtained, the test is requested without those involved having considered the likely impact of the result on all concerned. It is important therefore for health professionals to discuss with the adults concerned why the test has been requested and the implications for family relationships of receiving the result. The information given must be clear and unambiguous, and should raise, for discussion, the possibility that the results may provide distressing information that those who are seeking the test do not want to hear, and which may have a profound effect, with possible lifetime implications, for those involved.

When a decision is made to proceed with testing, patients would be well advised to use an approved service provider, which gives assurances about standards. An up to date list of approved paternity testing services in England and Wales can be obtained from the Family Division at the Lord Chancellor's Department.

"Motherless" testing

The code of practice on paternity testing states that tests that do not involve testing the mother's DNA (motherless testing) should take place only when the mother consents to the child being tested, or when the father has parental responsibility (see Chapter 4, pages 144–5). In addition, motherless testing may be undertaken if a court in England, Wales, or Northern Ireland considers the test to be in the child's best interests and authorises testing of the child on that basis. The Human Genetics Commission points out that motherless testing could have serious consequences for family life if large numbers of men decide to check whether or not the child they are supporting is genetically theirs.[63] When the putative father has parental responsibility for the child, such testing could be undertaken without the knowledge of the mother. The BMA believes that this could be very harmful to the child, as well as to the family unit as a whole, and would prefer to see a situation in which the consent of the mother and the putative father (and the child, if sufficiently mature) is required for paternity testing. In the absence of such a requirement, when doctors are consulted they should encourage those seeking testing to discuss their plans with the child's mother and the BMA would advise doctors not to become involved if that advice is rejected. Irrespective of the outcome, confidentiality must be respected and no information about the discussion should be passed to the mother or the child without the man's consent.

Testing without consent

As mentioned above, owing to the ease with which a DNA sample can be obtained unobtrusively and sent off for testing, the Human Genetics Commission has advised that there should be a new criminal offence of the non-consensual or deceitful obtaining and/or analysis of genetic material for non-medical purposes.[64] The BMA supports this recommendation in principle.

Forensic use of genetic information

In 1995 the Government set up the UK National DNA Database. This initially recorded, as numerical representations, the DNA profiles of individuals who had been charged with, informed they would be reported for, or convicted of a recordable offence. With the appropriate authorisation, samples could also be taken from those suspected of being involved in a recordable offence when it was believed that this would tend to confirm or disprove the individual's involvement by comparison with samples left at the crime scene. At the time of writing the Government is proposing to extend police powers to take DNA from anyone arrested for a recordable offence, including when there is no crime scene sample; the profiles could then be used for speculative searches against samples found at both past and future crime scenes.[65]

The profile recorded does not provide medical information about existing or future health and, although the original samples could, in theory, be used to obtain such information, the legislation under which they were taken does not permit such use. When the database was first set up, the sample and profile had to be destroyed if someone was acquitted of a crime, or if it was decided not to proceed with the case. This was amended, for England and Wales, by the Criminal Justice and Police Act 2001, to allow the profiles and samples to be retained even if the individuals are acquitted of the crimes for which they were taken, or if the case is dropped. Similar changes have been made for Northern Ireland. These provisions were unsuccessfully challenged under the Human Rights Act 1998 (see below).

Retention of DNA samples and the Human Rights Act

S was a 12-year-old boy, with no previous convictions, who was arrested and charged with attempted robbery. During the investigation his fingerprints and DNA samples were taken. On 14 June 2001 he was acquitted of the charge. Despite requests from his solicitor that the DNA sample be destroyed, it was retained and the profile was added to the DNA database. S's solicitor argued that this breached Articles 8 and 14 of the Human Rights Act.

Similar arguments were made by the solicitor acting for a 38-year-old man who was arrested and charged with harassment of his partner. The partner decided not to pursue the case and it was dropped, but the DNA sample was retained and the profile added to the database.

Both cases were dismissed by the High Court.

(Continued)

The Appeal Court held that the interference with the Article 8 right to privacy was real but not significant, and that the level of interference was proportionate and justified. It also held that there was a clear objective difference between individuals from whom samples had been taken and those from whom they had not been taken, which was wholly different from the categories mentioned in Article 14 and the case did not, therefore, fall within that Article.

R (on the application of S) v Chief Constable of South Yorkshire, R (on the application of Marper) v Chief Constable of South Yorkshire[66]

Those who volunteer samples for elimination purposes may be asked to sign a consent form for their profile to be added to the database. This consent cannot subsequently be revoked and any stored profile may later be used for speculative searches against samples left at scenes of crime (including both serious and more minor offences).

It is a matter for society as a whole to decide what safeguards are required to ensure these powers are not abused. However, there are two issues that are relevant to health professionals and these are discussed briefly here. The process of taking samples uses mouth swabs that are taken by police officers. Forensic medical examiners may, however, be involved with assessing or providing treatment to the person from whom a sample is being taken, or the person may be a patient in hospital at the time the sample is required. The treating doctor should object if any part of the process of taking the sample would be detrimental to the patient's care, but it is not the role of the doctor to assess whether the patient is competent to give consent.

When required for elimination purposes, consent is required for the taking of the sample and for its use for the current crime under investigation. A clear distinction should be made between this consent and that sought for the future addition of the profile to the DNA database.[67] It is possible that the individual – who may be the victim of, or a witness to, a crime – may be under the influence of drugs or alcohol or, because of his or her experience, may be very nervous or distressed. In such cases, although a sample may be needed quickly in order to expedite the investigation, there are good arguments – because of the irrevocable nature of the decision – for delaying seeking consent for the retention of the sample until the individual is able to make a more objective and informed decision. In deciding about future retention and use, people need to be given sufficient information to make an informed decision. In order for the consent to the retention and future use of the sample to be valid, the individual would need to know:

- that they have the option to refuse
- that it is possible to consent to the taking and use of a sample in relation to the crime currently being investigated, but to refuse consent for retention and subsequent use

- that, once given, the consent to retention can never be revoked
- what the sample may be used for in the future, including comparison with samples obtained in connection with any other crime, not just serious crime.

The second area of concern to health professionals is the possibility that, in future, additional information may be sought from the DNA samples for forensic purposes. Research is currently being undertaken with a view to identifying common characteristics so that, in the future, a "genetic photofit" could be derived from a DNA sample left at the scene of a crime.[68] This may include identifying sex, race, skin, hair and eye colour, stature, weight, age, and facial characteristics. It has also been suggested that in the future this could extend to behavioural traits and possibly to medical information.[69] The Forensic Science Service, which runs the database, is not, at the time of writing, contemplating the use of medical information for forensic purposes, but the BMA would have concerns about any future move in that direction.

Summary – controversial uses of genetic information

- The BMA welcomes the opportunity for rational and informed public debate about the use of genetic information by insurance companies. One of the issues that needs to be addressed is whether there are sound logical and objective reasons for treating genetic information differently from other medical information in the context of insurance.
- The BMA supports the principle that pre-employment medical reports should focus on the individual's current ability safely to carry out the work in question and believes that genetic information should be used by employers only for that purpose.
- It is important for health professionals who are asked to assist with paternity testing to ensure that the adults concerned have considered the implications of testing, including those for family relationships, of receiving the result. Health professionals should be involved only when they consider this to be in the best interests of the child.
- The BMA has concerns about "motherless" paternity testing and believes that the consent of the mother and the putative father (and the child if sufficiently mature) should be required for paternity testing.
- When DNA samples are taken for forensic testing, the BMA believes that the two types of consent – consent for the taking of samples from volunteers and their use for the current investigation, and consent for their retention and future use for other crimes – should be clearly separated. Sufficient information should be given for the individual to give valid consent.

Regulation of genetics in the UK

For many years it has been recognised that, in order to realise the huge potential benefits that genetic technology has to offer while protecting against the potential harms, a clear and coherent regulatory mechanism is required. Although there is no statutory body for genetics in the UK, a series of voluntary and advisory bodies have been established that each have a clearly defined remit. In 1999 the Government undertook a strategic review of the framework for overseeing developments in biotechnology and genetics, and subsequently rationalised the existing structure. After that review, the Human Genetics Commission was established to advise the Government on how new developments in genetics would impact on people and on health care. Information about the Human Genetics Commission and other bodies that oversee developments in genetic technology can be obtained from the Department of Health's website. The BMA's Medical Ethics Committee believes that there are strong grounds for the establishment of a statutory regulatory body for genetics along the lines of the Human Fertilisation and Embryology Authority and hopes that further consideration will be given to this option.

Other developments

Gene therapy

For many years there have been high hopes that gene therapy will provide a cure for many genetic diseases, cancers, and infections such as HIV. The basic principle of gene therapy is to correct defective genes. This could be done in the following ways.

- If a gene is missing, it could be added.
- Part of an abnormal gene could be changed to make it function correctly.
- The abnormal gene could be removed and replaced with a normal one.
- A normal gene could be inserted to supplement the abnormal gene, which would be left in the cell.

Of these options the one considered most likely to succeed is the insertion of a gene, either where the gene is missing or to augment an existing defective gene. This is far more complicated than it sounds and, so far, only limited success has been achieved. First, a method must be found for transporting the new gene and for ensuring that it reaches only those cells that need to be treated. Ideally, although even more difficult technically, it should be inserted into the stem cells so that, when new cells are generated, they already have the correct gene in place. If the gene is inserted into other cells, the effect lasts only as long as those cells survive and the treatment needs to be repeated at regular intervals. As with all experimental treatments, things could go wrong: the new gene could go into the wrong cell, it may not work appropriately, or it could disrupt the normal working of another gene, causing unexpected side effects. For this reason, careful research and monitoring is needed. For those with serious genetic disorders such as cystic fibrosis, however, gene therapy may offer the best hope of a cure. The potential benefits of gene therapy are not restricted to single gene disorders and much of the research undertaken has been aimed at developing new forms of treatment for cancer. This work has focused on trying to reverse the basic changes in cells that lead to them becoming cancerous, by finding ways of inducing the body's natural defences to kill the cancerous cells, or by inserting a gene that can convert a harmless chemical into one that destroys cancer cells but does not affect other cells in the body, thus removing the usual side effects of cancer treatment. Similar investigations are being undertaken into the possible use of gene therapy for treating infections such as HIV. In the UK all clinical trials are assessed, approved and monitored on a voluntary basis by the Gene Therapy Advisory Committee. By the end of 2000, more than 60 gene therapy trials were completed, under way, or in the process of being approved.[70]

Death of patient in gene therapy trial

Jesse Gelsinger was 18 years old when he volunteered to take part in a gene therapy trial at the University of Pennsylvania. He had a mild form of ornithine transcarbamylase deficiency, which was being managed by a drug regimen and a strict, non-protein diet. During the trial his liver was infused with genetically engineered adenoviruses, one of the viruses that cause the common cold, to correct a defective gene. A few days later, on 17 September 1999, he died of multiorgan failure, believed to have been triggered by a severe immune reaction to the infusion of corrective genes. The trial was immediately suspended and an inquiry was undertaken to establish the facts surrounding the death, which was believed to be the first directly resulting from gene therapy.

An inquiry by the Food and Drug Administration identified 18 areas in which the university had failed to meet the protocol and to provide proper supervision and monitoring of the trial. These findings led to calls for the approval and monitoring systems for gene therapy trials in the USA to be improved.[71]

Theoretically it would be possible to perform gene therapy using either somatic cells or germ cells. Alteration of the genes in the somatic cells affects only the individual treated, whereas altered genes in the germ cells would be passed on to the next generation. Although the two types of gene therapy would be very similar in technique, from an ethical perspective, they are quite different.

Somatic cell gene therapy

In 1989 the Government established a committee to consider the ethics of gene therapy. This committee, chaired by Sir Cecil Clothier, reported in 1992 and concluded that "somatic cell gene therapy will be a new kind of treatment, but it does not represent a major departure from established medical practice; nor does it, in our view, pose new ethical challenges".[72] Other commentators since that time have reached the same conclusion and this view is shared by the BMA. The issues raised by somatic cell gene therapy are essentially the same as those raised by the development of other new medical techniques. As with any new treatment, research results must show that the procedure is safe and efficacious before the shift is made from research to clinical practice, and those seeking treatment must give valid consent, having been informed of the inherent risks and uncertainties (this is discussed further in Chapter 14 on research and innovative treatment). The Committee on the Ethics of Gene Therapy recognised, however, that there may be particular public concern about techniques designed to alter an individual's genetic makeup and, for this reason, recommended additional safeguards. This recommendation was accepted by the Government and the Gene Therapy Advisory Committee was established to approve all gene therapy research and clinical trials in the UK.

Germ cell gene therapy

Alteration of a defective gene in a germ cell or in an early embryo would enable future generations to benefit from the treatment, but the safety of these procedures is not proven and cannot be proved in the short term. In view of these concerns about the effect on future generations, there is widespread agreement that germ cell gene therapy should not be undertaken. The Report of the Committee on the Ethics of Gene Therapy concluded "we are clear that there is at present insufficient knowledge to evaluate the risks to future generations of gene modification of the germ line. We therefore recommend that gene modification of the human germ line should not yet be attempted".[73]

Genetic manipulation of the early embryo, for treatment, is prohibited in the UK by the Human Fertilisation and Embryology Act 1990, which states that: "a [treatment] licence ... cannot authorise altering the genetic structure of any cell while it forms part of an embryo."[74] The same restriction is applied to research licences, but the option has been left open for regulations to be made to permit such research at some time in the future.

The Council of Europe's Convention on Human Rights and Biomedicine also addresses this issue, stating that: "an intervention seeking to modify the human genome may only be undertaken for preventive, diagnostic or therapeutic purposes and only if its aim is not to introduce any modification in the genome of any descendants".[75]

This part of the Convention prohibits germ cell gene therapy in treatment, but does not prohibit somatic cell gene therapy or *in vitro* research into germ cell gene therapy.

It is often stated that germ cell gene therapy is unethical. This is true insofar as it is unethical to perform a technique that has not been properly assessed and the safety of which is unknown. However, were it ever to be possible to give reasonable assurances about the safety of the technique, it is unclear whether it would still be judged unethical. It could be argued, for example, that decisions should not be made that affect an individual prior to his or her conception. The same argument could be used, however, against other techniques performed routinely for the benefit of a future child such as ensuring that the mother has been vaccinated against rubella. It has also been pointed out that "if we have the scientific capacity to alter the germ-line and do not do so, we are also making a decision about the health of future generations".[76] Some, such as Harris, argue not only that it would be ethical to use germ cell gene therapy, if it were proved safe and efficacious, but that there may be an obligation to do so. Parents have obligations and responsibilities to their unborn and potential children, including that to avoid harm, a duty that can include both not causing harm and taking steps to avoid harm.[77] This debate, although interesting, is likely to be academic because evidence of the safety and efficacy of germ cell gene therapy, particularly in the longer term and in future generations, is likely to remain elusive.

Cloning

Since the birth of Dolly the cloned sheep in February 1997,[78] the possibility of human cloning has been the topic of regular debate both in scientific circles and in the popular press. In the early days, much of the discussion was sensationalist, predicting the imminent and inevitable use of the technique to create genetically identical individuals and the consequent slide into moral decline. Sensible debate was frequently hampered by confusion caused primarily by the terminology used: the phrase "human cloning" was used both in its conventional sense, to refer to the deliberate creation of genetically identical individuals, but also as a generic phrase to refer to a much broader range of research activities. The BMA, like many other organisations, was concerned that the negativity associated with our commonsense understanding of "cloning" may have a detrimental effect on the development of important and worthwhile scientific research. (Stem cell research is discussed in Chapter 14, pages 518–20.) For this reason, the BMA produced a discussion paper for the World Medical Association,[79] which called for an informed and rational debate about the range of activities that had been included under the broad heading of "cloning". It also called for the phrase "human cloning" to be used only in its conventional sense.

Dolly, the cloned sheep

On 27 February 1997, a group of scientists from the Roslin Institute in Edinburgh announced in *Nature* the birth of Dolly the sheep.[80] Dolly was born after the transfer of the nucleus of a cell from the mammary gland of a 6-year-old Finn Dorset ewe into an unfertilised oocyte with its own nucleus removed. In total, the nuclei from 277 cells were transferred into 277 unfertilised eggs. The oocytes were then stimulated to begin cell division and the resulting embryos were replaced in the uteri of adult sheep for gestation. In total, 29 viable embryos were derived and transferred into surrogate Blackface ewes. This led to just one birth – Dolly – who was the first example of an adult vertebrate being cloned from another adult (the same technique had been used previously to clone cells from sheep embryos). Dolly subsequently gave birth to lambs conceived normally. She died in 2003.

The BMA is opposed to the deliberate creation of genetically identical individuals and welcomed the passage of the Human Reproductive Cloning Act 2001, which put its illegality in the UK beyond any doubt. The BMA also believes that the Government should take an active part in moves to negotiate an international ban on human reproductive cloning. Despite this, the BMA recognises that many of the arguments expressed in opposition to human cloning are based on popular misconceptions and instinct rather than clearly articulated robust and logical arguments. It may be the case that the very serious safety concerns about human cloning are never satisfactorily overcome or that the level of benefit to be derived from using it are not sufficiently high to surmount the inherent risks associated with any new technique. If that is the case then, although interesting from an academic perspective, debate about the ethical acceptability of human cloning loses its urgency because the safety concerns alone are sufficient to justify a prohibition. If in the future, however, it became possible to say, with a reasonable degree of certainty, that human cloning was safe, it would be essential to explore in more detail the motives of those who wish to use this technique and to consider the benefits, harms, and likely consequences of allowing it. If we ever reach that stage, detailed consideration will be required to ensure that continued opposition to cloning is based on careful analysis rather than relying on ill defined notions of "human dignity", and that decisions are made on the strength of the arguments rather than simply on the strength of public opinion.

Preparing for the "genetic revolution"

Despite the major developments seen over the last decade, there is a sense in which the "genetic revolution" has just begun. Early indicators show huge potential benefits and changes in the provision of health care, in terms of the way society perceives and manages illness and disability. The Government has been explicit about its desire to be at the forefront of developments in genetics, both from technical and ethical perspectives. Its white paper has been promoted as aiming to prepare the NHS to maximise the benefits of genetic advances in improving patient care.

References

1   See, for example: Rose P, Lucassen A. *Practical genetics for primary care*. Oxford: Oxford University Press, 1999.
2   Human Genetics Commission. *Inside information. Balancing interests in the use of personal genetic data*. London: HGC, 2002:30.
3   British Medical Association. *Human genetics: choice and responsibility*. Oxford: Oxford University Press, 1998.
4   Human Genetics Commission. *Inside information. Balancing interests in the use of personal genetic data. Op cit:* pp. 37–8.

5   Marteau TM. Communicating genetic risk information. *Br Med Bull* 1999;**55**:414–28.
6   This definition was drawn up by the American Society of Human Genetics in 1974 and is discussed in: Fraser FC. Current issues in medical genetics: genetic counseling. *Am J Hum Genet* 1974;**26**: 636–59.
7   McLean SAM. *Review of the common law provisions relating to the removal of gametes and of the consent provisions in the Human Fertilisation and Embryology Act 1990.* London: Department of Health, 1998:5–6.
8   Human Genetics Commission. *Inside information. Balancing interests in the use of personal genetic data. Op cit:* pp. 83–4.
9   Lord Chancellor's Department. *Who decides? Making decisions on behalf of mentally incapacitated adults.* London: The Stationery Office, 1997:39. (Cm 3803.)
10 Lord Chancellor's Department. *Making decisions. The government's proposals for making decisions on behalf of mentally incapacitated adults.* London: The Stationery Office, 1999. (Cm 4465.)
11 See, for example: Genetic Interest Group. *Confidentiality guidelines.* London: GIG, 1998.
12 General Medical Council. *Confidentiality: protecting and providing information.* London: GMC, 2000: para 14.
13 Harper PS, Clarke AJ. *Genetics, society and clinical practice.* Oxford: Bios Scientific Publishers, 1997:38–9.
14 Husted J. Autonomy and a right not to know. In: Chadwick R, Levitt M, Shickle D, eds. *The right to know and the right not to know.* Aldershot: Avebury, 1997:57.
15 Laurie G. *Genetic privacy. A challenge to medico-legal norms.* Cambridge: Cambridge University Press, 2002:209.
16 *Ibid.*
17 Laurie GT. Obligations arising from genetic information – negligence and the protection of familial interests. *Child Fam Law Q* 1999;**11**:109–24.
18 Balfour-Lynne I, Madge S, Dinwiddie R. Testing carrier status in siblings of patients with cystic fibrosis. *Arch Dis Child* 1995;**72**:167–8.
19 Harper PS, *et al. Genetics, society and clinical practice. Op cit:* p. 22.
20 Jarvinen O, Hietala M, Aatto AM, *et al.* A retrospective study of long-term psychosocial consequences and satisfaction after carrier testing in childhood in an autosomal recessive disease: aspartylglucosaminuria. *Clin Genet* 2000;**58**:447–54.
21 *Ibid.*
22 Harper PS, Lim C, Craufurd D, on behalf of the UK Huntington's Disease Prediction Consortium. Ten years of presymptomatic testing for Huntington's disease: the experience of the UK Huntington's Disease Prediction Consortium. *J Med Genet* 2000;**37**:567–71.
23 Almqvist EW, Block M, Brinkman R, Craufurd D, Hayden MR on behalf of the International Huntington Disease Collaborative Group. A worldwide assessment of the frequency of suicide, suicide attempts, or psychiatric hospitalization after predictive testing for Huntington disease. *Am J Hum Genet* 1999;**64**:1293–304.
24 Bird TD. Outrageous fortune: the risk of suicide in genetic testing for Huntington disease [editorial]. *Am J Hum Genet* 1999;**64**:1289–92.
25 Marteau TM, Croyle RT. The new genetics. Psychological responses to genetic testing. *BMJ* 1998;**316**:693–6.
26 Siggins S, Whyte P, Huggins M, *et al.* The psychological consequences of predictive testing for Huntington's disease. *N Engl J Med* 1992;**327**:1401–5.
27 Wright S. It's a yo-yo-type existence. In: Marteau T, Richards M, eds. *The troubled helix.* Cambridge: Cambridge University Press, 1996:5–7.
28 Harper PS, *et al. Genetics, society and clinical practice. Op cit:* pp. 31–48.
29 Marteau TM, *et al.* The new genetics. Psychological responses to genetic testing. *Op cit.*
30 Advisory Committee on Genetic Testing. *Report on genetic testing for late onset disorders.* London: Department of Health, 1998.
31 Michie S, Bobrow M, Marteau TM. Predictive genetic testing in children and adults: a study of emotional impact. *J Med Genet* 2001;**38**:519–26.
32 *Ibid.*
33 Easton DF, Ford D, Bishop DT, Breast cancer linkage consortium. Breast and ovarian cancer incidence in BRCA1-mutation carriers. *Am J Hum Genet* 1995;**56**:265–71. Easton DF, Steele L, Fields P, *et al.* Cancer risks in two large breast cancer families linked to BRCA2 on chromosome 13q12-13. *Am J Hum Genet* 1997;**61**:120–8.
34 Thorlacius S, Struewing JP, Hartge P, *et al.* Population-based study of risk of breast cancer in carriers of BRCA2 mutation. *Lancet* 1998;**52**:1337–9.

35 Marteau TM, *et al*. The new genetics. Psychological responses to genetic testing. *Op cit*.

36 Marteau TM, Lerman C. Genetic risk and behavioural change. *BMJ* 2001;**322**:1056–9.

37 Holtzman NA, Marteau TM. Will genetics revolutionize medicine? *N Engl J Med* 2000;**343**:141–4.

38 Lucassen A, Parker M. Revealing false paternity: some ethical considerations. *Lancet* 2001;**357**: 1033–5.

39 Bekker H, Modell M, Denniss G, *et al*. Uptake of cystic fibrosis testing in primary care: supply push or demand pull? *BMJ* 1993;**306**:1584–6.

40 Mitchell J, Scriver CR, Clow CL, Kaplan F. What young people think and do when the option for cystic fibrosis carrier testing is available. *J Med Genet* 1993;**30**:538–42.

41 Laurie G. Better to hesitate at the threshold of compulsion: PKU testing and the concept of family autonomy in Eire. *J Med Ethics* 2002;**28**:136–7.

42 House of Commons Science and Technology Committee. *Human genetics: the science and its consequences*. London: HMSO, 1995: para 92.

43 Department of Trade and Industry. *Government response to the third report of the House of Commons Select Committee on Science and Technology 1994–95 session*. London: HMSO, 1996: para 42. (Cm 3061.)

44 Meek J. Cancer gene tests "will destroy private health". *The Guardian* 2002 Aug 5:1.

45 Clarke AJ. Population screening for genetic susceptibility to disease. *BMJ* 1995;**311**:3–8.

46 Human Genetics Commission. *Genes direct. Ensuring the effective oversight of genetic tests supplied directly to the public*. London: HGC, 2003.

47 The HIV Testing Kits and Services Regulations 1992. (SI 1992 No. 460.)

48 Human Genetics Commission. *Inside information. Balancing interests in the use of personal genetic data. Op cit*: pp. 60–2.

49 *Ibid*: p. 62.

50 Department of Health. *Our inheritance, our future. Realising the potential of genetics in the NHS*. London: The Stationery Office, 2003: para 6.31.

51 Human Genetics Commission. *Inside information. Balancing interests in the use of personal genetic data. Op cit*: pp. 123–4.

52 British Medical Association. *Human genetics: choice and responsibility. Op cit*: pp. 153–69.

53 Human Genetics Commission. *Inside information. Balancing interests in the use of personal genetic data. Op cit*: p. 138.

54 Human Genetics Advisory Commission. *The implications of genetic testing for employment*. London: Department of Trade and Industry, 1999.

55 *Ibid*: p. 4.

56 *Government response to HGAC report on genetic testing and employment. Letter from Lord Sainsbury and Yvette Cooper to Baroness Helena Kennedy, Chair, Human Genetics Commission*. London: Department of Health, 2000 Jul 24.

57 UK Health Departments. *Code of practice and guidance on genetic paternity testing services*. London: Department of Health, 2001.

58 Family Law Reform Act 1969 s20. Law Reform (Miscellaneous Provisions) (Scotland) Act 1990 s70. Family Law Reform (Northern Ireland) Order 1977 art 8.

59 Child Support (Pensions and Social Security) Act 2000 s82. Child Support, Pensions and Social Security Act (Northern Ireland) 2000 s65(3).

60 H and A (children) (paternity: blood tests) [2002] 1 FLR 1145: 1146.

61 S v McC; W v W [1970] 3 All ER 107: 123.

62 H and A (children) (paternity: blood tests) [2002]. *Op cit*.

63 Human Genetics Commission. *Inside information. Balancing interests in the use of personal genetic data. Op cit*: p. 167.

64 *Ibid*: pp. 60–2.

65 Criminal Justice Bill (Report Stage). *House of Commons official report (Hansard)*. 2003 May 19: col 713.

66 R (on the application of S) v Chief Constable of South Yorkshire, R (on the application of Marper) v Chief Constable of South Yorkshire [2003] HRLR 1.

67 Home Office. *Police and Criminal Evidence Act 1984 code D: code of practice for the identification of persons by police officers*. London: Home Office, 2003.

68 Human Genetics Commission. *Inside information. Balancing interests in the use of personal genetic data. Op cit*: pp. 155–7.

69 *Ibid*: p. 155.

70 Gene Therapy Advisory Committee. *Seventh annual report January 2000 – December 2000*. London: Health Departments of the United Kingdom, 2001:iii.

71 Ciment J. Gene therapy experiments put on "clinical hold". *BMJ* 2000;**320**:336. Gene therapy under cloud [editorial]. *Lancet* 2000;**355**:329.

72   Committee on the Ethics of Gene Therapy. *Report of The Committee On The Ethics Of Gene Therapy.* London: HMSO, 1992:21. (Cm 1788.)

73   *Ibid.*

74   Human Fertilisation and Embryology Act 1990 Schedule 2, para 1(4).

75   Council of Europe. *Convention for the protection of human rights and dignity of the human being with regard to the application of biology and medicine: Convention on human rights and biomedicine.* 1996: art 13.

76   House of Commons Science and Technology Committee. *Human genetics: the science and its consequences. Op cit:* para 122.

77   Harris J. *Wonderwoman and superman.* Oxford: Oxford University Press, 1992:178.

78   Wilmut I, Schnieke AE, McWhir J, Kind AJ, Campbell KHS. Viable offspring derived from fetal and adult mammalian cells. *Nature* 1997;**385**:810–3.

79   British Medical Association. *Human "cloning". A discussion paper for the World Medical Association.* London: BMA, 1999.

80   Wilmut I, *et al.* Viable offspring derived from fetal and adult mammalian cells. *Op cit.*

10: Caring for patients at the end of life

The questions covered in this chapter include the following.

- What factors should be considered when deciding whether to withhold or withdraw life-prolonging treatment?
- Can artificial nutrition and hydration ever be withdrawn?
- What steps can, and should, health professionals take to help patients to achieve a "good death"?
- How does the relationship between the patient and the healthcare team change when the patient's condition is recognised as incurable?
- What skills and qualities are needed to provide good quality care to dying patients?
- How should doctors respond to requests from relatives to keep information from the patient?
- How can doctors help patients to maintain control over aspects of their life and death?

Breaking the taboo

Attitudes towards death have shifted through the ages. In earlier decades most people died at home, surrounded by their family, friends, and neighbours, who may have been actively engaged in caring for them and who would subsequently be involved with laying out the body. People were accustomed to the experience of death, whereas, by the latter part of the twentieth century death had become medicalised, sanitised and, to an extent, hidden in hospitals. Around the turn of the millennium, however, the pendulum began to swing back, with calls for greater acknowledgement and acceptance of death and to break "the final taboo of the 20th century".[1]

Although developments in some areas of medicine have saved and prolonged lives, they have also led increasingly to death being seen as a failure, often for which someone must be to blame, rather than as a natural and inevitable event. The notion that death can be delayed almost indefinitely can also lead to pressure on doctors to prolong treatment long past the stage where it is able to offer any benefit for the patient. For many patients with serious conditions there comes a stage where no more can be done to save or prolong life and the aim of medicine shifts from curative treatment to keeping the patient comfortable and free from pain. This shift is not an acceptance of failure, but a recognition of the natural progression of the care of that individual. This needs to be recognised and accepted by the patient, the treating team, and those close to the patient. If this is not so and "death is seen as a failure rather than as an important part of life then individuals are diverted from preparing for it and medicine does not give the attention it should to helping people die a good death".[2]

There is a large professional literature on managing death, and the mass media and popular television dramas and documentary programmes now more often discuss dying openly and show how patients and their friends and relatives cope with impending death. Such moves are to be welcomed because greater acceptance of death is needed if health professionals are to be able to fulfil their role to provide good quality care for their patients to the very end of their lives, including, wherever possible, helping them to achieve a good death. The aim of medicine is not, and should not be, to avoid death for as long as possible, but to recognise and accept when it is inevitable and to make the dying process as positive as possible for all concerned.

General principles

The following general principles apply when caring for patients at the end of life.

- The aim of medicine is not to avoid death for as long as possible, but to recognise when it is inevitable and to help patients to prepare for their death.
- Virtues such as compassion and sensitivity are particularly important in those caring for dying patients.
- Honest and clear communication is essential, while recognising that people's needs and desires for information vary.
- Care should be centred around the dying patient and the usual rules of confidentiality apply.
- Patients should be given the opportunity to maintain control over as many aspects of their life and death as possible.
- Health professionals should be sensitive to patients' cultural and religious backgrounds and needs.
- An important part of the care provided to dying patients is to help their relatives and loved ones to come to terms with the situation and to cope with their bereavement.

Decisions to withhold or withdraw life prolonging treatment

Being able to prolong life artificially has led to the difficulty of knowing when to stop. With all patients there comes a stage when further attempts to prolong life will not be successful and the aim of medical care should shift to keeping the patient comfortable and free of pain. In some cases, treatment may achieve its physiological aim but fail to provide a net benefit. Decisions about the benefits of treatment are made after discussion between competent patients and the healthcare team (see pages 354–5). When patients are not competent, these decisions are made by the healthcare team on the basis of whether providing treatment would be in the patient's best interests (see pages 356–8). Benefit accrues not only when progress can be made or recovery achieved; in some cases the patient will benefit from treatment that is able to maintain the *status quo* and prevent further deterioration. In other cases, the treatment may keep the patient alive but be unable to stop the progression of the disease or provide any hope of the person achieving any level of self awareness or awareness of others and the ability intentionally to interact with them. In many such cases it is decided that curative treatment should cease and the focus should shift to the palliation of symptoms and preparing for death. Such decisions are taken on a regular basis, when it is decided, for example, that the burdens of further aggressive chemotherapy outweigh the benefits for the particular individual. Similarly, a decision may be made that, in the event of cardiac arrest, a patient should not be subjected to cardiopulmonary resuscitation because the chance of recovery or the level of recovery that could reasonably be expected would not provide a net benefit to that patient (see pages 361–3). In some cases, decisions about continuation or withdrawal of artificial nutrition and hydration are needed (see pages 358–61). Such decisions are never easy but they form an important part of good quality care at the end of life. In law, a doctor may foresee that the patient will die if treatment is not provided, but this is not the same as withholding or withdrawing treatment with the intention of ending the patient's life.

It has been argued by some that a decision to withdraw life prolonging medical treatment necessarily involves a judgment that the patient's life is not worth living and that such a decision is, therefore, morally equivalent to euthanasia.[3] This argument is based on the assumption that, once it has been decided that withdrawing treatment is in the best interests of the patient, then this must be because it is judged to be in the best interests of the patient no longer to live. It is said, therefore, that it is not possible to separate the concept of net benefit, in this context, from that of the value of the patient's remaining life. The BMA takes a different approach to this question, however, focusing not on the value of the patient's life but rather on the justification, or otherwise, for continuing to provide treatment that has the effect of prolonging the patient's life artificially. For every proposed or actual medical intervention, a judgment should be made about whether that intervention would be worthwhile, in the sense of providing net benefit to the individual patient, recognising that each patient has his or her own beliefs, values, wishes, and philosophy. If the patient is known to have held the view that there is intrinsic value in being alive, then life prolonging treatment would, in virtually all cases, provide a net benefit for that particular individual. Most people, however, do not take that view. When the treatment is able to restore or maintain the patient to a level of health that he or she would find acceptable, then active treatment is clearly appropriate. As the expected benefits of the treatment, from the patient's perspective, decrease, however, so does the justification for providing it. To decide that the benefits of treatment for a particular individual are not sufficient to justify active intervention to prolong life is not, in the BMA's view, equivalent to saying that the patient's life is not worth living and therefore treatment should be stopped so that the patient will die. Rather it is to say that medical intervention is not indicated because it does not provide net benefit for the patient, which is the primary moral objective of medical practice. This distinction was summed up by Lord Goff, when considering the case of Tony Bland (see page 359), who said, "the question is not whether it is in the best interests of the patient that he should die. The question is whether it is in the best interests of the patient that his life should be prolonged by the continuance of this form of medical treatment or care".[4] The BMA recognises, however, that this is a philosophically contentious issue.

Advances in technology have not only presented ethical dilemmas about assessing when treatment ceases to benefit the patient, but have also raised the issue of withholding or withdrawing potentially beneficial treatment on grounds of cost. The BMA is concerned that patients who have lost or never attained competence and those who are severely physically disabled should not be excluded from potentially beneficial, but costly, treatment options solely by reason of their incapacity or disability. Doctors must therefore be able to show that all materially relevant criteria, such as the patient's ability to benefit from therapy, have been considered in deciding whether to offer treatment. They also need to take special care to ensure that such decisions can be justified and are not considered discriminatory. This is not only an ethical duty but is also a legal obligation, including that placed on all public authorities by the Human Rights Act 1998 not to discriminate unjustifiably in the protection of the rights of patients.

Any decision to withhold or withdraw life prolonging treatment, and the reasons for it, should be properly documented in the patient's notes and doctors must be willing to justify their decisions in every case. This section summarises the main factors to take into account when considering whether to withhold or withdraw life prolonging medical treatment. Those involved with making these decisions, or others seeking more detailed advice, should refer to the specific guidance on this subject from the BMA[5] and the General Medical Council (GMC).[6]

Competent adults

Competent patients should be encouraged to discuss their wishes about future treatment; in order to do this they need information. This requires honest and sensitive discussion between the patient and those providing treatment (see pages 368–74). After discussion, patients sometimes decide that the stage has been reached beyond which, for them, continued treatment aimed at prolonging life, although possible, would be inappropriate. As stated in Chapter 2, it is now well established in law and ethics that competent adults have the right to refuse any medical treatment, even if that refusal results in their death. Patients are not obliged to justify their decisions, but health teams need to discuss such refusals with them in order to ensure that they are acting free from pressure and have based their decisions on accurate information. When the health team considers that treatment would provide a net benefit, that assessment should be sympathetically explained to patients but they should not be pressured to accept treatment they do not want. As discussed on pages 84 and 225–6, the same rules apply to pregnant women even if a woman's refusal of treatment would put the life of her fetus at risk as well as her own. The refusal of a particular life prolonging treatment does not imply a refusal of all treatment or all facets of care. The health team must continue to offer other treatments and all procedures that are solely or primarily intended to keep the patient comfortable and free from severe pain or discomfort.

Advance refusals

Patients may refuse treatment in advance by means of an advance directive (see Chapter 3, pages 113–6), which comes into force when competence is lost. Advance directives that refuse particular treatments are legally binding if the patient was over the age of majority and competent at the time the directive was made, was acting voluntarily and free from pressure, and the circumstances that have arisen are those that were envisaged in the directive. Advance directives do not need to be in writing and, particularly with patients who have a progressive disease, discussion frequently takes place throughout the illness and decisions about future medical care are made jointly by the patient and the healthcare team. Such decisions should be documented in the medical records. All of those involved with the patient's care should be made aware of his or her wishes, which should be acted upon when the time comes. Occasionally, people with terminal illness attempt suicide and leave an advance directive refusing treatment to resuscitate them; see Chapter 15.

Children and young people

As with adults, an assessment of the benefits and burdens of treatment, and the wishes of the patient where these can be ascertained, are key factors in considering whether treatment should be provided or withdrawn. Those with parental responsibility for a baby or young child are legally and morally entitled to give or withhold consent to treatment. Their decisions are usually determinative, unless they conflict seriously with the interpretation of the child's best interests by those who are providing care. Parents' powers to withhold consent for a child's treatment are likely to be curtailed, however, when the treatment refused would provide a clear benefit to the child, when the statistical chances of recovery are good, or when the severity and burdens of the condition are not sufficient to justify withholding or withdrawing life prolonging treatment. If parents and doctors do not agree after discussion has taken place, and a second opinion obtained, the matter may have to go to court. Children with insufficient maturity and understanding to make treatment decisions for themselves are, nonetheless, often able to express views or opinions about their care, and they should be encouraged to discuss their views and wishes as much as they can.

A young person who has sufficient competence and understanding of the proposed treatment may give a valid consent to treatment, but his or her decision to *refuse* life prolonging treatment may not be determinative. In England, Wales, and Northern Ireland, the courts have held that a person with parental responsibility for the child, or the courts, may override even the informed refusal of a person under the age of 18 (see Chapter 4, pages 140–2). In Scotland, however, it appears unlikely that the refusal of a competent young person under that age could be overridden by either parents or courts, although this point cannot be regarded as settled in Scots law (see Chapter 4, pages 142–3).

Incompetent adults

In England, Wales, and Northern Ireland, nobody can give consent on behalf of adults who lack the capacity to make decisions for themselves, but the clinician in charge of their care may provide any treatment that is in the patient's best interests. In Scotland, a proxy decision maker may be appointed to give consent to medical treatment on behalf of an incapacitated person over 16 years of age. When such a proxy has been appointed, he or she must be consulted (when reasonable and practicable) about proposed medical treatment.[7] When a proxy has not been appointed, the doctors may do what is reasonable in the circumstances to safeguard or promote an incapacitated patient's physical or mental health. For more information about the provision of treatment to incompetent adults see Chapter 3.

Assessing best interests

When patients are unable to express their own wishes, the healthcare team is required to make an assessment of the individual's best interests (see pages 108–9). Views differ about what factors should be considered in deciding whether the provision of life prolonging treatment would be a benefit for the patient. Some people believe that there is intrinsic value in being alive and therefore that prolonging life always provides a benefit. In this absolute form, this is not a view the BMA shares. The vast majority of people with even very severe physical or mental disabilities are able to experience and gain pleasure from some aspects of their lives. In extreme cases, however, where the disability is so profound that individuals have no or minimal levels of awareness of their own existence and no hope of recovering awareness, or where they suffer severe untreatable pain or other distress, the question arises of whether continuing to provide treatment aimed at prolonging that life artificially would provide a benefit to them.

The types of factors that should be taken into account in assessing whether the provision of life prolonging treatment would provide an overall benefit to the patient include:

- the patient's own wishes and values (where these can be ascertained)
- clinical judgment about the effectiveness of the proposed treatment, including its likely benefits and harms
- the likelihood of the patient experiencing severe unmanageable pain or suffering
- the level of awareness the individual has of his or her existence and surroundings as demonstrated by, for example, an ability to interact with others (however expressed), the capacity for self directed action or the ability to take control of any aspect of his or her life
- the likelihood and extent of any degree of improvement in the patient's condition if treatment is provided

- whether the invasiveness of the treatment is justified in the circumstances
- the views of the parents, if the patient is a child
- the views of people who are close to the patient, especially near relatives, partners, and carers, about what the patient is likely to see as beneficial
- in Scotland, the views of an appointed health care proxy.

Discussion within the healthcare team

Although ultimately the responsibility for treatment decisions rests with the clinician in charge of the patient's care, it is important, when non-emergency decisions are made, that account is taken of the views of the rest of the healthcare team. Seeking agreement within the team about the most appropriate course of action can help to reduce the possibility of subjectivity or bias in cases of uncertainty. All involved healthcare professionals have an important contribution to make to the assessment; nurses often have a particular insight into the patient's wishes and may have spent considerable time with the patient and his or her relatives. Depending upon the type of treatment under consideration, it may be appropriate to involve a dietician, speech therapist, psychologist, or physiotherapist. The patient's GP is also often able to provide valuable information about the patient's wishes and values.

Discussion with those close to the patient

Even when their views have no legal status in terms of actual decision making, those close to the patient are often able to provide important information to help to ascertain whether the patient would have considered life prolonging treatment to be beneficial. It is important to be clear, however, that the information sought relates to any views the patient expressed when competent, which may help to ascertain what he or she would have wanted in the circumstances, as opposed to what those who are consulted would like for the patient, or what they would want for themselves if they were in the same situation. In practice, the extent to which friends and relatives are able to inform the doctor's decision is likely to depend upon whether the patient has discussed the issues with them. Knowing the patient, however, they may be able to give a clearer picture of the types of values the patient held and the things that were important when he or she was competent. Useful information may also be available from social workers or other carers.

In talking to those who are close to the patient, a balance must be sought between preserving confidentiality and obtaining sufficient information to make an informed assessment. Where a patient has, when competent, expressed a specific wish that his or her condition should not be discussed with relatives or friends, this must be respected. This should not, however, prevent the healthcare team from seeking information from them about the patient's wishes and values.

Although the views of those close to the patient are important to take into account in reaching treatment decisions, it is essential in England, Wales, and Northern Ireland that those who are consulted are clear that, under current law (see Chapter 3, pages 126–7), the treatment decision is not their right or their responsibility. The same applies in Scotland to those who are close to patients but who are not formally appointed healthcare proxies.

Withdrawing or withholding conventional treatment

When a patient presents with a sudden or unexpected medical event, such as after an accident, injury, or stroke, there is likely to be initial uncertainty about the diagnosis, the likely effectiveness of treatment, and the long term prognosis. In these cases, the initial efforts should be focused on stabilising the patient, so that a proper assessment of the condition may be undertaken and the likelihood and extent of any expected improvement can be assessed. Where insufficient information is available about the severity of the condition or the likelihood of recovery at the time a decision is needed, treatment should be provided, although this may be for a trial period with a prearranged review. If, after the review, it is decided that the treatment has failed or has ceased to be of benefit to the patient, consideration should be given to its withdrawal. Although emotionally it may be easier to withhold treatment than to withdraw that which has been started, there are no legal, or morally relevant, differences between the two actions. Nevertheless, many health professionals, as well as patients, perceive a psychological difference between withholding and withdrawing treatment. This is likely to be linked to the largely negative impression attached to a decision to withdraw treatment that can be interpreted as "giving up on the patient". There is a risk, however, that this perceived difficulty of withdrawing treatment could lead to some patients failing to receive treatment that could benefit them, or some patients being subject to continuing treatment that is no longer in their best interests. Treatment should never be withheld simply because withholding is considered to be easier than withdrawing treatment when there is a possibility that it will benefit the patient.

Any decision to withhold or withdraw treatment must be based on the best available clinical evidence; where relevant guidelines exist for the diagnosis and management of the condition (such as guidance from the Royal Colleges), these should be consulted. When guidelines are not available and there is reasonable doubt about the diagnosis or prognosis, or when the healthcare team has limited experience of the condition, advice should be sought from another senior clinician with experience in the relevant field before making decisions. Except when the patient's imminent death is inevitable, a decision to withhold or withdraw *all* treatment is likely to be inappropriate and potentially unlawful. Assessments should be based on whether each potentially available treatment would benefit the patient.

Withdrawing or withholding artificial nutrition and hydration

The guidance above applies to all decisions to withhold or withdraw life prolonging treatment, but when the treatment to be withdrawn or withheld is artificial nutrition and hydration (for example, nasogastric tubes, feeding by percutaneous endoscopic gastrostomy, and total parenteral nutrition) the BMA believes that additional safeguards are required. The classification of artificial nutrition and hydration as medical treatment was confirmed by the House of Lords in the case of Tony Bland (see below). Although this view coincided with the BMA's published opinion, the Association accepts that this is a controversial area in which views differ. Some people regard the provision of artificial nutrition and hydration as basic care that should always be provided unless the patient's imminent death is inevitable or the patient has refused it. In the case of Tony Bland it was held that it would not be unlawful to withdraw artificial nutrition and hydration even though this would lead to his death. It has subsequently been confirmed that when withdrawing or withholding artificial nutrition and hydration is in a patient's best interests, there is no breach of the patient's rights under Article 2 of the European Convention on Human Rights (the right to life).[8]

Withdrawal of artificial nutrition and hydration

Tony Bland was 17 years old when he was involved in the Hillsborough football stadium disaster in April 1989. As a result, his lungs were crushed and punctured and the supply of oxygen to his brain was interrupted. He suffered catastrophic and irreversible damage to the higher centres of the brain, leaving him in a persistent vegetative state. Bland could breathe unaided, but he had no cognitive function. He was unable to see, hear, taste, smell, speak, or communicate in any way or feel pain. Being unable to swallow, Bland was fed artificially by a nasogastric tube. In 1992 an application was submitted to the court for a declaration that it would be lawful to withdraw all life sustaining treatment, including artificial nutrition and hydration. The application had the support of Bland's family, the consultant in charge of his care, and two independent doctors.

In approving the application the House of Lords was satisfied that there was no therapeutic, medical, or other benefit to Tony Bland in continuing to maintain his nutrition and hydration by artificial means. It was also held that the provision of artificial feeding by means of a nasogastric tube was "medical treatment".

Airedale NHS Trust v Bland[9]

In view of the sensitive nature of such decisions, the English courts decided that a court declaration should be sought in each case where it was proposed to withdraw artificial nutrition and hydration from a patient in a persistent vegetative state. The guidance from the courts referred only to patients in persistent vegetative state, however, without making reference to patients with other serious conditions, such as those who have suffered a serious stroke or have severe dementia, in which a decision to withhold or withdraw artificial nutrition and hydration could also arise. In other serious cases where such a decision is needed, the decision is based, as for other forms of treatment, on whether providing the treatment would be in the best interests of the patient. In the absence of any clear statement from the court about how these cases should be handled, the BMA believes that there should be in place standard policies and guidelines to ensure that proper and transparent procedures are followed. Doctors need to be aware, however, that until clear guidance has been provided by the courts for such cases, their discretion to make decisions to withdraw artificial nutrition and hydration in these circumstances could be challenged. Particular care needs to be taken, therefore, when making such decisions.

Although the BMA believes that it is appropriate in some cases to withhold or withdraw artificial nutrition and hydration, oral nutrition and hydration – by the placing of food or nutritional supplements into the patient's mouth – should always be offered, but not forced upon those who resist or express a clear refusal. This is part of the basic care that is essential to keep patients comfortable and which the BMA believes should always be provided unless it is actively resisted.

Competent adult patients

Competent adult patients may refuse artificial nutrition and hydration, either contemporaneously or in advance, and such refusals must be respected.

Patients for whom death is imminent

Although not always easy to determine, once an individual's condition has reached the stage where death is considered to be imminent, such as in the final stages of an incurable illness, the focus of care changes from attempting to prolong life to keeping the patient as comfortable as possible until death occurs.[10] In these final stages the provision of many treatments, including artificial nutrition and hydration, may become unnecessarily intrusive rather than offering a benefit to the patient. In such patients, artificial nutrition and hydration should be withdrawn.

Patients who are in a persistent vegetative state

For patients in England, Wales, and Northern Ireland who are in a persistent vegetative state, a court declaration should be sought for each patient in whom it is proposed to withdraw artificial nutrition and hydration. In Scotland, it is not necessary to apply to the court in every case, but the Lord Advocate has stated that, when such authority has been granted, the doctor would not face prosecution.[11] This leaves open the possibility of prosecution should the doctor not seek authority from the Court of Session.

Other patients

As mentioned above, decisions about artificial nutrition and hydration sometimes arise in connection with more common conditions that are not taken to court, but around which a body of practice has evolved. Such cases arise, for example, when elderly patients suffer from profound dementia or have suffered a stroke that has left them similarly irreversibly brain damaged and unable to swallow. An assessment must be made in each case of whether the provision of artificial nutrition and hydration would provide a net benefit to the patient, taking account of the burdens of the treatment in relation to the possible benefits. As mentioned above, the requirement to seek a court declaration applies only to patients in persistent vegetative state, but the BMA and the GMC have advised that further safeguards should be in place for those cases that do not need court approval.

The GMC's guidance advises that, in cases where artificial nutrition and hydration are to be withdrawn from a patient whose death is not imminent

> as well as consulting the health care team and those close to the patient, ...[the doctor] must seek a second or expert opinion from a senior clinician (who might be from another discipline such as nursing) who has experience of the patient's condition and who is not already directly involved in the patient's care.[12]

The BMA supports this advice and recommends that this should involve the senior clinician reviewing the patient's notes, examining the patient, and discussing the circumstances with the treating doctor. The views of this person should be documented in the medical record. In addition, all cases in which artificial nutrition and hydration have been withdrawn should be available for clinical review to ensure that appropriate procedures and guidelines were followed.

Cardiopulmonary resuscitation

Cardiac or respiratory failure is a part of the dying process and cardiopulmonary resuscitation (CPR) can theoretically be attempted on every individual prior to death. Because for every person there comes a time when death is inevitable, however, it is essential to identify patients for whom cardiopulmonary arrest represents a terminal event in their illness and in whom attempted CPR is inappropriate. It is also essential to identify those patients who do not want CPR to be attempted. All establishments that face decisions about attempting CPR, including hospitals, general practices, residential care homes, and ambulance services, should have in place a policy about resuscitation attempts. The guidance on pages 352–8 of this chapter is also relevant to decisions about CPR, but this section summarises some of the specific factors to take into account when considering these decisions. (More detail can be found in the BMA's specific guidance on CPR.[13])

When no advance decision has been made

When no explicit advance decision has been made about the appropriateness or otherwise of attempting resuscitation prior to a patient suffering cardiac or respiratory arrest, and the express wishes of the patient are unknown and cannot be ascertained, there should be a presumption that health professionals will make all reasonable efforts to attempt to revive the patient. Although this is the general assumption, it is unlikely to be considered reasonable to attempt to resuscitate a patient who is in the terminal phase of illness or for whom the burdens of treatment clearly outweigh the potential benefits.

Making decisions in advance

Ideally, decisions about whether to attempt to resuscitate a particular patient should be made in advance as part of the overall planning for that patient and, as such, are discussed with the patient together with other aspects of future care. An advance decision that CPR will not be attempted (a "do not attempt resuscitation" or "DNAR" order) should be made only after the appropriate consultation and consideration of all relevant aspects of the patient's condition. These include:

- the probable clinical outcome, including the prospect of successfully restarting the patient's heart and breathing, and the overall benefit likely to be achieved from achieving resuscitation
- the patient's known or ascertainable wishes
- the patient's human rights, including the right to life and the right to be free from degrading treatment.

The views of patients, all members of the medical and nursing teams, and, with due regard to confidentiality, those who are close to such patients, are valuable in forming decisions, which must be made on the basis of individual circumstances rather than by applying the same decision to whole categories of patients.

Written information about resuscitation policies should be included in the general literature provided about healthcare establishments, to help patients, and their families, to understand and consider the issues.[14] Patients' own views about the level of burden or risk that they consider acceptable carry considerable weight in deciding whether treatment is given, so it follows that decisions about whether the likely benefits from successful CPR outweigh the burdens should usually be discussed with competent patients. Thus, when competent patients are at a foreseeable risk of cardiopulmonary arrest, or have a terminal illness, there should be sensitive exploration of their wishes regarding resuscitation. This normally arises as part of general discussions about that patient's care. Information should not be forced on unwilling recipients, however, and if patients indicate that they do not wish to discuss resuscitation this should be respected. When a DNAR order is made and there has been no discussion with the patient, because he or she has indicated a clear desire to avoid such discussion, this must be documented in the health records and the reasons for the decision given. A patient's initial refusal of information, like the DNAR order itself, should be sensitively reviewed on a regular basis. It should be made clear to patients that this is not a one off decision and that they can discuss the issue with the healthcare team at any time. The wishes of competent patients who refuse CPR must be respected.

Some patients may ask for CPR to be attempted, even if the clinical evidence suggests that, in their case, it will not effectively restart the heart and breathing or that it cannot provide any overall benefit. Sensitive efforts should be made without alarming the patient to convey a realistic view of the procedure and its likely success. If patients still ask that no DNAR order is made, this should be respected; in the event of cardiopulmonary arrest, there should then be a general presumption that

CPR will be attempted unless the burdens clearly outweigh the potential benefits for the patient. Doctors cannot be required to give treatment that is contrary to their clinical judgment but should, whenever possible, respect patients' wishes to receive treatment that carries only a very small chance of success or benefit. When patients are not competent to make decisions, the same criteria apply as for other treatment decisions and, in England, Wales, and Northern Ireland, decisions should be based on an assessment of the patient's best interests. In addition, in Scotland, the views of any appointed health care proxy should be sought.

When is it appropriate to consider making a DNAR order?

Some circumstances in which it may be appropriate to consider making a DNAR order for a particular patient are set out below, but those involved in making such decisions should refer to the more detailed guidance provided by the BMA.[15] A DNAR order may be appropriate where:

- a competent patient has refused CPR
- the healthcare team is as certain as it can be that attempting CPR would not restart the patient's heart and breathing, therefore the patient cannot gain any clinical benefit from an attempt
- there is no benefit in restarting the patient's heart and breathing, for example if only a very brief extension of very poor quality life can be achieved and the patient's comorbidity is such that imminent death cannot be averted
- the expected benefits to be gained from the prolongation of life are outweighed by the burdens of the treatment to the patient.

The overall responsibility for decisions about CPR and DNAR orders rests with the consultant or GP in charge of the patient's care, but that person should always be willing to discuss the decision with other involved health professionals. Once a decision has been made this should be effectively and sensitively communicated to the patient, those close to the patient, and those involved in providing care. Decisions should be reviewed regularly and in the light of changes in the patient's condition or wishes. All decisions not to attempt resuscitation and the reasons for them should be recorded in the patient's notes.

Summary – decisions to withhold or withdraw life-prolonging treatment

- For every proposed medical intervention, a judgment should be made about whether that intervention would be worthwhile in the sense of providing net benefit to the individual patient.
- Competent adult patients have the right to refuse any medical treatment, even if that refusal results in their death.
- In England, Wales, and Northern Ireland, decisions about whether to give or withhold treatment should be based on an assessment of that patient's best

interests. In addition, in Scotland, any appointed health care proxy should be consulted.

- The decisions of those who have parental responsibility for a baby or young child are usually determinative unless they conflict seriously with the views of those providing care about the child's best interests.

- In England, Wales, and Northern Ireland a young person's refusal of treatment may, in some circumstances, be overridden. In Scotland, a competent young person's refusal of treatment may be binding and legal advice should be sought.

- Discussion with the patient, other members of the healthcare team and (with due respect to confidentiality) those close to the patient are an important part of the decision making process.

- When the treatment to be withdrawn is artificial nutrition and hydration, additional safeguards should be in place.

- Ideally, decisions about whether to attempt CPR for a particular patient should be made in advance, with appropriate consultation and consideration of all relevant aspects of the patient's condition.

- Any decision to withhold or withdraw life prolonging treatment, together with the reasons for that decision, must be carefully documented in the patient's medical record.

Helping patients to prepare for "a good death"

For some, death comes quickly, and perhaps unexpectedly, but for others there is a period of time during which the patient, and his or her family know that death is approaching. In this period, the focus of care shifts to keeping the patient comfortable and free from distressing symptoms, and helping the patient and his or her family to come to terms with and prepare for death. Part of the role of the healthcare team at this time is to listen to the patient's hopes, wishes, and fears, and to help the patient to achieve a good death. In modern times, one of the first people to espouse the notion of "a good death" was Elizabeth Kubler-Ross in the 1970s. Having interviewed more than 200 dying patients in the space of 2½ years, she documented extracts from the interviews and the insights she and her colleagues had gained about the anxieties, hopes, frustrations, and fears of these patients.[16] One of her key findings, which remains relevant today, is the importance of both talking and listening to the dying patient. From her interviews, Kubler-Ross identified five stages that patients move between when they are told that they are dying:

- denial and isolation
- anger
- bargaining
- depression
- acceptance.

Others have developed this theme further[17] and it is now widely acknowledged that patients express a variety of emotions and reactions at different times in their illness, and may move between these stages rather than go sequentially through them. Understanding that such feelings are natural and common throughout a person's illness can help the patient, the relatives and health professionals to manage the situation and to provide the support needed for the patient as death approaches. Many of the lessons learnt from the work of Kubler-Ross, particularly about listening to what patients want in their final days, have had a lasting impact and have shaped modern thinking about caring for dying people.

Greater emphasis on what constitutes a good death and how health professionals, patients, and their families can work together to achieve this aim, signifies a major step forward and forms an intrinsic part of the care owed to dying patients. Often, it is not just death itself that people fear, but the manner, time, and place of their death. This distinction has been neatly summed up as follows:

> Most people fear death, or perhaps more accurately – most people fear dying. The prospect is often one of dying in hospital, perhaps in great pain, wired up to equipment and enduring uncomfortable interventions, suffering indignities and having little or no privacy, being sedated in such a way that there is little or no awareness of circumstances or surroundings, and, no opportunity to say goodbye.[18]

On the other hand, many older people are fearful of dying alone and unsupported at home, and not being found for days or perhaps weeks. The context of their death is what many people fear.

In the late 1990s, Age Concern England established a project, *The debate of the age*, to consider the future of the health and care of older people. The final report of this project articulated a set of principles for a good death, which should form the basis of the care of all terminally ill patients.

- To know when death is coming, and to understand what can be expected
- to be able to retain control of what happens
- to be afforded dignity and privacy
- to have control over pain relief and other symptom control
- to have choice and control over where death occurs (at home or elsewhere)
- to have access to information and expertise of whatever kind is necessary
- to have access to any spiritual or emotional support desired
- to have access to hospice care in any location, not only in hospital
- to have control over who else is present and shares the end
- to be able to issue advance directives which ensure wishes are respected
- to have time to say goodbye, and control over other aspects of timing and
- to be able to leave when it is time to go, and not to have life prolonged pointlessly.[19]

Health professionals caring for terminally ill patients work in accordance with these fundamental principles and, as far as possible when working within the limited resources available, apply them in individual cases. This requires particular attention to be paid to the provision of information and good quality care, and the need to discuss and, as far as possible, meet individuals' wishes about the circumstances of their death.

Palliative care

Hospice and palliative care services have made a major contribution to helping people to achieve a good death. Their emphasis on providing specialist care for those with life threatening illness has shown that the period leading up to death can be one of personal development, strengthened relationships, and spiritual and psychological growth. With effective symptom relief, good communication, and psychologically supportive care, patients can live out their lives to the fullest possible extent and, when death approaches, can prepare themselves for it. Palliative care is not just about terminal care. Rather, it "is an approach that improves the quality of life of patients and their families facing the problems associated with life-threatening illness, through the prevention and relief of suffering by means of early identification and impeccable assessment and treatment of pain and other problems, physical, psychosocial and spiritual".[20]

The philosophy of palliative care

Palliative care does not seek to cure patients but, recognising that a patient's condition is incurable, it offers relief from pain and distressing symptoms, and provides support for the patient and his or her family. Recognition of this change in focus, by patients, relatives, and staff, facilitates discussion of the management of death and bereavement. Some patients put the phase of struggling behind them and come to a different perspective. The approach of palliative care is based on the following core principles:

- focus on quality of life, including good symptom control
- a whole person approach, taking account of the person's past life experience and current situation
- care encompassing both the patient and the people close to the patient
- respect for patient autonomy and choice
- emphasis on open and sensitive communication with patients, informal carers, and professional colleagues.[21]

The development of palliative care

The modern hospice movement was established in the 1950s and, although still providing actual care for a very small minority of terminally ill patients, has exerted a positive influence and has raised the standards of terminal care more generally. In

1995 a Government report (the Calman–Hine Report) declared skills in a palliative care approach to be a core requirement of every health professional.[22] The GMC has identified "palliative care, including care of the terminally ill" as a core part of the undergraduate medical curriculum.[23]

General palliative care services are provided by primary care teams, caring for dying patients in the community and, in hospital, by the healthcare teams that treat patients throughout their illness. Such teams have varying degrees of expertise and knowledge of palliative care. The skills needed include being able to assess the palliative care needs of individual patients, to deliver general palliative care services, and to identify when additional specialist support is needed.

Specialist palliative care services are delivered by multidisciplinary teams, which are likely to include palliative medicine consultants, palliative care nurse specialists, social workers, counsellors, and other staff who are able to provide both the psychological and social support needed. Specialist palliative care teams may provide advice to those who are responsible for care, or may take the lead in a patient's care – whether in the community, hospital, or hospice – depending on that individual's needs. They also have an important role in education and training of the wide range of generalist staff who care for patients at the end of life.

A number of the problems that arise in relation to palliative care relate to the scarcity of resources. Traditionally, funding for hospices and palliative care services has come from the voluntary sector and in 2001 less than a quarter of inpatient hospices were managed by the NHS; for the rest, the NHS provided about one third of the funding.[24] This lack of comprehensive funding and of a strategic approach to the provision of services has inevitably led to wide variation in their nature and availability across the country. In 2000 the Government announced that "for too long the NHS has regarded specialist palliative care as an optional extra" and announced its plan to increase future funding in order to "end inequalities in access to specialist palliative care".[25] In December 2002 the Government announced a £50 million ring fenced funding package to improve care for terminally ill people in England.[26]

The expansion of palliative care principles

While historically focusing on the care of cancer patients, the general philosophy of palliative care has gradually been adopted for others, including patients with HIV/AIDS, heart disease, Creutzfeldt–Jakob disease, and other incurable diseases. Over the last few years there has been debate about the most appropriate way of meeting the terminal care needs of patients with non-malignant diseases.[27] One option would be to encourage those providing care for these patients to develop services based on the principles of palliative care, while another option is for existing hospices and palliative care teams to expand their service to incorporate these patients. Although the latter option may be acceptable in some areas, it has been questioned by some on the grounds that many hospices lack staff with the necessary skills, as well as the resources, to extend their care to non-cancer patients. The development of general palliative care services within hospitals, primary care, and nursing homes has illustrated that the integration of palliative care principles into existing services is a viable and appropriate response, and should be encouraged. It is hoped that, with additional funding for palliative care, this broadening of the availability of palliative care services to other categories of illness and to other settings, such as primary care, will continue.

Summary – palliative care

- Palliative care does not seek to cure the patient but, recognising that the patient's condition is incurable, it offers relief from pain and distressing symptoms and provides support for the patient and his or her family.
- The increased availability of palliative care for patients suffering from incurable diseases other than cancer should be encouraged.
- The adoption of palliative care principles in other healthcare settings such as hospitals, primary care, and nursing homes, should be further developed.
- It is essential that the benefits of education and research in palliative care are extended to the care of those dying in all settings.

Communication

Provision of information

In order for patients to contribute to discussions about their care, make informed decisions about future treatment offered, and take steps to prepare for their death, they need to know that they are dying. For this reason, and out of respect for patient autonomy, honesty and frankness combined with sensitivity and compassion are needed when providing information about life threatening illness. This emphasis on honesty and openness is a relatively new development in the history of medicine. In 1951, 90% of doctors did not disclose the truth to cancer patients; by 1977, 90% did so as a general policy.[28] This shift in attitude demanded considerable new skills for doctors, yet it is only fairly recently that communication skills in general, and techniques for breaking bad news in particular, have formed part of the medical curriculum. The skills needed to break bad news in a sensitive way are not something that doctors simply acquire from practice; they are skills that need to be taught.

A study of gastroenterologists from different parts of Europe found wide variations in whether they would tell their patient about a diagnosis of colonic cancer.[29] Those in northern Europe would usually reveal the diagnosis to the patient and, with the patient's permission, to his or her spouse. Those in southern and eastern Europe, however, would usually conceal both the diagnosis and the prognosis. This is likely to reflect cultural differences of which health professionals need to be aware. Care must be taken, however, not to assume that patients from parts of the world where information is usually not provided do not want to receive it.

The amount of information that individuals want and need is frequently underestimated. In a study of patients, doctors, and nurses in an acute-care hospital in New York, for example, a statistically significant difference was found between the percentage of patients who said they wanted to be told all the details of their condition (72%) compared with the proportions of doctors (42%) and nurses (40%) who said that patients would want to be given full information.[30] Similar results have been obtained from studies in the UK.[31] Many studies have found that virtually all patients want to know their diagnosis, although there is more diversity with regard to the *amount* of information that patients want about the likely progression of the disease and their prognosis.[32] Despite relatives' frequent requests that information is withheld from elderly patients, the same desire to know of a diagnosis of cancer was found in 88% of patients who were aged from 65 to 94 years.[33]

Honesty and truth telling

The BMA believes that honesty between doctor and patient is a key element in the partnership. It therefore stresses frankness and the need to explore issues gently with the patient rather than brutally confronting an unprepared patient with the truth. There is a school of thought, however, which places values such as beneficence above truth telling, particularly in relation to news of terminal illness. Patients or their relatives occasionally complain to the BMA that information, especially about degenerative illness, has been given prematurely, before the onset of acute symptoms, and has thus deprived the patient of a period of "blissful ignorance". A major problem with such an approach is that it assumes the ability on the part of the doctor to know what is best for the patient. The view taken throughout this book is that individuals are best placed to make that assessment for themselves and need information in order to make it. In some cases patients need to know in order to take appropriate health measures to delay the progress of the disease. Information at an early stage may allow the patient time to accomplish plans that would be impossible later. Therefore the BMA strongly recommends that health professionals should sensitively explore with the patient his or her particular wishes regarding the amount of information to be provided. The aim should be to encourage patients to receive information at a pace that suits their own needs and enables them to take part in the decision making process.

Among any group of people, however, there will be some who do not wish to know the full implications of their prognosis or need time to assimilate and accept the information they have been given. Doctors therefore need to be sensitive to cues from their patients about how much information they want to receive at any particular time. When a doctor decides to convey to the patient something less than the full implications of the illness, such a decision must be based on the genuine perception that such withholding of information is the patient's clear desire rather than the doctor's interpretation of what is best for the patient. The patient's wishes in this respect should be sensitively reviewed at regular intervals and the aim must be to prepare the patient to receive the information. Refusal to receive information is discussed further in Chapter 2 (pages 80–1).

Sometimes relatives let it be known that, in the event of a life threatening disease being diagnosed, they do not wish the patient to be fully informed of it. Doctors faced with such requests must explain that their primary duty is to their patient, both in terms of that person's right to information and to confidentiality. If the patient is competent, information should not be given to his or her relatives without consent. The healthcare team may also need to explore with the relatives the fears that lie behind such a request, in the hope that these can be overcome and, with the patient's consent, lead to communication and discussion between all concerned.

Facing reality and maintaining hope

With terminal illness it is not uncommon for an atmosphere of collusive disregard of reality to develop, which has characterised the final months of life for many people, as the patient and relatives try to protect each other from the truth. Even when doctors are willing to assist the patient and the family to face up to the inevitability of death, they often encounter strong social pressures to preserve an overly optimistic, rather than an honest, approach. Although it is important to try to prepare patients to receive information about their illness, it is also necessary to recognise the important place that denial has in the psychological process of coming to terms with an illness. From her studies, Kubler-Ross observed that "the need for denial exists in every patient at times, at the very beginning of a serious illness more so than towards the end of life".[34]

Information and false optimism

In their study of cancer patients' information needs, Leydon and her colleagues found that hope was indispensable for survival and that this interacted with information seeking in a complex way. Some patients searched avidly for information, while others limited their requests and frequently avoided any new information. Interviews with all patients in the study included a sense of hope and patients created a façade of hopefulness, even when suffering from advanced disease.[35] A group of researchers in the Netherlands studied the origins of this type of hopefulness, or "false optimism", in a group of patients with incurable small cell lung cancer by observing the communication process from the initial diagnosis to death of 35 patients over a 4 year period.[36] The researchers found that virtually all of the patients showed false optimism after the first course of chemotherapy and the patients' interpretation of their prognosis was considerably more optimistic than that of their doctors.

An interesting finding was that doctors appeared to collude with this false optimism by not discussing the poor prognosis openly, but instead focusing on

(Continued)

treatment options and timetable (what the researchers refer to as "medical activism"). They point out that what they observed was not only the result of doctors withholding information from patients, but of patients gratefully accepting the opportunities offered by doctors to "forget" the future and concentrate on the present. Although it was generally felt that this "adherence to the recovery plot" helped patients and their relatives to cope with the situation during treatment, it also made it more difficult for those patients to accept and prepare themselves for death; some of the relatives, interviewed after the patients' death, regretted this. Another interesting finding was the ambiguities around language and the way certain phrases were interpreted differently by the doctor and the patients. The authors of this article point out that the statement "this tumour can be treated" meant, to the doctor, that the patient's life could be prolonged, but to the patients, it meant that they could be cured.

It has been suggested that doctors collude with patients to maintain false optimism and that "solutions to the problem of collusion between doctor and patient require an active, patient oriented approach from the doctor".[37] But to what extent is this collusion "a problem"? A group of oncologists from Glasgow who responded to this suggestion, argued that false optimism is not a problem that needs to be overcome, but a common coping strategy frequently adopted by patients and one that is rarely regretted. They stated that "for any patient faced with life threatening disease, it is hope and the triumph of optimism over reality which makes life bearable. It is wrong to suggest that this optimism needs to be taken away from patients for their own good".[38]

This situation requires doctors to tread a careful path. It is important to give the patient as much information as he or she wants and needs to be able to retain control over the situation and to make appropriate decisions about future health care. At the same time, it is important not to impose unwanted information in a way that could have the effect of removing a valuable coping strategy for the patient and could cause great harm. There are no easy answers to this dilemma and, as stated earlier, the crucial factor is for doctors to take their cue from the patients themselves. Pressure to prevaricate should be resisted, but at the same time it must be recognised that individuals require varying degrees of time and support to assimilate what they are told. Care is needed to assess whether the patient has genuinely misunderstood the information provided or is not ready to accept it and is adopting the strategy of false optimism. The role of the health team in such situations includes attempting to help these patients and those who are close to them to face the reality in a compassionate way and within a timescale that is appropriate for them, bearing in mind that there may be very limited time available. As discussed in Chapter 2, however, the BMA believes that patients must be given basic information in order to make valid decisions.

Admitting uncertainty

The dialogue between doctor and patient should include informing the patient when there is medical uncertainty, for which there may be a number of reasons.

Perhaps there is no "best treatment" for the patient's condition, or it is not clear how much the disease process has advanced. It must be recognised, however, that both doctors and patients sometimes feel ambivalent about total frankness. Doctors may feel that by acknowledging uncertainty they are undermining the patient's confidence in them at a time when he or she most needs reassurance. At the same time, they may think that, by presenting an appearance of certainty that the circumstances do not justify, they are able to give a sense of hope and optimism, which may help the patient to cope with the situation. The difficulty for each doctor is how to evaluate the implicit messages from the individual patient in the face of a perhaps more generalised pressure from relatives to paint an optimistic picture.

Different members of the healthcare team can sometimes contribute unwittingly to confusion and uncertainty by giving different advice and information to the patient and relatives. Good communication between members of the healthcare team is essential and minimises the risks of conflicting messages being given.

Sharing information with those close to the patient

Although doctors may often find it easier to talk to those who are close to the patient rather than directly to the patient, this is a breach of confidentiality. While the patient remains competent, extension of the doctor–patient dialogue to include relatives and others should not take place without the patient's agreement. Some patients may not wish those close to them to be aware of the prognosis. In such circumstances, although confidentiality should be maintained, the doctor usually counsels the patient about the desirability of preparing those close to him or her. Vital last opportunities for communication or reconciliation may otherwise be lost. Part of the general perception of a "good death" involves patients and those close to them sharing the experience as fully as possible and supporting each other. There may also be situations in which informal carers need to know information in order to avoid the risk of serious harm, either to themselves or to the patient. This should be discussed with the patient, who should be encouraged to allow some necessary information to be shared; if permission is refused, the healthcare team should consider whether the risks of harm are sufficiently great to justify breaching confidentiality. If, in exceptional cases, confidentiality is to be breached, only the minimum amount of information necessary to achieve the aim should be provided and the patient should be informed of this in advance.

Occasionally patients request that information is given to their relatives rather than to themselves. This should be accepted, but it is appropriate to continue to offer the patient the opportunity to receive information at a pace and in a manner that is acceptable to him or her. It may also be appropriate to discuss, with the patient, the stress that such a request could place on the relatives.

Preparing for death

In addition to medical information, patients who are dying also need to know about what to expect in the period leading up to their death, in terms of their own feelings and those of people close to them. They may also need practical advice about the services and support mechanisms available to them and advice about the type of practical steps they need to take to put their affairs in order, such as making a will, sorting out finances, and making known any wishes about funeral arrangements. A number of booklets are available for patients that address these issues in a sensitive and constructive manner, which can be a useful aid to discussion.[39] A range of support groups also exist for conditions such as cancer and HIV, and for those who have suffered the loss of a child. These groups provide both information and support, and frequently the opportunity to talk to other families who have been through similar experiences, which can also be helpful for both patients and families.

Spiritual and pastoral care

As death approaches, doctors and other health professionals should explore whether the patient has a need for spiritual support. When patients wish to talk to a hospital chaplain or other religious or spiritual adviser, every effort should be made to accommodate this. The dying person may also wish to discuss personal, moral, or spiritual problems with health professionals, knowing that they will not only safeguard the confidence of discussions but also refrain from imposing their own moral or religious advice. The confidentiality aspects of spiritual and pastoral care are discussed in Chapter 5 (pages 186–7).

For many people, one facet of a peaceful death is the knowledge that their religious or personal beliefs concerning appropriate treatment of their bodies after death will be respected. It is important that health professionals should discuss with the patient, if appropriate, or with those close to the patient, how the body will be handled after death while it remains on hospital or hospice premises in order to conform with the individual's cultural or religious customs. Some patients may also wish to discuss whether their organs or tissue would be suitable for donation or research after their death. These issues are discussed in more detail in Chapter 12 (pages 416–8 and 431–5).

Summary – communication

- In order for patients to contribute to discussions about their care, make informed decisions about future treatment offered, and take steps to prepare for death, they need to know that they are in the terminal or dying phase of their illness.

- Honesty and frankness combined with sensitivity and compassion are needed when providing information about life threatening illness.
- When considering how much information to provide, the cue should always be taken from the patient. The aim should be to encourage the patient to receive information at a pace that suits his or her own needs and enables participation in the decision making process.
- Although it is important to try to prepare them to receive information about their illness, it is also necessary to recognise the important place that denial has in the psychological process of patients coming to terms with their illness.
- If the patient is competent, information should not be shared with relatives without the patient's consent. Relatives who do not want the patient informed about the diagnosis should be asked about the reasons for their request, but should be advised that the doctor's primary duty is to the patient.
- As death approaches, doctors and other health professionals should explore whether the patient has a need for specialist spiritual support. When patients express a wish to talk to a hospital chaplain or other religious or spiritual adviser, every effort should be made to accommodate this wish.

Maintaining control

For many patients with a terminal illness, being able to maintain control over some aspects of their life and death can provide significant relief and can help them to achieve a good death.

Listening to the patient

For as long as patients are competent to do so, they should be encouraged to discuss their wishes about both medical and personal aspects of their care. This may involve deciding whether to continue to receive active treatment or who should be involved in discussions about treatment. Encouraging such involvement and discussion is important both out of continuing respect for the patient's autonomy and dignity and as a way of increasing the likelihood of the patient achieving a good death. For many people the loss of control over events at the end of their life is one of their main fears. Consciously giving patients the opportunity to take control of even relatively minor aspects of their care can have a positive psychological effect on their overall sense of wellbeing.

Decisions about medical care

A competent patient should be involved in decision making about future medical treatment to the greatest extent that he or she wishes. Discussion should be encouraged about the likely progression of the disease in order to ascertain the patient's wishes about future treatment once competence has been lost. Some patients may wish, at this stage, to make a formal, written advance directive (see Chapter 3, pages 113–6), although others will be sufficiently reassured by the doctor making a note of the discussion in the medical record.

Dying patients do not, however, acquire greater rights than others and cannot make unreasonable demands on health professionals, for example, to be given futile treatment or for assistance to end their life (see Chapter 11 on euthanasia and physician assisted suicide). When doctors believe unreasonable demands are being made, they should examine why they appear unreasonable and what lies at the root of the request. Such demands often arise from an unexplored anxiety or concern that needs to be addressed. There may be strong arguments for complying with reasonable requests from competent patients for treatment considered to be futile to be continued for a limited period to allow them to achieve particular goals or to sort out their affairs. What is "reasonable" needs to be judged on an individual basis, taking account of factors such as the patient's ability to achieve the goal, the time it would take to do so, and the potential opportunity costs for other patients. Nevertheless, there may be situations where doctors have a responsibility to tell patients that their rights and authority are limited. This presents a challenge to those who are caring for terminally ill people.

There may be circumstances, however, in which patient preferences may appropriately determine the treatment to be given. The patient may, for example, prefer a course of treatment that does not necessarily give the best clinical outcome but is most compatible with the patient's lifestyle and values. In such cases the patient's personal interests should usually take precedence over their strictly medical interests. Similarly, pain relief and sedation can sometimes reduce the patient's overall level of awareness. Some people choose to tolerate a degree of pain in order to remain more alert.

Dilemmas can arise when patients have exhausted all the treatment possibilities of conventional medicine and place their last hopes in an unproven therapy. This is not a problem if the clinician is willing to take responsibility for supervising such therapy, either because it alleviates symptoms or because it provides a psychological benefit to the patient and does no harm. It is immensely more difficult when the clinician believes that the therapy in question is harmful or if its implementation causes a delay in more useful treatment being given. After advising patients of the reasons why they cannot support the proposed therapy, clinicians should continue to provide all those aspects of care that lie within their control. It is important, if the healthcare team cannot support the request of the patient, that the reasons for this are carefully explained and ongoing support continues to be given.

Expressing wishes about the circumstances of death

Once it has been recognised by all concerned that the condition is incurable, the opportunity arises to discuss the patient's wishes concerning the circumstances of his or her death. It is important, even at this stage, that the patient should be able to retain some control over the situation and is encouraged to think about what he or she wants. This requires careful and sensitive handling at a time and pace that suits the patient, but it is an important part of helping to ensure that the dying process is as positive as possible for all concerned. One question that can be raised with the patient is whether he or she wishes to stay in hospital or to go home to die. The latter option will not be possible in all cases, because of the resource implications or because the family simply could not cope, but if arrangements can be made for appropriate care to be provided, many patients would prefer to die at home. Although it is important not to raise the patient's expectations if this would not be feasible, it is something that could be explored in many cases. It is also important for discussion to take place, in advance, about whom the patient would want to be contacted when the time of his or her death appears imminent. It is important for patients to have the opportunity to say goodbye to their loved ones; advance planning can ensure that the relevant contact numbers are available and easily accessible when the time comes.

Summary – maintaining control

- For many people the loss of control over events at the end of life is one of their main fears. Consciously giving patients the opportunity to take control of even relatively minor aspects of their care can have a positive psychological effect on the patient's overall sense of wellbeing.
- A competent patient should be involved in decision making about future medical treatment to the greatest extent that he or she wishes.
- Dying patients do not acquire greater rights than other patients and cannot make unreasonable demands on health professionals, for example, to be given futile treatment or for assistance to end their life.
- Dying patients should be given the opportunity to discuss the circumstances of their death, including, if possible, where they want to die. If suitable arrangements can be made, many patients may prefer to die at home rather than in hospital.

Good quality care

How individuals, and their relatives, perceive the quality of care received at the end of life depends upon a combination of the medical and personal skills of the members of the healthcare team. In addition to mastering techniques to control pain and distressing symptoms, doctors also need to be able to develop a relationship with the patient and offer emotional and psychological support as well as physical help. Dying patients have sometimes complained that they are avoided and feel "written off" by doctors who may feel threatened by their inability to offer a cure. Such patients need and deserve reassurance that their doctor is interested in them as individuals right up to death and it is hoped that the greater emphasis placed on caring for dying people in the medical curriculum will help to equip doctors to deal with such situations.

Dying patients may show a wide range of emotions and doctors must be able to respond appropriately, listen, and develop care plans that meet the needs and wishes of individual patients. In the past, medical training, reflecting wider attitudes in society, tended to promote the view that attempts to extend life should be made almost regardless of the circumstances. Such views have undergone reappraisal alongside increasing recognition that the primary goal of medicine is not to prolong life for as long as possible; rather it is to benefit the individual patient by offering treatment where appropriate, but also by knowing when to stop. Many patients still fear that a full battery of medical technology will be gratuitously employed to prolong their dying. Callahan describes this as "the fears, anxieties, and indignation of a public that has become increasingly terrorised at the prospect of a life that will end stripped of dignity, the victim of a raw and cruel nature, or impersonal medical bureaucracies, or nervous doctors, or guilt-ridden families, or all of them together".[40]

At the other end of the spectrum, however, are those who fear that treatment may be withdrawn prematurely, when it could still provide benefit to them. Reports of treatment being withdrawn inappropriately from elderly patients, based on age rather than an individual assessment of the benefits of the treatment, have given particular cause for concern.[41] Growing recognition of the harms of overtreating must not lead to treatment being withdrawn prematurely.

Personal skills and qualities required when caring for dying patients

The care of dying patients must be founded on the same ethical principles as the treatment of all other patients. Health professionals caring for dying patients are aware of the continuing importance of respect for patient autonomy, provision of information for decision making, and the safeguarding of patient confidentiality. Patients, however, may need reassurance that these fundamental concepts will not be glossed over. Some people argue that medical ethics is excessively dominated by these issues of consent and confidentiality, and by the individual's competence to make decisions, to the virtual exclusion of other values such as care and commitment. At the end of life in particular, respect for all of these values should blend together in order to treat the whole patient by seeking to alleviate both physical and mental anguish.

Doctors are sometimes criticised for concentrating only on acquiring a high level of technical skills and failing to give enough attention to listening to and establishing rapport with the patient. Notions of "a good doctor" include values such as compassion, empathy, advocacy, beneficence and a willingness to be involved, as well as excellent medical and communication skills. These traits of a good doctor are particularly relevant and potentially therapeutic in the treatment of dying patients. This is not a denial of rights-based or duty-based ethics, but a recognition that the provision of medical treatment is considerably more complicated than providing patients with information and a list of options. The vulnerability and dependence of the sick person at the end of life makes it all the more important that there is trust and confidence as well as the observation of rights and duties. Doctors should, and generally do, approach dying patients with a deepened sense of how crucial it is to respond with sensitivity and feeling to patient need. Virtues of character such as veracity, honesty, integrity, humility, and courage are important, in addition to the requisite diagnostic and technical skills, in order to practise medicine optimally. Such virtues are complementary to, rather than in conflict with, notions of consent and confidentiality and help to develop the supportive context within which patients have the right to make choices and doctors have duties to empower their patients.

Respect for privacy

Privacy in the sense of confidentiality is discussed fully in Chapter 5, but there are also other aspects of privacy, such as the freedom from interference by others or patients' rights to be heard and to have their beliefs respected. For many patients the lack of privacy and private space afforded to them in hospital can be very distressing. Recognising the physical limits imposed by crowded facilities, the healthcare team should make whatever provision they can for patients to have some privacy either for discussions with family or doctors or simply to allow people to have some personal space. Those caring for patients should also do their utmost, within the constraints imposed, to respect the dignity and privacy of the patient when providing medical, nursing, or personal care. The right to privacy is not only an essential part of good quality care but is increasingly being articulated as a fundamental human right underwritten by the Human Rights Act.

Pain and other symptom relief

An essential part of good quality care of dying patients is adequate and appropriate pain and symptom relief. This is sometimes hindered, however, by doctors' concerns that their attempts to relieve their patients' suffering and distress may lead to an earlier death and doctors' motives being called into question. This concern is based on debate about the validity of what is often referred to as the principle of double effect.

Doctors are legally permitted to give sedatives and analgesics to sick patients with the intention of, and in proportion to, the relief of suffering, even if as a consequence the patient's life may be shortened. The moral distinction is between intending and foreseeing the harm. The intention of giving the drugs is to relieve the pain and distress of a dying patient; the harmful, but unintended, effect is the risk of shortening life, which the doctor may foresee but not intend.

Although the legal situation is clear, much fear has been engendered by a common perception that double effect is, in fact, "euthanasia by stealth"[42] and is used by doctors deliberately, but covertly, to practise euthanasia. This perception is reinforced by the fact that high profile cases, such as that of Annie Lindsell,[43] which rest on the principle of double effect, are promoted by the media as being "euthanasia cases".

Double effect

Ms Annie Lindsell had motor neurone disease and, in 1996, sought a declaration from the court that it would not be unlawful for her GP to administer drugs for the relief of her mental distress when she became unable to swallow. She asked the High Court to confirm that mental distress, as well as physical pain, could be treated with medication that could have the incidental effect of shortening her life. Ms Lindsell withdrew her application after her doctor's plans for her care were supported by all of the medical experts involved in the case; a declaration was therefore not required.[44] This case merely restated the already existing legal position on double effect.

The National Council for Hospice and Specialist Palliative Care Services points out that the choice many doctors and carers fear, between leaving the patient at a safe dose of analgesic but in discomfort or giving an "overdose" and deliberately precipitating death, is largely an illusion.[45] Guidance on pain control issued by the Royal College of Physicians confirms that "correctly used, morphine and other opioid analgesics are very safe, and so allow doctors to relieve pain and ensure a comfortable death without shortening life".[46] This point has also been confirmed by a retrospective study of the case notes of 238 patients who received opioids in the last week of their life.[47] Comparison of the patients who received a marked increase in opioids at the end of their lives with those who received no increase showed no significant difference in survival from admission, frequency of unexpected death, or description of death. The authors of that study warn that, while double effect may be a useful principle that can offer reassurance to health professionals, its role should not be exaggerated.

Fears that one's motives may be misinterpreted should not stand in the way of providing good quality symptom control. If the intention is clearly to relieve pain and distress and the dosage provided is commensurate with that aim, the action will not be unlawful. If, once pain has been relieved, the dose is increased, however, the motive in taking this step must be seriously questioned. When doctors are unable to relieve pain and are concerned about increasing the dose further, specialist advice should be sought from the local hospice or palliative care team.

Summary – good quality care

- Dying patients may show a wide range of emotions and the doctor must be able to respond appropriately, listen to patients, and develop care plans that meet the needs and wishes of individual patients.
- Principles such as respect for autonomy and confidentiality are important in the care of dying patients, but these need to be complemented by sensitivity, empathy, and compassion in order to provide a supportive environment within which the patient can begin to prepare for death.
- Every effort should be made to allow patients to have some privacy, either for discussions with family or doctors, or simply to allow them to have some personal space.
- An essential part of good quality care of dying patients is adequate and appropriate pain and symptom relief.

Caring for specific groups

The principles and guidance set out above apply to the care of all patients at the end of life but there are specific issues that arise in relation to children and elderly people. These are discussed briefly in this section.

Caring for dying children

Talking to dying children

Talking to dying children presents particular difficulties from both an emotional and a practical perspective. In the past a protective attitude was adopted and children were not told of their impending death. There is now considerable evidence, however, to show that, as with adults, from a very young age, children need to be given information in order to have the opportunity to talk about their fears and anxieties and to receive appropriate support.[48] In the BMA's view, information about illness and its treatment should not usually be withheld from people who want to have it, regardless of their age, although in this case it may need to be provided gradually over a long period of time by somebody who is skilled in communicating with children. This allows the child or young person to adjust to specific issues before being told the full gravity of the situation. It is not unusual for families to request secrecy, particularly in the case of young patients, in order to spare the sick person from having to cope with distressing information. Health professionals can also find it difficult to be frank with patients whose prognosis is poor. In practice, however, secrecy, bad communication, and the patient's suspicion that important questions are being avoided can contribute to and exacerbate fear and anxiety. In some circumstances, parents, carers, and health professionals may agree that it is not in a young person's best interests to be told precise details of his or her diagnosis, although this is the exception rather than the rule. The child or young person's willingness or need to talk is paramount as well as his or her level of understanding. The age at which a child is able to understand the concept of death, including its finality, varies depending on the development and past experiences of the individual child.

Talking to dying children

A senior ward sister described her approach to discussions with children before surgery as follows:

> I usually say to the child, "what do you want to be told?" Sometimes the teenagers say, "everything", but then you can see them edge away as if what I am saying is too much for them. I don't leave it at that. I say, "What is it upsetting you?" I make sure that before the day of surgery they have an opportunity to voice their fears and uncertainties. These girls can be very protective of their mothers. They don't want to upset them by showing how worried they really are, and they put on a brave face when others are around.

> Sometimes it is important that they know more than they have asked for. I try to edge them forwards to accept a little more information each time we have a chat. I watch carefully to see how successful this is being – and I ration it out, particularly if they seem very anxious, only telling them one main thing at a time.[49]

Communication with children needs to be appropriate to both their age and their development. With younger children, this may involve communicating through play such as with toys, books, or drawing pictures. As with adults, health professionals need to take their cue from the patient in deciding how much information he or she is ready and able to accept at any particular time. With young children, communication is a three-way process involving the child, the parents, and the healthcare team. More information about talking to children, and guidance on assessing competence and understanding, can be found in the BMA's book on children's consent.[50]

Supporting the child's parents

Although the death of a loved one is always difficult, losing a child is particularly traumatic and parents may need specialist support to help them to cope with their loss. In addition to the usual manifestations of grief experienced by most bereaved people, parents often feel intense guilt and anger at the unnaturalness of the death of a child. Although referral for specialist bereavement counselling may be appropriate, it is also essential that members of the healthcare team are able to provide clear and concise information in a sensitive and appropriate manner. As with other situations of dealing with dying patients, excellent communication skills are required to ensure that the information is presented honestly but with compassion. In a study of parents' experiences of treatment withdrawal from infants,[51] communication problems – in terms of both what was said and the way the information was given – were by far the commonest cause of dissatisfaction.

Caring for the parents of dying children

The parents of one preterm baby said:

> In all honesty I don't see you're being nice to somebody by not telling them the whole truth because it's got to come out some way. You're just delaying what's going to happen and I felt the hospital did that with us. In a way I'm actually glad [the junior paediatrician] thought we knew everything because she just came out with it and just said everything in a way we understood it. She said, "Your daughter's got chronic brain damage, she's got hydrocephalus, she's blind. You're never ever going to get her home" ... How hard that was at the time [but] when we look back now that was a relief because at long last somebody'd said to us what was [*really* happening rather than trying to describe the] worst case scenario ... If you think things are going to be bad, tell it, don't hide it because at the end of the day your "kindness" isn't going to work [in our interests].[52]

The mother of a preterm baby said about the care she received at the time of her daughter's death:

> [It was supportive] because they read what we needed. They said things to us: we *could* sit all night with her once she had died. But we just didn't [want to]. It's always been my belief that once you're dead your spirit's gone from your body and that's just this little shell there. And I just think that there could have been nothing worse for us than sitting all night with a dead baby. And I think they realised that. They seemed to judge. Because [the consultant] came in and he said that to us and then he went outside saying, "Right, we're going to let you discuss it. We know you want this over quickly, you want her to stop suffering. ... You tell us when you want the ventilator out." But when they went away ... she died – which took about an hour and a half I think – he came in and he said, "I can see you just want to go home, don't you?" So they didn't push – they didn't say, "Well, some people stay with them and maybe you should." It was just a case of, "What's good for you."[53]

Discussions with parents sometimes involve difficult issues such as providing information about postmortem examinations or raising the issue of organ or tissue donation. This is discussed in Chapter 12.

Paediatric palliative care

Although the principles that emerge from adult palliative care are equally important for terminally ill children, the special needs of children are increasingly being recognised. The Association for Children with Life-threatening and Terminal Conditions and their Families (ACT) and the Royal College of Paediatrics and Child Health have issued guidance on the development of children's palliative care services, which emphasises the following points.

- The continuing physical, emotional, and cognitive development of children sets them apart from adults and influences all aspects of their care.
- Parents are usually the main carers for children, and children are more frequently cared for at home.
- Parents and the child's siblings need support during the child's illness and after the child's death.
- Many professional and voluntary agencies are involved in different aspects of the care of a dying child and these services need to be properly coordinated.
- Many children have prolonged illnesses and the transition between active and palliative care is often less clear than with adults.[54]

The provision of palliative care services designed specifically for children highlights growing recognition of the particular care needs of dying children.

Caring for older people at the end of life

In 2001, 64% of all registered deaths in England and Wales were among people aged 75 years of age or over.[55] This fact, together with the knowledge that older patients are frequently disempowered, requires particular attention to be paid to the care needs of this group. This is not only about avoiding ageism in the provision of treatment, but also about finding ways to meet the particular needs of older people and to help them to maintain their dignity and autonomy in the healthcare setting. Older people have the same rights to information and confidentiality as younger patients. As discussed on page 370, relatives sometimes request that information is withheld from the patient – in order to avoid distress – but health professionals must always make patient care their primary concern. If the person is competent, information should not be shared with relatives without his or her consent. Older patients may, however, need additional support in terms of advocacy, in order to assist them to participate in decisions about their care.

The National Service Framework for Older People provides a 10 year programme of action to ensure fair, high quality, and integrated health and social care services for older people.[56] It focuses on rooting out age discrimination, providing person centred care, promoting older people's health and independence, and fitting services around people's needs. In addition, attention is being given to the development of local partnerships to support older people. Guidance on the care of older people is available from the BMA and the Royal College of Nursing.[57]

Summary – caring for specific groups

- In the past, a protective attitude was adopted whereby children were not told of their impending death, but there is now considerable evidence to show that, from a very young age, children need to be given information in order to have the opportunity to talk about their fears and anxieties, and to receive appropriate support.
- Communication with children needs to be appropriate to both their age and their development. With younger children, this may involve communicating through play such as with toys, books, or drawing pictures.
- Although the principles that emerge from adult palliative care are equally important for terminally ill children, the special needs of children are increasingly being recognised.
- Older patients are frequently disempowered in the provision of health care, but they have the same rights to information and confidentiality as any other patient.
- It is necessary to find ways to meet the particular needs of older people and to help them to maintain their dignity and autonomy in the healthcare setting.

Training and support

Training

In addition to their technical medical expertise – which should include competence in pain and symptom control – doctors who care for dying patients also need training in a range of skills, including communication and providing emotional support; this need is becoming increasingly recognised.[58] Regardless of how well-intentioned doctors may be, their relationships with their terminally ill patients and their families can be severely and irrevocably damaged by inadequate communication skills. It is imperative that all doctors receive training in recognising patients' needs for comfort, counselling, more or less detail, or simply a breathing space prior to receiving more information. Such training recognises the importance of the doctor's role in dealing with the patient's psychological pain as well as his or her physical symptoms. Senior clinicians who have developed the appropriate skills, such as consultants in palliative medicine, are invaluable role models. They have an ethical duty to share this expertise, just as much as their other clinical skills, with less experienced colleagues. In this context, doctors may also profit from the high levels of expertise acquired by other health professionals, including groups like the Macmillan palliative care clinical nurse specialists.

Support for those close to the patient

Providing support for those who are close to the patient to help them to come to terms with their bereavement is a routine part of caring for dying patients. Good communication and team care at an early stage can help to ease the pain of bereavement. It is important to remember, however, that although expected deaths do not represent a shock to the staff who have been caring for the patient, the death of a loved one, however expected, is often a shock for friends and family. Much preparatory work falls to the nursing staff or to GPs. After the patient has died, it is usual and comforting to see death as a release for the patient, but a sense of guilt and fear of criticism often prevent people from also admitting beforehand that the death of the patient may represent a relief for them. The family should be encouraged to discuss any concerns and, if appropriate, should be offered counselling. The situation in which relatives are suddenly confronted by unexpected death is discussed in Chapter 15 (page 553).

Support for the healthcare team

It is increasingly recognised that caring for dying and bereaved people can also take its toll on health professionals at all levels. Forming necessarily impermanent, although rewarding, relationships with patients is draining and being constantly exposed to suffering, helplessness, uncertainty, anger, and loss can be hard for healthcare staff. Employing bodies and colleagues of those caring for dying patients need to be sensitive to the possibility of "burnout" and to the need for adequate support mechanisms to be in place, which are easily accessible to all staff. Staff at all levels should have access to counselling and support both within and outside the healthcare team.

Summary – training and support

- Regardless of how well-intentioned doctors may be, their relationships with their terminally ill patients and their families can be severely and irrevocably damaged by inadequate communication skills.
- It is imperative that all doctors receive training in symptom control and communication skills as well as recognising patients' needs for comfort, counselling, and for more or less information.
- Providing support for those close to the patient to help them to come to terms with their bereavement is an essential part of caring for dying people.
- It is increasingly recognised that caring for dying and bereaved people can also take its toll on health professionals at all levels. All staff should have access to counselling and support both within and outside the healthcare team.

References

1   Debate of the Age. *The future of health and care of older people: the best is yet to come.* London: Age Concern England, 1999:41.
2   Smith R. A good death [editorial]. *BMJ* 2000;**320**:129–30.
3   Doyal L, Doyal L. Why active euthanasia and physician assisted suicide should be legalised. *BMJ* 2001;**323**:1079–80. Doyal L. The case for physician-assisted suicide and active euthanasia in

amyotrophic lateral sclerosis. In: Brown R, Meiniger V, Swash M, eds. *Amyotrophic lateral sclerosis*. London: Martin Dunitz, 1999. Harris J. Euthanasia and the value of life; The philosophical case against the philosophical case against euthanasia; Final thoughts on final acts. In: Keown J, ed. *Euthanasia examined: ethical, clinical and legal perspectives*. Cambridge: Cambridge University Press, 1995. Harris J. The moral difference between throwing a person at a trolley and throwing a trolley at a person: a reply to Frances Kamm. *Proceedings of the Aristotelian Society Supplementary Volume* 2000:41–58.

4   Airedale NHS Trust v Bland [1993] 1 All ER 821: 869.
5   British Medical Association. *Withholding and withdrawing life-prolonging medical treatment, 2nd ed*. London: BMJ Books, 2001.
6   General Medical Council. *Withholding and withdrawing life-prolonging treatments: good practice in decision-making*. London: GMC, 2002.
7   British Medical Association. *Medical treatment for adults with incapacity: guidance on ethical and medico-legal issues in Scotland*. London: BMA, 2002.
8   NHS Trust A v M; NHS Trust B v H [2001] 1 All ER 801.
9   Airedale NHS Trust v Bland [1993]. *Op cit.*
10 Ellershaw J, Ward C. Care of the dying patient: the last hours or days of life. *BMJ* 2003;**326**:30–4.
11 Law Hospital NHS Trust v Lord Advocate (1996) SLT 848.
12 General Medical Council. *Withholding and withdrawing life-prolonging treatments: good practice in decision-making. Op cit:* para 81.
13 British Medical Association, Resuscitation Council (UK), Royal College of Nursing. *Decisions relating to cardiopulmonary resuscitation*. London: BMA, 2001.
14 The BMA has produced a model patient information leaflet: British Medical Association, Resuscitation Council (UK), Royal College of Nursing, Age Concern. *Decisions relating to cardiopulmonary resuscitation. Model information leaflet*. London: BMA, 2002.
15 British Medical Association, et al. *Decisions relating to cardiopulmonary resuscitation. Op cit.*
16 Kubler-Ross E. *On death and dying*. London: Tavistock, 1970.
17 See, for example: Stroebe M, Schut H. The dual process model of coping with bereavement. *Death Studies* 1999;**23**:197–224. Parkes CM. Grief: lessons from the past, visions for the future. *Bereavement Care* 2002;**2**:19–22.
18 Debate of the Age. *The future of health and care of older people: the best is yet to come. Op cit.*
19 *Ibid:* p. 42.
20 World Health Organization. WHO Definition of Palliative Care. In: World Health Organization. *National cancer control programmes: policies and managerial guidelines, 2nd ed*. Geneva: WHO, 2002.
21 Addington-Hall J. *Reaching out: specialist palliative care for adults with non-malignant diseases. Occasional paper 14*. London: National Council for Hospice and Specialist Palliative Care Services and Scottish Partnership Agency for Palliative and Cancer Care, 1998.
22 Department of Health, Welsh Office. *Report of the Expert Advisory Group on Cancers to chief medical officers of England and Wales*. London: The Stationery Office, 1995.
23 General Medical Council. *Tomorrow's doctors. Recommendations on undergraduate medical education*. London: GMC, 2002:6
24 O'Neill J, Higginson IJ. Palliative care in the age of HIV/AIDS [foreword]. *J R Soc Med* 2001;**94**:429.
25 NHS Executive. *The NHS cancer plan: a plan for investment, a plan for reform*. London: The Stationery Office, 2000:68.
26 Department of Health press release. *Action to ensure £50 million investment in palliative care delivers the best services for patients*. 2002 Dec 23. (2002/0531.)
27 Addington-Hall J. *Reaching out: specialist palliative care for adults with non-malignant diseases. Op cit.*
28 Buckman R. *How to break bad news a guide for health care professionals*. London: Papermac, 1994.
29 Thomsen OO, Wulff HR, Martin A, Singer PA. What do gastroenterologists in Europe tell cancer patients? *Lancet* 1993;**341**:473–6.
30 Sullivan RJ, Menapace LW, White RM. Truth-telling and patient diagnoses. *J Med Ethics* 2001; **27**:192–7.
31 See, for example: Jenkins V, Fallowfield L, Saul J. Information needs of patients with cancer: results from a large study in UK cancer centres. *Br J Cancer* 2001;**84**:48–51.
32 See, for example: Meredith C, Symonds P, Webster L, et al. Information needs of cancer patients in West Scotland: cross sectional survey of patients' views. *BMJ* 1996;**313**:724–6. Leydon GM, Boulton M, Moynihan C, et al. Cancer patients' information needs and information seeking behaviour: in depth interview study. *BMJ* 2000;**320**:909–13.
33 Ajaj A, Singh MP, Abdulla AJJ. Should elderly patients be told they have cancer? Questionnaire survey of older people. *BMJ* 2001;**323**:1160.

34 Kubler-Ross E. *On death and dying. Op cit:* p. 37.
35 Leydon GM, *et al.* Cancer patients' information needs and information seeking behaviour: in depth interview study. *Op cit.*
36 The AM, Hak T, Koeter G, van der Wal G. Collusion in doctor–patient communication about imminent death: an ethnographic study. *BMJ* 2000;**321**:1376–81.
37 *Ibid:* p. 1376.
38 O'Rourke N, Barrett A, Jones R, Featherstone C, Hughes V. Collusion in doctor–patient communication. Patients rarely regret optimism. *BMJ* 2001;**322**:1062.
39 See, for example: CancerBACUP. *Dying with cancer.* London: CancerBACUP, 2000.
40 Callahan D. *The troubled dream of life. In search of a peaceful death.* New York: Simon and Schuster, New York, 1993:17.
41 Anonymous. NHS ageism row sparks action. *BBC Online* 2000 Apr 13. http://news.bbc.co.uk (accessed 2 May 2003).
42 National Council for Hospice and Specialist Palliative Care Services. *Voluntary euthanasia: the Council's view.* London: NCHSPCS, 1997.
43 The Voluntary Euthanasia Society. *Sanctity of life and the law: Annie Lindsell's case.* London: VES, 1998.
44 Wilkins E. Dying woman granted wish for dignified end. *The Times* 1997 Oct 29:3.
45 National Council for Hospice and Specialist Palliative Care Services. *Voluntary euthanasia: the Council's view. Op cit.*
46 Royal College of Physicians. *Principles of pain control in palliative care for adults.* London: RCP, 2000.
47 Thorns A, Sykes N. Opioid use in last week of life and implications for end-of-life decision-making. *Lancet* 2000;**356**:398–9.
48 Judd D. Communicating with dying children. In: Dickenson D, Johnson M, eds. *Death, dying and bereavement.* London: SAGE, 1993.
49 Alderson P. *Children's consent to surgery.* Buckingham, PA: Open University Press, 1993.
50 British Medical Association. *Consent, rights and choices in health care for children and young people.* London: BMJ Books, 2001.
51 McHaffie HE. *Crucial decisions at the beginning of life. Parents' experiences of treatment withdrawal from infants.* Oxford: Radcliffe Medical Press, 2001.
52 *Ibid:* p. 66.
53 *Ibid:* p. 191.
54 Association for Children with Life-threatening and Terminal Conditions and their Families (ACT), Royal College of Paediatrics and Child Health. *A guide to the development of children's palliative care services.* Bristol: ACT, 1997.
55 Office for National Statistics. Deaths: age and sex, numbers and rates, 1976 onwards. In: *Health Statistics Quarterly 17.* London: ONS, 2003.
56 Department of Health. *National service framework for older people.* London: The Stationery Office, 2001.
57 British Medical Association, Royal College of Nursing. *The older person: consent and care.* London: BMA, 1995.
58 British Medical Association Board of Medical Education. *Communication skills education for doctors: a discussion paper.* London: BMA, 2003.

11: Euthanasia and physician assisted suicide

The questions covered in this chapter include the following.

- What are the differences between withdrawing and withholding treatment, refusal of treatment, euthanasia, and physician assisted suicide (PAS)?
- Why does the BMA oppose euthanasia and PAS?
- May doctors tell patients about the quantity, or combination, of medication that would kill?
- How should doctors respond to patients who ask for advice about going abroad for euthanasia or assisted suicide?

End of life: what are the issues?

The previous chapter focused on what most health professionals see as the important discussion about the end of life: the provision of a high standard of palliative care and support that aims to sustain and prepare patients and their families for the approach of inevitable death. Although palliative care and its values are central to health care, medical ethics debate has tended to focus more on areas of controversy. Euthanasia and PAS are illegal in the UK, but they continue to raise profound and fascinating social questions about personal and societal values, autonomy and its limits, the purpose of medicine, and the duties owed to patients who want to die. The way in which the health professions and society resolve the dilemmas posed by life or death cases reflect deeply held moral beliefs about the value of life and the qualities that make it valuable, the scope and limits of individual autonomy, and the balancing of benefit for one patient with the possibility of causing harm to others. Legal and practical considerations also apply. What, if any, would be the legal ramifications of weakening the ban on intentional killing? Would patients nearing the end of their lives view their doctor in a different light, knowing that they could ask the doctor to kill?

This book's main focus is on the types of questions people ask the BMA's ethics department. For euthanasia and PAS, the questions from doctors are relatively few because doctors know these acts are illegal, but it is not always clear where the boundaries lie and some practising doctors do find themselves in very difficult situations when they know that a seriously ill patient is accumulating medication with the intention of committing suicide. Other doctors are asked for assurances from patients that they will be "seen right" at the end of their lives. This chapter addresses these practical questions, and explains the scope and limits of legal and ethical practice.

The majority of questions sent to the BMA about euthanasia and PAS come from the media, academics, students, and others with an interest in the BMA's views. This chapter therefore sets out the BMA's policy opposing euthanasia and PAS, together with the Association's reasoning. In doing so, the chapter touches on the experiences of jurisdictions that permit euthanasia or assisted suicide. It does not try to recreate all of the arguments that are relevant to these issues, but mentions the key points. There is a vast literature on euthanasia and PAS for those who are interested in the detailed philosophical debate.[1]

General principles

The previous chapter identified the key principles that underpin the care of dying patients. Many overlap with those that also underpin the BMA's views on euthanasia and PAS.

- Doctors must listen to patients, try to understand their fears about dying and act within the law to help them to achieve a good death.
- A goal of medicine is to relieve suffering and a good death has an important place in medicine, but these should not be achieved by intentionally bringing about death.
- Autonomy has limits, and patients' choices are, rightly, curtailed where there is an unacceptable impact on others.
- Patients can refuse medical treatment that they do not want to receive.
- Withdrawing or withholding treatment differs fundamentally from intentionally ending life. Doctors must analyse their own actions and be certain of their motives when considering withdrawing or withholding treatment.
- The BMA is opposed to euthanasia and PAS, both of which are illegal in the UK.

Definitions and distinctions

Definitions in this area are often imprecise. The purpose of this section is to explain how the BMA uses terms such as euthanasia and PAS, and to demonstrate where it believes the distinctions lie between these illegal acts and areas of legitimate medical practice, including decisions to withdraw life prolonging treatment and the doctrine of double effect.

Euthanasia

By "euthanasia", we mean deliberate, active steps to end a patient's life. Although euthanasia literally means a gentle or easy death, it has come to signify a deliberate intervention with the intention to kill, often described as the "mercy killing" of people who are in pain or with terminal illness. In law, such deliberate taking of life is categorised as murder.

The term euthanasia is sometimes qualified by the terms "voluntary", "involuntary", and "non-voluntary", used to indicate the degree of patient involvement. Many advocates of euthanasia limit their support to the "voluntary" category, where death is brought about at the patient's request. "Non-voluntary euthanasia" is used to describe the mercy killing of a patient who does not have the capacity to request or consent to it, including, for example, severely disabled babies. "Involuntary euthanasia" describes the mercy killing of competent people against their will or without their consent. All categories are legally prohibited.

All of these categories, where there is a positive intervention such as lethal injection, are sometimes referred to as "active euthanasia". This is contrasted with situations where death occurs as a result of an omission to provide treatment, for example when life prolonging treatment is withheld or withdrawn, which is sometimes termed "passive euthanasia". The qualifiers aim to identify the nature of the doctor's involvement and are often used by those who wish to equate non-treatment with active killing. As is discussed in Chapter 10 (pages 353–4) and also on pages 391–2, the BMA believes that there is a fundamental difference between avoiding treatment that cannot provide an overall benefit to the patient and deliberate killing. It shares the view of the House of Lords Select Committee on Medical Ethics that the qualifiers "active" and "passive" are unhelpful.[2]

Physician assisted suicide

Physician assisted suicide differs from euthanasia in that the patient undertakes the final act. The doctor may not even be present, but might have provided equipment, advice, or a lethal substance. What constitutes the "final act" may not be clear cut, however, especially when patients are physically incapacitated and need considerable help in getting to the stage where the final step can be taken.

Euthanasia and PAS were legal in Australia's Northern Territory for a brief period between July 1996 and March 1997.[3] During this time, a computerised machine was used that allowed patients to commit suicide by instructing it to deliver a lethal injection. A doctor attached the needle into the patient's arm, and the lethal injection was delivered after the patient had responded to the computer's three questions, confirming that death was his or her true wish. The final act that instructed the computer to deliver the lethal dose was taken by the patient, but such considerable assistance was needed to set up the machine and connect patients to it that, arguably, this activity fell more within the definition of euthanasia than PAS.

It is illegal for any person in the UK to assist suicide: "A person who aids, abets, counsels or procures the suicide of another, or an attempt by another to commit suicide, shall be liable on conviction on indictment to imprisonment for a term not exceeding fourteen years."[4]

Assisting suicide is not an activity that is necessarily restricted to health professionals and could be done by anybody with the appropriate expertise and access to the means to kill. In practice, jurisdictions that permit assisted suicide almost invariably give doctors a clear role, for example in determining the patient's condition and prognosis, and providing a prescription for lethal medication. This chapter is concerned primarily with the role of doctors, although some legal cases are also mentioned where people have sought assistance from their loved ones because these raise important matters of principle.

Intention

As shown in the detailed discussion of withholding and withdrawing lifeprolonging treatment (see pages 352–64), it is not only the nature of an act but the intention, purpose, or objective behind it that is a key factor in end of life decisions. The health professional's intention in prescribing a medication or withdrawing treatment may be the least demonstrable facet of a case, but may ultimately be what tips the balance between an act being legally and morally permissible or unlawful and, in the BMA's view, unethical. To summarise the BMA's advice, a doctor may withhold or withdraw life prolonging treatment if the purpose of doing so is to withdraw treatment that is not a benefit to the patient and is therefore not in the patient's best interests. The BMA thus supports the legal position that, although a doctor may foresee that a patient will die if treatment is not provided, he or she may withdraw or withhold treatment only if the overriding purpose or objective is to ensure that treatment that is not in the best interests of the patient is avoided.[5]

It has also been shown in the previous chapter (see pages 378–9) that the BMA and the law embrace the principle of "double effect", which provides the justification for the provision of medical treatment that has bad effects when the intention is to provide an overall good effect. An example is the use of pain relieving drugs that risk shortening life.

Significant differences between withdrawing or withholding treatment, double effect, treatment refusal, euthanasia, and PAS

Some argue that when withdrawing or withholding life prolonging treatment is the morally right thing to do (because the treatment provides no benefit or its burdens outweigh the benefits), and death is the inevitable outcome, there are no morally relevant differences between not providing the treatment and taking active steps to end life.[6] The argument may be taken further to say that active steps to end a patient's life that are carried out in a way that is dignified, quick, and painless is the morally right thing to do because unnecessary suffering is avoided.

However logically appealing this argument may appear, the BMA does not believe that it leads to the conclusion that, if one accepts the withdrawal of life prolonging treatment, or the doctrine of double effect, one must also accept euthanasia and PAS. The BMA believes that it is unhelpful to look at these ethical arguments in isolation from the additional issues that society and the health professions must consider in relation to deliberate killing. These include the likely impact that allowing doctors to kill could have on the practice of medicine, as discussed below, and the justification for allowing the withdrawal of life prolonging treatment in limited circumstances, as discussed in the previous chapter.

It was noted in Chapter 10 that some argue that a decision to withdraw life prolonging medical treatment necessarily involves a judgment that the patient's life is not worth living and that the withdrawal is, therefore, morally equivalent to euthanasia. It was also explained that the BMA does not believe that deciding to withdraw life prolonging treatment, or to provide treatment to relieve suffering in the knowledge that it may shorten life, means that death is necessarily "in the patient's best interests". The BMA believes that there is a fundamental distinction between decisions about the value or worth of the *patient*, and those about the value of the *treatment*. Although it is entirely appropriate to make decisions about the value of treatment in terms of its ability to benefit the patient (and this is an essential part of good medical practice), it is not acceptable to make decisions about the value of the patient. It is not for doctors to decide that certain patients are better off dead, but doctors, in consultation with patients and people close to them, are well placed to decide about whether a particular treatment can provide any benefit for a patient. Few believe that doctors must strive to prolong life at all costs, with no regard to the benefits or burdens to the patient. Balancing benefits with burdens in this way is the basis of most, if not all, decisions in medicine.

As well as there being, in the BMA's view, ethical distinctions between the types of legitimate medical decisions discussed above, and euthanasia and PAS, there are also legal distinctions. The former, provided that there is no suggestion of negligence, are lawful. Euthanasia and PAS are not. In the former it is not the doctor who causes death but the patient's illness or injury. Such acts or omissions by a doctor have "an incidental effect on determining the exact moment of death" but the law does not consider them to be "the cause of death in any sensible use of the term".[7] In contrast, the law makes clear that "no doctor, nor any man, no more in the case of the dying than the healthy, has the right deliberately to cut the thread of life".[8]

Euthanasia and PAS have been defined separately above, and there is some evidence that health professionals perceive a moral difference between the two. A detailed survey of health professionals' attitudes to PAS in 1996 found that, among those who supported the option of intentional killing, there was a preference for PAS over euthanasia, by a margin of around 2:1.[9] Doctors may consider that less responsibility or culpability attaches to the act of participating in another's suicide where that seems to be the individual's sustained and reasoned wish.

Philosophers, on the other hand, may argue that there is no moral difference between injecting a patient, at his or her request, with lethal medication, and watching a patient drink a lethal cocktail having provided the drugs. Additionally, they may cite the argument that, if able bodied citizens can legally commit suicide, it is discriminatory not to offer severely disabled people a means to end their lives. (A legal challenge to the UK's prohibition of assisted suicide that argued in part on the basis of this right was lost in 2002; see pages 399–400.) The BMA's approach is that, although there may be some distinctions, euthanasia and PAS are inextricably linked and the moral arguments for and against each are similar. To avoid repetition, wherever possible this chapter addresses the two together.

BMA policy and the views of UK doctors

The previous chapter identified the factors that contribute to a good death. Although a "good death" has an important place in health care, the BMA does not consider that this should ever be achieved by deliberately bringing about death. Such end of life issues have been firmly on the BMA's agenda since the Association's first rejection of the concept of euthanasia in 1950. BMA policy opposing euthanasia was established in 1969, when the Association's annual meeting affirmed the fundamental objective of the medical profession as the relief of suffering and the preservation of life. By 1997, PAS was also the subject of policy. The early policy statements categorically rejected the notion of euthanasia. Later statements have acknowledged the existence of a wide spectrum of views within the membership, but also the consensus that the law should not be changed to permit euthanasia or PAS for the time being.

The General Medical Council (GMC) too reminds doctors that they must act within the law.[10] In 1992 the Council stated that treatment whose only purpose was to shorten the patient's life was wholly outside the doctor's professional duty and fell short of the high standards that the medical profession must uphold.[11]

Individually, some doctors believe that euthanasia and PAS acts are morally justified in some exceptional circumstances. In the largest survey of the views of health professionals in the UK, just under 50% of the 804 doctors surveyed were in favour of a change in the law to allow PAS in specified circumstances.[12] Despite this, however, BMA policy and the outcome of a consensus conference on PAS held in 2000 reflect considerable agreement among BMA members that the Association should not press for legal change.[13] Like any profound shift in public policy there would first need to be very significant public pressure for such change.

The debate within the BMA about euthanasia and PAS has also encompassed discussion of whether the Suicide Act 1961 should be amended to reduce the maximum penalty for assisting suicide. Those in favour of reducing the penalty draw attention to the gap between the penalties available to the courts and those they actually impose. The courts are entitled to pass sentence of up to 14 years' imprisonment for assisting suicide, but use discretion and often give much lower sentences.

Sentencing

Charlotte Hough had been a regular visitor of an 84-year-old woman who was partially blind, partially deaf, and suffered from arthritis.[14] Ms Hough was described by the court as being a woman "of unblemished character, who was opposed to the taking of life and euthanasia" who had tried to dissuade the elderly woman from taking her life. Nevertheless, when the elderly woman was found dead with a suicide note pinned to her clothing, Ms Hough pleaded guilty to attempted murder. She had provided the woman with sodium amytal

(Continued)

tablets and placed a plastic bag over her head once she became unconscious after taking the tablets. It was not clear whether the elderly woman was already dead when the bag was placed over her head, and therefore whether Ms Hough had actually caused her death. The charge, to which Ms Hough pleaded guilty, was therefore "attempted murder".

Although Ms Hough's conviction was of attempted murder, the Court of Appeal noted that her actions fell to a great extent within the scope of the Suicide Act. She was sentenced to nine months' imprisonment, which the Court felt was appropriate in relation to a charge of attempted murder or assisted suicide.

R v Charlotte Helen Hough[14]

In 2002, although rejected as BMA policy, 44% of the BMA's Representative Body believed that, in the light of high profile media cases where people had wanted assistance to commit suicide, the Suicide Act should be changed "to take account of mentally competent individuals who wish to take their own lives but are physically incapable of so doing".[15] Again, however, this is an area where public policies need wide societal debate before change is envisaged.

Moral, legal, and pragmatic arguments

The key principle underpinning the BMA's views on euthanasia and PAS is that this is an area where it is unacceptable for individuals' choices to impinge pejoratively on others. Although there may be, and many believe that there are, cases in which euthanasia or PAS is the morally best option for the individual concerned, the BMA currently holds that the impact of a general lifting of the ban on intentional killing by doctors would have detrimental effects on society and medical practice that outweigh the benefits for the small number of people who would use these types of legal provisions. Although there is consensus within the BMA that the balance is currently in favour of not changing the law, members hold a wide spectrum of opinions and it is important that the Association's views are analysed carefully and open for public debate.

This section takes the ethical and practical issues, where there is often overlap with the law, to discuss the arguments supporting the BMA's position. It begins with a summary of some of the arguments for and against euthanasia and PAS.

Summary of arguments

The notion of ending a human life deliberately is obviously a profound and disturbing concept. The large and scholarly literature on the subject of euthanasia and PAS reflects continuing attempts by philosophers, judges, lawyers, and others to marshal the arguments on either side of the debate and draw firm boundaries. This is an area in which establishing coherent limits is complicated. It may, therefore, appear simplistic to attempt to summarise briefly the bare bones of such arguments here. Nevertheless, medical students in particular often ask for a quick overview of the key issues that the BMA has debated and this is what the following section provides. A fuller explanation of the points is given in the sections that follow.

- In support of euthanasia and PAS
  - Autonomy and human rights mean that patients are entitled to exercise control over aspects of their death, and that those who need assistance to do so must be provided with it (pages 395–7 and 399–401).
  - Doctors have a duty to benefit patients by relieving pain and suffering; for some patients euthanasia or PAS is the only way to achieve this (page 397).
  - Empirical evidence from jurisdictions that permit euthanasia or PAS do not provide convincing evidence that their acceptance begins a slide down a "slippery slope" (pages 397–9).
  - Society should not fail to pursue options that would be beneficial for fear of being inadequately equipped to resist the dangers (pages 397–9).
  - Permitting euthanasia or PAS would show sympathy for patients who find living intolerable for various reasons (pages 401–3).

- Opposed to euthanasia and PAS:
  - Autonomy should be limited when its exercise would have an unacceptable impact on others (pages 395–7 and 399–401).
  - Permitting euthanasia and PAS would undermine patients' ability to trust their doctor's role as healer (page 397).
  - The "slippery slope" argument suggests that euthanasia and PAS could come to be seen as desirable not only for people able to choose for themselves but for others who cannot (pages 397–9).
  - Permitting euthanasia and PAS would weaken society's prohibition of intentional killing, and thus weaken the safeguards against non-voluntary euthanasia (pages 397–9).
  - A convincing justification for euthanasia or PAS in an individual case is distinct from justifying their availability (pages 401–3).

Autonomy and the impact on others

Supporters of PAS and euthanasia usually argue on grounds of autonomy, empowerment, self determination, and the right to choose. Throughout this book, however, ethical dilemmas are often found where autonomy ceases to be the trump card because of the impact of an individual's choices on others. Confidentiality, which is discussed in Chapter 5, is a good example: information about an individual may be disclosed without consent in order to prevent serious harm to somebody else. The rights of one person cannot be permitted to undermine disproportionately the rights of others. The case of Dianne Pretty (see pages 399–400) showed that the law is clear that autonomy has its limits, and that the rights of one group cannot be permitted disproportionately to undermine the rights of others. This was also a key argument of the House of Lords Select Committee.[16]

As well as the potential impact on the doctor–patient relationship, the BMA believes that there is a danger that even a limited change in the legislation would bring about a profound change in society's attitudes. By removing legal barriers to the previously "unthinkable" and permitting people to be killed, society would open up new possibilities of action and thus engender a frame of mind whereby some individuals may well be pressured to explore fully the extent of those new options. The choice of exercising a right to die at a chosen and convenient time could become an issue all individuals would have to take into account, even though they might otherwise not have entertained the notion.

It is frequently argued that if a patient's desire to be killed by a doctor was recognised as a legitimate right, some elderly or disabled people could see their lives as burdensome to others and feel pressured to choose to end them. The UN Human Rights Committee,[17] when it considered the Dutch criteria for euthanasia and PAS in detail, reported that the Dutch system "may fail to detect and prevent situations where undue pressure could lead to these criteria being circumvented". Willingness by society to supply or condone euthanasia could confirm patients' sense of worthlessness, resulting in a society in which individuals are not deemed valuable unless they are demonstrably useful.

There are, of course, inevitable pressures that influence people's choices. Some, however, society decides are too great to permit. If euthanasia or PAS were permitted, some people may well voluntarily choose to take account, for example, of being a burden on their families. The BMA believes, however, that it would be unacceptable if patients felt pressured to consider precipitating the end of their lives. People should be assured of their worth and efforts made to avoid the impression that their lives lack value. Of patients who made use of Oregon's Death with Dignity Act during its first five years, 44% cited their fear of being a burden to their family, friends, and carers as part of their reasoning for wanting to end their life.[18]

The BMA fears that, if the law in the UK were relaxed, euthanasia and PAS would become an option for anybody facing death. Not only might that put pressure on people to consider a premature death, but some could realistically fear that others would choose it for them. In the debates before the brief legalisation of euthanasia and PAS in Australia's Northern Territory, there was evidence of considerable disquiet from the indigenous Aboriginal population. The Australian Select Committee on Euthanasia reported that some Aborigines were afraid to attend health clinics and hospitals for fear of doctors having "the power to kill".[19] In the Netherlands, families request euthanasia more often than patients[20] and studies there too show that some elderly people fear their lives will be ended without their consent.[21] This is likely to be a continuing suspicion among patient groups who feel particularly marginalised within the system of health care provision.

The BMA believes that there is also a danger that people close to patients who choose suicide will be harmed. At a consensus conference on PAS in March 2000,

BMA members agreed that an important factor was the impact on doctors' relationships with people who are close to their patients, and the potential for distress among those relatives, friends, and carers.[22]

The doctor–patient relationship

Some believe that providing euthanasia or PAS would be a natural extension of the medical profession's role as relievers of suffering. Since doctors may cease to strive to prolong life in certain limited circumstances (see pages 352–64), knowing that the patient will inevitably die as a result, why not achieve that result by active steps to kill? The BMA's views on this are discussed in detail on pages 353–4 and 391–2. The BMA believes that the debate is not about whether there is a difference of omission or commission – killing and letting die – but it is rather about the intention behind the doctor's actions. When treatment is withheld or withdrawn, the intention is not to kill but to avoid providing a treatment that cannot benefit the patient.

If doctors are authorised to kill or to help to kill, however carefully circumscribed the situation, they acquire an additional role that the BMA believes is alien to the one of caregiver and healer. The traditional doctor–patient relationship is founded on trust, which risks being lost if the doctor's role also encompasses intentional killing. In a famous quote, Capron summed this up:

I never want to have to wonder whether the physician coming into my hospital room is wearing the white coat ... of a healer – concerned only to relieve my pain and to restore me to health – or the black hood of the executioner. Trust between patient and physician is simply too important and too fragile to be subjected to this unnecessary strain.[23]

In some circumstances it may be that neither patient nor carers, and perhaps not even the doctors themselves, can be quite certain which role has been adopted.

"Slippery slope" arguments

In this area, "slippery slope" arguments are commonly invoked. Once a previously prohibited action becomes allowed, according to the "slippery slope" argument, it may come to be seen as desirable not only for people able to choose for themselves, but also for others who cannot. In other words, the reasoning underpinning claims for a right to voluntary euthanasia could easily be extended to those who are incapable of making any claim for themselves. The fear is that those "others" will typically be elderly people, which is a particular worry at a time when an ageing population is raising the question of imbalance between financial providers and financial dependants in many developed countries.

In 2001 the UN Human Rights Committee considered the Dutch criteria for euthanasia and PAS in detail, and reported its concern "that, with the passage of time, such a practice may lead to routinization and insensitivity to the strict application of the requirements in a way not anticipated".[24] This is another of the concerns about "slippery slopes", that permitting voluntary euthanasia may result in non-voluntary euthanasia because the safeguards against the latter would have been weakened.

In contrast, some philosophers argue that not all slopes are necessarily slippery but may reflect reasoned choices about changing moral boundaries. It could be considered irrational or immoral to decide not to pursue options that would be beneficial for fear of being inadequately equipped to resist the dangers outlined throughout this chapter.[25]

It is worth looking to the Netherlands, whose 30 years' experience with euthanasia and PAS has been subjected to continuous scrutiny, for evidence of slippery slopes. Guidelines, which were later to be given statutory force by the Termination of Life on Request and Assisted Suicide Act 2001, were published by the Royal Dutch Medical Association in 1984, when the Dutch Supreme Court ruled that euthanasia and PAS were lawful in certain circumstances. It is clear that over the years, the rules were sometimes neglected.

Due care criteria for euthanasia and assisted suicide in the Netherlands

Doctors must:

(a) be satisfied that the patient has made a voluntary and carefully considered request

(b) be satisfied that the patient's suffering was unbearable, and that there was no prospect of improvement

(c) have informed the patient about his or her situation and his or her prospects

(d) have come to the conclusion, together with the patient, that there is no reasonable alternative in the light of the patient's situation

(e) have consulted at least one other, independent physician, who must have seen the patient and given a written opinion on the due care criteria referred to in points a–d above

(f) have terminated the patient's life or provided assistance with suicide with due medical care and attention.[26]

Breaches of the rules included involuntary euthanasia, failure to consult another practitioner before carrying out euthanasia, and certifying the cause of death as natural.[27] Some may see this as lending credence to the view that even careful circumscription of the practice cannot guarantee observance of the rules. The existence of rules permitting euthanasia in some circumstances may well have the effect of making instances of non-voluntary euthanasia, or even medical error, harder to detect.

Similarly, of course, rules prohibiting euthanasia and PAS may be ignored in countries that ban these activities completely. Evidence supports the claim that these acts undoubtedly occur clandestinely everywhere. In a survey of UK doctors in

1996, 4% reported providing a patient with the means to kill himself or herself and 12% reported personally knowing another health professional who had assisted a patient to kill himself or herself.[28]

Keown claims that the lack of adherence to the rules in the Netherlands "lends weighty support" to the slippery slope argument.[29] Griffiths and colleagues, on the other hand, claim that Keown's work does not show evidence of a slope at all, much less one that is slippery.[30] Looking specifically at non-voluntary euthanasia, they claim that there is no evidence that its incidence increased in the 30 years during which euthanasia was practised openly, nor that the rates are higher in the Netherlands than elsewhere, although data can be hard to compare, especially where the practice is clandestine and definitions unclear.

The empirical evidence about other jurisdictions' experiences cannot tell us whether permitting euthanasia or PAS in the UK would begin a slide down a slippery slope towards deliberately ending the lives of patients who have not chosen this for themselves. The BMA believes, however, that this risk cannot be ruled out.

Human rights and assistance in dying

Supporters of a right to die often present this issue as one of personal liberty, maintaining that individuals should be entitled to end their lives at the time and in the manner they choose, and to be given the assistance they need. During 2001 and 2002, Dianne Pretty sought to persuade the domestic[31] and European[32] courts of her entitlement to these things by reference to the Human Rights Act 1998. She claimed that the UK's prohibition on assisted suicide infringed her rights.

Assisted suicide – a human right?

Dianne Pretty suffered from motor neurone disease. No treatment can prevent the progression of the disease, and respiratory failure and pneumonia are the usual causes of death. Mrs Pretty told the courts that she was frightened and distressed at the suffering and indignity that she would endure if the disease ran its course, and that she very strongly wanted to be able to control how and when she died. The nature of the disease prevented her from taking her own life. Although she wanted assistance primarily from her husband, he made it clear that he wanted medical advice in order to be able to do so. Mrs Pretty sought an undertaking from the Director of Public Prosecutions that her husband would not be prosecuted under the Suicide Act 1961 if he assisted her suicide.

Losing her case in the domestic courts, Mrs Pretty took her human rights arguments to the European Court of Human Rights. Her case rested on a number of Human Rights Act points. She claimed that the right to life in Article 2 of the European Convention on Human Rights[33] guaranteed her the right to choose whether or not to live, and that failure to guarantee this right breached

(Continued)

her Article 3 right to be free from inhuman or degrading treatment. Throughout her legal battle, the individual judges were sympathetic to her position, but they dismissed claims that Article 2 protected not only the right to life but also the right to choose whether or not to go on living. Mrs Pretty argued that allowing her assistance to commit suicide could not conflict with Article 2 because, otherwise, those countries in which assisted suicide was lawful would breach this provision. The European Court of Human Rights acknowledged that the extent to which a state permits, or regulates, the possibility for the infliction of harm on individuals raised conflicting considerations of personal freedom and public interest that could be resolved only on examination of the concrete circumstances of the case. It concluded, however, that, even if the circumstances prevailing in a particular country did not infringe Article 2, the proposition that the UK breached its obligations by not permitting assisted suicide was a different issue.

Article 8 of the Convention protects people's private lives. Mrs Pretty argued that the state was unduly interfering with her right to choose to die. Interference with a person's Article 8 right is acceptable in some circumstances, where it is in accordance with the law, has a legitimate aim, and is necessary in a democratic society. Although the European Court found that Mrs Pretty's Article 8 right had been engaged, it did not consider the UK's blanket ban on assisted suicide in order to protect the vulnerable was a disproportionate interference with this right.

The European Court also considered whether Mrs Pretty's Article 14 right to be free from discrimination in her enjoyment of other Convention rights had been breached. She argued that she was prevented from exercising a right enjoyed by others who could end their lives without assistance and were not legally prevented from doing so. The relevant provisions of the 1961 Act existed to protect the weak and vulnerable, but Mrs Pretty argued that she was not in that category. The court noted that there are clear risks of abuse if assisted suicide is permitted, and that it is for states to assess these risks. The risk of abuse of those who are vulnerable was a reasonable justification for treating people in analogous situations differently (or treating people in different situations the same way) so there was no breach of Article 14.

Pretty v United Kingdom[34]

In all, 15 judges in the domestic and European courts found that the UK's prohibition on assisting suicide was not incompatible with the European Convention on Human Rights. Dianne Pretty's initial approach to the courts was to ask for a declaration that the Director of Public Prosecutions (DPP) would not take action against her husband if he assisted her suicide. The European Court's judgment focused on whether the Convention required the UK to permit Mrs Pretty's request, rather than whether it would have been within the remit of the DPP to grant immunity. It has been suggested that this is unfortunate because this is an area in which states take different approaches, all of which may well be compatible with the Convention.[35] That the courts often give relatively minor, even non-custodial, sentences to people involved in mercy killings could suggest that a declaration from the DPP would not have been incompatible with the law's approach.

Dianne Pretty's case also highlights the definitional problems in this area. Although her challenge was to the prohibition of assisted suicide, circumstances forced her to need euthanasia, not just assistance.

Compromising principles to suit the circumstances?

Doctors have a duty to try to provide patients with a peaceful and dignified death with minimal suffering but, as is indicated throughout this chapter, the BMA considers it contrary to the doctor's role to kill patients, even at their request. Requests may come from patients with terminal illness, people with severe and intractable physical and emotional suffering, or those with progressive neurological disease. Despite the patients' condition, assisting their suicide remains deeply controversial, particularly when a psychological rather than a physical problem is concerned.

Assisted suicide in a case of psychological suffering

In the mid-1990s, the Dutch courts found that psychological suffering, even in the absence of terminal illness, was legitimate grounds for a doctor to assist suicide. Dr Chabot had helped a 50-year-old woman to commit suicide. The woman's two sons had died: one from cancer, and the other had committed suicide. She had been abused by her alcohol dependent husband. Dr Chabot, a psychiatrist, came to know his patient well over several months and concluded that she was not suffering from any diagnosable psychiatric disorder. Notwithstanding this, he recommended antidepressants and psychotherapy, but her wish was to commit suicide in a foolproof and painless way. Dr Chabot thought that her condition fell within the Royal Dutch Medical Association's rules of due care, and provided her with a lethal drink, which she took in her own home. He reported the death to the coroner, and was subsequently charged under article 294 of the Dutch Penal Code. His case went to the Supreme Court in 1994.

The court ruled that psychological suffering could fulfil the necessary criteria to make assisted suicide lawful, since what mattered was the amount of suffering, not its origin. Dr Chabot, however, had failed to obtain the opinion of an independent medical expert, as required in the rules of due care, and accordingly was found guilty of an offence. The Supreme Court declined to impose a penalty, although in February 1995 Dr Chabot received a reprimand from a Medical Disciplinary Tribunal.

Although the Dutch accept that psychological suffering may be grounds for euthanasia and PAS, in almost all its cases the patients are terminally ill; in 58% the shortening of life was estimated to be one week at most and in 83% less than one month.[36]

Supreme Court of the Netherlands. Arrest-Chabot[37]

Clearly, doctors have a very profound sympathy for patients who find living intolerable for various reasons, and arguments in favour of legalisation often use moving examples of patients in this situation. Timothy Quill describes in detail the response of one of his patients to the offer of treatment for acute myelomonocytic leukaemia that offered her a 25% chance of long term survival: "it became clear that she was convinced she would die during the period of treatment and would suffer unspeakably in the process (from hospitalisation, from lack of control over her body, from the side-effects of chemotherapy, and from pain and anguish)".[38] His patient, Diane, chose to end her life with barbiturates, which he provided to her together with information about the amount needed to commit suicide. His account is profoundly moving. Many people believe that euthanasia or PAS would be morally justifiable in cases such as this. As Beauchamp and Childress put it, however, "to justify an act is distinct from justifying a practice or a policy that permits or even legitimises the act's performance".[39] The BMA strongly supports this view, and believes it is right that this issue is fought not only on ethical grounds but also on grounds of public policy.

It is obvious that the profession must hope soon to arrive at the situation where skilled management of pain and distress is available and effective for everyone. The BMA and others[40] believe that this will minimise the number of requests for euthanasia and PAS from people near the end of their lives, although it will not eliminate them altogether. Many requests for euthanasia are not based on the presence of pain, but on patients' increasing sense of worthlessness and distress about their dependence on others.

Reasons for requests for physician assisted suicide – experience from Oregon

Oregon's Death with Dignity Act came into force at the end of 1997. It permitted doctors to prescribe lethal medication for competent patients over the age of 18. The action to end life, if it is taken, is carried out by the patient.

Of the patients who sought a lethal prescription in the first five years of Oregon's Death with Dignity Act, fear of inadequate pain control was a factor for only 22%.[41] Only the financial implication of treatment was reported less frequently as being a factor. Aspects that patients reported as more relevant included being a burden on their family, friends, or carers, losing their autonomy, a decreasing ability to participate in activities that make life enjoyable, and losing control of bodily functions.

Skilled and compassionate palliative care, with good communication and patient involvement, can help with these issues. There will always be people, however, for whom palliative care does not meet their needs and wishes, for example those who believe that they have a civil right to choose when and how to die. Requests for euthanasia and PAS are therefore unlikely to be eliminated entirely.

Evidence suggests that the current numbers who actually want assistance in dying are very small. Between 1998 and 2002, 38 Oregonians died after ingesting legally prescribed lethal medication, an average of less than 9/10 000 deaths per year. During this period, 198 lethal prescriptions were written.[42] Although the cases of the individuals who did choose to die in this way may, to many, justify euthanasia or PAS, the BMA remains swayed by the public policy argument that the risks of harm to the vast majority are too great.

The House of Lords Select Committee on Medical Ethics concluded similarly. Although it had been profoundly moved by the people and arguments in favour of euthanasia, ultimately it did not believe the arguments to be sufficient reason to weaken society's prohibition of intentional killing. The Committee acknowledged that "there are individual cases in which euthanasia may be seen by some to be appropriate. But individual cases cannot reasonably establish the foundation of a policy which would have such serious and widespread repercussions".[43]

Summary – moral, legal, and pragmatic issues

- A line is drawn between an active decision not to continue with futile treatment and so allow a patient to die as "nature takes its course", on the one hand, and any affirmative action undertaken with the intent of ending life, on the other. The former, unless an omission resulting from negligence, is both ethical and legal, whereas the latter is both illegal and ethically unacceptable.
- In the BMA's view, legalising euthanasia and PAS would have a profound and detrimental effect on the doctor–patient relationship.
- Although people's right to choose is important, it must be limited where offering choice would cause harm to others.
- Not all slopes are slippery, but there is little evidence on which to base an assessment of whether permitting euthanasia and PAS would lead to non-voluntary acts. We do know, however, that where it is allowed and regulated, the rules are sometime disregarded. This danger should not be dismissed.
- It would be unacceptable to put vulnerable people in the position of feeling they had to consider precipitating the end of their lives.
- Widespread and equitable availability of palliative care services will minimise the number of requests for euthanasia and PAS.
- The BMA acknowledges that there are some patients for whom palliative care will not meet their needs and wishes, but considers that the risks of significant harm to a large number of people are too great to accommodate the needs of very few.
- Despite the wide range of views among its membership, there is consensus within the BMA that the law should not be changed to permit euthanasia or PAS in the UK.
- Because these issues are complex and fascinating, the BMA welcomes open and transparent discussion.

Practical issues for doctors in the UK

This section covers the kinds of questions with which practising UK doctors approach the BMA. As has already been noted, doctors know that euthanasia and PAS are illegal. With euthanasia, the boundary of the law is fairly clear. With PAS, however, it may be less so. Handing somebody a cup containing a lethal cocktail of drugs knowing he or she was going to drink it would clearly be assisting suicide, but what about writing a prescription for a quantity of medication that could be fatal or advising about how much medication, and in what combination, would kill?

Identifying legal boundaries

In the early 1980s, the Voluntary Euthanasia Society (or Exit as it had formerly been known) produced and distributed a booklet entitled *A guide to self-deliverance*. Its preface said:

> When people talk of "the fear of death", they often fail to distinguish between two types of fear which may be combined in experience but are separate in origin. One is the fear of the state of death (or non-existence); the other the fear of the process of dying, the agony of the transition to that state. The aim of this booklet – and of the society which, after much soul-searching, decided to publish it – is to overcome the second of these fears.

The booklet claimed not to encourage suicide, and indeed to discourage it for frivolous or ill thought out reasons. It advised that a decision to commit suicide should be taken over a substantial period – months rather than weeks – and that alternative solutions should be considered. It claimed to aim to reduce the number of unsuccessful suicides, described "how not to do it" and set out five separate methods of "self deliverance".

Whether it was lawful to publish and distribute the book was considered in 1983 in the High Court.[44] The case centred around the Suicide Act 1961, which made aiding, abetting, counselling, or procuring the suicide of another unlawful.[45] The court considered all four parts of the offence together, and drew on academic writings[46] to identify the following criteria for an offence:

- that the accused knew that suicide was contemplated
- that he or she approved or assented to it and
- that he or she encouraged the suicide attempt.

The court found that there was nothing objectionable about the booklet's content, and that it could deter many a would-be suicide, but in some cases it would assist people to commit suicide when they may not otherwise do so. The Society was therefore found to have the intent necessary for an offence. It intended the booklet to be used by somebody who was contemplating suicide and to help that person to do so. It knowingly distributed the booklet to people in this position. Finally, an offence would be committed when the booklet assisted or encouraged people to take their own lives. It was subsequently withdrawn.

Attorney General v Able and others[44]

Many patients are articulate and vocal about their wishes for the end of their life. Against this background, doctors can feel more insecure and morally uncertain. Not least among these dilemmas is the degree to which a doctor can be frank and open with a patient about the effects of medication while not endorsing or facilitating a patient's implied or explicit intention to commit suicide. By attempting to do what they perceive to be the best for patients and to comply with their wishes, doctors can very easily fall foul of the law. It is essential to remember that assisting suicide carries a legal penalty of up to 14 years' imprisonment. Clearly, if a patient is depressed or suffering from a mental disturbance, therapy and counselling should be recommended. In any case, when the patient could enjoy more years of life, all reasonable efforts should be made to achieve that. Patients who are terminally ill or feel that their quality of life is irretrievably low present a dilemma. Doctors should listen to patients who ask for assistance to commit suicide, and give them control of their decision making as far as possible, in the hope that they will not resort to an extreme act. Doctors must not, however, advise patients about the quantity or combination of medication that would kill. Prescribing or supplying drugs with the intention of enabling patients to shorten their lives could lead to prosecution for assisting suicide. As the case above shows, so could the provision of advice or literature on the subject. For example, a doctor who makes drugs available knowing that the patient is likely to take a fatal overdose could be committing a crime.[47] The courts have also held that putting people in touch with someone who will help them to end their life is an offence.[48] Doctors have to be honest with patients and explain that they will not act illegally but will do all they can to provide the care and support they need at the end of their lives.

Medical tourism

Oregon chose to prohibit non-residents from using the provisions of its PAS legislation. Other jurisdictions do not have equivalent conditions, but arguably some do prevent people travelling to the country specifically for the purpose of having their life ended, by including a requirement that there is a close relationship between the doctor and the patient. In the Netherlands, for example, the legal procedure for the notification and assessment of each case of euthanasia requires the patient to have made a voluntary, well considered request, and to be suffering unbearably without any prospect of improvement. The Dutch Government claims that, in order to be able to assess whether this is indeed the case, the doctor must know the patient well.[49] This implies that the doctor has treated the patient for some time. The Government also notes that granting a request for euthanasia places a considerable emotional burden on the doctor. Doctors do not approach the matter lightly. From this point of view too, longstanding personal contact between the doctor and the patient plays an important role.

In Switzerland, euthanasia is illegal, but the penalty may be mitigated if the actor's motives are honourable, for example, in a case of mercy killing at a person's request. Assisted suicide is unlawful too, but only where the assistance involves a selfish motive.

Swiss right to die organisations provide assistance with dying in accordance with these aspects of Swiss law. There is nothing to require a longstanding doctor–patient relationship, nor for the person seeking assistance to be resident in the country.

Suicide tourism

In 2002 a 74-year-old man from Liverpool died after travelling to Switzerland for assisted suicide using barbiturates supplied by the right to die organisation Dignitas. Mr Reginald Crew, who had motor neurone disease, was accompanied to Switzerland by his wife and a television crew.[50]

Merseyside police investigated the circumstances of Mr Crew's death and concluded that there was insufficient evidence of an offence to seek the consent to pursue a prosecution under section 2(1) of the Suicide Act 1961.[51]

This high profile case reportedly caused alarm within the Swiss authorities because of Switzerland being seen as a centre for "suicide tourism".[52]

Travelling abroad for procedures that are prohibited in the UK is an issue in several areas of medical practice (see Chapter 8, pages 302–3). As the case of Mr Crew shows, however, travelling abroad for assisted suicide may have implications for the people involved. In the BMA's view it would be unethical, as well as unlawful, for UK doctors to provide information about the availability of euthanasia or assisted suicide in other jurisdictions. If patients ask, doctors should explain that they cannot advise about such matters.

Views of the public

Opinion polls provide some indication of the views of the public, and how these change over time. Polls tend to show considerable public support for euthanasia. In 1996 the British Social Attitudes Report noted that 82% of the British population said that individuals should have the right to ask a doctor to end their life if they are suffering from an incurable and painful disease.[53] Opinion polls in other countries where euthanasia and PAS are illegal appear to show similar levels of support: 70–85% in Germany, the USA, Spain, and France.[54] Where voters are given the opportunity to register their views about proposed legal change, there is also considerable support. In 2002, 72% of Belgians were in favour of changing the law to permit euthanasia.[55] In 1994, 51% of Oregon's voters were in favour of changing the law to permit assisted suicide. A move to repeal Oregon's legislation in November 1997 was defeated by a margin of 60% to 40%.[56] These figures give some indication of society's views, although it is notoriously difficult to gain a clear picture of support for euthanasia and PAS because much depends on the way in which the questions are put, definitional overlap, and confusion with other end of life issues such as withdrawing and withholding treatment.

This substantial public support does not translate into large numbers of people who actually seek these forms of assistance in dying. In Oregon, for example, less than 1 in 1000 deaths involve a lethal prescription.[57] Some patients who obtain a prescription for lethal medication do not use it. Again, in Oregon, of the 58 people who received prescriptions in 2002, 16 had died from their underlying disease by the end of the year (six were still alive).[58] The fact that not all people who receive a prescription go on to use it could show that even those who are apparently determined to end their lives may change their minds or never reach the stage when they feel the need. Alternatively, it may reinforce the view that personal control is what is really at stake.

The future?

Despite significant public[59] and professional[60] interest in the possibility of doctors intervening to end life, there is little indication that lawmakers would welcome change. Bills brought before the UK Parliament have failed to progress,[61] the legal problems associated with undermining the law of homicide being as likely a cause for this as ethical reasoning. The House of Lords Select Committee on Medical Ethics, appointed to consider the likely effects of a change in the law on euthanasia, also rejected law reform.[62]

In its concluding remarks the Committee said that, despite the very moving cases of deaths that were far from peaceful or uplifting, and the moral arguments in favour of euthanasia, ultimately it did

> not believe that these arguments are sufficient to weaken society's prohibition of intentional killing. The prohibition is the cornerstone of law and of social relationships. It protects each one of us impartially, embodying the belief that all are equal. We do not wish that protection to be diminished and we therefore recommend that there should be no change in the law to permit euthanasia.[63]

In the months preceding the implementation of the Human Rights Act there was considerable speculation about its likely impact on medical practice. Even after the courts ruled in Dianne Pretty's case (see pages 399–400) that the UK was not required to permit assisted suicide, legal commentators challenged the courts' findings and argued that the prohibition is incompatible with the Convention.[64] Others remarked that the courts' conclusions were inevitable.[65]

Debate within the healthcare professions and society about legalising euthanasia and PAS will continue. It is essential that society's decisions are made on the basis of a thorough examination of the values it wants to uphold. In relation to euthanasia and PAS, this involves looking at notions of harm and benefit, autonomy and its limits, how to benefit patients while at the same time avoid harming others, whether stepping beyond one legal boundary would lead inevitably to further steps, whether permitting an action trivialises it and makes it easier to undertake, and how important that ultimately is. Although the medical profession has an important voice in the debate, ultimately these decisions are for society as a whole, not just doctors.

References

1   Books that focus wholly or primarily on euthanasia and PAS include: Battin MP, Rhodes R, Silvers A. *Physician assisted suicide. Expanding the debate.* London: Routledge, 1998. Dworkin R. *Life's dominion. An argument about abortion and euthanasia.* London: Harper Collins, 1993. Griffiths J, Bood A, Weyers H. *Euthanasia and law in the Netherlands.* Amsterdam: Amsterdam University Press, 1998. Keown J. *Euthanasia, ethics and pubic policy. An argument against legalisation.* Cambridge: Cambridge University Press, 2002. McLean SAM, ed. *Death, dying and the law.* Aldershot: Dartmouth, 1996. Quill TE. *A midwife through the dying process. Stories of healing and hard choices at the end of life.* Baltimore: Johns Hopkins University Press, 1996. Weir RF, ed. *Physician assisted suicide.* Bloomington, IN: Indiana University Press, 1997.

2   House of Lords. *Report of the Select Committee on Medical Ethics.* London: HMSO, 1994. (HLP 21-I.)

3   Rights of the Terminally Ill Act 1995. The Northern Territory's legislation was repealed by federal legislation that removed the power of territories (but not states) to make legislation that has the effect of permitting euthanasia or assisted suicide.

4   Suicide Act 1961 s2(1). In Northern Ireland, "A person who aids, abets, counsels or procures the suicide of another, or an attempt by another to commit suicide, shall be guilty of an offence and shall be liable on conviction on indictment to imprisonment for a term not exceeding fourteen years." Criminal Law (Suicide) Act 1993. Assisting suicide in Scotland could lead to a charge of murder or culpable homicide. For discussion see: Ferguson PR. Killing "without getting into trouble"? Assisted suicide and Scots criminal law. *Edinb Law Rev* 1998;**2**:288–314.

5   R v Woollin [1998] 4 All ER 103.

6   For a discussion from a pro-euthanasia perspective, see: Doyal L. Why active euthanasia and physician assisted suicide should be legalised. *BMJ* 2001;**323**:1079–80. For a discussion from an anti-euthanasia perspective, see: Keown J. Part IV. Passive euthanasia: withholding/withdrawing treatment and tube-feeding with intent to kill. In: Keown J. *Euthanasia, ethics and public policy. An argument against legalisation.* Cambridge: Cambridge University Press, 2002.

7   Mr Justice Devlin in the case of R v W Adams [1957] CLR 365. Quoted in: Devlin P. Easing the passing. *The trial of Dr John Bodkin Adams.* London: The Bodley Head, 1985:171–2.

8   *Ibid*: 172.

9   McLean SAM, Britton A. *Sometimes a small victory.* Glasgow: Institute of Law and Ethics in Medicine, 1996:table 22. The survey was funded by the Voluntary Euthanasia Society of Scotland and carried out by an independent agency.

10   General Medical Council. *Withholding and withdrawing life-prolonging treatments: good practice in decision-making.* London: GMC, 2002: para 8.

11   General Medical Council Professional Conduct Committee hearing, 16–26 November 1992.

12   McLean SAM, *et al. Sometimes a small victory. Op cit.*

13   Details of the BMA's consensus conference, and a complete report of its outcomes, are available on the BMA's website.

14   R v Charlotte Helen Hough (1984) 6 Cr App R (S) 406.

15   BMA. Annual Representative Meeting. Harrogate, 2002. Motion 636.

16   House of Lords. *Report of the Select Committee on Medical Ethics. Op cit.*

17   United Nations Human Rights Committee. *Concluding observations of the Human Rights Committee: Netherlands.* Geneva: UN, 2001. (CCPR/CO/72/NET.)

18   Department of Human Services. *Fifth annual report on Oregon's Death with Dignity Act.* Oregon: DHS, 2003:20.

19   Select Committee on Euthanasia. *Report of the inquiry on the right of the individual or the common good? Vol. 2.* Darwin: Legislative Assembly of the Northern Territory, 1995.

20   Fenigsen R. Mercy, murder and morality: perspectives on euthanasia. A case against Dutch euthanasia. *Hastings Cent Rep* 1989;**19**(1)(suppl):S22–30.

21   Segers JH. Elderly persons on the subject of euthanasia. *Issues Law Med* 1988;**3**:429–37.

22   British Medical Association. *Physician assisted suicide: statements from a conference to promote the development of consensus.* London: BMA, 2000.

23   Capron AM. Legal and ethical problems in decisions for death. *Law Med Health Care* 1986;**14**:141–4:144.

24   United Nations Human Rights Committee. *Concluding observations of the Human Rights Committee: Netherlands. Op cit.*

25   Harris J. *The value of life.* London: Routledge, 1985.

26   Review procedures of termination of life on request and assisted suicide and amendment of the Criminal Code and the Burial and Cremation Act (Termination of Life on Request and Assisted Suicide (Review Procedures) Act) 2(1).

27 For a detailed discussion of how the guidelines were breached, see: Keown J. *Euthanasia, ethics and public policy. Op cit:* Chapter 10.
28 McLean SAM, *et al. Sometimes a small victory. Op cit.*
29 Keown J. Euthanasia in the Netherlands: sliding down the slippery slope? In Keown J, ed. *Euthanasia examined. Ethical, clinical and legal perspectives.* Cambridge: Cambridge University Press, 1995.
30 Griffiths J, *et al. Euthanasia and law in the Netherlands. Op cit:* pp. 26–8.
31 R v Director of Public Prosecutions (Respondent) ex parte Dianne Pretty (Appellant) and Secretary of State for the Home Department (Interested Party) [2002] 1 All ER 1.
32 Pretty v United Kingdom (2002) 35 EHRR 1.
33 *Convention for the protection of human rights and fundamental freedoms.* (4. ix. 1950; TS 71; Cmnd 8969.)
34 Pretty v United Kingdom (2002). *Op cit.*
35 Tur RHS. Legislative technique and human rights: the sad case of assisted suicide. *Criminal Law Rev* 2003;(Jan):3–12.
36 Medische beslissingen rond het levenseinde. I. *Rapport van de Commissie Onderzoek Medische Praktijk inzake* [I. Report of the Committee to Study Medical Practice Concerning Euthanasia] The Hague: Ministry of Justice and Ministry of Welfare, Public Health and Culture, 1991. (In Dutch.)
37 Supreme Court of the Netherlands. Arrest-Chabot, HR 21 juni 1994, nr 96 972.
38 Quill TE. A case of individualized decision making. *N Engl J Med* 1991;**324**:691–4: 692.
39 Beauchamp TL, Childress JF. *Principles of biomedical ethics, 5th ed.* New York: Oxford University Press, 2001.
40 See, for example: National Council for Hospice and Specialist Palliative Care Services. *Voluntary euthanasia: the Council's view.* London: National Council for Hospice and Specialist Palliative Care Services, 1997.
41 Department of Human Services. *Fifth annual report on Oregon's Death with Dignity Act.* Oregon: DHS, 2003:20.
42 *Ibid.*
43 House of Lords. *Report of the Select Committee on Medical Ethics. Op cit:* p. 48.
44 Attorney General v Able and others [1984] 1 All ER 277.
45 Suicide Act 1961 s2(1).
46 Cecil Turner FW, ed. *Russell on crime, 12th ed.* London: Stevens, 1964.
47 Montgomery J. *Health care law, 2nd ed.* New York: Oxford University Press, 2003:468.
48 R v Reed [1982] Crim LR 819.
49 Netherlands Ministry of Foreign Affairs International Information and Communication Department in cooperation with the Ministry of Health, Welfare and Sport and the Ministry of Justice. *Euthanasia. A guide to the Dutch Termination of Life on Request and Assisted Suicide (Review Procedures) Act.* The Hague: Netherlands Ministry of Foreign Affairs, 2001.
50 *Tonight with Trevor McDonald.* Reg's last journey – a Tonight special; ITV1, 2003 Jan 24.
51 The Solicitor-General. *House of Commons official report (Hansard).* 2003 Apr 10: col 346W.
52 Anonymous. Swiss to stop entry of "mercy death" Britons. *The Observer* 2003 Jan 26:5.
53 Jowell R, Curtice J, Park A, Brook L, Thomson K, eds. *British Social Attitudes: the 13th Report.* Aldershot: Dartmouth, 1996.
54 Voluntary Euthanasia Society. *Public opinion: factsheet.* London: VES, 2002.
55 Hovine A, Piret P. 72 pc de "oui" à la proposition euthanasie. *La Libre Belgique* 2001 Mar 28.
56 Oregon Public Health Services Center for Health Statistics (and Vital Records). *Oregon's Death with Dignity Act.* Oregon: Oregon Public Health Services, 2001.
57 Department of Human Services. *Fifth annual report on Oregon's Death with Dignity Act. Op cit.*
58 *Ibid:* p. 4.
59 Public support for doctors being allowed to end life on request was shown to be at levels of 82% in: Jowell R, *et al.,* eds. *British Social Attitudes: the 13th Report. Op cit.*
60 Support for a change in the law was shown to be at around 54% among health professionals in: McLean SAM, *et al. Sometimes a small victory. Op cit.*
61 Bills seeking to legalise voluntary euthanasia in 1936, 1969 and 1993 failed to progress.
62 House of Lords. *Report of the Select Committee on Medical Ethics. Op cit:* p. 48.
63 *Ibid.*
64 Tur RHS. Legislative technique and human rights: the sad case of assisted suicide. *Op cit.*
65 Freeman M. Denying death its dominion: thoughts on the Dianne Pretty case. *Med Law Rev* 2002;**10**:245–70.

12: Responsibilities after a patient's death

The questions covered in this chapter include the following.

- Why do the public and health professionals have differing expectations?
- What obligations do health professionals have for their deceased patients?
- Do relatives have a right to deceased patients' medical records or tissue samples?
- Should benefit for the living take precedence over protecting the dead as a general principle?
- Can relatives control what happens to a deceased person, including organ donation?
- Can cadavers be tested for infectious diseases to protect pathology staff?

Scope of this chapter

In this chapter, we look at ethical and legal issues that arise after a patient has died, mentioning a range of publications from authorities such as the Royal College of Pathologists, health departments, and the Retained Organs Commission. Discussion focuses on matters of principle because at the time of writing in 2003 much of the law in this area is set to change. Changes were expected on issues such as the coroners' system, death certification, the seeking of relatives' consent to postmortem examination, and the use and retention of human tissue. This means that there is only limited value in setting out the terms of current legislation and existing law is only briefly summarised.

A period of upheaval and public discussion about the values that underpin postmortem practice has occurred. Throughout the UK, public inquiries[1] into past organ retention practices challenged public confidence and created a legacy of distress and anger. At the same time, these inquiries recognised the essential nature of appropriate postmortem investigation and research. Nevertheless, "pathologists have felt under siege to the extent that some have left the service and new doctors have not chosen to specialise in the field".[2] This trend needs to be reversed and efforts made to restore public confidence in the service. This chapter includes a summary of some of the events that have focused public attention on this area and highlights some of the tensions involved. It does not address in any detail, however, societal attitudes to death, its rituals, or measures for coping with bereavement. Nor does the chapter explore comparative religious or cultural attitudes to death, although health professionals need to be aware of such factors in the communities they serve. A series of public consultations[3] have attempted to map out general societal expectations in relation to interventions on deceased people and these are mentioned here. Aspects of the management of deceased patients generate frequent queries to the BMA from doctors and medical students. Some of the most common questions are set out on pages 439–44.

General principles

The general ethical principles applicable to this sphere of practice include:

- the duty to show respect for people, living and dead
- the need to have clear and effective communication with people who were close to the deceased person
- the obligation to offer relatives as much information as they need about any medical procedure
- the duty to balance this openness with the duty of confidentiality owed to the dead patient
- the responsibility of demonstrating cultural awareness and sensitivity in relation to the existence in the community of differing attitudes to death
- the duty to bear in mind the public good and to promote ethical ways of maximising knowledge
- the duty to involve the public more in informed debate on matters pertaining to death and its management
- the duty to minimise harm and distress
- the need to have concern for justice.

The implementation of these principles is discussed on pages 422–6.

Terminology

Death and the handling of human remains after death are sensitive matters, particularly for bereaved people. Much of the traditional medical terminology relating to postmortem practice has undergone review, not only to make clear to the public what is involved but also to avoid insensitive language. Terms such as "disposal" are not ideal to describe human material because of the connotations, but such explicit terminology makes clear what is intended. In 2000 the interim report of *The inquiry into the management of care of children receiving complex heart surgery at the Bristol Royal Infirmary*[4] (Interim Bristol report) criticised the fact that, when families had previously been approached about hospital postmortem examinations, much information was left too vague. Consent forms, for example, "employed such unfamiliar terms that they were not understood or remembered".[5] They did not say what a postmortem examination involved or even what was meant by "tissue". Retention of "tissue" or "samples of human material" was sometimes mentioned when the actual intention was to keep entire organs. Sometimes, however, the need for unambiguous clarity and the search for sensitivity are in conflict. Individuals need to know what they are being asked to authorise, but there are circumstances in which they may choose not to have all the information that is available (although it should be offered). Although recognising the importance of sensitivity to relatives' feelings, the BMA is emphatic about the necessity for transparency and openness.

"**Consent**", "**authorisation**", and "**best interests**": Among the issues highlighted by the Independent Review Group on Retention of Organs at Post Mortem were some problems with the usual language of consent in this context.[6] The group's report argued that it is more appropriate to talk of relatives' "authorisation" rather than their "consent" and noted that parents have legal authority to consent only when the particular decision is in the "best interests" of their child. When the child has died, the notion of best interests is hard to apply. The semantics of "consent" and "authorisation" remain problematic, not least because many people see advantages in continuing to use "consent" (even if not strictly correct) because it is a term that is well understood by both health professionals and the public. As Brazier makes clear, however, the central ethical point is unambiguous. "However we define consent (or authorisation), its central feature is an entitlement to say no".[7] Also, whichever terminology is used, it is essential that it conveys the sense that bereaved families must be offered information in order to make a decision.

"**Next of kin**": We refer to "families" or "relatives" as a shorthand way of indicating that people emotionally close to the deceased person need to be involved in decisions. For many adults without close family ties, cohabiting partners, carers, or friends may be more in tune than blood relatives with the individual's values and intentions. Ideally, patients should have made some prior indication of whose views should be consulted. Where they have not done so, decisions have to be made on a case by case basis. In terms of discussing postmortem examinations, for example, doctors need to be aware that identifying the most appropriate person to give permission may not be straightforward and must be careful not to make assumptions.[8]

"**Postmortem examination**": The purpose of a postmortem examination is to discover the cause of death. The Royal College of Pathologists describes it as the final step in the investigation of an individual's illness, indicating that many health professionals perceive it as a continuation of the care process.[9] There are two types of postmortem examination: those which are a legal requirement and those that are elective ("hospital" postmortem examinations). Concerning the first type, in England, Wales, and Northern Ireland, a coroner can order a postmortem examination; in Scotland, a procurator fiscal has the same powers. These are the most common kind of postmortem examinations in the UK and the agreement of relatives is not required, although the family should be informed. (The common reasons for requiring a coroner's postmortem are listed on pages 441–2.) The second kind of postmortem examination is one requested by the doctor or health team who previously cared for the deceased person. This can be done only with the permission of the relatives unless the deceased person has already given prior consent. In either kind of postmortem examination – elective or legally obligatory – the prior consent of the deceased person or that of relatives is needed for the continued retention or use of organs or tissue after the examination. In the past, this requirement was not sufficiently clear, leading to the erroneous assumption that indefinite retention was permissible.

The "**gift relationship**": In the sphere of organ and tissue retention and use, considerable effort is made to shift the emphasis away from past language and culture to a situation where society understands better the importance of altruistic organ donation.[10] Such a gift relationship is already well understood in the context of donation for transplantation, but there is a need for much greater public information to be available about the benefits of tissue donation for research. In addition, families need more information about the benefits for future patients, as well as possibly for themselves, of agreeing to allow hospital postmortem examinations.

Changing expectations

The way in which deceased people are treated must reflect changing societal values. In 2000, however, it became clear that discrepancies had developed, particularly between public expectations and traditional medical practice regarding tissue and organ retention after autopsy. The chairman of the NHS Retained Organs Commission, Margaret Brazier, was one of many experts who referred to a "gulf between families' expectations and medical practice".[11] Early in 2000 professional guidance was already attempting to address such discrepancies. The Royal College of Pathologists[12] and the Department of Health,[13] for example, published guidance on the retention of tissues and organs.

Soon after, in May 2000, the Interim Bristol report[14] was the first of several drawing attention to the fact that, in the past, families of deceased patients had often been unaware of the retention of human tissue after postmortem examination. The Royal Liverpool Children's Inquiry report (the Alder Hey Inquiry)[15] documented the fact that body parts from deceased children had been retained at Alder Hey hospital without parents' knowledge. Although this is contrary to the legal obligations to make enquiry about whether relatives object to the body being retained for education or research,[16] the law in this area has long been unclear. "The 1961 (Human Tissue) Act does not expressly require that identifiable next of kin authorise autopsy or retention. It sets up a fuzzy no-objection rule",[17] which has universally been judged to be unsatisfactory and in need of legislative reform. (This is discussed further on page 420) As a result, a variety of inadequate consent mechanisms were in use prior to 2000, when a census by the Chief Medical Officer of England indicated that over 54 000 organs, body parts, stillborn children, or fetuses retained since 1970 were still held by English pathology services.[18] In Wales, Scotland, and Northern Ireland, there were similar findings. Later, in 2003, a subsequent investigation by HM Inspector of Anatomy discovered that large numbers of human brains had been retained for research without the knowledge of relatives, after coroners' postmortem examinations.[19] A Scottish review group set up in September 2000 to review past portmortem practice, particularly organ retention, developed a code of practice emphasising consent issues and recommended legal change.[20] In Northern Ireland, the Human Organs Inquiry was established in March 2001.[21] Also in 2001, the NHS Retained Organs Commission was set up to oversee the return of retained tissue and organs to relatives who wished to have them back.

Its remit also included providing advocacy for families and advising ministers about changes needed in the law relating to organ retention.

A major theme of all the reports was the lack of transparent process by which people could be informed of what was happening to bodies. Many families indicated that they would have supported the appropriate use of some of the retained material if they had been asked, but there was also particular anger among relatives about the retention of whole organs, particularly those with emotive connotations such as the heart or brain. When organs or tissue had been removed as part of a legal need to establish the cause of death (and relatives' authorisation to the actual removal was therefore not legally required), families had not even been informed that organs had been kept. Nor had their permission been sought for continued retention once the legal investigation was completed. Many of the recommendations from the public inquiries echoed the same key points. They set the tone for political debate and wide ranging proposals for reform of the law and pathology practice.

Some key recommendations from the public inquiries

- The Human Tissue Act 1961 and Human Tissue Act (Northern Ireland) 1962 should be urgently reformed.
- Families must be asked for permission for the retention of tissue after postmortem examination (except when deceased adult patients had previously made a decision to donate tissue).
- In particular, the rights of parents of minors must be fully respected.
- Staff in obstetric, neonatal, and paediatric units should have mandatory training in dealing with bereavement.
- Clear and uniform consent forms should be introduced.
- Good practice must be consistently enforced and consideration given to introducing penalties for non-consensual use of human material.
- Procurator fiscal services should improve liaison with bereaved relatives, such as by "next of kin interview clinics".
- Coronial rules should clarify the lack of any rights for pathologists to retain, use, or dispose of human tissue, except on the authority of the coroner or with families' agreement.
- Standard codes of practice should set out how to communicate with families about postmortem examinations.
- Public education and information programmes are needed to increase public understanding of postmortem procedures.
- Such information programmes should be explicit about different potential uses of human tissue, distinguishing clearly between donation for transplantation and other purposes.
- Elective hospital postmortem examinations should be seen as part of a continuum of care.
- Formal controls on the import and export of body parts are needed.
- Health professionals should have training in the law and good practice in this area.

Completely separate to the debate about reform of the law on the use and retention of human material, significant flaws in the systems of death certification, coronial investigation, and the issuing of cremation certificates were highlighted by the case of Dr Harold Shipman, whose murders of his patients remained undetected for decades. This raised questions about the safeguards intended to detect such patterns of abuse and triggered legal review of all these areas.

Some effects of the Harold Shipman case

In January 2000, a Manchester GP, Dr Harold Shipman, was sentenced to life imprisonment for the murder of 15 patients. In July 2002 the independent inquiry into the case found that he had begun killing patients in 1975 and had murdered at least 215.[22] It concluded that the true number of his victims could be far greater, but in some cases the evidence was inadequate to form an accurate view retrospectively. The inquiry sought to learn why Shipman had escaped detection for so long. Many of the deaths occurred suddenly without prior life threatening illness and so should have been reported to the coroner. By carrying out death certification himself and persuading relatives that no postmortem examination was needed, Shipman managed to avoid the involvement of coroners in all but a few cases. The inquiry found that a major weakness of the system had been the lack of exchange of information between those involved in the various stages of death certification, registration of the death, and preparation for cremation. This meant that no person had an overview of the circumstances of the death. Relatives were neither able to find out what had been written nor asked to give their own views about the death. The death certification review was initiated and the inquiry also examined the system of cremation certificates.

In March 2001, a review was commenced of the coroner system and the concept of introducing a new post of "medical examiner" was proposed. In addition, a new system of death certification involving such medical examiners began to be explored.

One effect of the debate around the Shipman case was to reinforce some pre-existing expectations that relatives should control what happened to dead people. In Shipman's case, if relatives had been able to access information easily after an individual's death, any inconsistencies regarding the diagnosis or treatment of his victims prior to death might have been identified earlier. The idea that families should have the final say in what happened to dead people was already widespread. For example, it was a common misperception among families in the mid-1990s that a postmortem examination invariably required permission from relatives.[23] Although the law has not traditionally recognised any "ownership" of bodies, there is a growing expectation that relatives should control the remains and also the medical information of deceased people. This expectation challenges the traditional view of health professionals that they owe duties of confidentiality to their deceased patients and have moral obligations to respect the wishes of deceased adults, even though these may clash with relatives' views.

Another separate change in this period was the establishment of a working group on human remains[24] to consider the legal status of collections of human material in publicly funded museums and art galleries. The fact that as a society we allow the exhibition of deceased people as mummies, for example, or their body parts as religious relics or objects of curiosity, appeared to clash with the sensitivity demanded for the care of our own relatives' remains. It was considered important to address such societal ambivalence and inconsistencies. Established in early 2001, the role of the working group included considering whether such collections gathered for artistic, educational, and cultural purposes should be brought within the same legislation as would be introduced to cover other stored human tissue.

Much of the subsequent ethical and legal debate about postmortem issues has taken place in the shadow of these events and changing expectations. Health professionals are sometimes confused about their own duties to deceased persons, especially if these seem to conflict with relatives' views, and tensions exist between professional and societal views. These need to be widely discussed. For example, a doctor's duty of confidentiality extends beyond the patient's death, restricting even what relatives can be told if that was the patient's former wish (see Chapter 5, page 168, and Chapter 6, pages 220–1). Similarly, the obligation for health professionals to respect adult patients' self determination, including through advance decision making, emphasises individuals' rather than relatives' wishes on issues such as organ donation. Sometimes, however, relatives argue that they should keep and own the records of deceased people in order to check that no negligence has occurred, or to help them to understand any inherited conditions in the family. A theme in this chapter is the need for clear frameworks to be in place to accommodate the potentially conflicting needs of relatives, the privacy of the individual, the requirements of the justice system, and society's desire for medical research and education. These need to be discussed and reflected in future legislation.

Society's and individuals' attitudes to deceased people

Individuals cope with loss in their own way. In her study of parents' response to the death of young children, McHaffie describes how "death and involvement mean different things to different people" by reference to the deep anger felt by one father on seeing a nurse cuddling his dead baby.[25] Another parent refused to show photographs of her dead child even to family members because they were too private for public scrutiny. In multicultural, multifaith settings, diverse views exist about the importance of the dead body and how it should be treated. Families are often intensely protective of deceased relatives, perceiving them still as loved individuals. Feelings about the moral presence of the dead fade only as time passes. Nevertheless, many decisions, such as the donation of organs for transplantation, have to be made quickly when families are likely to feel least ready to consider them. Knowledge of the deceased individual's own intentions are therefore vitally important.

Dignified, respectful, and culturally appropriate treatment of dead people is an essential requirement. Although the fundamental cause of distress for the relatives involved in the Alder Hey case was the lack of consent to organ removal, this was compounded by the unsatisfactory conditions in which some of the human material had been stored.[26] The inquiry strongly criticised the manner as well as the fact of tissue retention. Subsequently, one of the pathologists was prosecuted and fined in Canada for the improper and undignified storage of children's remains in a warehouse.[27] Public sensibilities were particularly shocked by the emotive nature of the case and the apparently major gap between public values and the attitude of that particular doctor, who was erroneously assumed to be representative of many pathologists. In simplistic terms, doctors were portrayed as treating cadavers as useful objects, whereas to the relatives they were still people. Society is shocked by any perceived lack of respect for the dignity of human bodies. In January 2001, for example, media criticism focused on the fact that some corpses had had to be placed on the floors of hospital mortuaries or chapels of rest.[28] Such treatment was perceived as unacceptable.

Religion, tradition, and moral intuition all lead us to show respect to dead people in order to honour the individuals they once were and in the hope that our own remains will be treated likewise. For those who are bereaved, the last acts of care and remembrance can be of vital importance in coming to terms with their loss. Parents continue to have very strong feelings of responsibility for a deceased child and therefore can experience guilt as well as distress if bereavement is compounded by what may appear as unjustified interference with the corpse. Other relatives too may feel that they have failed in their protective duty if arrangements after death seem to be wrong. Death after invasive treatment often evokes the response from relatives that the deceased person "has been through enough" and should not be exposed to further interventions such as a postmortem examination. Although people who donate their bodies for scientific purposes often describe the corpse as organic waste, rubbish, or an empty container, they may still worry about whether they will be treated respectfully.[29] Brazier reminds us that:

> Death, especially sudden or untimely death, leaves the funeral of a relative or friend as the last service those who loved him or her can render to them. The reality of death, or loss, takes time to come to terms with. The dead infant, the wife succumbing to breast cancer at 35, the elderly father dying suddenly of a heart attack do not change their nature for their mother, husband or daughter. They remain Susannah, Lucy and Dad. How each bereaved mother, husband or daughter grieves will differ dramatically ... The image of the newly dead person remains fixed in the mind of most bereaved families. Mutilation of the body becomes a mutilation of that image. Reason may tell the family that a dead child could not suffer when organs were removed. Grief coupled with imagination may overpower reason. Families grieve differently just as they live their lives differently. Respect for family life requires respect for such differences.[30]

Maintaining the integrity of the body is an important issue for some people and, even within specific religious faiths, individuals' views may differ. Disfigurement or mutilation of cadavers arouses particular anxiety. Distress about the notion of their child's body being cut is a primary reason for parents to refuse an autopsy, for example, and reassurance about lack of disfigurement of the body is a potent factor in their agreement to it.[31] Similarly, in 2001 an Australian inquiry[32] into limitations on the research use of donated cadavers argued that some valid distinction could be made between scientific activities that left the corpse seriously disfigured and acts that did not.

Historically, society reserved procedures such as anatomical dissection for people about whom there was little societal concern: condemned criminals for whom it was part of a punishment extending beyond death, inmates of institutions, or destitute persons.[33] A lingering sense of this view remains in some cultures. In 1991, for example, when the BMA objected to the linking of organ donation to execution in Taiwan, the National University Hospital defended the practice saying that cultural and religious requirements for bodies to be buried intact made donation morally unacceptable to many people. For prisoners, however, automatic organ donation after execution was "an act of contrition".[34] For the public, the notion of dissection has long involved a mixture of repulsion and fascination. Such societal ambivalence was manifest when in 2002 a public anatomical dissection was broadcast on television, provoking calls for the anatomist to be prosecuted.[35] Many people objected to the manner in which this took place, perceiving it as a misuse of the human body for entertainment. Others saw it as an educational experience, a reminder of our mortality and an attempt to demystify death for a public increasingly unfamiliar with the sight of dead people. Such ambivalence needs wider discussion.

Although, in purely practical terms, dead people cannot be physically harmed, profound societal abhorrence is generated by failure to respect human remains and any failure to consider the effect on relatives. Furthermore, even though dead people are not attributed rights, the use of improperly obtained cadavers or human material is increasingly recognised as a violation of accepted standards. Their improper provenance is often seen as nullifying any benefits that may be gained for living people. For example, the retention of historical collections of human samples from aboriginal people has become unacceptable in the same way as the use of material or data from Nazi concentration camps was investigated and denounced in the postwar period.[36] The morality of retaining ancient bodies in museums is questioned and many such remains have been returned to their descendants. In May 2003, for example, the remains of 300 aboriginal Australians of the Ngarrindjeri tribe, which had been held in museums in Edinburgh, London, and Sydney, were returned to tribal elders for burial.[37] The acceptability of importing human anatomical samples from developing countries is also in doubt unless donor consent is documented.[38] Wishes that donors expressed in their lifetime should help to elucidate the boundaries of acceptable usage of their cadaveric material but, even so, society retains reservations about measures such as the use of donated human bodies to test safety systems in car crashes. Similarly, the plastination of bodies as art exhibits not only raises fundamental questions of consent and appropriate usage of human material, but also its potential commodification as saleable merchandise. Society as a whole will increasingly have to consider such issues.

The law

Legal issues concerning the handling of dead bodies are covered only briefly here because significant changes to some aspects are anticipated.

Legislation in force in 2003

Human Tissue Act 1961 and Human Tissue Act (Northern Ireland) 1962[39]

The legislation allows individuals in their lifetime to designate that their bodies be used for therapeutic purposes, medical education, or research. On death, the person "lawfully in possession" of the body can comply with the donor's advance request unless there are grounds to believe the bequest was withdrawn. The person lawfully in possession of the body can also authorise removal of tissue for therapy, education, or research, or authorise a hospital postmortem examination (as opposed to a compulsory coroner's postmortem) as long as there is no reason for believing that the deceased or close relatives would have objected. In order to check this fact, "such reasonable enquiry as may be practicable" must be made.

Anatomy Act 1984

The Anatomy Act enables adults to bequeath their bodies for anatomical examination by dissection for teaching, study, or research purposes. The request to donate must be specific, in writing or, exceptionally, a witnessed oral request. The bequeathed body must be buried or cremated within 3 years.

Human Rights Act 1998

Various inquiries considered whether issues of human rights were likely to be infringed by any lack of consent in relation to interventions carried out on dead people. The Interim Bristol report mentioned the possibility that relatives who had suffered great distress could have a potential claim under the Act.[40] This was echoed by some other reports. In Scotland, for example, it was noted that the rights and freedoms provided by the human rights legislation cannot be invoked by dead persons but that "there may well be rights and freedoms a living person may wish to enforce arising out of, or after the death of, another person".[41] The chairman of the NHS Retained Organs Commission also considered that actions to prevent the burial or cremation of a body intact could violate religious beliefs and, if not done with good cause, could infringe the human right to religious freedom.[42] At the time of writing, however, no cases relating to the treatment of deceased people have been brought under the Act. In Northern Ireland, it was believed that the Human Rights Act did not add substantially to the postmortem and organ retention debate but that it certainly reiterated the "standards which can be reasonably expected and required as a matter of medical ethics and good practice".[43]

The Access to Health Records Act 1990, the Access to Health Records (Northern Ireland) Order 1993, and Data Protection Act 1998

Statutory rights of access to the health records of deceased patients is contained in the Access to Health Records Act 1990 and the Access to Health Records (Northern Ireland) Order 1993 (see Chapter 6, pages 220–1). The Data Protection Act 1998 does not extend to data relating to deceased people, although the BMA, the General Medical Council (GMC), and the Department of Health emphasise that the ethical obligation of confidentiality endures beyond the patient's death (see Chapter 5, page 168).

Legal need for consent to postmortem examination

The current human tissue legislation is seen as seriously flawed in not making a clear requirement for consent or authorisation for hospital postmortem examinations, but relying on the absence of reason to believe that the individual or family had objections. After the public inquiries in 2000–2002, much debate focused on this interpretation gap between "making reasonable enquiry" about potential objections and positively seeking specific "consent". Future legislation will focus on the latter. Indeed, many people had long assumed that this was what the law had always intended, even though it was not clearly articulated. When the Northern Ireland Human Organs Inquiry examined the evolution of the Human Tissue Act (Northern Ireland) 1962, for example, it noted that Northern Ireland Senators speaking in support of the Act in 1962 envisaged that there would invariably be a clear and specific request to relatives for a postmortem examination.[44] It was apparently expected that doctors would approach the nearest relative, explain the facts, and ask for permission to carry out the postmortem examination. "Such a request should be addressed directly to the surviving relatives and it should not be just a question of a member of the hospital committee thrusting one of these stereo-typed forms to a surviving relative for his signature".[45] The inquiry report emphasised that:

> doctors need to realise and accept, both as a matter of law and a matter of ethics, that the public are entitled to know what they are in fact consenting to when their consent is sought for postmortems. Doctors also need to realise and accept that offering more information in an open and sensitive way is as likely as not to result in that consent being given.[46]

Issues of ownership

An extensive literature exists on the law relating to ownership of the human body. The common law has declined to recognise such a notion of ownership of bodies or of human material as property. Control of what happens to them has been based on notions of appropriate custody ("lawful possession"). Relatives or executors and administrators of an estate have limited possessory rights to a corpse, mainly related to its burial or disposal.[47] Nevertheless, whole bodies or body parts that have been modified in some way may constitute property. Legal cases such as R v Kelly[48] indicate at least that "parts of the body may become the object of legal protection (whether this is based on the notion of property protection or on some other basis) provided that they have been subjected to processes or treatment (usually to enhance their value for a particular purpose)".[49] An example is the method of plastination pioneered by Dr Gunther von Hagens at Heidelberg University in 1978 and subsequently applied to cadavers displayed as art objects.

In Scotland, the Independent Review Group on Retention of Organs at Post Mortem considered that, in law, there was no reason in principle why human tissue could not be sold or otherwise transferred in ownership, provided that it is not an organ.[50] Nevertheless, it recognised that a court could declare that such tissue should not be seen as a commercial object on principle. This, however, "would have the result of effectively excluding the legal protection of the sale of any medicinal product which was manufactured from human bodily materials, unless the critical factor was not the origin of the materials, but rather the way in which they had been processed or treated".[51] This legal debate continues and is clearly important for medicine because other preservation techniques for teaching or research purposes could also convert human material into "property", capable of being stolen or sold. In order to do so, human tissue would need to be substantially modified so that it acquires different attributes, notwithstanding the general "no property" in a corpse rule.

It has been problematic in the past that the law on matters such as who must be consulted and to what extent about use of human remains has been imprecise and open to interpretation. It was partly because the law had been so unclear that it was decided after the Alder Hey Inquiry that collections of human material, ranging from whole organs to small tissue samples in blocks and slides, should be returned on request to the relatives of the deceased on compassionate grounds.[52] Medical organisations understood that many relatives would wish the return of symbolic or emotive human material, but were also deeply concerned that medical research and teaching would be seriously and adversely affected, particularly by the loss of blocks and slides comprising tiny fragments of tissue. Many of the families were highly supportive of research and education, but distressed by the previous lack of discussion. It therefore became clear that greater transparency was essential and that any new legislation should reflect this.

Attitudes of health professionals

Health professionals are expected to be both sensitive and stoic. Accustomed to dealing with death, they are also expected to remain compassionate, caring, and open in their dealings with families for whom death may come as a shocking event. Traditionally, early medical training has sought to inculcate a dispassionate detachment and scientific interest in the cadaver, which make it hard to see it as the remains of a real person (see Chapter 18, pages 667–8). Nevertheless, dissecting human bodies or analysing human bones and tissue cannot occur in an ethical or cultural vacuum but must reflect society's moral intuitions. Jones reminds doctors that even "subcellular and molecular work should be viewed with human considerations in mind".[53] Such scientific work was previously regarded by professionals as ethically neutral, but after 2000 it emerged as the focus of ethical debate. Interventions such as postmortem examinations represent "an intrusion into the intimacy and privacy normally reserved for the dead, and where societies tolerate these activities, they do so only within given parameters".[54] It is obviously important for health professionals to be aware of these parameters and sensitive to changes.

Summary – changing expectations

- Families can rightly expect to be consulted about interventions involving deceased people.
- Doctors must be ready to provide as much information as families require to make a decision.
- The public needs more information, however, about how data from autopsies can bring huge benefits for living people.
- Sensitive publicity also needs to be given to how human tissue and organs, retained with appropriate authorisation, are vital for teaching and research.
- The assumption may have been too readily made in the past that postmortem interventions are devoid of any potential for harm and are beneficial to society. In retrospect, it seems that only the second assumption is accurate.
- In assessments of harm and benefit, attention needs to be given to the potential distress to people who are emotionally close to the deceased person.

Implementing good practice

Respect for people: what duties do doctors have to dead persons?

Respect for persons is a fundamental part of medical ethics, but it is not obvious how it applies to dead people. Harris points out that, although differences of opinion exist about how to define a "person" or when a person begins or ceases, two aspects of respect for persons are widely accepted: respect for autonomy and concern for welfare.[55] In most respects, neither of these can be usefully applied to dead people. Autonomy "as the ability and the freedom to make the choices that shape our lives, is quite crucial in giving to each life its own special and peculiar value".[56] Concern for welfare provides the conditions under which autonomy can flourish. Personal consent is normally an important facet of autonomy, but Harris argues that such concepts are applied in any meaningful way only to those who are living. Advance consent or refusal by a now deceased person about posthumous interventions is something to be taken into consideration, but this is different from other paradigm cases of consent in medical contexts.

Nevertheless, doctors believe that they have a strong moral duty to respect such wishes. Those who have had a relationship of care with a patient often express the sense that the moral duties owed to that relationship extend beyond the patient's death. Part of this almost retrospective duty of care may involve obligations to determine whether patients had received the best treatment, whether their diagnosis and treatment regimen were correct, or whether avoidable errors that should be acknowledged were made. Doctors audit all of these things to improve practice for future patients and to promote the public interest, and give informed explanations to relatives, but they often also have a sense of "owing" it to the deceased person. This sense of unfinished business may be a strong motive in asking for a hospital postmortem examination, without which, in some cases, the presumed cause of death will be wrong or incomplete. Although it may not fall within the usual understanding of "respect for persons", health professionals do feel a duty to respect the person's known wishes and the relationship that formerly existed. Ethical duties, such as that of confidentiality, also continue even though the patient is dead. From an ethical perspective, doctors are encouraged to assess what the deceased person would have wanted concerning disclosure. Even though it can be argued that dead people have no interests, public and professional expectations are that deceased patients' cultural and religious values should be respected, for example in the handling of the body and its disposal. Relatives also have a strong interest in ensuring that dead persons are handled appropriately and health professionals have an obligation to avoid harming them.[57]

Do doctors have responsibilities to patients' families?

It is clear that doctors do have responsibilities to the families of deceased people, although such duties were rarely thoroughly articulated prior to the public inquiries of 2000–2002. Among other obvious duties to offer support and information, the medical profession as a whole has an obligation to raise awareness about the benefits to be gained from procedures such as autopsies. Clearly, it can be difficult to convey this to bereaved families, but doctors need to discuss with them the reasons why an autopsy is recommended, the information that may be revealed, and how this information will be handled. Health professionals often continue to have contact with the family after a patient's death, especially in the primary care setting or as part of bereavement support or counselling. As we discuss further below, advance thought needs to be given not only to who should be consulted about postmortem interventions, but also to how the confidentiality owed to the deceased person can be balanced with the needs for information of a surviving partner or relative.

In the BMA's view, when duties owed to people close to deceased persons are discussed, some distinction should be made between health professionals' obligations to parents, who are the main decision makers for young children, and the duties to relatives of adult patients. Parents have rights and duties to protect the welfare of their children and there are good arguments for requiring that they be consulted about anything affecting a child's remains. In their lifetime, adults have the liberty to decide matters for themselves and, in our view, who decides for deceased adults should depend in large part on the prior wishes of the deceased person and the closeness of the emotional attachment to other people. Nevertheless, the difficulties of trying to argue that dead people are harmed by having their wishes or their confidentiality overturned by their relatives are obvious. On a practical level, individuals can neither be harmed nor helped once they are dead, although arguably some intangible harm may be done to their reputation and symbolic benefit may be derived from the implementation of their known wishes. The most immediate harms and benefits, however, are experienced by people who are close to the deceased and who have the satisfaction or distress of knowing that the dead person's values continue or fail to have an influence. Other people too may be distressed to become aware that their own wishes may not be respected after their death.

Duties to benefit and not harm

Medical training is focused on prolonging life, maximising its quality, relieving suffering, and minimising the effects of disabilities. When a premature death occurs, both health professionals and families often seek to make sense of it by obtaining some benefit for other people by, for example, ensuring that any errors are recognised and avoided in future. It could also be argued that where cadaveric material can help to achieve benefits for living people, there are good moral reasons for saying it should be used. This means that, unless the individual expressed in life a clear wish about postmortem interventions, relatives should have opportunities to consider what that person would have wanted. People close to the deceased person must be involved and have a chance either to agree or to say, as Brazier suggests, that they "remain unconvinced that the moral arguments advanced about benefits to the living" outweigh other considerations such as religious beliefs or personal desires to bury a loved one intact.[58]

Traditional medical practice may have assumed that benefits could be obtained without any harm through the use of cadavers in research or teaching. If achievable, benefit without harm would be consistent with ethical principles. In this context, however, living people were shielded from potentially distressing information in a way that is now seen as outdated. In the past, it was deemed acceptable to protect relatives from uncomfortable knowledge, such as facts about postmortem examinations or research involving cadaveric material. It is now recognised that the views of people close to deceased persons must feature prominently in decision making, although they cannot override legal requirements and may not automatically supersede instructions left by the deceased person. Balancing notions of harm and benefit has become more complex.

The hope of achieving practical benefits for science must be balanced against a variety of risks of less tangible harms. People who are emotionally close to the deceased person suffer the effects if an individual case is mishandled. So does the wider community if the result is a loss of public trust. Research benefits, for example, do not necessarily outweigh the overall harm associated with unauthorised tissue collection. Cadavers and human material should be treated with respect, not solely in deference to the deceased individual, but also as a comfort to bereaved relatives and to reassure the community about professional integrity in this sensitive area.

Concern for justice and the public good

There are various ways in which postmortem examinations promote the concept of justice. They help to identify, for example, when patients' disease has not been treated correctly and can also contribute evidence to the legal system. Correcting previous miscarriages of justice in homicide cases often depends upon the evidence obtained by pathologists. The responsibilities of doctors involved in such enquiries may extend beyond the provision of evidence at the time to include alerting the courts to any important and relevant information they subsequently obtain.

Provision of evidence in legal cases

Sally Clark was convicted in 1999 of murdering her two baby sons but was released in 2003 when the postmortem evidence was re-examined. The children died in 1996 and 1998. Postmortem examinations were carried out on both. Microbiological tests at the time of the postmortem examination indicated that the second child, Harry, had probably died in reaction to a *Staphylococcus aureus* infection, but the pathologist judged the infection to be irrelevant to the legal case and failed to disclose it at the trial. In 2000 the evidence was re-evaluated and Sally Clark's conviction was quashed after it was revealed that the Home Office pathologist had not disclosed such vital information to other doctors prior to the trial or later. In 2003 the GMC said that it would look into the role played by the pathologist and other medical experts.[59]

Maximising useful knowledge in an ethical manner is an obligation of doctors. This means, for example, that when a postmortem examination is carried out, it should be done in a manner that is technically adequate to yield accurate information that is useful to relatives and to the way that future patients are managed. Among its purposes are:

- the need to ascertain or confirm the cause of death
- the classification of disease or condition so as to explain biological behaviour to relatives
- the collection of information about the extent of the disease or condition in the patient's case
- to contribute to a better understanding of the disease and the biological responses to it
- the assessment of the patient's response or otherwise to the treatment provided
- the detection of other relevant pathology not established in life
- the need to contribute to audit of patients' medical management, including the value of investigations and treatment and the accuracy of diagnosis
- the detection of genetic or other heritable conditions relevant to other family members
- the provision of reliable data on which to base death certification.

In 2003 the review of death certification in England, Wales and Northern Ireland recommended that, as routine practice, a copy of the autopsy report should be sent to the doctor who had been responsible for treating the patient at the time of death.[60]

Clearly, it is in everyone's interests that medical research, education, and transplantation programmes are carried out. A range of human organs and tissues are needed for such purposes. (This is discussed in Chapter 14 on research and innovative treatment.) The public is generally aware of this, but individuals also want to be asked about their own role or that of people close to them. In the past, doctors felt bound to pursue what seemed beneficial for society and to protect grieving relatives from difficult knowledge. Pre-empting their choice, however, denied people the opportunity to decide whether they wanted to be altruistic and derive consolation from knowing that some good would come from their loss. A repeated message from intending donors and families of deceased people is the desire to retrieve some meaning and value from death or bereavement through helping others. For some, this is a facet of their religious and spiritual beliefs, whereas for others it is part of a general desire to benefit mankind. It is in the public interest that such altruism should be encouraged and plentiful information provided about various facets of donation.

The ethics of consent and authorisation

In this section, we consider the importance society attaches to obtaining personal consent and the way in which it may need to clarify further the rules governing interventions on deceased persons for whom no advance permission has been given. It can be argued that "consent" is simply a misplaced notion when talking about dead persons because the reasons for valuing consent are to promote individual autonomy in a way that is inapplicable to deceased people. Partners and relatives may give their agreement or authorisation to procedures involving the dead person, but this proxy procedure is not "consent" as we normally understand it (i.e. people agreeing to things being done to themselves). Nevertheless, the general language of consent is well understood by most people and it is likely to continue to be used in this context.

Society expects that the advance wishes of people now deceased should carry some weight unless there are strong reasons to the contrary. Such reasons can include the public interest in conducting a postmortem examination to ensure that the cause of death is identified and homicide is revealed. Harris reminds us that "the public interest serves principally the interests of existing and future individuals" rather than the past wishes of the deceased person.[61] He draws an analogy to how, in some areas, society feels entitled to overrule the prior wishes of dead people by, for example, demanding the payment of death duties, which are usually very much against those prior wishes. Nevertheless, in some other areas, the question of whose wishes should dominate is left vague. In the BMA's view, in the absence of an overriding societal need or if the anticipated risks and benefits of an intervention are finely balanced, the wishes of the deceased person should be respected. Assessing risks and benefits can be complex. If the deceased individual carried an organ donor card, the removal of organs for transplantation could clearly benefit other people as well as respect that individual's former intent. On the other hand, if relatives know that the individual carried a donor card but still adamantly oppose donation, proceeding will cause them distress and alienation. If they cannot be persuaded to accept the wishes of the deceased person, their opposition may generate a difficult confrontational situation or a backlash leading other people to refuse to donate. By this reasoning, some would argue that there may even be grounds for disregarding the wishes of the deceased person because the overall harm could outweigh any benefit from implementing them.

Practising procedures on newly deceased people

It is clearly desirable that future practitioners are adequately trained in the techniques they will need in emergency care, but it is sometimes less clear how they will obtain their practical training. A complex question is whether we should carry out certain procedures only on consenting living people – even though this may carry some risks for them and for future patients – rather than on deceased individuals who have not consented. In the USA, for example, intubation and the placing of catheters into major veins of the body have been carried out as training procedures on recently deceased corpses. Both procedures involve essential skills that emergency professionals must acquire and can be done respectfully. Future patients may suffer if such techniques are not thoroughly mastered because "emergency clinicians do not spring fully trained into the medical world" but "must be patiently taught those lifesaving skills society expects them to have".[62] In Australia, surgeons have sometimes practised plastic surgery on bodies in a mortuary (although this has been labelled as clearly inappropriate).[63] In the UK, fresh cadavers have been used for health professionals in training to practise tracheal intubation in accident and emergency and intensive care departments, as well as on wards after failed resuscitation. In the BMA's view, this is now likely to be unacceptable unless some form of valid authorisation has been provided for the body to be used in teaching, either in advance by the deceased individual or by the bereaved relatives. The practical obstacles also need to be considered. People may donate their bodies for teaching purposes to medical schools and the latter have advance notice that they have future donors "on their books". The context in which intubation training has traditionally arisen is rather different, being carried out at short notice when the deceased's intentions regarding donation for research or teaching are less likely to be known.

The BMA has long argued that, for most professionals, sufficient experience of intubation should be obtainable through training on mannequins and animals. An alternative option is for live patients who are undergoing routine general anaesthetic to be asked to allow a trainee to carry out intubation in the anaesthetic room under expert supervision. The reluctance to use dead people, even though they cannot be harmed as living volunteers could be, indicates how highly consent is valued and how great is the fear that any unnecessary intervention on a dead person will be seen as disrespectful. These kinds of dilemmas need to be understood and discussed by society as a whole.

Testing for communicable diseases

The GMC advises that testing cadavers for communicable diseases should be done only when it is likely to be relevant to the cause of death and a postmortem examination has been authorised or ordered.[64] Clearly, in many instances testing is necessary for these purposes. If this is not the case, the GMC says that testing should not be done routinely simply to protect healthcare workers. In any instance where there are grounds for believing that a serious communicable disease is present, the GMC advises doctors to assume that the body is infectious and take precautions accordingly.[65] Pathology teams often have only imprecise information about the deceased individual and so this means they probably need to take full precautions in every case. It may be useful to consider, however, the moral reasons why we seek to apply the same rules about testing to the dead as we do to the living. Clearly, for living patients there can be serious personal and financial implications in having a communicable disease such as HIV and, as a result, individuals often take steps to avoid knowing their own infection status. This is not true for dead people and, even if information about them was discovered, through testing, which might impinge on their posthumous reputation, it would still be governed by the ethical obligation of confidentiality. It can be argued that obtaining some tangible benefit in terms of protecting living people should take precedence over notions of symbolic harm to dead individuals. To sustain such an argument, however, would require evidence that the difficulties involved in protecting the health team were great and the risk of infection to them serious. There would also need to be societal consensus that the aim of protection is more important than the privacy of deceased persons. At present, there is no such consensus and doctors are clearly obliged to abide by the GMC's advice.

Patients in whom death has been confirmed by brain stem tests may be assessed as suitable organ donors. This should be explained to the relatives or people close to the patient who need to be aware that assessment includes testing for certain infections, including HIV. Health professionals and people close to the deceased person need to consider in advance how the resulting information should be handled. Here the GMC makes clear that information about a living or dead patient may be disclosed to protect a person from death or serious harm but it should not normally be disclosed to relatives who are not at risk.[66] Therefore, it could be appropriate to disclose the deceased's positive HIV status to a spouse or partner, for example, but not to parents or siblings.

Postmortem DNA testing

The length of time a person has been dead may affect the suitability of the cells for testing but, in some cases of historical research, DNA has been tested from people who died centuries ago. Other reasons for testing include to establish kinship or involvement in criminal cases. Internationally, guidance has been produced by organisations such as the International Committee of the Red Cross to identify remains of "the missing" in conflict situations or through the excavation of mass graves.[67] Ethical aspects in such cases include ensuring that relatives who donate DNA are not given unrealistic expectations about what is achievable in individual cases, and consideration of how data will be made public.[68]

A common medical situation is for a need to test tissue samples obtained while the patient was still alive in order to gain information for relatives, for example about possible hereditary breast or ovarian cancer. Stored blood or tissue from deceased patients may also be used in family linkage studies. In many families where there is thought to be a genetic disorder, patients request the storage of samples for future use when a reliable test has been developed. If samples have been stored, but specific consent was not given for testing, the question arises about whether it would be appropriate to test them. In the BMA's view, if they were to consider it in advance, most people would wish to help family members and this is also an instance in which the potential benefits in terms of useful knowledge for living people may outweigh other considerations. The Human Genetics Commission takes a similar approach, suggesting that, in the absence of evidence to the contrary, a "benevolent intent" and, therefore consent, can be presumed.[69] Individual cases should be considered on their merits and advance thought be given to the use and disclosure of the information.

In its published advice[70] on diagnostic genetic testing after death, the BMA notes that this may occur when it is suspected that death was caused by a genetic disorder or if it is thought that an unborn fetus died from a genetic or chromosomal disorder. In either case, a postmortem examination (either with the family's permission or at the behest of the coroner or procurator fiscal) may be carried out to clarify the cause of death, but the results can have profound implications for other family members. Prior to testing, thought should be given to how the results will be handled and who should have access to them, including the fact that some family members may not want to know. When a test is proposed for a deceased child or fetus, the issues should be discussed in advance with the parents, whose agreement should be sought.

DNA testing for identification

Another purpose of DNA testing is to establish kinship. Parentage testing using a sample from a dead person can have serious consequences for families and can be divisive, so that those likely to be affected need to agree to it. Cases need to be considered on their merits. In general, this is an instance where the interest that living people have in knowing the identity of their relatives is seen as more important than other considerations. In particular, people may have a strong desire to identify their deceased biological parents or children.

Consent in the context of postmortem examinations

In this section, the focus is on elective postmortem examinations (autopsy or necropsy) when families must be asked to authorise the procedure. Legally required examinations are covered later (pages 442–3). As briefly mentioned on pages 418–9, under the terms of the Human Tissue Act 1961 and the Northern Ireland equivalent, hospitals approach relatives to authorise such an examination and they cannot proceed if the family objects.[71] If there are no known relatives and no evidence that the deceased had objected, a hospital administrator who is legally in possession of the body can authorise the procedure. The primary intention is to discover more about the deceased person's illness and, when the subject of the autopsy is a deceased child, information may also be gained about genetic conditions and the risks for subsequent pregnancies and children.

The World Health Organization has stated that:

> It is generally agreed that an autopsy is a procedure of considerable ethical significance as it interferes with the body. The significance is such that the community has a right to expect that systems are developed, within legal and resource constraints, and with community input and understanding, to ensure that the substantial potential benefits of performing an autopsy are realised and that the autopsy is not meeting only narrowly defined needs.[72]

This, however, can be problematic. The pathologist's aim may appear vague when explained to relatives, although part of the importance of postmortem examinations lies in the unexpected information they can provide beyond the original narrowly defined purpose.

Seeking consent from relatives

- Sensitive communication skills are essential.
- It can be helpful for the health professionals who have cared for the deceased person and developed a relationship with the family to raise the issue of an autopsy, but whoever explains the autopsy process needs to be well informed.
- The presence of the pathologist who would perform the examination is also helpful and can clarify misunderstanding.
- Bereavement counsellors advising families should also be aware of the reasons why autopsy is proposed in individual cases.
- Talking to other families who have previously been through the process can also be helpful.
- Anxieties about the body being mutilated or disfigured are a key factor in families' refusal, and reassurance on the sensitivity of the process should be provided.
- When families object strongly to the body being cut, an examination may be acceptable through an existing incision, by a needlecore necropsy, or by radiography (see minimally invasive methods on page 446).
- Families need to know how and why the information gained will help them or other families in the same situation because some fear that "doctors were doing it for themselves to confirm their diagnosis".[73]
- Follow up meetings in which families can discuss the findings should be established without a lengthy delay in relatives receiving information.
- Families may fear that funeral arrangements will be delayed and need reassurance about this.

An important issue raised by many studies is the need to increase general awareness in society about the importance of postmortem examinations. Well before the inquiries into retained organs, it seemed that the public had a good awareness of the need for postmortem examination for forensic purposes because these were often portrayed in popular television programmes and the press.[74] Its importance for the improvement of patient care, research, and education, however, was poorly understood. The accuracy or otherwise of the deceased person's certified cause of death is verifiable by such an examination and it can be argued that, in the past, unwarranted clinical confidence in the assumed cause of death contributed to the decline in postmortem examination rates.

In the 1990s, researchers found that:

> many members of the medical community, including allied professions such as nursing, appeared unaware of the importance of the necropsy and misconceptions regarding the procedures are common. The influence such negative attitudes can have on the public should not be underestimated and any measures to improve public awareness must also address this issue.[75]

In 2002, after the inquiries in Scotland and England and Wales, a significant amount of helpful guidance was produced for both health professionals and the public. In Scotland, for example, a clear explanatory leaflet for relatives was drawn up by the Independent Review Group, detailing background information about postmortem examinations.[76] The Department of Health also drafted guidance and a series of model forms.[77]

Consent to organ and tissue donation for research and teaching

During their lifetime, people can give advance permission for tissue samples, organs, or their entire body to be kept and used for research or teaching purposes. In addition, if either an elective or a mandatory postmortem examination is carried out, relatives should be aware that some body samples could be usefully retained and used for such purposes if they give permission. Studies indicate that people who bequeath their bodies express a strong desire to help others and contribute to medical progress, but some worry that their wishes will be countermanded by relatives.[78] In our view, if the donor's intentions were clear they should be respected except in rare cases where great distress would be caused to relatives who disagree with the donor's values and therefore the harms associated with retention could outweigh the benefits. Many donors are well aware that donated cadavers are used for a variety of purposes, such as dissection, demonstrations, or experimentation.[79] In all cases, the altruism of their gift should be appropriately recognised and their remains treated with respect by those who make use of them. The ability to see an echo of a real person in donated human material and gain an understanding of the hopes of donors and relatives may help to bridge the gap between the expectations of families and those of health professionals.

A doctor's views

"Our cadaver was a 62-year-old (ex-sailor) ... When we reached it, the cancer in his lung felt like sand under the blade. I felt it in my hands long after the lesson was over. It was strong and frightening, because even as we reduced him to pieces I knew that he was real, that he had stories to tell, that he had looked out at the sea from the decks of ships."[80]

"She was dead now, though you wouldn't have known it to look at her ... So now it was her organs we were taking care of. She was the best of donors, young, strong, undamaged in every other way, with decades left in her heart and lungs and kidneys. A young woman in her prime. That morning there were pictures in her room. A family portrait. A child on the grass. A girl in a white dress, smiling in the kitchen. She looked happy, excited. I've often seen these photographs. It's the nurses who do it. They tell the family, bring pictures, it will help us to see her for what she is."[81]

Would-be donors' views

"If by donating my body I can help future surgeons and physicians to acquire the skills so necessary for them to bring healing to those who are suffering, what better way to end one's life?"[82]

"I would like to have read medicine. By body donation I somehow slip in by the back door, and am curiously present with students and anatomy teacher. I hope the anatomical pieces are always carefully put into a marked and labelled container ready for cremation. Can you assure me about this? Are the students always taught respect?"[83]

In the past, human material was sometimes retained without authorisation for research purposes after a coroner's or fiscal's postmortem examination. (Research using human material is discussed in detail in Chapter 14, pages 523–4.) In 2000 the Royal College of Pathologists published guidance on the retention of tissue and organs.[84] Subsequently, in the Interim Bristol report,[85] a new code of practice was called for, backed by appropriate enforcement mechanisms. Two fundamental principles were identified that should be prominent in retention of human material for research. The first was the need to show respect for families; the second was that the value of continued access to human material for the advancement of medical care and treatment should be acknowledged. Later, after the Alder Hey Inquiry, the Chief Medical Officer made 17 specific recommendations regarding the removal, retention, and use of human organs and tissue.[86] In Scotland, the Independent Review Group on Retention of Organs at Post Mortem produced 52 recommendations, almost half of which specifically covered aspects of organ retention and use.[87] Therefore, in addition to the guidance from the Royal College,[88] a range of other detailed advice is available,[89] including the 2003 guidance from the Central Office for Research Ethics Committees (COREC).[90] Researchers in this area need to be familiar with these guidelines and, in particular, must be aware of the need for transparency and appropriate authorisation. Discussing such issues with bereaved relatives is a difficult task that requires training.

Consent to other procedures

Research indicates that by far the most common motives quoted by people who are willing to bequeath their body is to aid medical science and teaching, help other people, or express gratitude to the medical profession.[91] Such reasons are dependent upon the perceived status of medical science, its discerned value for society, and the trust placed in doctors. These reasons may change. Furthermore, few people, including some pathologists, have always fully understood the kinds of activities that can fall within the definitions of "research", "education", or "anatomical examination". This was highlighted by the cases investigated in an Australian report, which examined the legal limits of the infliction of trauma on donated cadavers.[92]

Australian examples of unacceptable uses of cadavers

In a coronial investigation, a pathologist at the New South Wales Institute of Forensic Medicine thought that a murder victim had died from bludgeoning by a hammer. He and the mortuary assistant carried out an experiment with a hammer on a donated corpse, which was then photographed for forensic use. Both the pathologist and the mortuary assistant believed that the research was permissible, lawful, and consistent with the definition of "anatomical examination". An inquiry, however, concluded that "their mistake illustrates a longstanding deficiency within the medical profession generally and among pathologists in particular of adequate legal instruction concerning the use of dead bodies and human remains".[93] In other cases, donated bodies were stabbed to provide instruction about the wounds caused by different blades, scissors, or a screwdriver, or scalded to replicate the burns on a murdered child. The inquiry judged that these activities were "scientific" but not authorised under the Anatomy Act passed in New South Wales in 1977. It noted that "the motivations and methods of all those involved were respectful of the donated bodies and sincere as to their beliefs that what they were doing was permissible".[94] The inquiry argued the need for a balance between the extent of the interference and disfigurement, the scientific methodology used, and the usefulness of the findings. It also noted that similar experiments had been carried out in the UK, but that the authority for their legality seemed unclear from the evidence presented.

Organ and tissue transplantation

Legally, in the UK, the removal of organs after death for transplantation depends either on the deceased person having previously indicated a positive desire to donate or, in the absence of any known desire or objection, the lack of objection from relatives.[95] If it is necessary to hold an inquest, or a coroner's or procurator fiscal's postmortem examination, however, organs or tissues may be removed only with the specific authorisation of those authorities. Over decades, the law on this matter came to be widely regarded as unsatisfactory and in need of reform.[96] After the various inquiries into organ retention, there was broad agreement that new legislation should replace it. At the time of writing, the shape of such legislation is still being debated. (See the BMA website for more recent information about the law.)

As previously mentioned, bodies cannot be owned, but are seen as in the custody of other people. It is generally accepted that when a patient dies in hospital, the hospital management is "lawfully in possession of the body" until the executors or relatives have it removed. When the person dies elsewhere, relatives or a partner may have lawful custody. As the law has been imprecise on whose views should be sought about possible donation, a pragmatic approach has been taken. In most instances, this consists of discussing the matter with those relatives who have been in close contact with the deceased in the period leading up to the death. These people are asked about their own views, those of the deceased patient, and whether any other relative is likely to object. Many potential organ donors have spent a short time in hospital before their death and the medical and nursing staff are already in contact with the close relatives. It has also become standard practice to seek the consent of the relatives for donation even though the legislation merely requires that the person lawfully in possession of the body makes enquiries to ensure that relatives do not object to the donation.

Although the UK currently operates an "opt-in system" for organ donation (with explicit consent from either the individual or the relatives), these procedures have developed by custom and practice rather than being a necessary requirement of the law. Arguably, it would be possible to operate a form of "presumed consent" (or "opt-out" system) under the current legislation, simply by changing the way in which relatives are approached. The BMA supports the concept of an opt-out system as one component in a broader strategy to improve organ donation rates, but strongly believes that any such change must be made explicit and with the support of the public and health professionals. An essential prerequisite to the BMA's proposals in relation to donation for transplantation is that efforts be made towards creating a culture in which voluntary donation is seen as the accepted norm for many people. In the BMA's view, however, in the absence of such societal expectation and ample opportunities to dissent, any automatic appropriation of corpses would be harmful in terms of contravening religious and cultural requirements, distressing relatives, and depriving people of the option of acting altruistically.

The BMA is among a group of organisations who have worked together to identify coherent strategies for increasing the voluntary donation rate. In 1999 this alliance of professionals and patient organisations formed the Transplant Partnership to lobby for change. The consensus view was that no single change would suffice and a multifaceted approach is needed. This is set out in the publication *Organ donation in the 21st century: time for a consolidated approach.*[97]

Public opinion

Public opinion surveys in the UK consistently report that around 70% of those interviewed say they are willing to donate organs after their death but only 20% of these make their views known by carrying a donor card or being listed on the organ donor register.[98] The importance of making known one's views about organ donation cannot be overstated and, where feasible, health professionals should sensitively encourage people to talk to those close to them about their wishes. When an individual dies without expressing views about donation, relatives are approached and, in practice, the responsibility falls to them at what is a difficult and emotional time. It is estimated that around 30% of relatives, when asked in these situations, refuse a request for organs to be used but rarely do so when they know that donation was the deceased's intention. Carrying a donor card gives a clear indication of intent and can act as a prompt to timely discussion within the family.

Advance consent in other situations

In some cases, despite the fact that apparent advance consent has been provided, doctors have reservations about fulfilling deceased patients' alleged wishes because the process seems tainted or the validity of consent is very dubious. Although it can be argued, for example, that prisoners should have the same opportunity as other people to act altruistically, the BMA has repeatedly objected to the use of organs from executed prisoners in countries such as China. The Association has a clear policy opposing the death penalty and opposes the use of capital punishment to provide a regular supply of organs for transplantation in China and Taiwan, even though prisoners are said to consent.[99]

The BMA is also occasionally asked about the acceptable limits of what may be done to a deceased person's body in order to conform with their advance wishes. Typical of this type of enquiry are concerns about the deceased person's former fear of being inadvertently buried alive or cremated while still living. In such cases, deceased patients may have left instructions that a vein should be opened or their heart removed prior to disposal of the body. In the past, such requests have sometimes been stimulated by media coverage of a misdiagnosis of death and "recovery" of a patient in the mortuary. While alive, patients can be counselled about the improbability of this happening, but if such instructions have been left by a person now deceased, health professionals are often unsure how to handle them. In the past, complying with the patient's wish was not seen as problematic. Nevertheless, health professionals are more likely to have reservations after the impact made by the Shipman case (see page 415). Doctors who are willing to implement such wishes should take legal advice. There could be potentially problematic implications if the doctor asked to carry out the patient's wish is also the person who certified death.

Cryonics is the practice of freezing the body of a deceased person for possible resuscitation in the future when a cure has been found for the disease that caused the individual's death. This procedure is dependent upon unpredictable future technology and its history in the USA has been tainted by fraud and mismanagement. (One of the first organisations promoting the practice in the 1960s froze and stored a number of corpses underground but owing to financial mismanagement failed to keep them in a frozen condition.) Biological death is a process rather than a single event, which causes particular problems for this type of preservation. Deterioration at cellular level occurs in the hours after cessation of the heartbeat. People wishing to be preserved for possible reanimation request that cryopreservation procedures be initiated as soon as possible after the legal declaration of death to minimise deterioration of cells. Currently, all the organisations offering cryonic suspension services are in the USA and some feature their protocols on their websites. Some European countries have legislation restricting the preservation of bodies, so some people make arrangements directly with American companies to circumvent such restrictions.

Legality of cryonics in Europe

In France in February 2002, Remy Martinot froze his father when he died at the age of 80. The father, Dr Raymond Martinot, had been a pioneer in the field of cryonics and had previously frozen his wife when she died of cancer in 1984. At that time, he had permission to bury her at the family's chateau but he had in fact injected anticoagulants into her veins and placed her body in a refrigerator. In March 2002, a French court ruled it illegal for bodies to be frozen for later reanimation and ordered that the frozen cadavers must be removed from their refrigerated chambers and either buried or cremated. At the time of writing, this decision is being appealed and was expected to go on to the Conseil d'Etat and, ultimately, to the European Court of Human Rights.[100]

Summary – consent issues

- People need to be involved in making choices in their lifetime about what should happen to their remains after death.
- Ideally, individuals should discuss their preferences with people close to them and the health professionals who care for them so that the right choices are made later.
- Families and other people close to deceased patients should be consulted about interventions such as postmortem examinations.
- When autopsies are legally required, people close to the patient should be kept informed.

Issues of confidentiality

The moral basis of the duty of confidentiality is primarily to protect patients' privacy and respect their wishes. A common argument is that individual patients will lose faith in doctors if their confidentiality is not protected. When they are no longer alive, patients cannot be harmed in the same way, although the trust of the public at large may be diminished if confidentiality is routinely breached. The GMC emphasises that the duty of confidentiality is not extinguished by the patient's death, but the extent to which it must be protected depends upon the circumstances. Factors to be taken into account include:

- the deceased person's former wishes
- the nature of the information
- whether it is already public knowledge
- the use to which the information will be put
- whether the objective could be attained by anonymised data.

Therefore the general principles, outlined in Chapter 5, should be observed. Disclosure should be kept to the minimum unless the patient indicated to the contrary.

Benefit and harm

As health professionals see themselves as owing a continuing duty to dead patients, doctors often have to make judgments about what the person might have wanted in a particular situation. The fact that the law says little about the confidentiality of deceased people does not mean that information or photographic records of dead individuals can be used in an unlimited way, nor does it mean that information cannot be disclosed for an appropriate purpose. Doctors have always had discretion to disclose information to a deceased person's relatives or others when there is a clear justification. In many cases, it is obvious that the deceased person would have wanted a partner or relative to have specific information. A common example is when the family requests details of the terminal illness because of an anxiety that the patient might have been erroneously diagnosed or there might have been negligence, or from a feeling of guilt that warning signs were missed within the family. Disclosure in such cases is likely to be what the deceased person would have wanted and may also be in the interests of justice. Refusal to disclose in the absence of some evidence that this was the deceased patient's known wish exacerbates suspicion and can result in pointless litigation. The statutory right of access to relevant parts of deceased patients' records by people with a claim arising from the death is discussed in Chapter 6 (pages 220–1). In other cases, the balance of benefit to be gained by the disclosure to the family, for example, of a hereditary or infectious condition, may outweigh the obligation of confidentiality to the deceased.

What can be problematic, however, is the apparently growing assumption that relatives (regardless of how emotionally close they were to the deceased person) should have more or less automatic access to aspects of the deceased person's health information. After the public inquiries into organ retention, for example, one of the proposals that emerged was that any reports prepared by pathologists during a postmortem examination should be made available to the deceased person's relatives.[101] In many cases, this may be entirely appropriate, but this is also one of the areas where the former instructions and wishes of the deceased person need to be taken properly into account. After the Shipman case (see page 415), it was also proposed that relatives should have routine access to more information about deceased patients' health management, including their visits to their doctor and more details of the cause of death.[102] The intention was to provide more monitoring, via the family, of any mismanagement of deliberate harm, but the potential effect was to reduce further the notion that dead people are owed confidentiality.

Thorough investigation of deaths can provide an early warning system of many hazards in the community. Patterns of preventable deaths may be identified in hospitals, on the roads, in the workplace, or in the home. Identifying such patterns over time and geographical areas while having regard to issues of confidentiality requires sophisticated information handling. Forensic pathology services accumulate information and experience that has importance in terms of public health and safety. It has been argued that forensic pathology systems have an ethical responsibility to contribute to the prevention of deaths and injuries by identifying such patterns. Some have argued that this responsibility is of even greater significance to society than the judicial role of forensic pathology.[103]

Information on death certificates

Death certification is an important source of data, not only for families but also for society (although without the availability of data from postmortem examinations, the reliability of death certificates cannot entirely be known). The law requires that death certificates be completed honestly and fully, but anyone can purchase the certificates, which are also used by families for a range of official purposes, such as redirecting mail or dealing with the Benefits Agency. In particular, information about the cause of death can be sensitive. In 1995 the BMA called for an abbreviated death certificate to be available for administrative purposes. In 2002 the Government agreed to this,[104] confirming that it intended to ensure that confidential information would be available only to families, people authorised by the family, and agencies with legally prescribed access. Nevertheless, this did not solve the potential problem of limiting disclosure when, for example, patients had not wished relatives to be informed of sensitive information relating to their illness. Much debate has occurred about how to describe the cause of death in relation to HIV infection. A system that has been used is for doctors to indicate for audit purposes that the death was HIV related without making that explicit. For example, the cause of death may be stated as pneumonia but an indication would be given that further information is available. This is an area where further debate is needed to ensure that a proper balance is achieved between society's need for accurate data and the duty of confidentiality owed to deceased people.

Pathology archives

Pathology archives include records, tissues, and semipermanent and permanent pathological preparations. Such materials, including microscope slides, provided with consent from living patients, are generally seen as an extension of their medical record. They need to be appropriately stored and available for review in connection with patient care or the need for a second opinion. After the patient's death, they may be retained for the benefit of patients' families, including for genetic testing. They may also be archived for education, teaching, research, or audit, or retained for legal purposes such as evidence in future litigation or allegations of fraud.[105] Health departments have issued guidance that makes it clear that the same principles apply to pathology materials and biological samples as to patients' medical records.[106] This is also the BMA's view since much material is acquired during patient's lives as an adjunct to their health record and is used for diagnostic purposes. Efforts need to be made at the time of obtaining samples with patient consent to identify materials likely to be particularly useful for medical research so that they can be permanently preserved beyond the normal retention period for patient records (see also pages 213–5).

Summary – confidentiality

- Ethically, the obligation of confidentiality extends beyond the patient's death.
- This duty needs to be balanced with other considerations, such as the interests of justice and of people close to the deceased person.
- Ideally, patients should indicate in their lifetime the kinds of information (if any) that they would prefer not to be known to their families after their death.

Common practical queries

Who should certify and confirm death?

As mentioned on page 415, the system for certifying death is likely to change and a new post of Statutory Medical Assessor may be introduced in England, Wales and Northern Ireland. In this section, however, we reflect the law current in 2003. Confusion has often arisen about the distinction between confirmation of death and its certification. Any health professional can confirm that death has occurred, but a certification of death can be completed only by a doctor who attended the patient during that person's last illness. This doctor provides an opinion of the cause of death and certifies the cause of death, not the fact.

The law does not require:

- a doctor to confirm that life is extinct
- a doctor to view the body of the deceased person
- a doctor to report the fact that death has occurred

but it does require the doctor who attended the patient during the last illness to issue a certificate detailing the cause of death.

Although only a registered medical practitioner can legally certify death, nurses and other health professionals can confirm that death has occurred. It is common for nurses to confirm death in cases where the death is expected and there is an explicit policy or protocol specifying the nurse's role in this context.[107] Clearly, any professional who is expected to carry out this task must have appropriate training and assessment to ensure that it is competently done. Even though it is not a legal requirement for a doctor to confirm death, hospital rules may require that a doctor do so before a deceased patient is moved from the ward.

The method for confirming death can give rise to anxiety for relatives when organ donation is envisaged. People who are close to the patient are sometimes unfamiliar with the term "brain stem death tests" or may believe that brain stem tests show a "special" form of death rather than simply measuring its clearest manifestation. The BMA uses the term "death confirmed by brain stem tests" to indicate the finality of the diagnosis and that recovery is impossible. Death confirmed by brain stem tests should be seen as the clearest indication of death rather than the stopping of the patient's heart or of breathing, both of which can be reversed in certain circumstances. Current guidance specifies that, when donation is envisaged, death should be confirmed by at least two doctors who have been registered for over five years, one of whom is a consultant. They should be competent in this field and not members of the transplant team.[108]

Who notifies stillbirths?

One of the measures for which the BMA had long lobbied was a simplified system for registering stillbirths. The duty of notifying a birth (whether the baby is born alive or stillborn) rests with the father or any other person present at the birth or present within six hours of the birth. Nevertheless, in many cases it is the midwife or attending doctor who actually does this. A baby born alive at any stage of pregnancy must be registered. If such a baby dies after birth, both the birth and the death must be registered. A baby born dead after the 24th week of pregnancy must be registered as a stillbirth. When a baby is born dead before the legal age of viability (before 24 weeks' gestation), the law does not require the birth to be certified or registered. If, however, parents wish to hold a funeral, they need a certificate or letter from the doctor or midwife stating that the baby was born dead before the legal age of viability. Funeral directors cannot accept a body without this.

When a registered doctor is present at a stillbirth or examines the body, he or she has a statutory duty to issue a certificate of stillbirth. If a doctor is not present but has accepted responsibility for maternity care, that doctor should be asked to examine the body and complete the stillbirth certificate. If a registered doctor is not involved, the midwife who attended the birth or examined the body can complete the certificate. A stillborn baby cannot be buried or cremated until a burial or cremation certificate has been obtained from the registrar of deaths or an order for burial has been issued by the coroner or, in Scotland, the procurator fiscal. In certain circumstances, a certificate from the registrar confirming that he or she has received notice of the stillbirth will serve the same purpose.

In the past, the BMA objected to the registration procedures that incorporated features of both birth and death registration. These were perceived as hindering the parents' grieving process. Proposed changes would bring registration into line with that for death and allow medical investigation to be carried out in appropriate cases. For example, individuals could agree to the re-use of information that had already been provided or which was already available within the health service.

Among the areas facing change is the registration of all deaths. In January 2001, in response to the Alder Hey Inquiry report,[109] the Chief Medical Officer recommended that further consideration be given to the proposal for a new post of medical examiner whose duties would include some tasks currently undertaken by the registrar of deaths.[110] The medical examiner would have responsibility for checking the medical certificate of cause of death and the statutory responsibility to refer deaths to the coroner in certain circumstances. In 2002 the Government noted strong support for an updated death registration system and proposed a central database of deaths, allowing electronic data exchange between doctors, coroners, and registrars.[111]

Which deaths should be referred to a coroner or procurator fiscal?

In England, Wales, and Northern Ireland any death suspected of being unnatural or which cannot be certified has to be reported to the coroner for investigation, as does the death of a person in custody.[112] All citizens, including doctors, have a duty to report such deaths to the coroner. In Scotland, such reports are made to the procurator fiscal, who fulfils a similar role in determining the precise cause of death and may order a postmortem examination.[113]

Violent deaths and accidents should also be reported to the police. Although there is no statutory duty for doctors to contact the coroner, it is usual practice for them to do so in the event of doubt or suspicion. GPs are not obliged to attend if a body is found by the police or ambulance service if that person was not the GP's registered patient. In any case where there are grounds for believing that the death was violent, unnatural, or unexpected and of unknown cause, coroners and fiscals must investigate if the body is lying within their district, even though death may have occurred elsewhere. Suicides and any deaths in prison must also be investigated. All such deaths may be the subject of a postmortem examination at the coroner's or procurator fiscal's direction. Generally, the death cannot be registered until the enquiries have been completed and notification of that fact has been sent to the registrar.

Summary – reportable deaths

All citizens, including doctors, have a duty to report certain deaths to the coroner. The common categories include any death:

- suspected of being unnatural, suicide for example
- in suspicious circumstances or where there is a history of violence
- linked to an accident including any traffic or workplace death
- due to industrial disease or linked to the deceased's occupation
- linked to an abortion, miscarriage or a pregnancy
- occurring during an operation or before full recovery from anaesthesia
- related to a medical procedure or treatment or prescribed medication
- where the actions of the deceased may have contributed (self neglect, drug or solvent misuse)
- in police, prison or military custody or asylum detention centre or when death resulted from an injury or illness sustained in custody
- within 24 hours of admission to hospital
- when the deceased was detained under mental health legislation.[114]

Who gives consent to a legally required postmortem investigation?

The coroner or procurator fiscal may order an autopsy in order to clarify the cause of death. Respectful and sensitive communication with bereaved families is essential and they should understand the reasons for the investigation, but they cannot prohibit it. Nevertheless, if they have specific cultural or religious objections to the procedure, this should be made known to the coroner or procurator fiscal.

Some general guidance applies to both types of investigation. In 2003 the Department of Health issued a code of practice concerning the involvement of families in decision making about postmortem examinations.[115] This sets out recommended practice for all those involved in talking to relatives about the procedure and with mothers of fetuses who may undergo autopsy. It seeks to ensure:

- that those close to the deceased person understand the reasons for the autopsy and their rights in relation to it
- that, where possible, the wishes of the deceased person and people close to that individual are ascertained and respected
- that organs and tissue are not retained after the postmortem examination without proper authorisation

- that the disposal of retained organs, tissue, body parts, stillborn or miscarried babies, and fetal remains is in accordance with either the known wishes of the deceased or of those close to that person.

Who should be informed about retained human material?

Advance requests to relatives concerning the potential desire to retain some tissue after a postmortem examination have already been discussed. If there is a foreseeable need for retention after a hospital autopsy to which relatives have consented, this should ideally have been discussed with the family in advance. The pathologist should have been contacted to determine what is likely to be retained so that the retention can be discussed and properly authorised by the family, when all the questions have been answered. At the time when the subject is raised with relatives, their views should also be sought about eventual disposal (regardless of whether the autopsy is for a coroner, procurator fiscal, or at the request of the hospital). Detailed advice is provided in the 2003 code of practice on postmortem examinations.[116]

In some cases, when a postmortem examination has been carried out on the instructions of a coroner or procurator fiscal, doctors may become aware that the pathologist has retained tissue or an organ. Relatives should already be aware that a legally obligatory examination is taking place and also of the likelihood of any tissue or organ retention. In a coroner's or a procurator fiscal's case, it is for the coroner, the procurator fiscal, or a person delegated by either of them, to tell the family what precisely has been retained and how long it will be retained.

Can members of the public attend an autopsy?

Doctors are sometimes asked if people such as a school student considering a medical career can observe an autopsy. The confidentiality of the deceased person and relatives' views must be taken into account. In a coroner's case, the coroner's permission must first be obtained. It is helpful if hospital trusts, coroners, and fiscals provide information leaflets for the public that mention the possibility of potential medical students attending the examination.

How do individuals donate their bodies for anatomical dissection?

A common enquiry concerns how individuals can donate their bodies after death to a medical school for medical research or education. Enquiries can be addressed to the Inspector of Anatomical Dissection at the Department of Health (for England, Wales, and Scotland) or at the Department of Health, Social

Services and Public Safety (for Northern Ireland), who can supply the relevant information. The appropriate medical school is then determined by the donor's residential postcode.

What are the rules about importing and exporting body parts?

Detailed guidance about the importing and exporting of human body parts and tissue for non-therapeutic uses was published in a UK-wide code of practice in 2003.[117] This notes that the importation of such material is primarily for training in new surgical techniques. The main purpose of the code is to ensure that accurate and formal records are kept of all imports and exports of human body parts for teaching, education, research, or other non-therapeutic uses. The code sets out fundamental ethical principles, such as the need for respect to be shown to all human material. It specifies the requirement for the specific and explicit consent of the donor if bodies or body parts are to be displayed to the public (but this does not apply to historical materials gathered before 1948). When bodies or body parts are intended for public display, consent from the next of kin after the individual's death is deemed to be insufficient.

Areas needing further debate

Doctors have obligations to their deceased patients and their relatives. They also have general duties to promote public health and the public interest. Often it is difficult to reconcile all of these responsibilities. This chapter highlights the importance of the patient's own views about matters such as the future retention of diagnostic materials or tissue donation being discussed during the person's lifetime. After the person's death, people close to them should be consulted about proposed interventions. More widely, considerable effort needs to be put into informing everyone in society about the immense benefits that can accrue from donation for transplantation, research, and education.

The remainder of this section highlights a number of areas where further debate is needed.

Resolving tensions between the former wishes of deceased individuals and the wishes of families

How doctors should approach cases in which people close to the deceased person may take a completely different view to that previously expressed by the deceased person has been discussed earlier in this chapter. There needs to be wider discussion within society, however, about the handling of profound disagreements or when families disagree among themselves.

Combining transparency with respect for people's refusal to receive information

In the past, the medical profession has not communicated clearly to the public the value and significance of postmortem examinations, and there needs to be some cultural change in order to bridge the gap that has existed between the profession and the public. From the evidence provided by families to public inquiries, it is clear that some families and sections of the community want detailed discussion about the procedures that make an autopsy valuable. Others do not want to be exposed to those details, and their desire not to know is equally valid. Practitioners have to be able to take their cue from the relatives, but there needs to be more debate about how the full importance of postmortem examinations can be better understood while at the same time not forcing information on bereaved people.

Discussing death and removing the mystique

In this chapter, we have emphasised that health professionals need to be aware and sensitive when talking to relatives, but this is an understatement of what is required from them. Perhaps the profession needs to be drawn into a wider debate about how best to manage death and its repercussions. For some health professionals, there may still be an impression that care resulting in death is a failure. A feeling of inadequacy to change the course of the disease can prevail and the availability of sophisticated technology can feed this perception, even though doctors themselves are generally too well aware of the limitations of what medicine can do. This is potentially unhelpful to families who could benefit from information and reassurance. This is discussed further in Chapter 10.

Should the retention of small tissue samples be routine in some cases?

Among the proposals put forward by the Department of Health and Welsh Assembly in 2002 was the suggestion that some small tissue samples should be routinely retained in the event of any sudden infant death or from other unexpected deaths.[118] It was noted that such blocks and slides could be vital to the public interest in identifying homicides and, in the long term, shed light on the causes of unexplained infant death. It was suggested that routine retention in such cases, irrespective of the views of relatives, pathologists, or coroners, could be the fairest system rather than appearing to cast suspicion on parents or relatives in an individual case. In its response to the proposal, the BMA saw merit in this idea and considered it to be in the interests of justice.

How important is confidentiality after death?

In 2002 views were sought by the Shipman Inquiry about proposed changes to the existing system of death certification. Among the suggestions were measures that would assist in the identification of abnormal trends and ensure that professionals involved in the various stages of certification have some information about the past health of the deceased person. It was envisaged that families too would receive more information about the cause of death and the medical consultations involving the deceased person in the period prior to death. Clearly, the interests of justice and the need to minimise any risk of the successful concealment of murder or medical error dictate that robust monitoring mechanisms are in place. Nevertheless, such proposals need also to take account of the fact that many adults do not have close relatives and may have objections to people having access to information on the basis of a blood relationship.

Is there a role for minimally invasive autopsies?

Among some patient groups there is strong religious or cultural opposition to the performance of autopsies. Nevertheless, the general consensus in the medical profession is that "judicial decisions based on conclusions about the cause and manner of death reached without the benefit of an autopsy will have a high rate of error".[119] In such circumstances, doctors must be frank about the limitations of any investigation that relies on the external examination of a body or circumstantial evidence. One of the recommendations of the Chief Medical Officer after the Alder Hey Inquiry was that attention be given to the concept of minimally invasive postmortem examinations using magnetic resonance imaging or postmortem laparoscopy.[120] The findings of such procedures have been accepted by some coroners as verifying the cause of death, but the literature on both types of intervention indicates significant error rates. Clearly, the precise purpose of the postmortem examination is relevant. Magnetic resonance imaging, for example, may be useful for identifying problems within the brain of the deceased person. Pathologists point out, however, that one of the significant benefits of full autopsies is the number of unexpected findings made that are unrelated to the initial question that the procedure set out to answer. Although there may be limited circumstances in which minimally invasive examinations are of use, the general view among practitioners appears to be that minimally invasive examinations are unlikely to be a valid alternative to a conventional autopsy.

References

1   The Bristol Royal Infirmary Inquiry. *The inquiry into the management of care of children receiving complex heart surgery at the Bristol Royal Infirmary. Interim report: removal and retention of human material.* London: The Stationery Office, 2000. The Royal Liverpool Children's Inquiry. *The Royal Liverpool Children's Inquiry report.* London: The Stationery Office, 2001. (HC12-II.) Independent Review Group on Retention of Organs at Post Mortem. *Retention of organs at post mortem: final report.* Edinburgh: Scottish Executive, 2001. The Human Organs Inquiry. *The human organs inquiry report.* Belfast: Department of Health, Social Services and Public Safety 2002.

2   The Human Organs Inquiry. *The human organs inquiry report. Op cit:* p. 5.

3   One of the key consultations was: Department of Health, Welsh Assembly Government. *Human bodies, human choices: the law on human organs and tissue in England and Wales: a consultation report.* London: DoH, 2002.

4   The Bristol Royal Infirmary Inquiry. *The inquiry into the management of care of children receiving complex heart surgery at the Bristol Royal Infirmary. Interim report: removal and retention of human material. Op cit.*

5   *Ibid:* p. 13.

6   Independent Review Group on Retention of Organs at Post Mortem. *Retention of organs at post mortem: final report. Op cit:* p. 16.

7   Brazier M. Retained organs: ethics and humanity. *Legal Studies* 2002;**22**:550–69.

8   This is discussed in detail in: Department of Health. *Families and post mortems: a code of practice.* London: DoH, 2003:5.

9   Royal College of Pathologists. *Examination of the body after death: information about post mortem examination for relatives.* London: RCPath, 2000:4.

10 Department of Health, *et al. Human bodies, human choices: the law on human organs and tissue in England and Wales: a consultation report. Op cit:* p. 7.

11 Brazier M. Retained organs: ethics and humanity. *Op cit:* p. 554.

12 Royal College of Pathologists. *Guidelines on the retention of tissues and organs at post mortem examination.* London: RCPath, 2000.

13 Department of Health. *Interim guidance on post mortem examination.* London: DoH, 2000.

14 The Bristol Royal Infirmary Inquiry. *The inquiry into the management of care of children receiving complex heart surgery at the Bristol Royal Infirmary. Interim report: removal and retention of human material. Op cit.*

15 The Royal Liverpool Children's Inquiry. *The Royal Liverpool Children's Inquiry report. Op cit.*

16 Human Tissue Act 1961 s1(2).

17 Brazier M. Retained organs: ethics and humanity. *Op cit:* p. 552.

18 Department of Health. *Report of a census of organs and tissues retained by pathology services in England.* London: The Stationery Office, 2001.

19 Department of Health. *Isaacs report: the investigation of events that followed the death of Cyril Mark Isaacs.* London: DoH, 2003.

20 Independent Review Group. *Retention of organs at post mortem: final report. Op cit.*

21 The Human Organs Inquiry. *The human organs inquiry report. Op cit.*

22 The Shipman Inquiry. *Developing a new system for death certification.* London: The Shipman Inquiry, 2002. (CP 29 0001.)

23 Start RD, Saul CA, Cotton DWK, Mathers NJ, Underwood JCE. Public perceptions of necropsy. *J Clin Pathol* 1995;**48**:497–500.

24 Department of Culture, Media and Sport press release. *Working group will consider potential return by museums of human remains.* 2001 May 8 (165/01).

25 McHaffie HE. *Crucial decisions at the beginning of life. Parents' experiences of treatment withdrawal from infants.* Oxford: Radcliffe Medical Press, 2001:409.

26 The Royal Liverpool Children's Inquiry. *The Royal Liverpool Children's Inquiry report. Op cit:* p. 30.

27 Anonymous. Organ doctor given probation. *BBC Online,* 2001 Jun 30. http://news.bbc.co.uk (accessed 4 May 2003).

28 Anonymous. New row over body dumping. *BBC Online,* 2001 Jan 18. http://news.bbc.co.uk (accessed 4 May 2003). Anonymous. Hospital chapel used as mortuary for years. *BBC Online,* 2001 Jan 31. http://news.bbc.co.uk (accessed 4 May 2003).

29 Richardson R, Hurwitz B. Donors' attitudes towards body donation for dissection. *Lancet* 1995;**346**:277–9.

30 Brazier M. Retained organs: ethics and humanity. *Op cit:* p. 561.

31 McHaffie HE. *Crucial decisions at the beginning of life. Op cit:* p. 172.

32 Walker B. *Inquiry into matters arising from the post mortem and anatomical examination practices of the Institute of Forensic Medicine report.* Sydney: Government of the State of New South Wales, 2001.

33 Richardson R. *Death, dissection and the destitute.* London: Routledge and Kegan Paul, 1987.
34 British Medical Association. *Medicine betrayed.* London: Zed Books, 1991:101.
35 Anonymous. Police report on public autopsy. *BBC Online*, 2002 Nov 21. http://news.bbc.co.uk (accessed 4 May 2003).
36 See, for example: British Medical Association. *The medical profession and human rights: handbook for a changing agenda.* London: Zed Books, 2001:229–31.
37 Anonymous. Aborigine remains return home. *BBC Online*, 2003 May 5. http://news.bbc.co.uk (accessed 7 May 2003).
38 Department of Health. *The import and export of human body parts and tissue for non-therapeutic uses: a code of practice.* London: DoH, 2003.
39 The Human Tissue Act 1961 covers England, Scotland and Wales. The Human Tissue Act (Northern Ireland) 1962 incorporated the same provisions.
40 The Bristol Royal Infirmary Inquiry. *The inquiry into the management of care of children receiving complex heart surgery at the Bristol Royal Infirmary. Interim report: removal and retention of human material. Op cit.*
41 Independent Review Group. *Retention of organs at post mortem: final report. Op cit:* p. 13.
42 Brazier M. Retained organs: ethics and humanity. *Op cit.*
43 The Human Organs Inquiry. *The human organs inquiry report. Op cit:* p. 25.
44 *Ibid:* p. 22.
45 Senator Donaghy speaking in debate on the Act in 1962. Quoted in: The Human Organs Inquiry. *The human organs inquiry report. Op cit:* p. 22.
46 The Human Organs Inquiry. *The human organs inquiry report. Op cit:* p. 5.
47 Dobson v North Tyneside Health Authority [1996] 4 All ER 741.
48 R v Kelly [1998] 3 All ER 741.
49 Independent Review Group. *Retention of organs at post mortem: final report. Op cit:* p. 65.
50 *Ibid.*
51 *Ibid.*
52 Retained Organs Commission. *Tissue blocks and slides: a consultation paper.* London: Department of Health, 2002.
53 Jones DG. *Speaking for the dead: cadavers in biology and medicine.* Aldershot: Ashgate Dartmouth, 2000:8.
54 *Ibid:* p. 1.
55 Harris J. Law and regulation of retained organs: the ethical issues. *Legal Studies* 2002;**22**:527–49.
56 *Ibid:* p. 530.
57 This is discussed in detail, especially in relation to the need to avoid infringing families' religious beliefs in: Brazier M. Retained organs: ethics and humanity. *Op cit.*
58 *Ibid:* p. 557.
59 Anonymous. Pathologists may face action over case. *BBC Online*, 2003 Jan 30. http://news.bbc.co.uk (accessed 4 May 2003). Anonymous. Clark case questions expert testimony. *BBC Online*, 2003 Jan 30. http://news.bbc.co.uk (accessed 4 May 2003).
60 The Review of Coroner Services. *Death certification and investigation in England, Wales and Northern Ireland. The report of a fundamental review 2003.* London: The Stationery Office, 2003.
61 Harris J. Law and regulation of retained organs: the ethical issues. *Op cit:* p. 535.
62 Iserson KV, Sanders AB, Matheiu D. *Ethics in emergency medicine, 2nd ed.* Tucson: Galen Press, 1995:124.
63 Walker B. *Inquiry into matters arising from the post mortem and anatomical examination practices of the Institute of Forensic Medicine report. Op cit.*
64 General Medical Council. *Serious communicable diseases.* London: GMC, 1997.
65 *Ibid:* para 8.
66 *Ibid:* para 22.
67 The project is discussed in: Coupland R, Cordner S. People missing as a result of armed conflict. *BMJ* 2003;**326**:943–4.
68 This is discussed in: British Medical Association. *The medical profession and human rights: handbook for a changing agenda. Op cit:* ch 6.
69 Human Genetics Commission. *Inside information: balancing interests in the use of personal genetic data.* London: HGC, 2002: paras 4·67–4·68.
70 British Medical Association. *Human genetics: choice and responsibility.* Oxford: Oxford University Press, 1998.
71 Human Tissue Act 1961 s1(2). Human Tissue Act (Northern Ireland) 1962 s1(2).
72 World Health Organization. *Ethical practice in laboratory medicine and forensic pathology.* Geneva: WHO, 1999:39.
73 McHaffie HE. *Crucial decisions at the beginning of life. Op cit:* p. 172.

74   Start RC, *et al. Public perceptions of necropsy. Op cit.*
75   *Ibid:* p. 499.
76   Independent Review Group. *Retention of organs at post mortem: final report. Op cit:* p. 118.
77   Department of Health. *Families and post mortems: a code of practice. Op cit.*
78   Richardson R, *et al.* Donors' attitudes towards body donation for dissection. *Op cit:* p. 278.
79   Murray TH. Gifts of the body and the needs of strangers. *Hastings Cent Rep* 1987;**17**(2):30–8.
80   Huyler F. *The blood of strangers.* London: Fourth Estate, 1999:10.
81   *Ibid:* p. 64.
82   Richardson R, *et al.* Donors' attitudes towards body donation for dissection. *Op cit:* p. 279.
83   *Ibid:* p. 278.
84   Royal College of Pathologists. *Guidelines on the retention of tissues and organs at post mortem examination. Op cit.*
85   The Bristol Royal Infirmary Inquiry. *The inquiry into the management of care of children receiving complex heart surgery at the Bristol Royal Infirmary. Interim report: removal and retention of human material. Op cit:* recommendation 7.
86   Department of Health, Department of Education and Employment, Home Office. *The removal, retention and use of human organs and tissue from post-mortem examination.* London: DoH, 2001.
87   Independent Review Group. *Retention of organs at post mortem: final report. Op cit:* pp. 16–25.
88   Royal College of Pathologists. *Guidelines on the retention of tissues and organs at post mortem examination. Op cit.*
89   See: Medical Research Council. *Human tissue and biological samples for use in research: operational and ethical guidelines.* London: MRC, 2001. Royal College of Pathologists, Institute of Bio-medical Science. *Retention and storage of pathological records and archives, 2nd ed.* London: RCPath, 1999.
90   Department of Health, Welsh Assembly, NHS Central Office for Research Ethics Committees (COREC). *The use of human organs and tissue: an interim statement.* London: DoH, 2003.
91   Fennell S, Jones DG. The bequest of human bodies for dissection: a case study in the Otago Medical School. *N Z Med J* 1992;**105**:472–4. Richardson R, *et al.* Donors' attitudes towards body donation for dissection. *Op cit.*
92   Walker B. *Inquiry into matters arising from the post mortem and anatomical examination practices of the Institute of Forensic Medicine report. Op cit.*
93   *Ibid:* para 148.
94   *Ibid:* para 152.
95   The law is discussed, along with a detailed discussion of presumed consent for donation, in: British Medical Association. *Organ donation in the 21st century: time for a consolidated approach.* London: BMA, 2000.
96   See, for example: Mason JK. Organ donation and transplantation. In: Dyer C, ed. *Doctors, patients and the law.* Oxford: Blackwell Scientific, 1992.
97   British Medical Association. *Organ donation in the 21st century: time for a consolidated approach. Op cit.*
98   See, for example, the results of three surveys discussed in: Kings Fund Institute. *A question of give and take: improving the supply of donor organs for transplantation.* London: Kings Fund, 1994:37–42.
99   This is discussed in detail in: British Medical Association. *The medical profession and human rights: handbook for a changing agenda. Op cit:* ch 8.
100   Anonymous. French court rules against frozen couple. *BBC Online,* 2002 Mar 13. http://news.bbc. co.uk (accessed 4 May 2003). Anonymous. Frozen couple saga rumbles on. *BBC Online,* 2002 Sep 9. http://news.bbc.co.uk (accessed 4 May 2003).
101   The Human Organs Inquiry. *The human organs inquiry report. Op cit:* recommendation 14.
102   The Shipman Inquiry. *Developing a new system for death certification. Op cit:* p. 15.
103   World Health Organization. *Ethical practice in laboratory medicine and forensic pathology. Op cit.*
104   Office for National Statistics. *Civil registration: vital change. Birth, marriage and death registration in the 21st century.* London: The Stationery Office, 2002.
105   Royal College of Pathologists, *et al. Retention and storage of pathological records and archives, 2nd ed. Op cit.*
106   See, for example: Department of Health. *For the record: managing records in NHS trusts and health authorities.* London: DoH, 1999. (HSC 1999/053.) National Assembly for Wales. *For the record: managing records in NHS trusts and health authorities.* Cardiff: National Assembly for Wales, 2000. (WHC(2000)71.)
107   Nursing and Midwifery Council. *Legislation relevant to midwives.* London: NMC, 2000.
108   Department of Health. *A code of practice for the diagnosis of brain stem death: including guidelines for the identification and management of potential organ and tissue donors.* London: DoH, 1998.
109   The Royal Liverpool Children's Inquiry. *The Royal Liverpool Children's Inquiry report. Op cit.*

110   Department of Health, *et al. The removal, retention and use of human organs and tissue from post-mortem examination. Op cit:* recommendation 11.

111   Office for National Statistics. *Civil registration: vital change. Birth, marriage and death registration in the 21st century. Op cit.*

112   Criminal Law Act 1977. Coroners Act 1988. Health and Safety at Work Act 1974 s19. Coroners Act (Northern Ireland) 1959 s7.

113   Crown Office. *Death and the procurator fiscal.* Edinburgh: Crown Office, 1998.

114   The Review of Coroner Services. *Death certification and investigation in England, Wales and Northern Ireland: the report of a fundamental review 2003. Op cit.*

115   Department of Health. *Families and post mortems: a code of practice. Op cit.*

116   *Ibid.*

117   Department of Health. *The import and export of human body parts and tissue for non-therapeutic uses: a code of practice. Op cit.*

118   Department of Health, *et al. Human bodies, human choices: the law on human organs and tissue in England and Wales: a consultation report. Op cit:* p. 56.

119   World Health Organization. *Ethical practice in laboratory medicine and forensic pathology. Op cit.*

120   Department of Health, *et al. Human bodies, human choices: the law on human organs and tissue in England and Wales: a consultation report. Op cit:* p. 168.

13: Prescribing and administering medication

The questions covered in this chapter include the following.

- Who is ultimately responsible for shared prescribing decisions?
- How should doctors respond to patients' requests for particular medication?
- What, if any, hospitality may be accepted from pharmaceutical companies?
- Should doctors prescribe for patients they have not seen?
- Should doctors inform patients about medication that could help them but is not available within the NHS?
- Are doctors in England and Wales obliged to follow guidance issued by the National Institute for Clinical Excellence (NICE)?

The challenges and dilemmas

A number of recent changes within the doctor–patient relationship, in the health service, and in knowledge and technology have led to new challenges and dilemmas in relation to prescribing. The traditional dilemmas – conflicts of interests, resource allocation, relations with pharmaceutical companies, and pressures on doctors' independence in prescribing – remain, but many of these have taken on increased importance or greater prominence. This has been partly the result of patients becoming more informed, sometimes asking doctors to prescribe particular drugs or treatments, the rise of so-called "lifestyle drugs", and the increasingly consumerist attitude towards health care. The more frequent use of private medicine and changes in the role of pharmacists and nurses have not only required modifications in traditional methods of working, but also increased the frequency of shared prescribing, which can cause tension and raise questions of responsibility and liability for prescribing decisions.

The introduction of bodies such as NICE in England and Wales have added another dimension to prescribing decisions and, in some ways, restricted clinical freedom. The rapid increase in knowledge and technology over the last decade has affected not only the range of products available, but also the way in which they are provided. Developments in information technology have offered an alternative to the traditional face to face consultation by introducing consultations and prescribing via the internet so that the doctor and the patient may never meet and may be in different towns, or even in different countries. Further changes are expected as knowledge develops of the role that genetic factors play in the success or otherwise of particular medicines. Pharmacogenetics will change significantly the way in which medication is prescribed in the longer term and it is important for doctors to be aware of the type of dilemmas that may arise. This chapter discusses the issues raised by such changes and offers practical advice.

General principles

The following general principles apply in relation to prescribing.

- The doctor who signs a prescription accepts clinical and legal responsibility for the decision.
- Doctors should prescribe medication only when they have sufficient knowledge and experience to be satisfied that it is appropriate for the patient.
- If the prescribing doctor is not the patient's GP, he or she should encourage the patient to allow communication with the GP in order to avoid any conflict with existing treatment.
- Doctors must not ask for or accept any inducement, gift, or hospitality from pharmaceutical companies or others that may affect or be seen to affect their judgment.
- It is generally unwise for doctors who prescribe to form business connections with companies that produce, market, or promote pharmaceutical products.

Responsibility for prescribing

A major part of medical practice is prescribing medicines, products, and treatments. Deciding which medication to prescribe for which patient and in what dose is a matter of clinical judgment based on experience and published guidance, which reflect the evidence base on factors such as efficacy, safety, and cost. Decisions are made on the basis of appropriateness, effectiveness, safety, and economy. The range of drugs available is constantly changing, so it is important that doctors should keep up to date with new products and guidance through regularly updated resources such as the *British National Formulary*,[1] *Clinical evidence*,[2] and the *Drug and Therapeutics Bulletin*.[3] Doctors are permitted to prescribe for individual patients drugs that have not yet been licensed or to use them in a way that is outside the scope of the product licence. This is usually known as use on a "named patient basis".[4]

Prescribing doctors accept clinical and legal responsibility for their prescribing decisions and must be prepared to justify them if called upon to do so. Doctors should, therefore, prescribe medication only when they have sufficient knowledge and experience to be satisfied that it is appropriate for the patient, and where they are willing to accept this responsibility. This can sometimes prove difficult when prescribing is shared between a GP and a specialist (see pages 472–4) or when a patient requests a particular form of medication that is unfamiliar to the doctor. If the prescribing doctor is not the patient's GP, he or she should ensure that the prescription does not conflict with other treatment provided by the patient's GP, with whom liaison is required, with the patient's consent, before any prescription is issued. If the patient refuses consent to the GP being consulted, then this should be respected. Whether the doctor should go on to prescribe in the absence of that information is a matter of clinical judgment and is likely to depend on the risks of the particular drug to be prescribed. Consultants who instruct junior doctors to prescribe particular medication are also likely to be liable for any resulting harm.

Common prescribing errors

In a survey of 1000 consecutive clinical negligence claims against GPs, 193 prescribing errors were identified.[5] The four most common errors were:

- giving the wrong dosage
- giving inappropriate medication
- failure to monitor the treatment for side effects and toxicity
- problems arising from poor communication between doctor and patient and between different doctors providing care for the patient.

In addition to the clinical and legal responsibilities of prescribing, doctors are also under a professional duty to prescribe in an appropriate and responsible manner. The GMC states:

> In providing care you must … prescribe drugs or treatment, including repeat prescriptions, only where you have adequate knowledge of the patient's health and medical needs. You must not give or recommend to patients any investigation or treatment which you know is not in their best interests, nor withhold appropriate treatments or referral.[6]

Failings in relation to prescribing

In 2002 a doctor was found guilty by the GMC of serious professional misconduct for a series of failings in relation to his prescribing of phentermine (the licence for which had been withdrawn in May 2001) to three women attending his private slimming clinic.[7] It was found that his decision to prescribe this drug had been inappropriate, unjustified, not in the best interests of the patients, and contrary to accepted medical practice. In addition, it was found that he had failed to:

- adequately, or at all, warn of the dangers of taking phentermine, in particular when it was an unlicensed drug
- take and record an adequate physical examination
- properly or adequately discuss the nature of obesity, its dangers or levels of severity
- enquire as to the identity of the patients' GPs and/or advise the patients of the benefits and importance of keeping their GPs informed of the treatment and seeking their agreement to do so
- properly discuss or make arrangements for adequate follow-up review or treatment
- record the dosage of phentermine.

The doctor's registration was restricted to practice within the NHS, and not in a single handed general practice either as a principal or a locum, for a period of three years.

Providing information to patients about medication

As with other forms of treatment, patient consent is required for the administration of medication. For that consent to be valid, patients must be provided with sufficient information about the products prescribed, including information about known side effects, to allow them to make informed decisions. They should be made aware of the risks of the medication prescribed and any alternatives available. The amount of information patients need depends upon a range of factors including the diagnosis, prognosis, the type of medication proposed, the level of risk associated with it, and the amount of information the patient is willing and able to accept. Doctors need to have an up to date knowledge of effectiveness, safety, and cost, and possess good consultation skills in order to assist individual patients in making informed choices about treatment.

Information should be comprehensible to individual patients, with special attention being given to the needs of those who may require particular assistance, such as elderly people and people who do not speak English. Written patient information leaflets must be provided for all marketed medication. Where the product is prescribed and dispensed as an original pack, then this is not a problem but, when the dispensing requires the pack to be split, it is sometimes difficult in practice always to supply either an original information leaflet or a copied version. Medicines used in hospitals fall into a special category and so medication dispensed for inpatients does not require an information leaflet to be provided, but one should be held either in the pharmacy or on the ward.[8] This is also a problem for GPs who are administering medication out of hours. Even when written information is given to patients, this does not diminish the duty of doctors to discuss the medication with them and to answer any questions. The primary responsibility for informing patients about prescribed medicines rests with the prescribing doctor, although pharmacists also share that responsibility, particularly in relation to how the medication should be administered. The pharmacists' code of ethics emphasises this role, stating that "pharmacists must ensure that the patient receives sufficient information and advice to enable the safe and effective use of the medicine".[9] Pharmacists also have a central role in providing information about over the counter medicines available from pharmacies.

Involving patients in "concordance"

Very serious problems can arise if patients do not fully understand aspects of their medication and fail to take it correctly or consistently. In 1997 an expert working group studied research in clinical pharmacology, health psychology, and medical sociology to try to understand why half the patients prescribed medicines for long term illnesses failed to take the medicine as directed.[10] The group found that these patients had a complex but coherent set of beliefs about medicines and illnesses. Some also had practical problems with medication that they had not discussed with health professionals. The remedy suggested by the group was called "concordance", which describes a way for prescribers and patients to discuss medication and agree a detailed plan about how it will be taken. It is based on the concept of partnership, highlighting not only patients' rights but also their responsibilities for maintaining their own health and not burdening the NHS unnecessarily. The aim is to reach an agreement, after negotiation between a patient and a health professional, that gives primacy to the beliefs and wishes of the patient in determining whether, when, and how medicines are to be taken.[11]

The problem of people failing to take their medication properly is not new. The working group's report gave details of a number of studies, over decades, that have indicated that significant numbers of patients consistently fail to follow their treatment regimen, jeopardising their life and health.[12] Two large studies carried out in 1989 and 1998, for example, indicated that one in five kidney transplant patients decided not to take their life prolonging medication as prescribed. Other studies published between 1979 and 1991, which are quoted in the report, showed that up to half the patients diagnosed with chronic diseases failed to take medication that could alleviate their symptoms and many people who had previously suffered heart attacks failed to keep to a treatment regimen even though it could double their chances of survival. The reasons why patients risk dying or suffering unnecessarily from the effects of conditions like asthma and diabetes that can be well controlled by medication have been poorly understood. Annually, however the NHS incurs significant avoidable costs as a result of patients failing to follow their treatment regimen.

Unfortunately, although the problem is well documented, the solution is not obvious. Experts conclude that in many cases patients have not properly assimilated the information in the first place and so fail to realise how vital the follow up procedures are. Part of the solution is perceived to lie in encouraging health professionals to embark on more detailed communication with patients. Both doctors and patients need to have a say and reach agreement on how medicines should be used to control the problem under discussion. It is well recognised that, in many senses, the most influential person in the transaction is ultimately the patient, whose decision is generally final. It is important, however, that doctors make notes of the discussions held and agreements made with patients. Doctors clearly cannot be considered negligent when they have done all that they could reasonably be expected to do to try to convince the patient to maintain an essential course of medication.

Summary – providing information to patients about medication

- Patients must be provided with sufficient information about any medication prescribed, including details about known side effects, to enable them to make informed decisions.
- Written information for patients is provided with all medication, but this does not diminish the duty of doctors to discuss the medication with patients and answer any questions.

- It has long been the case that many patients do not take their medication as directed. Doctors should discuss with patients the importance of taking the medication and should encourage them to ask any questions. Efforts should be made to work towards agreeing a plan with the patient about how the medication will be taken.

Pressure from patients

It is usual for doctors' prescribing decisions to be informed by colleagues, the medical literature, and established guidelines. Patient preference must also be considered. Ethical dilemmas may arise, however, when substantial additional expenditure for the NHS results from acceding to such preferences, thus affecting the resources available for other patients, or when patients request particular drugs.

Requests for particular medication

Increasing public access to medical information, particularly on the internet, has empowered patients and enabled them to contribute to a greater extent in medical decision making. It has also, however, led to the more frequent practice of patients asking their GPs to prescribe a particular drug or treatment, some of which may be of unproven efficacy or may be requested outside the scope of the drug's licence. Doctors faced with such requests are not obliged to comply and should do so only if they are satisfied that the treatment requested is the most appropriate option for the particular patient. If the doctor is concerned about the safety or efficacy of the drug, this should be explained to the patient and the doctor should refuse to prescribe. It is always important to explain the reasons for refusing to comply with the patient's request. This may be because the patient has obtained inaccurate or misleading information. A number of studies have raised concerns about the accuracy of even apparently credible websites containing health information.[13] In response to such concerns, the NHS Information Authority set up the National Electronic Library for Health,[14] which, together with NHS Direct Online[15], NHS Direct Wales[16] and NHS24 in Scotland,[17] aims to meet the needs of both health professionals and patients for accurate and up to date medical information. The Medicines and Healthcare Products Regulatory Agency – formerly the Medicines Control Agency – also has a website, which includes information on the safety of herbal medicines and their interaction with other medication.[18] Patients who present with inaccurate information should be informed of that fact and encouraged to access websites, such as those mentioned above, where there is a higher degree of control over the accuracy of the material published. The BMA's General Practitioners Committee publishes a leaflet giving tips for patients who are searching the internet for medical information.[19]

Pressure can also arise from inaccurate or incomplete information that patients have received from the media. A particular problem has arisen in England and Wales from the way in which the decisions of NICE have sometimes been reported. Headlines stating that a particular medication has been "approved" by NICE have resulted in all patients assuming they have an immediate and automatic right to that particular product in the NHS. In reality, guidance may restrict treatment to certain categories of patients or there may be a time lag between guidance being given and the funding for treatment becoming available. Also, the consultative process that NICE follows in developing guidance includes publishing preliminary findings on its website. The media sometimes report these preliminary findings as final guidance without explaining that initial decisions may change after consultation.

The BMA considers that it is the doctor's ethical duty to use the most economical and efficacious treatment available when the patient is receiving treatment within the NHS. Therefore, choosing a more costly product is unethical unless it can be expected to produce a superior outcome. Patient preference and compliance may be elements that constitute superior outcome. Implicit in this view is the assumption that objective assessment should be made of the factors that could justify prescribing the more expensive product. When patients are being treated privately, there can be no objection to them choosing a more expensive option that they prefer and are prepared to pay for, provided the doctor is willing to accept clinical responsibility for the prescription requested. However, private insurance companies are very unlikely to be willing to cover options that are more expensive than they consider necessary.

Dealing with patient expectations

A common problem faced, particularly by GPs, is dealing with patients' expectation that they will leave the surgery with a prescription for some form of medication irrespective of the nature of their complaint. Some doctors may opt for the easier and quicker option of writing a prescription rather than spending time assessing the root of the problem or explaining why medication is not the answer. Patient demand and the placebo effect have been put forward as a justification for prescribing drugs acknowledged by the doctor to be pharmacologically ineffective for the condition diagnosed. This is not good practice and undermines the ideal of a doctor–patient relationship based on honesty and trust. A good example of this has been the inappropriate use of antibiotics. In the past, doctors frequently reported coming under pressure from patients to prescribe antibiotics for self limiting illnesses against which antibiotics are ineffective, such as the common cold. Public education campaigns have been helpful in reducing the demand for antibiotics in such cases.

Requests to continue medication

Other dilemmas arise from patients insisting on the continuation of a prescription that the doctor feels can no longer be justified. Common examples include hypnotics and anxiolytics, which may have been prescribed to enable the patient to deal with a painful situation such as bereavement. Similarly, centrally acting appetite suppressants are often sought by patients who want to lose weight. Patients may underestimate or disregard the possibility of creating a physical or psychological dependence, particularly when they are feeling in control of their drug use. Dealing with the situation requires time for doctors to listen to patients' views and for doctors to explain their clinical understanding of the situation. Some doctors have proposed that if counselling fails to convince the patient of the undesirability of the requested treatment, the patient should be asked to sign a document accepting responsibility for insisting upon a prescription. Such a document is unlikely to carry any weight in law. Ethically it would not be justifiable for doctors to issue such prescriptions, contrary to their clinical judgment, in response to pressure from patients.

Requests for repeat prescriptions

In an increasingly consumerist society where individuals are seen as consumers of doctors' services, patients' demands for easy and convenient solutions to their health problems has led to some reluctance to take the time to visit a doctor. This is reflected in many ways, including the greater demand for email consultations (see pages 479–80) and drop-in health centres. For those who receive ongoing medication, there is often a feeling that a consultation is an unnecessary obstacle to obtaining their repeat prescription. This view was recognised, and to an extent endorsed, by the Government, which identified one of its key aims as "making sure that people can get medicines or pharmaceutical advice easily and, as far as possible, in a way, at a time and at a place of their choosing".[20] Although there is a role for repeat dispensing, whereby patients obtain a prescription from their GP that is dispensed in several instalments by pharmacists, pressure from patients for continuous repeat prescriptions, without a consultation, must not be permitted to undermine the quality of care that patients receive. The importance of regular clinical assessment for those taking ongoing medication should be explained to patients, and doctors must resist pressure from patients to prescribe larger doses of medication than they consider clinically appropriate or for repeat prescriptions to be issued repeatedly without clinical review.

Requests for "lifestyle drugs"

It is generally accepted that doctors should prescribe medication only if they consider it necessary for the patient, but views of what is "necessary" differ. More frequent requests from patients for what have been termed "lifestyle drugs", such as antiobesity drugs, antidepressants, and hair loss treatments, illustrate the way in which perceptions of "clinical need" have changed. Although there are certainly those for whom antidepressants and appetite suppressants are clinically indicated and cannot be considered as lifestyle drugs, for many others they are seen as a quick and easy solution. When in search of a quick fix, it is easier to take medication than to spend time and energy on diet and exercise, or to spend time exploring, through counselling, the root of anxiety or depression.

What constitutes a lifestyle drug has been the subject of debate in the medical literature. It is defined in the Concise Oxford Dictionary as: "a pharmaceutical product characterised as improving quality of life rather than alleviating or curing disease". Improving quality of life is, however, a legitimate aim of the health service, so the fact that products such as oral contraceptives fall within this definition does not mean they should not be prescribed within the NHS. Where the boundary lies between what is and what is not acceptable to prescribe with NHS funding, however, is a matter for debate. Until clear guidance is issued, cases should be considered on an individual basis. An analysis of the prescribing of 5 mg of norethisterone in Oxford over a three year period identified clear peaks during the holiday seasons (a similar pattern was found throughout England), which the researchers concluded was most likely to be caused by patients wishing to delay menstruation during their holidays. The researchers questioned whether this meant that norethisterone was a lifestyle drug, or was being used as such, and whether such "lifestyle or convenience prescribing" was appropriate for the NHS.[21] This suggestion was challenged by many of those who responded to the article arguing, for example, that "health is not merely the absence of disease, but a positive concept of wellbeing. Norethisterone used to delay a period is no more a 'lifestyle treatment' than other activities of the NHS aimed at promoting health".[22]

It is important that doctors should give some thought to how to respond to requests for medication intended to be used in a way that could lead to them being described as lifestyle drugs. NICE guidance may be available, and access to some of these drugs within the NHS may be either prohibited (schedule 10) or restricted (schedule 11).[23] In other cases it is for the individual doctor to decide whether it is appropriate to prescribe as requested. In addition to the financial considerations, there are also questions of safety. There are inherent risks with virtually all medication and part of the doctor's role is to balance those risks against the anticipated benefits for the patient. When the drug is not clinically indicated, the benefits the patient will, or believes he or she will, derive need to be weighed against the risks. Doctors must be willing to justify their decisions to prescribe in these circumstances; patient demand or preference, on its own, is unlikely to provide sufficient justification.

Summary – pressure from patients

- When faced with patients' requests for particular medication, doctors are not obliged to comply and should do so only if they are satisfied that the treatment requested is the most appropriate option for the particular patient.
- Doctors have an ethical duty to use the most economic and efficacious treatment available when the patient is receiving treatment within the NHS.

- Doctors must resist pressure from patients to prescribe larger doses of medication than they consider clinically appropriate or for prescriptions to be issued repeatedly without clinical review.
- "Lifestyle drugs" should be prescribed only when the doctor considers them clinically appropriate for the patient and where the actual, or perceived, benefits outweigh any risks.

Pressure from employers

A doctor employed by a private organisation bears responsibility for prescribing and must be able to exercise independent clinical judgment, regardless of the policies of the clinic's management. In the past a practice developed whereby some establishments, particularly slimming clinics, appeared to have a predefined policy concerning the product and dose that doctors should supply to all patients. Prescriptions must not be influenced by factors such as the convenience of a clinic or hospital management, and any pressure from employers for doctors to practise according to such predefined prescribing policies must be resisted.

Clinical freedom and resources

Doctors can prescribe whatever approved medicine they consider appropriate for a patient but, in practice, clinical autonomy is not absolute. Within the NHS, the state takes an interest in prescribing habits and studies have identified tremendous variations in the volume and cost of prescribing between different geographical areas and between individual prescribers. Inevitably, resources are limited and there are various ways in which this fact can create ethical dilemmas for doctors.

Explicit rationing within the NHS

The prescribing of sildenafil (Viagra) was the first example of explicit rationing within the NHS. Sildenafil was licensed in the UK on 15 September 1998, for use by patients with erectile dysfunction. The Government anticipated a huge demand for the drug and was fearful of the financial implications of making it freely available within the NHS. It had been estimated that the annual drug bill for Viagra would exceed £1 billion a year if all men who might benefit were prescribed the drug.[24] As a result of these fears, the Standing Medical Advisory Committee of the Department of Health advised doctors not to prescribe the drug until definitive guidance had been drawn up.

After many months of intense debate, both in the media and among professional groups, and a six week period of formal consultation,[25] final guidance was issued. For the first time the Government was rationing access to a drug explicitly, not on the basis of clinical need or through the use of the

(Continued)

waiting list system, but on the basis of the aetiology of the condition. From 1 July 1999 the availability of sildenafil and other treatments for impotence within the NHS was restricted, by extending schedule 11 of the GMS Regulations, to patients who:

- were receiving NHS treatment for impotence on 14 September 1998
- were suffering from: diabetes, multiple sclerosis, Parkinson's disease, poliomyelitis, prostate cancer, severe pelvic injury, single gene neurological disease, spina bifida, or spinal cord injury
- were receiving treatment for renal failure by dialysis or
- had had the following surgery: prostatectomy, radical pelvic surgery, renal failure treated by transplant.[26]

In addition, treatment was to be made available, in exceptional cases of severe distress, through specialist care.

The BMA has opposed this form of rationing – on the basis of the cause of the underlying condition rather than on the basis of clinical need – which, it has argued, makes "a cruel, unethical, and inequitable distinction between 'acceptable' and 'unacceptable' forms of impotence".[27]

"Uneconomic" patients

Some NHS GPs have been accused of removing patients from their lists for so-called economic reasons, such as the need for expensive drug treatment. The BMA considers that removing a patient from a practice list for financial reasons would be unethical, but also believes that this is more of a perceived than an actual problem. In fact, where the costs of treating an individual patient are higher than anticipated, adequate mechanisms exist to enable doctors to seek and be granted an increase in their prescribing budget to cover the higher costs. Media reports have, however, highlighted cases in which the reason for removal was considered by the patient to be financial. This emphasises the importance of doctors informing patients of the reasons for their removal (even though this is not a requirement) so that the motives for such action are not misinterpreted. The General Medical Council (GMC) makes it clear to doctors that "you should not end relationships with patients solely because they have made a complaint about you or your team, or because of the financial impact of their care or treatment on your practice".[28]

Truth telling and resources

Although truth telling is generally advocated, some doctors have expressed concern about the implications of telling patients that there is medication available that could potentially help them, but that it is not available within the NHS or in the area in which they live. This has raised particular concern where the doctor believes that paying for the treatment privately would be beyond the financial means of the patient. Although it is only by having information that patients can make an informed choice about the options open to them, when the treatment option is clearly not open to them for financial reasons, is there any obligation to discuss it? Concerns have been raised that discussing the option of private treatment simply adds to the patient's burden, raises unreasonable hopes that treatment is available, and puts pressure on the patient and his or her family somehow to find the money to pay for the treatment. Although NICE was intended to remove inequalities in access to treatment (see page 464), it may have the effect of making this type of situation more common if potentially beneficial drugs are judged not to be cost effective.

In the past, some doctors have expressed concern about being instructed by their commissioning body to inform patients only of the treatments that are available within the NHS. The BMA does not consider that this is an appropriate position for commissioners to take and believes that doctors should be free to provide as much information as they consider to be appropriate for each patient. The right to impart information also gains support from Article 10 of the Human Rights Act 1998, which guarantees freedom of expression. This protects communication from any unjustified interference by a public authority, including NHS policy makers. In addition to health professionals' rights and ethical duties to give relevant information to their patients, patients also have rights to know the information if it is available.

The BMA has supported the view that patients should be told about the existence of potentially beneficial treatment options, but has recognised that providing such information can be problematic. In the BMA's view, part of the role of doctors is to ensure that decision making is returned as much as possible to the patient, rather than pre-empting the choice by withholding potentially important information. The BMA therefore believes that, as a general rule, patients should be given information about other treatment options that may benefit them, even if the doctor does not believe that the patient could afford to pay for the treatment. There may be rare cases, however, in which such information would clearly be unwelcome, when doctors should take their cue from patients as to the amount of information to impart. When information is to be provided, the manner and timing of its provision needs to be carefully considered and may need to be supported by professional counselling. If the treatment cannot be funded, patients should have access to information about the factors leading to the rationing decision and it should be made clear whether the treatment is unavailable because it is unproven or solely on grounds of cost.

Summary – clinical freedom and resources

- The BMA considers that removing a patient from a practice list for financial reasons would be unethical, but also believes that this is more of a perceived than an actual problem.
- The BMA believes that, as a general rule, patients should be given information about treatment options that are not available within the NHS but which may

benefit them, even if the doctor does not believe that the patient could afford to pay for the treatment.

- If treatment cannot be funded by the NHS, patients should be informed whether it is not available because it is unproven or solely on grounds of cost.

Clinical freedom and official guidance

A fairly common enquiry to the BMA is about the clinical freedom doctors have to prescribe what they consider appropriate for the patient, regardless of local or national guidelines. Since the late 1990s new (and some established) treatments, devices, and drugs have been subject to formal assessment for clinical efficacy and cost effectiveness. Separate bodies carry out this role in England and Wales, Scotland, and Northern Ireland, with differing levels of influence over decision making. In England and Wales, NICE[29] issues guidance that commissioning bodies are required to fund and doctors are expected to take into account in decision making (see pages 463–8).

In Scotland, this assessment role has been adopted, since 1 January 2003, by NHS Quality Improvement Scotland (NHS QIS),[30] part of whose responsibility is to provide advice to health boards about new and existing technologies. This guidance is sometimes based on a review of the recommendations of NICE and sometimes on separate NHS QIS health technology assessments. NHS QIS also supports the Scottish Medicines Consortium, which advises NHS boards about the efficacy of all newly licensed medicines, all new major formulations of existing medicines, and any major new indications of established medicines. Health boards in Scotland are expected to ensure that the drugs or treatments recommended by NHS QIS are made available to meet clinical need, but doing so is not mandatory. Doctors in Scotland also have the benefit of guidance from the Scottish Intercollegiate Guidelines Network (SIGN). The aim of SIGN is to improve the quality of health care for patients in Scotland, by reducing variation in practice and outcome, through the development and dissemination of national clinical guidelines containing recommendations for effective practice.

In Northern Ireland, the Department of Health, Social Services and Public Safety assesses guidance produced by NICE and decides whether it should be implemented in Northern Ireland. Proposals have been made to formalise these links with NICE.

Clinical freedom and NICE

Although the remit of NICE formally extends only to England and Wales, as noted above, its decisions and guidelines are clearly influential throughout the whole of the UK. For this reason, NICE is discussed in some detail below in order to provide clarification about its role and function and the way in which its work affects and relates directly to doctors' practice.

The role of NICE

The main function of NICE is to produce authoritative national guidance in order to create consistent clinical standards across the NHS. Guided by evidence-based practice, NICE is responsible for collecting and evaluating all relevant evidence and considering its implications for clinical practice, with reference to both clinical and cost effectiveness.[31] Confusion has arisen about whether affordability is also a factor that NICE should take into account in its appraisals. Giving evidence to the House of Commons Health Committee, both Lord Hunt, on behalf of the Department of Health, and NICE were clear that affordability for the NHS was not an issue for NICE and should not form part of its assessment.[32] This view was repeated in the Government's response.[33] The BMA welcomes the Government's assurance that NICE's recommendations on clinical and cost effectiveness should be made separately from considerations of affordability.

NICE provides health professionals, patients, and the public with authoritative, robust, and reliable guidance on current best practice. It produces *technology appraisals*, primarily of pharmaceutical products but also of medical devices, diagnostic techniques, health promotion, and surgical procedures, which result in recommendations in the form of guidance as to whether, and, if so, in what circumstances, it would be appropriate to use the technology in the NHS. It also produces *clinical guidelines*, which give broad guidance on the management of particular diseases and clinical conditions, and cover several different treatment options (e.g. for myocardial infarction, induction of labour, and fetal monitoring). Some of the issues addressed by NICE, such as the prescribing of cannabinoids,[34] raise questions of public policy in addition to those of clinical efficacy and cost effectiveness.

The status of NICE guidance

Funding and prescribing in line with NICE guidance

Since 1 January 2002, commissioning bodies in England have had a statutory obligation to provide funding to meet recommendations in NICE's technology appraisals (this does not apply to clinical guidelines).[35] Funding must be made available within three months of the publication of the guidance, unless separate direction is provided by the Department of Health. The same obligation has applied in Wales since 1 March 2002.[36] Implementation of NICE guidance after technology appraisals has not, however, been subject to systematic monitoring. The House of Commons Health Committee, in its review of the work of NICE, recommended that this should change.[37] The Government agreed, in its response, that the Commission for Healthcare Audit and Inspection should be the principal external inspector of the implementation of NICE recommendations.[38]

Survey on implementation of NICE guidance

In January 2001 NICE produced guidance recommending that donepezil, rivastigmine, and galantamine should be made available in the NHS as one component of the management of people with mild to moderate Alzheimer's disease. In February 2002 Mace and Taylor sent a questionnaire to 91 prescribing advisers for health authorities in England and Wales, to investigate the implementation of this guidance.[39] Responses were received from 69% of the health authorities contacted. Of these, only 76% provided formal funding for these drugs. Although nearly a quarter were not complying with the guidance, it had clearly been influential since this represented a significant increase in the number of health authorities funding the use of anticholinesterases for Alzheimer's disease. In May 2000 a similar survey, carried out by the same authors, had found that funding was provided by less than half of the health authorities questioned.

The BMA has received anecdotal reports of doctors being criticised by commissioning bodies for prescribing drugs that have been approved by NICE, and of doctors being pressured to limit their prescribing of expensive but NICE-approved drugs. Any BMA member faced with such pressure should contact their BMA regional office for advice and support.

Diverging from NICE guidance

Although in England and Wales funding must be provided for treatments recommended by NICE, this does not imply that the guidance is mandatory on health professionals or that approved medicines, products, or treatments are necessarily available to all patients. There is still some, although more limited, scope for clinical discretion in the provision of treatment to individual patients.

NICE explains the status of its guidelines as follows:

The guidance represents the view of the Institute which was arrived at after careful consideration of the available evidence. Health professionals are expected to take it fully into account when exercising their clinical judgment. The guidance does not, however, override the individual responsibility of health professionals to make appropriate decisions in the circumstances of the individual patient, in consultation with the patient and/or guardian or carer.[40]

Although NICE guidance is not binding on health professionals, the latter are "expected to take it fully into account" – a fairly strong statement. When a doctor decides, on clinical grounds, not to follow the guidance for a particular patient, it would be advisable to document this fact and the reasons for the decision in the patient's notes. Decisions not to follow guidance on other than clinical grounds, for example because the doctor does not agree that a particular treatment should be provided by the NHS, are unlikely to be considered acceptable. Thus, although doctors are not legally or contractually obliged to provide treatments that have been approved by NICE, there is strong pressure on them to do so.

NICE and clinical freedom: nicotine replacement therapies

In 2002 NICE recommended that nicotine replacement therapies (patches, chewing gum, lozenges, tablets, inhalators, or nasal sprays) and bupropion should be available on prescription to patients who expressed a wish to stop smoking.[41] It recommended that ideally an initial prescription should be sufficient to last two weeks after the target stop date and a second prescription should be given only to those who demonstrated their continuing effort to quit. If a smoker's attempt to quit is unsuccessful with treatment, the NHS should not normally fund any further attempts for six months unless there are external factors making it reasonable to provide the treatment sooner.

The BMA received calls from some of its members who were unhappy with this guidance, believing that nicotine replacement therapies should not be provided with public funding and that those who wished to quit smoking would have more commitment to their decision if they had funded the treatment themselves. Some doctors considered the pressure exerted on them to prescribe nicotine replacement therapies, against their judgment, represented inappropriate interference in their clinical decisions. The BMA, however, welcomed this development, recognising that drug therapies represent "an important step forward in helping patients to kick the habit, and improve their health".[42]

Given the status of NICE guidance, a doctor could legitimately decide in an individual case that prescribing was not appropriate (and should record and be prepared to justify the reasons for that decision), but a blanket refusal to prescribe nicotine replacement therapies and bupropion would not be acceptable.

At some time in the future, NICE guidelines are likely to be taken to set the standard and quality of care that a patient is entitled to expect[43] and failure to comply with the guidelines could be challenged in the courts. Departure from what NICE recommends is therefore likely to require the health professional or NHS body to demonstrate justification relating to the individual patient and the individual circumstances of that patient's case.

Doctors are legally able to prescribe any medicine within the NHS except those listed in the drug tariff as schedule 10 (prohibited) and, other than in specified circumstances, those listed in schedule 11 (restricted) or on the borderline substances list. In addition, some drugs may be prescribed only under special licence in the treatment of addiction. Doctors are not prohibited from prescribing drugs that NICE has assessed and rejected. It is likely, however, that strong pressure would be applied on doctors, from both clinical governance and financial perspectives, not to prescribe such drugs. When patients have been taking a particular medication for some time, however, the doctor should assess the needs of individuals and the impact of withdrawing or changing the treatment. In some cases, particularly relating to chronic conditions, if the treatment is not recommended but has been on the market for a long time, and it is likely that there are a significant number of patients taking it, NICE gives advice for handling the situation. For example, NICE guidance on drugs for multiple sclerosis states:

it is likely that patients currently receiving beta interferon or glatiramer acetate for MS, whether it be as routine therapy or as part of a clinical trial, could suffer loss of well-being if their treatment is discontinued at a time that they did not anticipate. Because of this all NHS patients who are on therapy at the date of the publication of this guidance should have the option to continue with treatment until they and their consultant consider it is appropriate to stop.[44]

NICE and rationing of resources

One of the aims behind the establishment of NICE was to provide NHS staff with clear and reasoned advice to meet patients' needs without draining a limited pool of resources. It was hoped that it would eliminate so-called "postcode prescribing" whereby different commissioners of health care had different policies on what types of treatment should be available and to whom.

Making the funding of NICE approved technologies mandatory could, however, simply shift "postcode prescribing" to areas of practice that have not been considered by NICE or divert funding away from care that is not subject to appraisal, such as nursing care. This was acknowledged by the House of Commons Health Committee in its review of NICE, which concluded that there was the potential for NICE approved technologies to be given priority over other, perhaps equally important, treatments and services that had not been considered by NICE.[45] It therefore recommended that "the government must work to achieve a comprehensive framework for health care prioritisation underpinned by an explicit set of ethical and rational values to allow the relative costs and benefits of different areas of NHS spending to be comparatively assessed in an informed way".[46] In its response, the Government pointed to its programme of National Service Frameworks as evidence that it had already developed a prioritisation framework at a broad level and said that there were not sufficient data available to produce a detailed framework in the short term.[47] In the meantime, commissioners are left with the dilemma of being required to fund certain treatments from a cost limited budget without clear guidance stating from where the money should be diverted. This is a growing problem given that, at the time of the Health Committee's review, NICE had recommended or partially recommended 28 out of the 31 treatments and interventions it had appraised at an increased cost of between £135·2 million and £154·8 million.[48]

Summary – clinical freedom and NICE

- Funding must be made available for the implementation of NICE recommendations.
- It is not mandatory for health professionals to follow NICE guidance in individual cases and there is some scope for clinical discretion. Health professionals are, however, expected to take the guidance "fully into account" and would be required to justify any departure.

- If doctors face local pressure to limit their prescribing of NICE approved drugs, they should contact their BMA regional office for advice and support.
- Decisions not to follow guidance on other than clinical grounds, for example, because the doctor does not agree that a particular treatment should be provided by the NHS, are unlikely to be considered acceptable.
- Although doctors are not prohibited from prescribing drugs that NICE has assessed and rejected, it is likely that strong pressure would be applied, from both clinical governance and financial perspectives, not to prescribe these drugs within the NHS.

Conflicts of interest in prescribing matters

Prescribing decisions should be made on the basis of the individual needs of the patient. Doctors must not be, or be seen to be, influenced in prescribing matters by the offer of any pecuniary or other incentives, or any personal financial interests. It is important, therefore, for doctors to be alert to any actual, or perceived, conflicts of interest and to take steps to avoid them; guidance is available for those working in the NHS.[49] The types of situation in which a conflict of interest could arise in relation to prescribing are discussed below.

Gifts or hospitality from pharmaceutical companies

The offer of financial or other incentives from the manufacturers of particular drugs would clearly raise questions about the motivation of a doctor who prescribed that drug in preference to one produced by a competitor. Even if the doctor sincerely believed the former drug to be the best option for the patient, it would be difficult to prove that his or her judgment had not been affected by personal gain. For this reason, doctors are not permitted to accept gifts or hospitality from pharmaceutical companies, and representatives of pharmaceutical companies are not permitted to offer them. The Medicines (Advertising) Regulations 1994 specifically forbid the offer or acceptance of "any gift, pecuniary advantage or benefit in kind, unless it is inexpensive and relevant to the practice of medicine or pharmacy".[50] The GMC's guidelines also state "you must act in your patients' best interests when making referrals and providing or arranging treatment or care. So you must not ask for or accept any inducement, gift or hospitality which may affect or be seen to affect your judgment".[51] The Association of the British Pharmaceutical Industry (ABPI) gives advice to the industry about the type of gifts that would fall within the permitted range.[52] In its 2001 code of practice it suggests that gifts should cost the company no more than £6 excluding VAT. The types of gift that would be acceptable include pens, pads, diaries, and surgical gloves, whereas items such as table mats or compact discs of music would not, because they would fail to meet the criteria of being "relevant to the practice of medicine or pharmacy".

There is nothing to prevent a doctor accepting travel costs for attendance at a meeting, or accepting hospitality at a meeting or event hosted by a pharmaceutical company provided that:

- the meeting has a clear educational content
- the hospitality offered is reasonable in level
- it is subordinate to the main purpose of the meeting and
- the hospitality applies only to those qualified to attend the meeting and does not, for example, extend to their spouses.

Pharmaceutical companies sometimes offer to provide a nurse or other member of staff to a general practice to undertake audit or a review of prescribing. It has been suggested that acceptance of such an offer could be interpreted as a gift or benefit in kind, since the company is effectively giving the practice the cost of the staff member's time. Concerns have also been expressed about the motivations of companies making such offers, with fears that there could be implicit pressure on the practice to change its prescribing patterns to the benefit of the company. The extent to which such concerns are justified is likely to depend upon the individual circumstances, but doctors must ensure that they are able to defend any decision to accept such offers and can show that their prescribing decisions have not been affected. Any practice planning to accept the offer of such assistance should ensure that there is a detailed written protocol specifying the terms of the agreement (see also Chapter 5, pages 180–1).

Payments for meeting pharmaceutical representatives

It is unacceptable for doctors to demand payment for meeting and listening to pharmaceutical representatives or to charge a fee for the use of a room for such a meeting. It is also contrary to the ABPI's code of practice for a medical representative to pay a fee in return for an interview.[53]

Financial involvement of doctors in external health related services

With some types of financial interest in health related services, such as doctors having a stake in private nursing homes or clinics, it is considered sufficient for the doctor to make the patient aware of his or her financial interest in the matter, and of any suitable alternatives. (The BMA's general advice on declaring financial interests is discussed in Chapter 16, pages 598–9.) The declaration of a financial interest, however, does not provide sufficient safeguard in the case of prescribing, since the patient is usually not in a position to exercise an informed choice about other medicines available as suitable alternatives to the one in which the doctor has a financial interest.

Common enquiries in this area concern the propriety of prescribing medicines marketed by companies in which the doctor or the doctor's family has a significant financial interest. Sometimes the financial interest is acquired after patients have been prescribed a long term course of a drug that suits them. In such cases, it has been thought unlikely that any objection would be raised to the doctor maintaining a patient's prescription. On the other hand, it would be questionable to consider changing a patient's medication from an already established pattern to a new medicine in which the doctor has a financial interest. It would certainly be unethical to do so if the doctor's decision was influenced by any financial benefit. Dilemmas arise, however, if doctors become convinced of the superiority of the product in which they have a financial interest. Genuine concern for the patient's benefit can easily be confused with self interest. For such reasons, the BMA believes it is generally unwise for doctors to form a business connection with companies producing, marketing, or promoting such products.

Participation in market research

Doctors are sometimes invited to participate in market research, carried out by an independent organisation on behalf of a pharmaceutical company. This can include questionnaires, interviews, or focus group work to ascertain doctors' views and practices in relation to certain generic drugs. Usually, the doctor participating does not know which company has sponsored the research. The ABPI code of practice makes it clear to pharmaceutical companies that market research simply involves the collection and analysis of information and must be unbiased and non-promotional.[54] There is no problem with doctors participating in such research provided that the personal health information of individual patients is not used without their consent. Doctors must also be able to demonstrate that their participation, and any remuneration received, has not in any way influenced, or could be perceived as influencing, their prescribing decisions. Those carrying out market research within, or on behalf of, the pharmaceutical industry are advised that "professional" respondents, such as doctors, should be given appropriate recompense, but that this "should be kept to a minimum level, proportionate to the amount of their time involved and should not be more than the normal hourly fee charged by that person for their professional consultancy or advice".[55]

Ownership of pharmacies

In the past the BMA advised that the independence of doctors and pharmacists was best demonstrated by their refraining from sharing premises or having a close financial connection, such as a doctor investing in, or owning, a pharmacy within the practice area. In the early 1990s, changes in the provision of primary health care led to some GPs offering a range of additional services on their premises, including dispensing facilities. Rural GPs had long been able to dispense for their own patients and this did not appear to give rise to unethical practices. The BMA withdrew its objection to GPs owning pharmacies, employing pharmacists, or sharing premises with pharmacists, providing doctors informed their patients of their financial interest in the pharmacy and that there was no direction of patients to the pharmacy in question. In fact, the relationship between doctors and pharmacists is changing, with pharmacists increasingly being integrated into the provision of NHS care, which has considerable advantages for patients (see pages 475–6).

Maintaining clinical objectivity

Doctors must not allow their personal beliefs to interfere with the treatment offered to patients. Doctors may explain their beliefs to patients, if invited to do so, and may suggest options such as complementary or alternative therapies, if they consider them to be appropriate for a particular patient. Information must, however, be provided objectively, giving a balanced view of the options available, and pressure must not be placed on the patient to accept the advice.

Failing to obtain consent for homeopathic treatment

In 2003 a GP was found guilty by the GMC of serious professional misconduct for failing to obtain the informed consent of patients before prescribing homeopathic or natural remedies for them. None of the patients had specifically requested homeopathic treatment. The GP also failed to explain the rationale for using dowsing in the process of the selection of a remedy. In addition, the GP was found to have put pressure on the mother of a young child to accept the services of a geopathic stress consultant (and did not inform her that the consultant was not medically qualified) by indicating that geopathic stress gridlines in the vicinity of her house could cause cot death.

The GP was suspended from the medical register for three months. The GMC's Professional Conduct Committee strongly recommended that she used the opportunity, during her suspension, to consider the effect on her patients of her use of alternative medicine, in order to ensure that, in future, her personal beliefs did not prejudice her patients' care.[56]

Summary – conflicts of interest in prescribing matters

- Doctors must not be, or be seen to be, influenced in prescribing matters by the offer of any pecuniary or other incentives or any personal financial interests. They should be alert to any actual or perceived conflicts of interest and take steps to avoid them.
- Doctors are not permitted to accept gifts or hospitality from pharmaceutical companies unless they are inexpensive and relevant to the practice of medicine or pharmacy.

- Subject to certain conditions doctors may accept hospitality to attend meetings or events hosted by pharmaceutical companies.
- The BMA believes it is generally unwise for doctors to form business connections with companies producing, marketing or promoting pharmaceutical products, but does not object to doctors owning pharmacies.

Shared prescribing

It is preferable for one doctor, usually the GP, to be fully informed about, and be responsible for, the overall management of a patient's health care. When a patient may be prescribed medication by different doctors, it is particularly important that one doctor is fully aware of the range of medication being taken in order to advise on any contraindications or adverse reactions. When more than one health professional is involved in aspects of the patient's care, effective liaison and communication is essential. All doctors should help to facilitate effective communication and should encourage patients to allow information about their treatment, and any medication prescribed, to be passed to others involved in their care. If patients refuse to allow information to be shared, for example with their GP, this should be respected, but the implications of their decision should be explained to them and, depending upon the level of risk, doctors may decide not to prescribe.

Prescribing shared between GPs and hospital doctors

There is a range of situations in which prescribing is shared between GPs and hospital doctors. General practitioners may be asked to take over the prescribing of long term medication or to continue ongoing medication after a patient's discharge from hospital. It is not unusual for a patient to present his or her GP with a list of medication recommended by the treating specialist with the expectation that the GP will issue a prescription. As mentioned above, if GPs prescribe this medication they accept full clinical responsibility for the decision. This means that GPs should comply with such requests only if they are satisfied that the recommended course of treatment is the correct medication and dose for the individual patient and they are willing to accept ongoing responsibility for monitoring the drug regimen. Shared prescribing happens quite frequently, but both parties need to be happy with the situation and the decisions made in each particular case. Sometimes this arises from the GP receiving a full and detailed report, which enables him or her to confirm that the drug recommended is appropriate. On other occasions, the hospital doctor discusses the case with the GP (with the patient's consent) and agreement is reached on the most appropriate course of action. Where there is disagreement about the appropriate medication, or dose, that cannot be resolved through discussion, the GP should refuse to participate in a shared prescribing arrangement and explain the reasons for this to both the requesting doctor and the patient. There are also financial implications for GPs who are asked to take over from hospital doctors the prescribing of what may be very expensive medication.

Guidance on the transfer of prescribing responsibility between hospitals and GPs was issued in 1991 by the Department of Health.[57] This guidance can help GPs to decide under what circumstances to accept prescribing responsibility, and hospital consultants to assess whether transfer of responsibility is appropriate. The following basic points should be borne in mind.

- Legal responsibility for prescribing rests with the doctor who signs the prescription.
- Hospital consultants have full responsibility for prescribing for inpatients and for specific treatments administered in hospital outpatient clinics.
- Responsibility for prescribing should rest with the consultant if the drugs are included in a hospital-based clinical trial and when it is more appropriate for the consultant to monitor the medication because of the need for specialised investigations, or where there are supply problems with the drugs.
- When a consultant considers that a patient's condition is stable, he or she may seek the agreement of the GP concerned to share the care. In proposing a shared care arrangement, a consultant may advise the GP which medicine to prescribe. When a new or rarely prescribed medicine is being recommended, its dosage and administration must be specified by the consultant so that the GP is properly informed and can monitor and adjust the dose if necessary. When a treatment is not licensed for a particular indication, full justification for the use of the drug should be given by the consultant to the GP. Where a hospital drug formulary is in operation and a recommended treatment is not included, the GP must be informed and given the option of prescribing alternatives.
- When an inpatient is discharged from hospital, sufficient drugs should be prescribed and dispensed by the hospital pharmacy for at least a seven day period. The GP to whose care the patient is transferred should receive notification in good time of the patient's diagnosis and drug therapy in order to maintain continuity. If that information cannot be transferred to the GP within the timescale, drugs should be prescribed by the hospital for as long a period as is necessary.
- When clinical, and therefore prescribing, responsibility for a patient is transferred from hospital to GP, it is of the utmost importance that the GP feels fully confident to prescribe the necessary drugs. It is essential that a transfer involving drug therapies with which GPs would not normally be familiar should not take place without full agreement between the hospital consultant (or any transferring doctor) and the GP, who must have sufficient information about the drug therapy. When drawing up shared care protocols, or when there is a professional disagreement over who should prescribe, it may be necessary for local discussion to take place between hospital managers and medical staff and the relevant local medical committee as a prelude to establishing agreement with individual GPs. A GP is obliged only to provide treatment that is consistent with GPs' terms of service.
- When a GP takes responsibility for prescribing or dispensing drugs that have not normally been dispensed in the community, there should be liaison between the transferring hospital and the community pharmacist to ensure continuity of supply.

In May 2003 a new categorisation system for specialist medicines was introduced in Northern Ireland.[58] Under this system medicines are divided into "red list drugs", for which prescribing responsibility should remain with the consultant, and "amber list drugs" for which responsibility may be transferred to primary care with the agreement of the individual GP. Shared care arrangements will be developed, in collaboration with GPs and consultants, for amber listed medicines.

Prescribing shared between the private sector and the NHS

In addition to questions of clinical responsibility, a frequent enquiry concerns the acceptability of a patient seeking private treatment but requesting that any medication recommended is supplied by the NHS. Even though individuals opt for private treatment or assessment, they are still entitled to NHS services. If the GP considers that the medication recommended is clinically necessary, he or she would be required under the terms of service to prescribe that medication within the NHS, even if the assessment from which the need was identified was undertaken in the private sector. This is subject to the comments above about whether the GP has sufficient information and is willing to accept clinical responsibility for the prescribing decision recommended by another doctor.

The same obligation to prescribe does not arise if the medication recommended is not clinically necessary or if it is generally not provided within the NHS. A common example is fertility treatment, where patients seek *in vitro* fertilisation in the private sector and ask their GP to issue NHS prescriptions for the drugs. The decision about whether to comply with such requests rests with the individual GP or commissioning body. In the past, these requests have caused some concern amongst GPs, who felt they were being placed in the invidious position of either appearing unsupportive of their patients or accepting legal, financial, and ethical responsibility for a course of medication that they had not initiated and which, in some cases, they may not consider to be clinically necessary. When the product is of a very specialised nature, requiring ongoing monitoring, some GPs may feel they have insufficient expertise to accept responsibility for the prescription and so refuse such requests. Others initiate discussions with the relevant specialists to reach a position with which all parties are content.

Many of the problems and concerns that arise in relation to prescribing shared between the private sector and the NHS could be avoided by improved communication between the parties concerned. In many cases patients are simply informed that their GP will prescribe the recommended medication rather than being advised to ask their GP. This is not simply a matter of etiquette. If the GP does not feel able to accept clinical responsibility or, in the case of medication that is not clinically necessary, financial responsibility for the recommended medication, this could cause difficulties for the doctor–patient relationship. Those requesting GPs to take over prescribing should bear these points in mind when discussing the matter with patients.

Prescribing shared with independent nurse prescribers

The range of medicines that can be prescribed by independent nurse prescribers has expanded over time. A complete and up to date list of the preparations nurses may prescribe for patients receiving NHS care can be found in the *Nurse prescribers' formulary*.[59] Independent nurse prescribers who have undertaken a longer, specific programme of training can also prescribe from the "extended formulary". As in any other circumstance in which prescribing responsibilities are shared, good communication between health professionals is essential.

Prescribing shared with pharmacists

The *NHS plan* set out the Government's aim to utilise the knowledge and experience of pharmacists to improve patient care by integrating them more into the provision of NHS care. This notion was supported by the Audit Commission, which recommended that medicines were so central to patient care that pharmacies should be seen as a core clinical service rather than as a technical support service.[60] A number of proposals were made to implement this shift including:

- more medicines being available direct from pharmacists, such as the provision of emergency hormonal contraception under patient group directions
- repeat prescriptions being available without the need to visit a GP
- the introduction of electronic prescribing
- the development of e-pharmacy to allow people to consult a pharmacist electronically, seek advice, and make arrangements for the delivery of their prescriptions
- NHS Direct referring more callers directly to their local pharmacy where appropriate
- pharmacists providing extra help for patients on how to use their medicines
- the establishment of "one stop primary care centres" where pharmacists work alongside other professionals such as GPs, dentists, and opticians.[61]

All of these proposals require major changes to the relationship between doctors and pharmacists. An integrated service requires closer liaison and sharing of responsibility for patient care. Pharmacists are independent practitioners, subject to statutory regulation by the Royal Pharmaceutical Society of Great Britain. The most significant change is likely to be in terms of pharmacists working alongside doctors rather than doctors delegating care to pharmacists. Increasingly, for example, pharmacists are working with GPs in primary care and many are employed as prescribing advisers. Changes in legislation in 2001 extended prescribing rights to pharmacists, to allow for "supplementary prescribing": when the patient has already been clinically assessed by an independent prescriber (a doctor, for example), supplementary prescribers (suitably trained pharmacists or nurses) may prescribe in line with an agreed clinical management plan.[62] Medicines legislation permits the introduction of supplementary prescribing across the UK, but the method and timing of its implementation is a matter for the devolved administrations in Scotland, Wales, and Northern Ireland. In England, it has been suggested that, in the future, this may be extended to full "independent" prescribing by pharmacists.[63]

Patient group directions

In most cases doctors retain responsibility for prescribing for their patients on an individual basis, although in some instances the way in which medicine is prescribed has changed. In England, for example, patient group directions, drawn up by multidisciplinary groups and signed by a senior doctor and a senior pharmacist permit certain named health professionals to supply medicines to patients within strict protocols, but without the need for an individual prescription.[64] The supply and administration of medicines under patient group directions are reserved for those limited situations where this method offers an advantage for patient care, without compromising patient safety; the provision of emergency hormonal contraception provides a good example of their use. As with individual prescriptions, doctors should not sign patient group directions if they have any doubts about the safety or efficacy of the medication, or uncertainties about the ability of the named health professional adequately to assess the patient's suitability for the treatment or to provide any necessary supervision.

Practitioners of complementary therapies

An area of concern about shared prescribing arises in connection with the treatments recommended by complementary practitioners to whom patients frequently self refer. Anxiety is often expressed by doctors about patients' decisions to suspend or postpone orthodox treatments while they explore other remedies. The evidence appears to suggest, however, that the predominant pattern is for patients to use complementary and orthodox medicine simultaneously.[65] Where treatment is being provided by more than one practitioner, it is important that there is good communication to ensure that any risk of harmful interaction between the preparations recommended is identified and avoided. It is important that complementary therapists should encourage patients to inform their GPs about any medication prescribed. (Information about herbal medicines and their interaction with other medication can be found on the Medicines and Healthcare Products Regulatory Agency website.) Similarly, when doctors are aware that patients are seeing a complementary therapist, they should ensure that the therapist has the relevant information about prescribed medication. Some patients are, however, reluctant to discuss complementary therapies with their GPs, fearing that their decision to seek alternative remedies may be derided or perceived as a lack of faith in the doctor's skills. GPs should adopt a non-judgmental approach to their patient's choices (except when these choices are detrimental to the patient's health) and should encourage the sharing of relevant information about the patient's treatment. Where the doctor considers the complementary therapy to be potentially harmful, however, either because of the treatment itself or the qualifications and experience of the practitioner, this should be sensitively explained to the patient. For more information on liaison with complementary therapists see Chapter 19 (pages 688–9).

Summary – shared prescribing

- Where a patient may be prescribed medication by different doctors, one doctor should be fully aware of the range of medication being taken in order to advise on any contraindications or adverse reactions.
- If patients refuse to allow information to be sought from their GP, this should be respected but the implications of the decision should be explained and, depending upon the risks and the seriousness of the condition, other doctors may decide not to prescribe.
- GPs should prescribe medication at the request of another doctor only if they are satisfied that the recommended course and dose of medication is appropriate for the individual patient and if they are willing to accept full clinical responsibility for the prescribing decision.
- Patients sometimes ask their GPs for NHS prescriptions for medication recommended during private consultations. If the GP believes the medication to be clinically necessary (and it is medication for which the GP is willing to accept clinical responsibility) the GP would be required to comply.
- The same obligation to prescribe does not arise if the medication recommended is not considered clinically necessary, or if the medication is generally not provided within the NHS.
- Doctors should not sign patient group directions if they have any doubts about the safety or efficacy of the medication or doubts about the ability of the named health professional adequately to assess patients' suitability for the treatment or to provide any necessary supervision.

Prescribing for children

The National Audit Office has reported that up to 90% of medicines prescribed to children in hospitals are not actually licensed for such use.[66] Other research has found that approximately 25% of medicines used in general paediatric wards, 40% in paediatric intensive care units, and 80% in neonatal intensive care units are unlicensed or used outside the terms of their licence approval.[67] Parents are sometimes understandably concerned that the medication their child has been prescribed is not licensed, or is not licensed for children. In order to address these concerns the Royal College of Paediatrics and Child Health has produced information leaflets for older children and for parents or carers.[68] These leaflets explain that often the clinical trials that led to the drug being licensed were restricted to adults and so the licence did not extend to children. It also explains why some medicines do not have a licence at all or are being used for conditions other than those originally covered by the licence. The leaflets provide reassurance that, based on the evidence available, the doctor in charge of the child's care believes that the medication in question is the best treatment for the child's condition, despite the drug's status with respect to licensing. The BMA supports moves by the Committee on Safety of Medicines and others to minimise the use of unlicensed medicines in children.

Children's formulary

In 1999 the Royal College of Paediatrics and Child Health and the Neonatal and Paediatric Pharmacists Group produced a paediatric formulary for the UK.[69] This gives general guidance and recommendations on treatment and prescribing for children, and information on individual drugs, dosages, contraindications, and licence status.

Self prescribing and prescribing for family members

The BMA and the GMC advise doctors against prescribing for themselves or for family, friends, and colleagues. There are clearly some cases, such as in an emergency situation, in which such action would be reasonable, but as a general rule it should be avoided. There is a risk that doctors who self treat may ignore or deny serious health problems or may simply treat symptoms without taking steps to identify the underlying cause. There is also a risk that self prescribing could lead to drug abuse or addiction; this is discussed further in Chapters 1 (page 53) and 21 (page 761).

Treating family, friends, and colleagues could raise questions about the objectivity of the advice provided and, although the same duty of confidentiality would apply, raises issues of privacy for the family members and friends. One-off prescribing for family and friends, except in exceptional circumstances, is also to be avoided because this could interfere with care or treatment being provided by the patient's usual doctor. There is also a risk that, if the patient is harmed by the medication, the doctor's motives could be called into question.

Prescribing for addicts

Doctors who are responsible for prescribing to drug addicts must be familiar with the relevant regulations[70] and guidance,[71] and ensure that their actions comply with the law. Their role extends beyond simply prescribing and may include health promotion, harm minimisation, and treatment or rehabilitation. Information and guidance about the role of health professionals in treating drug addicts can be found in the report, *The misuse of drugs*, produced by the BMA's Board of Science and Education.[72] GPs should not refuse to accept patients on to their list solely on the grounds of their addiction, although they are not required to provide specialist treatment for a patient's drug addiction. In fact, only those doctors who hold a special licence may prescribe, administer, or supply diamorphine, dipipanone, or cocaine in the treatment of drug addiction; other practitioners must refer addicts requiring these drugs to a treatment centre.

Prescribing at a distance

Consulting by internet, email, or telephone

One of the changes that has taken place in the way medicine is practised in the UK is the adoption of an increasingly consumerist attitude towards health care. Patients are requesting easier and more convenient methods of obtaining medication; developments in information technology have facilitated email consultations and internet prescribing as facets of that general trend.

Prescription-only medicines marketed over the internet

In 2003 the National Audit Office reported that 1% of the public it surveyed had purchased prescription-only medicines over the internet, saying it was the easiest way to obtain the medicine and that it cost less than with a prescription.[73] At that time, the top 10 prescription-only medicines marketed over the internet in the UK were:

1. Xenical – obesity
2. Proscar – prostate disorders
3. Propecia – hair loss
4. Viagra – erectile dysfunction
5. Uprima – erectile dysfunction
6. Reductil – appetite suppressant
7. Zyban – antismoking
8. Relenza – influenza
9. Phentermine – obesity
10. Meridia – obesity.

In some limited circumstances, providing medical advice and treatment over the telephone or by email can be a useful addition to the services offered to existing patients, but there are serious concerns about prescribing to new patients over the internet. The GMC advises that consultations and prescribing by telephone, email, or online may seriously compromise standards of care where:

- the patient is not previously known to the doctor
- no examination can be provided
- there is little or no provision for appropriate monitoring of the patient or follow up care.[74]

Doctors are advised to consider very carefully whether prescribing in this way would be in the best interests of their patients.

Internet prescribing

In 2002 the GMC found a doctor guilty of serious professional misconduct for inappropriately prescribing Viagra and Xenical via the internet. In relying on the answers given on an online questionnaire, it was found that the doctor had not taken adequate steps to:

- assess prospective patients to ascertain their condition, based on their medical history and clinical signs
- conduct an appropriate examination or
- ensure the information provided by the patient online was truthful and correct.

He could therefore not satisfy himself to a sufficient standard that prospective patients had a clinical need for Viagra or Xenical. The doctor also failed to take steps to arrange for the patients' GPs to be informed about the drugs prescribed, or to provide appropriate monitoring and follow up care. By prescribing in this way, it was held that the doctor was not acting in his patients' best interests.

The doctor was suspended from the medical register for three months.[75]

Guidance for GPs is also provided by the BMA's General Practitioners Committee, in the document *Consulting in the modern world*, which discusses the advantages and disadvantages of using a range of electronic means of communication. It highlights the difficulty for doctors who are seeking to justify the prescription of medication to patients:

- whose identities they could not verify
- in geographical jurisdictions they could not identify
- using a system that severely constrains both parties' ability to communicate
- whom they had been unable to see, hear, touch, or examine
- to whom they are unable to provide follow up care.

It concludes that "other than for requesting repeat prescriptions ... drugs should never be prescribed as a result of an on line consultation".[76]

Prescribing for patients in other countries

A very difficult question concerns prescriptions for patients who live in other parts of the world. Relatives in this country sometimes approach their own GP with a request for medication for a seriously ill patient living abroad where appropriate drugs are unobtainable. As with any other prescription, the prescribing doctor would retain full clinical responsibility for prescribing such medication and this can prove particularly difficult when he or she cannot examine the patient personally, but is relying on information obtained from others. There is no obligation on doctors to comply with such requests and many refuse because of the obvious risks of prescribing for a patient they have not seen. Some doctors, however, feel impelled by humanitarian considerations to look into the case and to offer some assistance if they can. Such situations are fraught with difficulty, but if doctors wish to pursue the matter, after considering the risks for the overseas patient, and for themselves if harm to that patient should result, the BMA gives the advice below.

It is unwise to rely solely on relatives' account of the patient's condition. Often the patient's own doctor abroad is willing to give a clinical report of the condition and recommendations for medication, as well as confirming that the medication is necessary and unobtainable by other means. Such cases virtually amount to a situation of shared prescribing, with the doctor who writes the prescription relying heavily on the medical opinion of the examining doctor. Some lives are probably saved by this arrangement and this is usually the factor that persuades the prescribing doctor to cooperate, on the grounds that in the particular situation the risks of not obtaining treatment at all are likely to be greater than the risks of prescribing error. The BMA has not heard of any cases in which a prescribing doctor subsequently suffered legal repercussions, although the possibility of erroneous prescribing in such situations cannot be ruled out.

Even when the prescribing doctor is willing to participate in such an arrangement, there are a number of further hurdles to be overcome and these may influence the doctor's view of the practicality of the proposal. For example, relatives have to consider how the drugs will be transported, including the rules governing the export and import of drugs that are not for their personal use. Many countries have their own restrictions on the drugs that can be taken into the country; even some that are available over the counter in the UK cannot be taken into other countries. Advice will need to be sought in individual cases from the relevant embassy for the country concerned. Any drugs posted overseas are subject to customs labelling and postage regulations. Any such prescriptions must, of course, be paid for privately as they are not covered by the NHS.

Summary – prescribing at a distance

- Prescribing by email or over the telephone could seriously compromise the standard of care provided to patients. Doctors should think carefully about whether prescribing in this way is in the best interests of their patients.
- There are serious safety risks of prescribing in cases where the patient is unknown to the doctor, there is no opportunity for examination, and the arrangements for monitoring and follow up are limited.

- Doctors are not obliged to comply with requests from patients to prescribe drugs for relatives in another country. Those who wish to assist, however, must be aware of the possibility of liability arising and should seek information from the patient's own doctor whenever possible in order to verify the information provided. They also need to give consideration to the practicalities of such an arrangement.

Drug administration

Responsibility for administering drugs in hospital

Doctors who are responsible for administering drugs must ensure that they have the necessary knowledge and expertise to do so safely and effectively. Those who are responsible for training doctors have an ethical responsibility to ensure that students are adequately supervised and trained in any procedures they may be required to undertake. Any doctor who is in doubt about the method of administration of a particular drug, or the correct procedures to be followed, should seek advice from a more senior member of the team or from a pharmacist. Similarly, the advice of a pharmacist should be sought if there is uncertainty about the appropriate dosage of a drug for a particular patient.

A study of the incidence and severity of intravenous drug errors on 10 wards in two UK hospitals found that errors occurred in almost half of the intravenous drug doses observed.[77] Of the 430 doses observed during the study, preparation errors occurred in 32 doses (7%), administration errors in 155 doses (36%), and both types of error in 25 doses (6%); these errors were potentially harmful in about a third of cases. Protocols should be in place in all hospitals, setting out clearly the checking procedures that must be followed to ensure that the dose and strength of a drug are those prescribed and that the drug is administered to the correct patient in the correct way. There have been a number of tragic cases of drugs being administered to the wrong patient or by the wrong route (between 1985 and 2001 at least 13 patients died or were paralysed as a result of accidental intrathecal administration of vincristine[78]). These cases have highlighted the importance of ensuring that adequate training, supervision, and safeguards are in place, as far as possible to guard against such errors. Doctors should not feel pressured to carry out procedures they feel are beyond their training or capability, and it is their responsibility to speak out about any concerns (see also Chapter 21, pages 749–54).

Error in drug administration

On 4 January 2001, an 18-year-old male patient, WJ, attended Queen's Medical Centre, Nottingham, for the administration of chemotherapy as part of his medical maintenance programme after successful treatment of

(Continued)

leukaemia. He was to receive cytosine by intrathecal (spinal) injection and, on the following day, he was to receive vincristine intravenously. Owing to a series of errors and the lack of training and experience of the doctors concerned, the vincristine was administered on the same day and also by intrathecal injection. This error is almost always fatal and, despite emergency treatment being provided, WJ died on 2 February 2001.

An external inquiry was carried out, which concluded that the death "was not caused by one or even several human errors but by a far more complex amalgam of human, organisational, technical and social interactions".[79] Among the failings highlighted in the report were the lack of explicit written protocols, the lack of formal training for the doctors concerned, and the unwillingness of the senior house officer to mention his doubts about the treatment to his senior colleague.

Special safeguards

Some drugs carry significant risks, require particularly rigorous safeguards, and should be administered according to standard operating procedures. Because of the potency of the drugs involved in chemotherapy, for example, a set protocol should exist for their use and the drugs should be administered only by those who have received specific training. This should include how to make up the drugs, the nature of the agents, including their danger to the administering health professional and other employees, and their administration. The individual administering the drug should also be aware of the appropriate procedures to follow in the event of spillage or a failure in clinical technique during administration, as well as procedures for the safe disposal of any unused drugs and the containers and instruments used in administration. Where necessary, supervision and advice should be available from a more senior colleague and doctors must not be afraid to seek help. Doctors have an ethical responsibility to be satisfied that they have the necessary competence and support to undertake these procedures.

Covert administration of medication

Competent patients have the right to refuse medication, as well as any other treatment, and must not be given medication against their wishes. When patients are not competent to take decisions about their health care, they should be treated in their "best interests" or, in Scotland, either under the general authority to treat or with the authorisation of an appointed healthcare proxy (see Chapter 3, pages 110–2). There may be exceptional cases in which doctors take the view that an incompetent patient requires medication and his or her interests would be best served by giving this in the least distressing manner, which could include covert administration. Any such decision must be made on an individual basis, and blanket rules must not be applied to particular categories of patient. Covert administration of medication is never justified for the convenience of those providing treatment. This is discussed further in Chapter 1 (pages 43–5).

Summary – drug administration

- Doctors who are responsible for administering drugs must ensure that they have the necessary knowledge and expertise to do so safely and effectively.
- Doctors should not feel pressured to carry out procedures they feel are beyond their training or capability, and it is their responsibility to speak out about any concerns.
- Competent patients have the right to refuse medication and must not be given medication against their wishes.
- In exceptional cases where an incompetent patient requires medication, it may be acceptable to administer the medicine covertly if this is in the best interests of the patient. Any such decision must be made on an individual basis, and blanket rules must not be applied to particular categories of patient.
- Covert drug administration is never justified for the convenience of those providing treatment.

Reporting adverse drug reactions

The Committee on Safety of Medicines relies on information from clinicians for the effective running of its Yellow Card Scheme. This scheme invites spontaneous reporting of suspected adverse drug reactions. Information is supplied on a voluntary basis by doctors, dentists, pharmacists, and coroners, and by pharmaceutical companies under statutory obligations.[80] Doctors should be alert to the possibility of side effects and are strongly encouraged to participate in this scheme, which seeks pseudonymised information: information that is not identifiable to the Committee on Safety of Medicines, but that can be traced back to an identifiable individual if necessary. From 2003 patients in England have been able to report suspected adverse drug reactions directly via NHS Direct.[81]

The National Patient Safety Agency has developed a National Reporting and Learning System in England and Wales, through which adverse incidents and near misses, including those involving medication, are collected. Using these data the Agency will develop solutions to try to ensure that the same errors are not repeated.

Pharmacogenetics

It is well known that individuals respond in different ways to medication: some patients do not respond at all to a particular drug, others require a higher than the usual dose to be effective, and some people suffer adverse effects. It is also known that some of this difference is due to genetic variation. Pharmacogenetics offers the potential to identify how individual patients will respond to certain types of medication, based on differences in their genetic makeup, so that this information can be taken into account in prescribing decisions. This could lead to a form of individualised treatment regimens for some conditions, whereby prescribing is preceded by a genetic test to ascertain whether the drug will be effective, the appropriate dose to administer, and whether the individual is likely to suffer adverse effects. This could have a very big impact on the way in which drugs are prescribed in the future in both primary and secondary care. Although the possibility of safer and more effective medication is to be welcomed, it is important to give some thought to the ethical dilemmas that could arise before pharmacogenetics is adopted into mainstream medical practice.

Many of the ethical issues raised are similar to those discussed in Chapter 9 about the implications of genetic information being available and, in particular, issues around consent, confidentiality, and privacy. There are some aspects, however, that are novel to pharmacogenetics. In addition to identifying those who are likely to experience side effects, testing the individual's response to a drug would also identify a group of patients for whom the treatment may not be effective. In most cases this would not give a certain answer about whether the drug will work or not, but is more likely to offer a probability of success. This leads to questions about where to draw the line in terms of prescribing and, in particular, when to restrict the use of public funds. If a genetic test indicates that an individual has only a very low chance of the drug being successful, is it appropriate for that to be provided within the NHS? That decision clearly depends partly on other factors such as the risks or side effects of the medication, the seriousness of the condition, and whether other treatments are available that may be more successful. As with other forms of treatment, however, ultimately some judgment is needed about what anticipated level of success is sufficient to justify providing the treatment. Should a patient who has only a 10% chance of success be offered that medication from public funds? Should there be limits to what people can pay for privately? This is not only a question of equity, but also of the extent to which it is reasonable for individuals who may be particularly vulnerable at the time to pay for treatment that is unlikely to be successful. Provided they receive sufficient information, is it for the individual to decide or should there be limits on what can be offered?

When the probability of success is low, this could mean informing the patient that, although there is a drug available, it is unlikely to work for him or her and therefore will not be provided. The advantage of knowing in advance that the drug is unlikely to work is that it is possible to avoid a trial and error approach in which a patient may be exposed to unnecessary risks or side effects. The disadvantage, for those who are unlikely to benefit, however, is the risk of psychological harm from removing the hope of recovery that can provide an important coping strategy for those faced with serious illness. Health professionals need to be prepared for the possible effect on patients of receiving this information, particularly for those individuals who are suffering from serious conditions for which no other effective treatment is available.

One major difference arising from the future development of pharmacogenetics will be the scale of genetic testing performed. At the time of writing, only a small number of people, primarily those who know themselves to be "at risk", have genetic testing. The expansion of testing to the rest of the population could present new problems. This is likely to be associated with the possibility and nature of any additional information being inadvertently discovered. If, for example, a test carried out to assess drug response was also capable of providing evidence of a high genetic risk of a serious disease, perhaps where there is currently no effective treatment available, this would need to be explained carefully to the patient who would need to take that into account when deciding whether to consent to the test. Problems could arise if the information available to assess drug response was later found to have relevance in terms of the risk of developing another condition, because the individual would be given no choice about whether to receive that information.

Although the potential for pharmacogenetics is great, there is a possibility that its application, and therefore its benefits, will be limited because of economic considerations. By identifying those patients for whom the drugs would not be effective, pharmaceutical companies would reduce the market for their products. This could lead to a reduction in the development of drugs that would be suitable for only a small group of the population unless incentives were provided for research into those conditions. Another possibility is that, by reducing the market for particular products, pharmacogenetics could lead to inexorable rises in the price of some medicines, which would raise serious questions about affordability within the NHS.

References

1 Joint Formulary Committee. *British national formulary*. London: British Medical Association and Pharmaceutical Press. (Published biannually.)

2 *Clinical evidence*. London: BMJ Publishing Group. (Published biannually; updated monthly online.)

3 *Drug and Therapeutics Bulletin*. London: Which? (Published monthly.)

4 Montgomery J. *Health care law*, 2nd ed. New York: Oxford University Press, 2003:220.

5 Panting G. Best practice: prescribing. *Doctor* 2002;(Apr 4):42.

6 General Medical Council. *Good medical practice*. London: GMC, 2001: para 3.

7 GMC Professional Conduct Committee hearing, 23–25 September 2002.

8 Medicines Control Agency, Department of Health Social Services and Public Safety, Northern Ireland, Department of Health. *Provision of patient information with dispensed medicines: guidance note*. London: DoH, 2002.

9 Royal Pharmaceutical Society of Great Britain. *Medicines, ethics and practice. A guide for pharmacists*. London: RPS, 2002:87.

10 Royal Pharmaceutical Society of Great Britain. *From compliance to concordance*. London: RPS, 1997.

11 Marinker M, Shaw J. Not to be taken as directed. *BMJ* 2003;**326**:348–9.

12 Royal Pharmaceutical Society of Great Britain. *From compliance to concordance*. *Op cit*.

13 See, for example: Meric F, Bernstam E, Mirza N, *et al*. Breast cancer on the world wide web: cross sectional survey of quality of information and popularity of web-sites. *BMJ* 2002;**324**:577–81. Kunst H, Groot D, Latthe PM, Latthe M, Khan KS. Accuracy of information on apparently credible web-sites: survey of five common health topics. *BMJ* 2002;**324**:581–2. Pandolfini C, Bonati M. Follow up of quality of public oriented health information on the world wide web: systematic re-evaluation. *BMJ* 2002;**324**:582–3.

14 National Electronic Library for Health: http://www.nhsia.nhs.uk/nelh

15 NHS Direct Online: http://www.nhsdirect.nhs.uk

16 NHS Direct Wales: http://www.nhsdirect.wales.nhs.uk

17 NHS24 in Scotland: http://www.nhs24.com

18 Medicines and Healthcare Products Regulatory Agency: http://www.mhra.gov.uk

19 General Practitioners Committee. *Searching the internet for medical information – tips for patients.* London: British Medical Association, 2000.

20 Department of Health. *Pharmacy in the future – implementing the NHS plan. A programme for pharmacy in the National Health Service.* London: DoH, 2000:3.

21 Shakespeare J, Neve E, Hodder K. Is norethisterone a lifestyle drug? Results of a database analysis. *BMJ* 2000;**320**:291.

22 Bryant G, Scott I, Worrall A. Is norethisterone a lifestyle drug? Health is not merely the absence of disease. *BMJ* 2000;**320**:1605.

23 Schedule 10 of the National Health Service (General Medical Services) Regulations 1992 (SI 1992 No. 635) provides for a list of drugs and other substances that are not to be prescribed within the NHS. Schedule 10 drugs are also frequently referred to as the "blacklist". Schedule 11 drugs are a small list within the drug tariff of drugs to be prescribed within the NHS only in certain circumstances.

24 Brooks V. Viagra is licensed in Europe but rationed in Britain. *BMJ* 1998;**217**:765.

25 Department of Health. *The use of sildenafil in the treatment of erectile dysfunction; consultation letter from the Secretary of State.* London: DoH, 1999.

26 NHS Executive. *Treatment for impotence.* Leeds: Department of Health, 1999. (HSC 1999/115.)

27 Chisholm J. Viagra: a botched test case for rationing. *BMJ* 1999;**318**:273–4.

28 General Medical Council. *Good medical practice.* London: GMC, 2001: para 24.

29 National Institute for Clinical Excellence. *A guide to NICE.* London: NICE, 2003.

30 Before 1 January 2003 this role was undertaken by the Health Technology Board for Scotland.

31 The National Institute for Clinical Excellence (Establishment and Constitution) Order. (SI 1999 No. 220.)

32 House of Commons Health Committee. *Second report of session 2001–02 volume 1 – National Institute for Clinical Excellence.* London: The Stationery Office, 2002: para 105. (HC515-I.)

33 Department of Health. *Government response to the Health Committee's second report of session 2001–02 on the National Institute for Clinical Excellence.* London: The Stationery Office, 2002:13. (Cm 5611.)

34 In 2003 NICE was in the process of developing guidance on the clinical and cost effectiveness of cannabinoids (cannabis derivatives) for the treatment of the symptoms of multiple sclerosis.

35 National Health Service Act 1977. Directions to Health Authorities, Primary Care Trusts and NHS Trusts in England, 11 Dec 2001.

36 National Health Service Act 1977. Directions to Health Authorities and NHS Trusts in Wales, 28 Feb 2002. Specific directions have been issued to extend the 3 month period for implementation to 12 months in some cases.

37 House of Commons Health Committee. *Second report of session 2001–02 volume 1 – National Institute for Clinical Excellence. Op cit:* para 76.

38 Department of Health. *Government response to the Health Committee's second report of session 2001–02 on the National Institute for Clinical Excellence. Op cit:* p. 9.

39 Mace S, Taylor D. Adherence to NICE guidance for the use of anticholinesterases for Alzheimer's disease. *Pharm J* 2002;**269**:680–1.

40 National Institute for Clinical Excellence. *Compilation. Summary of guidance issued to the NHS in England and Wales. Issue 5.* London: NICE, 2002: inside front cover.

41 National Institute for Clinical Excellence. *Guidance on the use of nicotine replacement therapy (NRT) and bupropion for smoking cessation.* London: NICE, 2002.

42 British Medical Association press release. *BMA welcomes go-ahead for therapies to help smokers.* 2002 Apr 11.

43 Kennedy I, Grubb A. *Medical law, 3rd ed.* London: Butterworths, 2000:125.

44 National Institute for Clinical Excellence. *Beta interferon and glatiramer acetate for the treatment of multiple sclerosis. Technology appraisal guidance no. 32.* London: NICE, 2002:1.

45 House of Commons Health Committee. *Second report of session 2001–02 volume 1 – National Institute for Clinical Excellence. Op cit:* para 80.

46 *Ibid:* para 135.

47 Department of Health. *Government response to the Health Committee's second report of session 2001–02 on the National Institute for Clinical Excellence. Op cit:* p. 16.

48 House of Commons Health Committee. *Second report of session 2001–02 volume 1 – National Institute for Clinical Excellence. Op cit:* para 127.

49 NHS Management Executive. *Standards of business conduct for NHS staff.* Leeds: NHS, 1993. Department of Health. *Commercial sponsorship – ethical standards for the NHS.* Leeds: NHS Executive, 2000.

50 The Medicines (Advertising) Regulations 1994 s21(1). (SI 1994 No. 1932.)

51 General Medical Council. *Good medical practice. Op cit:* para 55.
52 Association of the British Pharmaceutical Industry. *Code of practice for the pharmaceutical industry 2001.* London: ABPI, 2001: supplementary information, clause 18·2.
53 *Ibid:* clause 15·3.
54 *Ibid:* clause 10·2.
55 British Healthcare Business Intelligence Association (BHBIA) in consultation with the Association of the British Pharmaceutical Industry. *Guidelines: the legal and ethical framework for healthcare market research.* St Albans: BHBIA, 2002: section 12.
56 GMC Professional Conduct Committee hearing, 13–17 January 2003.
57 NHS Management Executive. *Responsibilities for prescribing between hospitals and GPs.* London: Department of Health, 1991. (EL(91)127.)
58 Department of Health, Social Services and Public Safety. *The regional group on specialist drugs – implementation of red/amber lists – 1 May 2003.* Belfast: DHSSPS, 2003. (HSS(MD)16/2003.)
59 Nurse Prescribers' Formulary Subcommittee. *Nurse prescribers' formulary.* London: British Medical Association and Pharmaceutical Press in association with Community Practitioners' and Health Visitors' Association and the Royal College of Nursing. (Published annually)
60 Audit Commission. *A spoonful of sugar. Medicines management in NHS hospitals.* London: Audit Commission, 2001.
61 Department of Health. *Pharmacy in the future – implementing the NHS plan. A programme for pharmacy in the National Health Service. Op cit.*
62 Department of Health. *Supplementary prescribing by nurses and pharmacists within the NHS in England. A guide for implementation.* London: DoH, 2003.
63 Department of Health. *Pharmacy in the future – implementing the NHS plan. A programme for pharmacy in the National Health Service. Op cit.*
64 NHS Executive. *Health service circular: patient group directions [England only].* London: Department of Health, 2000. (HSC 2000/026.)
65 Stone J, Matthews J. *Complementary medicine and the law.* Oxford: Oxford University Press, 1996.
66 National Audit Office. *Safety, quality, efficacy: regulating medicines in the UK.* London: The Stationery Office, 2003:24. (HC 255.)
67 Nunn T. Using unlicensed and off-label medicines. *Pharm Manage* 2002;**18**(4):64–7.
68 Royal College of Paediatrics and Child Health, Neonatal and Paediatric Pharmacists Group Standing Committee on Medicines. *Medicines for children. Information for older children.* London: RCPCH, 2000. Royal College of Paediatrics and Child Health, Neonatal and Paediatric Pharmacists Group Standing Committee on Medicines. *Medicines for children. Information for parents and carers.* London: RCPCH, 2000.
69 Royal College of Paediatrics and Child Health, Neonatal and Paediatric Pharmacists Group. *Medicines for children. 2nd ed.* London: RCPCH, 2003.
70 See, for example, the drug misuse pages on the Department of Health website at: http://www.doh.gov.uk/drugs.
71 See, for example: Department of Health, The Scottish Office Department of Health, Welsh Office, Department of Health and Social Services, Northern Ireland. *Drug misuse and dependence – guidelines on clinical management.* London: The Stationery Office, 1999.
72 British Medical Association. *The misuse of drugs.* Amsterdam: Harwood Academic, 1997.
73 National Audit Office. *Safety, quality, efficacy: regulating medicines in the UK. Op cit:* 26.
74 General Medical Council. *Providing advice and medical services on-line or by telephone.* London: GMC, 1998.
75 GMC Professional Conduct Committee hearing, 7–9 January 2002.
76 General Practitioners Committee. *Consulting in the modern world – guidance for GPs.* London: British Medical Association, 2001:10–11.
77 Taxis K, Barber N. Ethnographic study of incidence and severity of intravenous drug errors. *BMJ* 2002;**326**:684–7.
78 NHS Executive. *Health service circular: national guidance on the safe administration of intrathecal chemotherapy.* London: Department of Health, 2001. (HSC 2001/022.)
79 Toft B. *External inquiry into the adverse incident that occurred at Queen's Medical Centre, Nottingham, 4th January 2001.* London: Department of Health, 2001:40.
80 Medicines for Human Use (Marketing Authorisations etc.) Regulations 1994 No. 3144: Regulation 7.
81 National Audit Office. *Safety, quality, efficacy: regulating medicines in the UK. Op cit.*

14: Research and innovative treatment

The questions covered in this chapter include the following.

- How does innovative treatment differ from research?
- Why have issues of consent been perceived as particularly crucial in this area?
- Is it ever acceptable not to tell patients about a research project that involves them?
- How can the public be made more aware of research?
- Is it wrong to exclude from research patients who cannot consent personally?
- What measures are in place to combat research fraud?

Range of issues discussed

In this chapter a discussion of research ethics is combined with an examination of some of the problems associated with innovative therapy because the same principles about truth telling, informed consent, and minimising harm are particularly pertinent to both. In relation to research, a large amount of published guidance – both general and highly specialised – is already available. Rather than duplicate it, sources of relevant advice are flagged up and the focus is particularly on those areas of medical research and experimental treatment that give rise to most practical queries to the BMA. These tend to concentrate on issues of valid consent, the inclusion of children and other vulnerable people in medical and pharmaceutical trials, and the use of stored human material. BMA policy on less common but potentially very controversial issues such as embryo and stem cell research is also set out in this chapter.

Definitions

Mechanisms for scrutinising research are well established and guidance for the monitoring of innovative therapies is evolving. Questions sometimes arise, however, about the boundary between research and innovative treatment or between research and audit. New treatments almost inevitably involve an element of both research and audit so that their efficacy and risks can be properly assessed. In all cases, the safeguards to be applied must be commensurate with the risks involved.

Research

The aim of research is to produce new knowledge; it is not intended to benefit research participants, although there may be some incidental benefit to them. They must be protected from harm, but future patients are the real beneficiaries. Wherever the intention is to acquire new knowledge rather than *solely* to care for individuals, the constraints applicable to the conduct of research apply. (These safeguards and regulatory mechanisms are discussed on pages 529–31.) When doctors initiate treatment that diverges from normal medical practice in order to gain information to help future patients, the recipients must be informed about the choices open to them. The activity must always be subject to review by an appropriately constituted research ethics committee.

"Research" can be defined as the attempt to derive generalisable new knowledge by addressing clearly defined questions using systematic and rigorous methods. All research must meet certain minimum standards. It must, for example, have a well designed protocol, constitute a well conducted project, involve statistically appropriate participant numbers, not unnecessarily duplicate previous research, and be subject to external review and continuing surveillance. In addition, research involving people who are somehow dependent or vulnerable must also take special account of their interests and priorities.

Since the 1960s, research has often been divided into two categories. Research combined with trying to improve patient care was termed "therapeutic" or "clinical" research, which is a concept that overlaps considerably with innovative treatment. Research that simply sought knowledge without claiming to benefit its participants was "non-therapeutic". The key early guidance on research ethics, the World Medical Association's Declaration of Helsinki (first adopted in 1964) perceived a fundamental distinction between the two. It emphasised that, in treating sick people, "the physician must be free to use a new diagnostic and therapeutic measure" if it seemed helpful in the doctor's judgment.[1] Thus, "therapeutic research" was perceived by many clinicians as something to be pursued at their discretion and which potentially required less stringent external scrutiny than projects that were purely and solely research. Its aim was to ensure that, in the absence of any satisfactory treatment, patients should be able to access experimental procedures without impediment. Although sounding reassuring, however, the "therapeutic" label merely reflected the intention of the researcher rather than the effectiveness of the intervention.

By 2000, it was more frequently argued that this therapeutic/non-therapeutic categorisation was outmoded and should be dropped. Not only were the terms increasingly seen as unhelpful, but they disguised the fact that some therapeutic research was considerably more hazardous than the non-therapeutic variety.[2] There was growing consensus that all research should be assessed according to the same criteria of risks and benefits. In 2000 the World Medical Association, which had originally introduced the terms to a wide audience, deleted them from its guidance. It also reversed the previous expectation that more allowance should be made for research combined with patient care by insisting that extra safeguards be applied in such cases. Sick people were thought more likely than healthy volunteers to be tempted into risky innovative treatments and research, or to misunderstand the extent to which they personally could expect to benefit.

Audit

Audit is a means of assessing whether actual clinical performance conforms to good clinical practice. Although research seeks to add to the knowledge base, routine audit ensures that the knowledge base is used, by observing what has been done and assessing the degree to which predetermined standards for any given healthcare activity are met. If they are not met, the reasons should be identified and changes implemented prior to re-audit. Audit methods can be similar to research. Both can involve survey sampling, questionnaire design, and statistical analysis. Like records-based epidemiology, audit does not involve disturbance to the patient beyond that required for normal clinical management. If patients are involved in audit, for example by the use of questionnaires or interviews, scrutiny of the questions by a research ethics committee is desirable to minimise the possibility of distressing topics being raised without appropriate support. As with research, patient consent and confidentiality are issues for consideration. The use of medical records for audit by the clinical team managing the patient's care does not require specific patient consent or review by a research ethics committee. The concept of implied consent can be relied upon provided that patients are generally aware that audit occurs and their records will be used by the professionals who already have legitimate access to them. Confidentiality issues and the limitations on implied consent are discussed in detail in Chapter 5.

Consent is not needed for any audit using anonymised data, but the use of identifiable information by people who do not already have access to it may be unlawful unless patient consent is obtained. In England and Wales, however, section 60 of the Health and Social Care Act 2001 allows for the development of regulations permitting certain limited uses of identifiable information without consent. Such use must be in the interests of patients or the wider public and is acceptable only when seeking consent is not practicable and where anonymised information will not suffice (see Chapter 5, pages 182–3). At the time of writing, regulations have been made to permit data processing without consent for audit, quality assurance, and anonymising data. For detailed advice, however, doctors should consult the Department of Health about whether particular uses of data fall within the scope of the regulations. If a specific use does not fall within these regulations, express consent is needed for any disclosure of information to anyone other than the health professionals who already have access to it.

Innovative treatment

Innovation embraces a wider range of activities than those managed formally as research. Doctors have always modified methods of investigation and treatment in the light of experience and so innovative therapy is a standard feature of care. In many cases, however, it is the same thing as what used to be called therapeutic research. Nowadays, it would be unacceptable for unproven remedies or new surgical techniques to be applied without ethical overview or independent assessment. New medicinal products require research ethics approval and it would be desirable for innovations such as new surgical techniques also to undergo ethical review, although as yet this is not the norm. Traditionally the monitoring of new treatment was part of the profession's own responsibility, but the importance of external, independent review has become increasingly recognised. In 2001 *The report of the public inquiry into children's heart surgery at the Bristol Royal Infirmary 1984–1995* (the Bristol report)[3] argued that, in any case of a new, untried invasive clinical procedure, permission should be sought from the local research ethics committee, thereby indicating that some innovative treatments differ little from research, especially when they involve an unknown or increased risk for the patient. In individual cases, the aim of innovative treatment is to achieve the best outcome for the patient, who must be informed of how and why the proposed treatment differs from the usual measures and have an opportunity to consider the risks involved. The Bristol report also said that patients are entitled to know what experience the doctor has in the technique before agreeing. The degree of digression from usual practice is an important consideration for patients, the research ethics committee, and the healthcare team. Conclusions reached from the implementation of changes in treatments should be shared with others. Since 1998, the National Institute for Clinical Excellence (NICE) has been operational and its role includes assessment of the efficacy of both existing and innovative therapies (see Chapter 13, page 464).

General principles

The general principles applicable to research and innovative treatment are:

- truth telling and effective communication
- informed consent and voluntariness of the participant
- the welfare of the individual as the primary consideration
- other health professionals involved in providing care being aware of the research (with patient's consent)
- proportionality: benefits and burdens must be appropriately balanced
- ensuring involvement of a representative population
- justice being considered in relation to vulnerable groups
- careful independent scrutiny of research and experimental treatment
- the confidentiality of participants
- health professionals acting only within their sphere of competence
- the accurate recording of results.

Implementation of these general principles is discussed in detail on pages 497–517.

Research governance

The use of new or unproven interventions, either in research or therapy, needs special care and consideration. It may require specific supervisory or governance arrangements.[4] Traditionally, however, good practice in both research and innovative treatment has been largely defined by guidance rather than law (although embryo research is an exception). Although this situation has not been tackled in relation to innovative therapy, the way in which research is regulated began to change when the European Parliament agreed in 2001 to implement uniform rules on clinical trials of medicinal products[5] and the UK drafted specific regulations to do this.[6]

Even prior to the legislation, however, the International Conference on Harmonisation Guidance on good clinical practice (GCP)[7] was observed for research projects in the UK from 1997 onwards. This defined:

- a comprehensive glossary of terms, including standardised definitions of "confidentiality", "informed consent", "independent ethics committee", "legally acceptable representative", and "vulnerable subjects"
- a set of ethical principles of good clinical practice, including the duty to weigh the benefits and burdens in advance, to protect the rights and welfare of the participant, to ensure the competence of those conducting the trial, to obtain freely given informed consent from participants, and to respect their confidentiality
- the responsibilities of the research ethics committee, including the obligation to safeguard the rights, safety, and wellbeing of all trial participants, especially those who are vulnerable, and to carry out continuing review of each ongoing trial at appropriate intervals
- the obligations of the investigator, including the duty to facilitate monitoring and audit, to ensure resources are adequate, to ensure medical care for any adverse event, and to inform patients' doctors about their participation in research, with patients' consent
- the obligations of the sponsor, including the provision of insurance, compensation if needed, continuing safety evaluation, and the prompt provision of information if the research trial needs to be terminated prematurely or suspended.

In 2001 the Department of Health's *Research governance framework for health and social care*[8] (and the parallel document in Scotland[9]) required that all research involving patients, service users, care professionals, or volunteers, or their organs, tissue, or data, be reviewed independently to ensure that it meets ethical standards. A quality and accountability framework for research in health and social care was set out. It emphasised the importance of obtaining informed consent from participants, and of researchers recognising the diversity of people who may be involved in research in terms of ethnicity, gender, disability, age, and sexual orientation. It also specified the need for clear agreements detailing the respective responsibilities and rights of all those involved in the conduct of research. The document not only spelled out the accountability of investigators, employers, and sponsors, but also of patients, saying that everyone who uses health and social care services should seriously consider agreeing to be involved in research.[10] Although at that time there was no clear legal obligation for researchers to submit their research for ethical review, in practice, access to NHS patients and data was contingent upon obtaining such research ethics committee approval. Subsequently, in 2003, the Government indicated that legal changes were afoot. Article 6 of the European Directive on the implementation of good clinical practice in trials on medicinal products for human use[11] required the UK to harmonise its legislation on clinical trials of medicinal products with that of other European countries. Draft regulations[12] published in early 2003 were intended to make it legally obligatory to obtain a favourable opinion from an ethics committee prior to starting a research trial on any medicine. At the time of writing, these draft regulations have not been finalised.

The functions and operation of research ethics committees were described in the Department of Health's 2001 document *Governance arrangements for NHS research ethics committees*.[13] This placed responsibility upon health authorities to set up, support, and monitor such committees. It provided a standards framework, including general ethical principles and regulatory standards, guidance on operating procedures, and current advice published by a range of medical bodies on particular ethical issues. It also covered questions such as legal liability of research ethics committee members and the need for initial and continuing education and training in research ethics, methodology, and governance. In 2003 the above mentioned draft regulations made provision for a new statutory system throughout the UK for establishing and recognising research ethics committees and a new supervisory body, the UK Ethics Committee Authority (UKECA).

Since the 1960s, a significant amount of international and national ethical guidance has been published about the kind of supervision that should be applied to research. It is impossible to do full justice here to this literature and, although we have summarised many of the salient points, researchers and members of research ethics committees need to be familiar with key publications in their entirety.[14] Internationally, the World Medical Association's Declaration of Helsinki[15] has been the foundation of all other guidance. Subsequently, UN agencies, including the World Health Organization[16] and the Joint United Nations Programme on HIV/AIDS (known as UNAIDS),[17] have built upon that. Although the UK is not a signatory to it, the European Convention on Human Rights and Biomedicine[18] set standards for research in the European Union. International guidance is also available for trials or joint projects in developing countries: core documents include those from the Council for International Organizations of Medical Science,[19] the European Group on Ethics in Science and New Technologies,[20] and the Nuffield Council on Bioethics.[21] In the UK, helpful detailed guidance is available from bodies such as the General Medical Council (GMC),[22] the Royal Colleges, the Medical Research Council, the Association of the British Pharmaceutical Industry, and organisations representing patients and carers, such as the Alzheimer's Disease Society. The charity Consumers for Ethics in Research (CERES) also provides guidance for people who are invited to take part in research.

Relevant legislation

Under the Medicines Act 1968, all trials of new medicinal products on people had to be notified to the Medicines Control Agency, which became the Medicines and Healthcare Products Regulatory Agency in April 2003. In February 2003, the Government published for consultation new draft legislation on clinical trials of investigational medicinal products for human use, including placebos used in trials. (Guidance on the legislation will be available on the BMA's website.) Its aim was to incorporate into law the European guidance, *Good clinical practice*, which had already been perceived as obligatory in practice since 1997 and which is summarised on page 493.

Medicines for Human Use (Clinical Trials) Regulations – some main points

- Good clinical practice guidance must be observed.
- The foreseeable risks and inconveniences must be weighed against the anticipated benefit for each participant in the trial, and other present and future patients.
- There must be provision for indemnity.
- The rights of each participant to physical and mental integrity, privacy, and protection of personal data must be safeguarded.
- Provision is made for involvement of individuals who cannot consent.
- A new statutory system for establishing and recognising research ethics committees is set in place.

In addition to the as yet still draft Medicines for Human Use (Clinical Trials) Regulations 2003, potentially relevant statutes include:

- Human Rights Act 1998
- Data Protection Act 1998
- Health and Social Care Act 2001.

All of this legislation is discussed in detail in other sections of this book and the purpose here is simply to flag up issues that researchers and research ethics committees need to bear in mind. For example, the lack of appropriately informed participant consent for involvement in research or experimental treatment could raise issues under the Human Rights Act. In X v Denmark,[23] the European Commission of Human Rights concluded that medical treatment of an experimental character and without the consent of the person involved may under certain circumstances be regarded as a breach of human rights under the prohibition on torture or inhuman or degrading treatment. Similarly, the use of personal health information without permission could be a breach.[24] Research ethics committees are likely to be recognised as "public authorities" under the Act, which means that they need to ensure that all their decisions are compatible with human rights legislation.[25]

As is discussed in Chapter 5, the Data Protection Act is a complex piece of legislation. Principle 2 of the Act requires that data be "processed for limited purposes and not in any manner incompatible with those purposes", but it does envisage some exceptions when personal data are processed for the purposes of research. These exceptions are set out in section 33 of the Act, which is commonly known as "the research exemption".[26] To be acceptable, the processing must be only for research purposes and the following criteria must be met:

- the data are not processed to support measures or decisions relating to particular individuals
- the data are not processed in a way that damage or distress is likely to be caused to anyone who is the subject of the data.

The exemption does not excuse the person holding the data from complying with the rest of the Act, including the requirement that personal data shall be obtained only for one or more specified and lawful purposes. The data processing must be lawful, which means that it must meet any common law requirements for consent (see Chapter 5, pages 168–9). At the time of giving the information, the individual should be made aware of how it will be used. If the data controller would subsequently like to use it for further research not envisaged when the data were collected, the "fair processing" requirements of the Act still need to be met (see Chapter 5, page 170). The exemption cannot be used to justify the retention of records longer than normal simply because they could be useful in future research. This means that the exemption applies only if research is actually about to be carried out or there is a firm intention to use the records for that purpose.

In England and Wales, the Health and Social Care Act 2001 potentially allows disclosure of personal health information for medical purposes without consent when that would be in the interests of patients or society, subject to regulations made by the Secretary of State. Regulations made under section 60 of the Act can allow the use of data for some research or public health purposes when seeking individual consent is not a viable option (see Chapter 5, pages 182–3). At the time of writing, there is no equivalent legislation in Northern Ireland or Scotland.

Why dilemmas arise in research and innovative treatment

In the past, many dilemmas arose because of differences in the priorities and expectations of the various parties. Advances in medical knowledge benefit everyone and so society has an interest in promoting research and innovative treatment within an acceptable framework. Over time, however, opinions change about what constitutes an acceptable framework. As some of the case examples featured in this chapter indicate, established practice has failed, at times, to reflect public opinion and has often not engaged people positively as responsible partners. Although we recognise that ethical review of research has improved significantly in recent years, researchers and clinicians still need to be constantly sensitive to changing societal views.

In order to be ethically acceptable, the potential benefits of any intervention must outweigh any inherent risks of harm. One of the problems with research and innovative treatment is the fact that the individuals who agree to undertake any potential risks are often not the people who reap the potential benefits. Healthy volunteers, for example, help to secure improvements for others and, when we evaluate such benefits, the gains for society as a whole form part of the equation. Similarly, however, when assessing potential disadvantages of research projects or innovation, it is also essential to avoid too narrow a definition of "harm" or one that relates only to physical damage. Less tangible harms such as loss of trust or damage arising from deception need to be considered; it is in failing to assess these risks that research and innovative treatment have sometimes run into trouble. Developing new techniques and gaining knowledge are subordinate to the main aim of medicine, which is to enhance the welfare of individual patients. Therefore, patients who agree to participate in extending knowledge must never be treated as simply a means to obtaining that end. For its part, the public needs to be informed about the benefits that can be obtained through small, incremental steps as well as by major scientific advances. The BMA also strongly encourages feedback from researchers and clinicians to participants on the general findings and implications of the research and new therapies in which they have participated. Clearly, in some contexts this may involve giving bad news and needs to be very carefully done, ideally after seeking advice from any patient representatives who were involved in the research design at the outset.

Not only must there be a balance between the desire to extend knowledge and the rights of individuals who participate in research and innovation, there must also be a balance of populations included in these activities. Although much publicity has been given to the harms for the people who take part in some research projects, less attention has centred on the harms of being excluded. Some patient groups, such as women of childbearing age, can be potentially disadvantaged by being excluded from research. The charity CERES, which provides advice for research participants, notes, for example, that people who have limited English language skills are often excluded. In order to try to tackle this, it has been involved in projects to translate information about health research into other languages. Owing to the rightly heavy emphasis on autonomy and personal consent, there can also be difficulties involved in research on young children and on adults with impaired capacity. (This is one of the issues covered by the regulations for clinical trials of medicinal products, discussed on pages 506–13.) This research deficit can result in a lack of proven treatments for some patient populations and, therefore, in this chapter the arguments for including them, with appropriate safeguards, are emphasised.

Implementing ethical guidance in research and innovative treatment

Truth telling and provision of information

Consent is a key concept in research and innovative treatment, and an essential prerequisite for valid consent is access to information. An absolutely fundamental point is that people should be told when there is any proposal to involve them in research or innovation. It would be unacceptable, for example, to recall patients for what they assume to be health monitoring for their own benefit when the actual intention is to carry out research on some aspect of their condition.

The American case of Mr Moore's leukaemia cells

As part of his treatment for hairy cell leukaemia, Mr Moore's spleen was removed. Although he appeared to have recovered, the patient was recalled to hospital repeatedly over subsequent years. Specimens of blood and bone marrow were taken during outpatient visits and, although Mr Moore consented, he was under the impression that these procedures were solely for the purpose of monitoring his health. Unknown to Mr Moore, a cell line had been developed from his extracted cells, which had a potential market value of millions of dollars. When Mr Moore discovered this, he sued all those involved in a series of actions through the Appeal Court and Supreme Court of California. A large part of the litigation concerned whether he had property rights in cells removed from his body and therefore had a claim to share any profit derived from their use. Another strand of argument, however, concerned the duty of the doctors to disclose all the relevant information to the patient in order to obtain his informed consent to participate in the research. This had plainly not occurred.

Moore v Regents of the University of California, 1990[27]

What is adequate information varies according to the requirements of the individuals involved and the complexity of the procedures proposed. General guidance has been published by the Central Office for Research Ethics Committees (COREC)[28] and by CERES.[29]

Patient information sheets are a useful way of providing reference material, and advice is available on drafting them[30] but, no matter how well written, these cannot replace discussion and the opportunity for patients to pose questions. Potential participants in research or innovative treatment need to know the likely benefits and risks involved, why the options are proposed, and what alternatives exist. They should know that they can withdraw without detriment to their rights to care. If asked to participate in research, they need to know how the project is expected to advance knowledge and the researcher's own stake (if any) in proposing it. Much routine research, including in general practice, is undertaken at the behest of the pharmaceutical industry and may involve testing new variants of existing drugs, so it is important that patients have an accurate perception of their contribution. It is not only an obligation that the potential significance of the research is not exaggerated when recruiting participants, but obviously also when the findings are reported.

Some innovative treatments and research involve discomfort or pain. It is important that this fact is not omitted from information sheets for volunteers. Obviously, participants should have a realistic impression of what is involved or their consent is likely to be invalid. Opinions frequently differ about how pain should be defined, especially in relation to research or innovative treatment involving children. From a child's perspective, routine procedures such as venepuncture can seem painful and frightening[31] and there need to be opportunities to discuss the patient's own perspective.

Research participants need to know:

- the purpose of the research and confirmation of its ethical approval
- whether the participant stands to benefit directly and, if so, the difference between research and treatment
- the meaning of relevant research terms (such as placebos)
- the nature of each procedure, and how often or for how long each may occur
- the processes involved, such as randomisation
- the potential benefits and harms (both immediate and long term)
- arrangements for reporting adverse events
- the legal rights and safeguards for participants
- details of compensation if harm results from their participation
- how their health data will be stored, used and published
- if samples of human material are donated, whether they will be used for any other research or purpose
- whether and how DNA will be extracted, stored or disposed of
- the name of the researcher whom they can contact with enquiries
- if the researcher stands to benefit (for example, financially)
- the name of the doctor directly responsible for their care
- how they can withdraw from the project
- what information they will receive about the outcome
- that withdrawal will not affect the quality of their health care.

Patients involved in innovative therapies need to know:

- why the therapy is proposed in their case
- the evidence to support its use and the areas of uncertainty about it
- whether it has had any form of ethical review
- the clinician's experience with it
- the alternatives, if any
- how it differs from standard treatment
- the likely risks and benefits for themselves
- the measures for safety monitoring and support that will be provided if things go wrong
- the likely future use of the therapy, if successful.

Is it ever acceptable not to inform patients?

As a general principle, failure to inform participants is unacceptable. One of the few circumstances in which patients cannot be properly informed that their treatment is innovative or part of research occurs when their mental capacity is impaired. The particular problems associated with research in the contexts of emergency treatment, resuscitation, and intensive care are discussed on pages 509–10.

As is discussed in Chapter 1, traditionally, doctors were advised against admitting to uncertainty when talking to competent patients; maintaining patient confidence and optimism were part of the treatment, but experience has shown that such efforts to protect patients from uncomfortable truths have the potential for backfiring. Patients are likely to become very mistrustful if they discover or suspect that accurate information has been withheld for any reason. In relation to research or innovative procedures, three common but unsustainable arguments are often put forward for not seeking consent from people who are involved.[32] These are that:

- patients would be distressed by information
- the risks of harm are negligible
- medical progress is in the public interest and would be undermined by emphasis on autonomy.

These arguments have now generally been rejected (although, as mentioned on page 496, the Health and Social Care Act recognises a limited discretion for the Secretary of State to permit data to be used without consent in the public interest).

Many studies in a large variety of research settings have identified major problems in the communication of the most basic elements of the informed consent process.[33] Explaining the full context of research and innovation can be particularly difficult because it necessarily involves discussing the limitations of current medical knowledge. Nevertheless, it has been argued that doctors have a stronger professional duty to communicate information about risks in the context of research than in normal clinical care.[34]

Research in which the patient's awareness of it could itself significantly affect the outcome obviously poses a particular challenge. The case examples below indicate this problem. In many cases, however, even though important knowledge is gained, this benefit is probably outweighed by the harm and distress caused by patients' loss of trust. In each case where it is being argued that specific patient consent need not be sought, it is important that health professionals and research ethics committees are clear about the robustness of the justification. As part of that assessment, consideration needs to be given to the wider harms to public confidence if research or innovative therapy is carried out in what appears to be a clandestine manner. When individuals cannot consent or when tissue is retained from deceased patients, families expect to be consulted. As indicated by the Alder Hey Inquiry[35] into the retention of paediatric cadaveric material for research and other purposes, genuine concern about upsetting families or patients is not an acceptable reason for keeping them uninformed.

Examples of controversial research

In the early 1980s, Mrs Thomas agreed to a mastectomy for breast cancer but subsequently noticed that her aftercare differed from that of the patient in the next bed.[36] Whereas the other patient received postoperative counselling and useful information from a special nurse, Mrs Thomas did not. It took her

(Continued)

four years to discover that she had been included in a trial to compare the effects of counselling with those of no counselling. The trials ran from 1980 to 1985 at 58 centres. Some 2230 women were involved but were not told of the research. Mrs Thomas complained to the Health Service Commissioner and her case was subsequently taken up by the Committee on the Parliamentary Commission for Administration, which expressed significant concern. Health professionals involved in the research, however, said that patients had not been informed because it would be upsetting for them to have to explain it. It was reported that health workers "found it very upsetting, very emotional to tell these patients all the facts".[37] In the light of this argument, the research ethics committee had waived the normal requirement for consent.

In the late 1990s, a study in Edinburgh aimed to discover whether stroke family care workers improve outcomes for patients with strokes and their families.[38] The researchers decided not to seek consent from patients and families because this could have biased outcomes that were basically subjective. They also argued that the intervention – providing care workers for some people but not others – was unlikely to be harmful. Families and patients could decline to see the care worker. It was counterargued, however, that these reasons were insufficient to deviate from the normal rule requiring consent and that, even if there were no physical harms, the implied failure to respect patients was a harm in itself.

In 1997 in South Africa, researchers sought to discover whether HIV infection affected outcomes for patients needing intensive care.[39] The issue was important because when patients were already known to be HIV positive, there was a tendency not to admit them to intensive care. In this case, patients were neither asked to be in the study nor to be HIV tested. The researchers argued that the question was of such importance that the need for consent could be waived and, in any case, most of the patients were too ill to consent. Furthermore, it was argued that no additional interventions had been carried out over and above what would have been considered necessary, and that the harm to patients was small. Nevertheless, the perception was that lower ethical standards had been applied to patients who were too disadvantaged to be able to complain effectively.

Information for "consumers"

It is not only patients and research participants who need a clear understanding of what is on offer, but other "consumers" also need information. In this context, this includes potential patients, carers, consumer organisations, members of the public targeted by health promotion programmes, and people requesting research because they may have been exposed to potentially harmful products or services. Research that "reflects the needs and views of consumers is more likely to produce results that can improve practice" and "the involvement of consumers in the research process is likely to lead to research that is more relevant and likely to be used".[40] Such community participation has sometimes been portrayed unhelpfully as essentially passive, involving inexpert people who are separated by a wide knowledge gap from health professionals.[41] Unfortunately, as a result, the public and research participants were not told much at all. Therefore, in addition to specific information for patients, research participants and their families, there should be more general information available and consultation with a range of non-health professionals on issues such as protocol design and dissemination of results. In medical facilities and public places, leaflets or notice boards could describe research taking place in local hospitals, for example, or improvements in care that have been achieved by previous research, making it clear that people are not entered into research projects without their consent.

Communicating the concept of risk

Assessment of risk is an important part of decision making in all forms of health care and is notoriously difficult to explain to patients. The increasing emphasis on both training and evaluation of doctors' communication skills seeks to address problems such as this. People enrolled in research projects should be clear that no payment offered, such as their expenses or compensation, is for undertaking a risk. Risk is relative rather than absolute, so, when innovative treatment is considered, the risks have to be assessed both in terms of the likely effects of the new procedure and the risks to the patient if it is not carried out. Obviously in all cases, the degree of risk must be in proportion to the expected benefit. Health professionals are sometimes criticised for apparently poor communication about some aspects of innovative treatment, so that patients or families lack adequate explanations.[42] When they are told that the treatment or research involves some uncertainty, the issue about which patients most often seek reassurance is the degree of risk of harm involved. Despite the existence of some guidelines, no generally applicable categorisation of "risk" is available and so it needs to be discussed on a case by case basis. Clinicians need to ensure that there is systematic review of the evidence base for the procedures they offer, so that the information they provide reflects accurately what is currently known about the risks and relative merits. They must make clear which aspects of a proposed treatment are innovative and answer honestly any questions about their own success rate. If new treatment involves significant risk, an independent and objective second opinion should be sought so that clinicians can be confident that they are not putting too positive a gloss on it. Patients should be informed if procedures are not standard treatment in other facilities. It is not acceptable to rely on the concept of implied consent on the grounds that an innovative treatment is "standard" when this is plainly not a widely shared view. Consent can never be implied or taken for granted in this situation.

Informed consent

Valid consent or refusal is at the very heart of research and innovative treatment. A focus on the aim of increasing medical knowledge – either as the primary research objective or as a by product of new treatment – means that more than in any other sphere of medical activity, people risk being seen as a means to an end. Only if they are engaged as partners in the project are the risks of exploitation minimised.

Consent and refusal by "healthy volunteers"

One of the major concerns with the recruitment of healthy volunteers is the voluntariness of the person's decision. Public advertisement is probably the most common recruitment method but, in the past, researchers often involved people who were in a dependent position, such as their students or employees, as a potential pool of volunteers. The International Conference on Harmonisation GCP guidelines include in its definition of "vulnerable subjects", anyone "whose willingness to volunteer in a clinical trial may be unduly influenced by the expectation, whether justified or not, of benefits associated with participation or of a retaliatory response from senior members of a hierarchy in case of refusal to participate".[43] It gives the example of any group with a hierarchical structure, such as medical, pharmacy, dental, and nursing students, laboratory personnel, employees of a pharmaceutical company, members of the armed forces, and detainees. Thus recruitment from such groups is seen as potentially problematic because of the risk of a perception of pressure being brought to bear on them. The BMA emphasises that the recruitment of students and junior staff from the same department as the researcher should be avoided. Nevertheless, there is an argument for offering employees an option to participate if they are likely to derive some benefit either from taking part or the results of the research. Laboratory staff, for example, who may be unavoidably exposed to some infective agents in specimens upon which they are working, could appropriately be offered the opportunity to participate in some vaccine trials. As with any research, the research ethics committee would need to reassure itself that no pressure or undue additional risk was involved. In other cases, financial incentives are generally used to attract volunteers. Payments must never be for undergoing risk and research ethics committees should monitor the level of financial incentives.

People in a situation of dependency

It is not only employees, students, and colleagues who are likely to be pressured in some way to participate in research or innovative treatment. Others, such as people living in institutions of various kinds may be seen as a captive pool of potential participants. A problem, however, is that while they should not be totally excluded from research or new therapy that could bring benefit to them and others in the same category, they must not be persuaded to take part in projects that are likely to be contrary to their interests. Most people in a situation of dependency are entirely able to give valid consent or refusal, but may still feel obliged to please others. Precautions to avoid coercion or inducement must be given particular attention by researchers, carers, and research ethics committees. There may be a risk that elderly people in care homes, for example, could feel pressured by wanting to keep the goodwill of their carers, but it would be wrong to exclude them from having choices about research or innovation. Even in research that is not designed to bring them any direct advantage, some patients benefit from the indirect consequences or side effects of being involved in research. This may be the result of renewed efforts by professionals to eliminate the minor health problems that could affect research findings or early access to potentially beneficial new drugs. The extra attention from health professionals and more frequent health monitoring for the purposes of research can be morale boosting and are not unfair inducements as long as individuals are given information and a choice, and are not exposed to uncomfortable or invasive interventions. In some cases the pressure may be more perceived than real, which highlights yet again the need for health professionals to explain fully that patients will not be viewed badly or treated less carefully if they opt out of research or innovative projects. Patients with long term conditions, for example, feel very reliant upon their health team and may worry that a refusal will alienate those health professionals. It needs to be made clear to them that their care entitlement is not affected.

People such as prisoners and inmates of institutions for those who are criminally insane should be involved only in projects that specifically address the health problems experienced particularly in that setting, such as the physical and psychological effects of detention. Careful consideration needs to be given by the relevant research ethics committee if incentives or special privileges are proposed to attract volunteers in such contexts. (General advice about care in custodial settings is given in Chapter 17.) Similarly, if included in research or new treatment, unconscious or brain damaged patients should not be exposed to measures contrary to their interests and included only when they or people in the same category stand to benefit. Many drug trials are carried out on antidepressants and other products for mentally ill people. Apart from those patients suffering from severe conditions, the vast majority of mentally ill people are able to give valid consent. This includes patients who are detained in psychiatric hospitals under mental health legislation, whose consent should be sought. It is unlikely that research that is not combined with some elements of treatment would be ethically acceptable for such patients, however, because, although they may understand the procedures, the very fact of their detention may make it difficult for them to give free consent.

Can anyone be obliged to participate in research or innovative treatment?

Normally no-one can be obliged to participate in either research or new therapies against their will, but there are some exceptional instances in which people are acknowledged to have little or no choice. Those who join the armed forces, for example, may forfeit their rights to opt out of some medical interventions, such as vaccination programmes. Where such programmes have not already been rigorously tried out on voluntary human participants, there is an element of both research and innovative therapy in their use. In such cases, the ethical justification is seen as consisting of the obligation to protect individuals against the risks of infection or injury, but also of the duty for all personnel to protect the welfare of the unit. Doctors still have a responsibility to maximise benefit and minimise risk but, obviously, this can be problematic in the absence of reliable evidence about potential risks and benefits. They also have duties to the individuals they treat and, wherever possible, should be willing to offer them whatever information they can. It is also important that there is ethical oversight of such programmes, for example, by Ministry of Defence research ethics committees.

Experimental treatment

In preparation for the first Gulf War in 1990, the requirement for informed consent for experimental vaccination was removed for American personnel who could be facing chemical or biological weapons.[44] The US Defense Department said that informed consent was important in peace time but "military combat is different".[45] Thousands of army personnel were given pyridostigmine bromide and a botulism toxoid vaccination, although both drugs had some known problems. Nevertheless, the aim was to use them therapeutically. It has been argued, however, that their use blurred the distinction between treatment and research because the drugs had not been established to be either effective or safe.[46] British service personnel were also vaccinated. Between August and December 1990, 52 300 British troops were sent to the Gulf and many were injected with a mixture of drugs, intended to protect them and their units.

Consent and patient preferences

In randomised controlled trials (RCTs), new treatments are tested with consent, but patients cannot choose which treatment they receive and are often alarmed at the prospect of deliberate randomisation. Clearly, patients who have treatment preferences should not participate in any study in which their treatment will be randomised. The prerequisite for establishing RCTs is the lack of a recognised optimum treatment for the condition or the presumption that a new product may be more effective than existing therapies. Thus, randomisation is ethical only if there is substantial uncertainty about the best treatment *for that patient*. Where some therapies with established effectiveness already exist they, rather than placebos, should normally be the comparator for new treatments. If the doctor considers that one of the treatments in the study is appropriate or inappropriate for a particular patient for any reason (including that patient's irrational fears or subjective preferences), then randomisation would be unethical. In such cases, the responsible clinician should talk to the patient about the options that are available outside the RCT and seek to identify those likely to reflect the patient's preferences.

Summary – informed consent to research or innovative treatment

In order to give valid and informed consent:

- participants must be mentally competent to consent
- consent must be voluntary and unpressured

- participants should have access to detailed information
- participants should know that they can withdraw without prejudice to future treatment.

People who cannot consent to research or innovative therapy

Wherever possible, research and innovative therapy should be carried out on competent and consenting adults. Unfortunately, however, research cannot be limited to people who can consent validly for themselves because the effect would be to deprive non-autonomous people of proven therapies for the conditions that specifically afflict them. Included within the scope of this term are people whose physical illness makes it impossible for them to give a valid consent or refusal, as well as those suffering from severe mental illness or a severe learning disability.

Clearly, within these patient groups are individuals with widely varying capacity to understand and communicate. Many patients with a mental disorder are able to consent to research or new treatment, if care is taken in explaining the procedures, but the risks of inadvertently exercising undue pressure or persuasion need to be borne in mind. If they are likely to be potential participants in research or new therapy, they must be helped to understand to the maximum of their ability. Families need to understand the implications of agreeing on behalf of someone else or trying to second guess the individual's own views. For instance, they need to understand that, by consenting to a double blind randomised trial, they have no choice regarding which treatment is given, and will not even know which treatment was given until the trial is over.

Non-autonomous patients should be involved only in projects likely to benefit them or designed to benefit people in the same category. Babies, children, and people with severe mental health problems should be involved only when, for example, a particular disease affects only this group or because people in these categories respond differently to therapies already proven effective in trials involving consenting adults. Developing new and effective treatments for neonates, for example, inevitably involves babies. Great care must be taken that a small population of patients is not repeatedly called upon to participate in studies around their illness.

In some exceptional cases the patient's chances of recovery with an unproven treatment are better than with standard therapies. In very serious situations with few other options there may be a justification for exposing people to some risk if they potentially have much to gain. In such cases, it is essential that the patient (where possible), families, and the healthcare team give careful consideration to all the evidence. Exceptionally, the prospect of success may be relatively low, but the value of the attempt for the patient and the family can be high, and then consideration would need to be given to the individual's wishes. Clearly, very sick people should not be exposed to experimental treatment if there is significant doubt about both the likelihood of success and the value of attempting it. In some cases advice may need to be sought from the courts.

Court authorisation for experimental treatment for variant Creutzfeldt–Jakob disease (vCJD)

In December 2002, the High Court was asked to decide whether it would be lawful to provide treatment that had not been tested on human beings to two young patients who were thought to be suffering from vCJD. Both patients, JS aged 18 and JA aged 16, lacked the capacity to make treatment decisions, but their parents argued that it would be in their best interests to have the new therapy. It involved intraventricular administration of pentosan polysulphate, which had been tested in Japanese research, but only on rodents and dogs infected with scrapie. It was due to be used, however, for Japanese patients with iatrogenic CJD. Although not expected to provide a cure, it was hoped that the treatment would improve patients' lives. The judge said that, although the patients would not recover, the concept of "benefit" to a patient suffering from vCJD would encompass:

- an improvement from the present state of illness
- a continuation of the existing state of illness without deterioration for a longer period than might otherwise have occurred or
- the prolongation of life for a longer period than might otherwise have occurred.

Given the possibility of some benefit being derived and the lack of any other alternative, it was held that this treatment would be in the best interests of both JS and JA and so could lawfully be provided.

Simms v Simms, PA v JA (Also known as: A v A, JS v An NHS Trust)[47]

The legality of involving individuals who cannot consent in projects not intended to benefit them directly has long been debated. In 1999, for example, the GMC noted that "in these cases the legal position is complex or unclear, and there is currently no general consensus on how to balance the possible risks and benefits to such vulnerable individuals against the public interest in conducting research".[48] It advised researchers to keep abreast of any guidance published by the Medical Research Council and Royal Colleges. It has been argued, however, that it could be legally permissible if such projects are not contrary to the personal interests of the participants, even though not strictly in their own best interests. Therefore, such projects should not involve more than minimal risk and safeguards must be in place to minimise the possibility of exploitation. Equity demands that all patients are treated fairly and non-participation in research should not cause any deliberate disadvantage for them. In some cases, inclusion in a pharmaceutical trial may bring advantages for some participants, such as early access to new therapy, more medical and nursing attention, or more regular health checks. For such reasons, relatives and carers are often keen to ensure that such patients are included in research, even though the views of the patients themselves are unknown. As with other research and innovation, the research ethics committee needs to weigh carefully the expected benefits and drawbacks and consider whether there is a means of knowing the patient's own wish.

Families and carers of mentally incapacitated adults are generally asked to consider what the individuals would want. In Scotland, since the implementation of the Adults with Incapacity (Scotland) Act 2000, proxy decision makers have been legally empowered to decide for incapacitated adults as long as the intervention agreed by the proxy meets the criteria set out in the Act. Section 51 of the Act states that surgical, medical, nursing, dental, or psychological research can permissibly involve incapacitated people only if it could not equally well be done on competent adults. The purpose of the research must be to obtain knowledge of the causes, diagnosis, treatment, or care of the adult's incapacity or to understand the effect of treatment that has been provided for it. The legislation says the research must be expected to produce benefit for the patient, reflect that person's wishes as far as these can be ascertained, and take account of the views of other relevant people who are close to that person. It must have research ethics committee approval, involve no more than minimal risk or minimal discomfort, and cannot proceed if the person indicates unwillingness to participate. The legislation goes on to say, however, that even when the research is not likely to provide any real and direct benefit for the adult, it may be carried out if it meets the other requirements and would contribute to bringing real and direct benefit to other people who have the same incapacity. Nevertheless, a concern that arose in relation to the Act was that it appeared to prohibit research without consent in emergency situations (see pages 509–10). In addition, in Scotland, provision has been made in law for the establishment of a specialised ethics committee to consider the issue of research involving incapacitated adults.[49] This has the advantage of ensuring that those involved in scrutinising such research are familiar with the problems of this patient group.

General guidance on consent and impaired capacity

- Individuals should be positively involved in decision making to the maximum of their ability.
- If apparently unwilling, they should not be included in research or new treatment.
- Any advance refusal made by the individual when competent must be respected.
- Extra safeguards must be in place when participants cannot consent personally.
- Assurances must exist that the research cannot feasibly be done by involving a less vulnerable group.
- The expected benefits must outweigh any foreseeable risk of harm.
- Information for proxy decision makers must be as detailed as for other persons.

The Department of Health published a consultation document concerning a system of proxy decision makers for incapacitated adults who may participate in research on medicinal products.[50] This specified that close relatives should be able to act as personal legal representatives and health professionals (if not connected with the research) could act as a professional representative for patients lacking close family members. This aimed to set in statute very similar guidance to the general advice on proxy decision making in Scotland given above. (Any subsequent BMA guidance will be available on the website.)

Proposals for consent on behalf of incapacitated adults by legal representatives

- As proposed in 2003, the provisions would apply only to clinical trials of medicinal products and not to other forms of research or experimental therapy.
- The clinician in charge of the patient's care must believe the intervention to be in that person's best interests.
- Any advance refusal of treatment made by the person prior to the onset of incapacity must be respected.
- In the absence of such evidence, for incapable adults in England, Wales, and Northern Ireland, there would be provision for two types of legal representative who could consent to interventions in the patient's interests:
  - "personal" representatives who have a relationship with the patient
  - "professional" representatives who can act if there is no suitable person to take the role of personal representative.
- In Scotland, prior legislation[51] already allows a guardian, welfare attorney, or nearest relative to provide proxy consent. In some cases, however, under the new regulations, it would be acceptable for a "professional" legal representative to consent as in the rest of the UK.
- The Government has promised to provide guidance for legal representatives.

Information about the outcome of this consultation can be obtained from the Department of Health.

Emergency research and innovation

Research and innovation in the context of emergency and acute care pose ethical problems. In the emergency care setting, there is often little time to contact families for their view of what an individual would want if that person is incapable of communication. Urgent action is often needed if, for example, a patient has suffered a cardiac arrest or a severe head injury. Similarly, very few patients in intensive care wards are able to give valid consent, although their relatives may be contactable and able to discuss the options. Any improvements in outcomes in these settings can be achieved only through research. In 2003 the Government made it clear that implementation in the UK of the European Directive on clinical trials of medicinal products involving human subjects was not intended to hamper research in emergency situations.[52] It suggested that ethics committees asked to authorise research in emergency care settings could consider the scheme for legal representatives set out in the box above (although this was intended legally to cover only research on medicinal products).[53]

In the USA, codes for exception from informed consent requirements for emergency research[54] have been developed. These allow for interventional studies in a life threatening situation for which present treatment is unsatisfactory. The requirements include the necessity of providing some treatment before it is possible to obtain consent and there must be a prospect of benefit for the patients involved. Clinicians must specify a therapeutic window of time and indicate how much of that time span can safely be taken up by trying to obtain consent. Furthermore, patients who are known to have previously expressed unwillingness to be involved in research cannot be included. When they recover the ability to communicate, patients have the option of either continuing or withdrawing. The process has to be authorised and monitored by an institutional review board (equivalent to a research ethics committee), which receives regular progress reports. Consultations are carried out in the local community before and after the project to assess its public acceptability.

In the UK, the Royal College of Paediatrics and Child Health has also grappled with the dilemmas inherent in any effort to develop new therapies for people who cannot give consent, while respecting the principle of seeking appropriately informed consent. The College has suggested a compromise in the form of "provisional" consent when research is needed on the emergency treatment of newborn babies.[55] Parents obviously have little or no time to reflect on their decision, but may be willing to agree in principle to an unproven intervention if it is likely that emergency care will be needed and clinicians are unsure of the best option. For example, parents would be asked to agree in principle to allow one of the potential methods of resuscitation or ventilation in conditions where the best method for the circumstances is still unclear. The proposal attempts to deal with the problems of pressured decision making or seeking only retrospective consent, as happened in the Resair-2 study.[56] This compared resuscitation at birth with either air or oxygen in 11 centres in six countries, but no advance consent was sought. Although the project was authorised by research ethics committees, the parents of children involved in that study were informed only after the resuscitation. With any proposals concerning ways of tackling the need for emergency research there needs to be advance public discussion.

Research and innovative treatment for children and babies

Children and babies should be eligible for inclusion in research and innovative therapy, with appropriate safeguards. It is often argued, for example, that it would be unethical not to do important clinical research on newborn babies and infants. To fail to do research would lead to stagnation of current practice and the continuation of medical management by using untried or unproven remedies on the basis of belief rather than best evidence.[57] The need for pharmaceutical products specifically designed for use by children has long been recognised. These need to be developed with the involvement of children and young people once initial studies involving adults have proved the safety and efficacy of the product. The final decision about participation rests with patients (when competent) and with parents.[58] Consensus also exists about the need for clear and candid explanations of the purposes, risks, and expected benefits of the research. Families also need support when making such decisions. The Royal College of Paediatrics and Child Health has published detailed advice on the involvement of children in research that points out that since "children are not small adults; they have an additional, unique set of interests".[59] Research on minors, therefore, must not only meet the minimum standards set for research on adults, but also take account of children's special interests and perspective. Researchers need to bear in mind that "many children are vulnerable, easily bewildered and unable to express their needs or defend their interests. Potentially with many decades ahead of them, they are likely to experience, in their development and education, the most lasting benefits or harms from research".[60]

Proxy consent by parents

Obviously, competent children must be consulted themselves, although it is generally good practice to obtain consent also from parents or a person with parental responsibility. With regard to clinical trials of medicinal products, proposed regulations[61] in 2003 stipulated that, for everyone under the age of 16, consent to participate in research would be needed from parents or legal representatives. Minors capable of understanding would also be given appropriate information. Neither patients nor their parents should be paid for participation in research, although any expenses they incur should be reimbursed.

When children lack competence, questions arise as to whether any person, including parents, can consent in law to a child being exposed to a procedure that carries no prospect of direct benefit and some (if only minimal) risk. It is clear that people with parental responsibility can consent to measures that are in the best interests of children, but cannot agree to any intervention contrary to the child's best interests. The duty to act *in* the child's interests can probably be interpreted as allowing parents to agree to procedures that are not *against* those interests. Much research on babies and young children involves relatively routine interventions such as the taking of blood samples. Where these are additional to the blood tests required for the child's own medical treatment, it is important that parents are fully aware that the samples are for research purposes and that they can refuse such procedures without any detriment to the child's treatment. The Royal College of Paediatrics and Child Health has devoted much attention to blood sampling and agrees that, as far as can be currently judged, parents can consent to venepuncture for non-therapeutic purposes as long as they have been given and understand a full explanation of the reasons, and have balanced the risks for their child. Regarding the viewpoint of children themselves, it states:

Many children fear needles, but with careful explanation of the reason for venepuncture and an understanding of the effectiveness of local anaesthetic cream, they often show altruism and allow a blood sample to be taken. We believe that this has to be the child's decision. We believe that it is completely inappropriate to insist on the taking of blood for non-therapeutic reasons if a child indicates either significant unwillingness before the start of the procedure or significant stress during the procedure.[62]

In practice, this answers the question of whether parental consent to children's participation in research can be overridden by children themselves. It would be hard to argue that a non-therapeutic procedure that the child rejected could be in the child's interests. It is increasingly accepted that, when the procedures are more intrusive than those required for ordinary clinical care, a child's (verbal or non-verbal) refusal is good reason not to proceed even if parental consent has been obtained. In some situations, parents may disagree about whether a child, who cannot express a view, should participate in research or experimental therapy. As is also discussed in Chapter 4, great caution is needed on the issue of whether it would be appropriate (even if legal) to proceed if parents disagree about the child's participation. Legally, the consent of one person with parental responsibility should suffice if the intervention is not contrary to the child's interests, and there are obvious circumstances when the consent of one parent has to be sufficient because, for example, the child is in contact with only one parent. Nevertheless, the reasons for one parent refusing would need to be taken very seriously.

Great caution is needed in cases where parents – who are ordinarily the best judges of what is acceptable for their children – may be too ready to give consent as a result of their reasonable concerns to achieve an effective treatment for the condition from which their child suffers.[63] A major problem is the difficulty of obtaining valid consent for research involving clinical trials testing the appropriateness of products or procedures for vulnerable groups such as sick babies. Similar problems apply to innovative treatments in these circumstances. Clearly, when children are ill, the family is likely to be under great stress. In some instances, no matter how often and how carefully a project is explained to parents or research participants, it is not possible to be completely sure that their consent is valid.[64] The risks of families making erroneous or premature decisions as a result of extreme anxiety and pressure is obviously something that research ethics committees and researchers need to consider when protocols involving very sick patients are put forward.

Summary – consent for children and young people

- If competent, the child must give unpressured and informed consent.
- Parental consent should also be obtained even if the child is competent.
- Parents cannot agree on a child's behalf to anything that is contrary to the child's interests.
- Pharmacological studies on children should be avoided, unless valid results can be obtained only by including children, in which case this should be done after adult studies have been completed.[65]

- There must be no financial reward to the child or parent (expenses are permitted).
- All projects must be carefully scrutinised by a research ethics committee.
- Families need support and independent advice about their options.

Welfare of individuals: the duty to achieve balance and minimise harm

Important among the core principles and duties is the responsibility to protect the welfare of participants, minimise risks for them, and ensure that these are offset by the expected benefits. Research guidelines, including the World Medical Association's Declaration of Helsinki, emphasise that the welfare of the research participant must be a primary concern. It is unacceptable to prioritise the expected benefits for society over the welfare of individual people. In the history of research, however, there have been multiple examples of known beneficial treatments being withheld from individuals, without their knowledge, in order for researchers to assess the effects of leaving diseases untreated. This is clearly unacceptable when a recognised treatment is available.

Failure to safeguard the welfare of research participants

In 1986 publicity was given to unethical research that had been conducted in New Zealand at the National Women's Hospital in Auckland.[66] The researcher believed that carcinoma *in situ*, when left untreated, would not lead to invasive cancer of the cervix. This was contrary to international opinion at the time. In order to test the premise, conventional treatment was withheld from some women diagnosed with carcinoma *in situ*. Some patients were given the standard treatment, which involved removal of the suspect tissue, but others were not. For many of them the disease progressed to an invasive cancer. An official inquiry found that at least 27 women in the non-treatment group had died prematurely and many others suffered the effects of non-treatment without being informed of their initial diagnosis.

Consent to participate in research or innovative treatment does not mean that the participants take away any of the responsibility of researchers and research ethics committees to ensure that all foreseeable risks are minimised. In research, assessment of risk is not limited to consideration of the particular study but must also take account of the background context in which it is likely to be implemented. People with rare conditions, for example, may be repeatedly asked to participate in research where the risks of serial involvement may differ from the risks of involvement in just one study.

The possibility of harm cannot be entirely eliminated from research or from new treatments. However, by insisting that participants have adequate information and choice about taking part, the possibility of exploiting them is reduced. By their nature, innovative treatments have less evidential support than conventional regimens. The benefit for the patient is harder to predict. At the same time, there is likely to be an intuitive wish to try anything that may help to save or improve a life. Clinicians may be more tempted to be over optimistic and to recommend treatment, especially if the patient is a child or young person who potentially has a long life ahead if therapy is successful. Parents and the patient often find it very hard to resist agreeing to any therapy – even unproven treatment – that doctors recommend.

Failure to minimise harm

In 1979 a Selectron afterloading machine was used in a Manchester hospital to test whether the established three-day radium treatment for cervical cancer could be replaced by a new one-day regimen using caesium. This was thought potentially to reduce the harm of the treatment for patients, but insufficient safeguards were incorporated. By early 1982, many women treated with caesium or combined caesium and radium were found to have injuries to the rectum, bowel, and vagina as a result of the treatment. The hospital's initial response seemed to be to minimise the harm for itself rather than for patients, by informing those injured that their cases were exceptional. In fact, as their injuries were publicised by the media it became evident that hundreds of women had been damaged and many had died.[67]

Inclusiveness

Inclusiveness and justice as important principles in research and innovation have already been identified. As discussed above, this means finding ethical ways to include people who cannot consent for themselves. It also means examining whether all sectors and cultural groups in the community have the opportunity to participate in projects and that none is marginalised. In the past, for example, ethnic minorities were underrepresented in projects examining their health and disease patterns. More recently, little research seems yet to have been done on the particular health needs of the very diverse people who become refugees and asylum seekers. In 2002 the BMA drew attention to the gaps in knowledge about the healthcare needs of this particular population, especially those of its children.[68]

Confidentiality

The importance of protecting individuals' confidentiality in all healthcare contexts is explained in detail in Chapter 5, which includes the duties of confidentiality owed to children, to mentally incapacitated adults, and to deceased people. The legal and ethical framework outlined there also regulates the use of identifiable data in research. In addition, the Medical Research Council has published very detailed guidance about the confidentiality and use of patient data in medical research.[69]

Wherever possible, research should use anonymised data and individuals should generally be aware of the research use of their medical records. As previously indicated, the Data Protection Act requires the fair and lawful processing of information, so patients need to know which organisations may process their data and why. They need to be aware, in general terms, of who may need to see their information and why, and know that they have a right to object. The BMA believes that, when individuals are invited to participate in research, there should be no disclosure of their details to researchers prior to them giving consent (unless disclosure is covered under regulations made in connection with section 60 of the Health and Social Care Act, see Chapter 5, pages 182–3). Usual recruitment methods are either for patients to be given information about a pharmaceutical study at the time of their consultation and be invited to participate, or for their doctor to identify potential participants from the medical records. In the latter case, the patient's GP or hospital doctor should be responsible for sending out invitations and giving some initial details of the project so that patients can decide whether or not to allow their names to be forwarded to researchers. Because the main point of carrying out such projects is to gain and share new knowledge, individuals agreeing to participate in them need to be aware of that goal and its implications for themselves.

As well as providing information to individuals who are potential participants in research, the general public needs to understand the reasons why information is collected, how it is used, and the extent to which they can control it. Measures such as public notices and patient leaflets help to raise awareness of research projects.

Confidentiality and records-based research

Some records-based research is carried out in parallel with the provision of treatment by health professionals who already have access to the records as part of their duty of care. In such cases, where researchers are working on data from their own patients, there is no breach of confidentiality, as only those who already have access to the information use it for research. Nevertheless, when it was provided by patients, the information was given for treatment purposes and so individuals need to be made generally aware that it may be used by their own health team for research and audit connected with their care. Clearly, the express permission of patients is a prerequisite if their information is disclosed to other people or any conclusions are published that contain any kind of identifiable information about them. Even anonymised case studies should not be published without permission of the person concerned. The GMC advises doctors that, if they are asked to disclose patients' personal health information for research, they must satisfy themselves that express consent has been sought from the participants wherever that is practicable.[70]

Much records-based research involves no contact with the patient, whose data should be anonymised. The general principles mentioned in the definition of "audit" at the start of the chapter apply here also. Unless regulations made under section 60 of the Health and Social Care Act specifically say otherwise, patient permission should be sought if the extraction of information from records, prior to anonymisation, is carried out by other than the patient's health team (see Chapter 5, pages 180–1). General guidance about the use of anonymised data is provided in Chapter 5 (pages 171–2). As with all research, express authorisation for the detailed research protocol should be obtained from an appropriately constituted research ethics committee. The fact that a research project is solely records based does not mean that it is exempt from the requirement for review.

Somewhat different confidentiality issues may arise when the implications of the data are not restricted to the person providing them. Obviously, particular care is needed when identifiable samples are used for genetic research that has implications for other family members.[71] The issues raised by genetics are discussed in more detail in Chapter 9.

Confidentiality and publication

The GMC advises that researchers have a duty to "publish results whenever possible, including adverse findings, preferably through peer reviewed journals" and "explain to the relevant research ethics committee if, exceptionally, you believe there are valid reasons not to publish the results of a study."[72] Patient consent must be sought for publication of case studies even if the person cannot be identified. Often, individuals who have participated in research or innovative treatment could be identified by themselves, or by people close to them, by means of some of the details described, even if the author does not believe that they would be more widely identifiable. Aggregated data, however, should not pose problems (see Chapter 5, pages 171–2).

The duty to self audit and to act only within one's sphere of competence

All doctors must be assiduous in monitoring outcomes from their treatment patterns and must investigate the reasons if their success rates fall below those achieved by other practitioners in similar circumstances. The emphasis on both self monitoring and peer review is increasing. As part of the GMC's revalidation process, all doctors should collect audit results, which should be fed back to patients in a sensitive manner if it is revealed that errors have been made (see also Chapter 1, pages 37–9). If standard treatment is adapted for particular patients and seems successful, a formal research protocol should be drawn up for appraisal by a research ethics committee. All doctors have a duty to know their own limitations and not exceed their knowledge or competence (but see also Chapter 15 on emergency care, where the priority to provide urgent care may justifiably lead doctors to act beyond what they would normally attempt). Innovative medical and surgical techniques are constantly developing and specialists need to learn to use them safely and, if necessary, adapt them for specific patients, including for children and babies. Clearly, however, it is unethical for doctors who are on a steep learning curve to fail to monitor their own mastery of the new technique and their own success rate in performing it in comparison with national rates or those of colleagues. Regular appraisal, audit, and external scrutiny by means of clinical governance and revalidation make it less likely that serious errors in practice will remain undetected. Nevertheless, the primary responsibility to ensure that their treatment is safe and ethical rests with individual doctors themselves.

Specialised areas of research

Highly specialised areas of research and innovative therapy involve only a small proportion of doctors on a day to day basis, but this section sets out BMA policies on issues that are frequently raised in debate.

Embryo research

Embryo research stands out as the only research in which there is clear legislation and a statutory regulatory body. After the recommendation of the Warnock Committee (see Chapter 8, page 272) that research involving human embryos should be permitted up to 14 days after fertilisation, there followed nearly a decade of fierce debate on the subject. The Human Fertilisation and Embryology Bill was published in 1989 with alternative clauses either allowing or prohibiting embryo research.[73] The Parliamentary vote was overwhelmingly in support of the use of human embryos for certain categories of research, with strict controls. The Human Fertilisation and Embryology Act 1990 requires that a licence must be issued for every research project in the UK that involves the creation or use of human embryos.

The source of embryos for research

Embryos used in research come from two sources. They may have been created as part of the research process or as part of an *in vitro* fertilisation (IVF) procedure, to which they are now surplus (and would otherwise be donated to other infertile people or allowed to perish). Those who believe that embryos have, or should have, equal moral status to that of living people believe that research on them can never be ethical. Others accept research on "spare" embryos but not the creation of embryos for research purposes. Adherents of this latter view assume that the creation of more embryos than is strictly necessary for IVF is unavoidable for medical reasons and argue that to use them for research is no worse than destroying them and may bring about some good. Both sources of embryos for research are permitted under the Human Fertilisation and Embryology Act.

In the mid-1980s, there was extensive discussion within the BMA about the ethics of research involving human embryos. Opinions were sharply divided on the question of whether human life could be created for the purposes of research, although there was wide acceptance of the need for such research into contraception, and the diagnosis and treatment of infertility and inherited diseases. There was less objection to research on "spare" embryos and, despite some concerns, it was recognised that there are some areas of research in which embryos must be created as part of the research process. For example, when new methods of infertility treatment are being developed, it is an essential part of the research carefully to assess the effect of the treatment on the development of the embryo, to ensure that the embryo itself is not damaged.

A good example of this need for research arises with the development of intracytoplasmic sperm injection, in which a single sperm is injected into the centre of an egg as a means of overcoming severe male infertility. Before embryos created by using this new technique were replaced in the uterus for development, it was necessary to assess the embryos for any damage caused by the procedure itself. The process of checking the development of the embryo meant that they were no longer suitable for replacement. A failure to permit this type of research would have resulted either in embryos created in this way being replaced without proper checks on their safety or an end to the development of such new treatments for infertility. After debate, the BMA confirmed its belief in the need for research involving embryos and refused to rule out the possibility that embryos could be created for this purpose, although it also stressed that "the prime objectives" of IVF concerned the provision of infertility treatment for those who are unable to have children naturally.[74]

Embryonic stem cell research

In 1998 stem cells from human embryos were isolated and cultured in a laboratory for the first time. The ability of embryonic stem cells to develop into almost any body cell type meant that this development raised the possibility of a new source of tissue for the treatment of diseased or damaged tissues or organs. Combined with the technique of cell nuclear replacement this could lead to the development of compatible tissue for transplantation, which would involve transferring the nucleus – containing the genetic material – from one of the patient's own cells into a donor egg that has had its own nucleus removed. The egg would then be stimulated so that it begins to divide, but it would be allowed to develop only to the stage needed to separate and grow embryonic stem cells.

It is believed that these embryonic stem cells could then be stimulated to develop into whatever tissue was needed by the patient, such as:

- neural tissue for the treatment of degenerative diseases such as Parkinson's disease
- bone marrow for leukaemia sufferers
- muscle tissue for the repair of a damaged heart or
- skin for treating burns.

It is possible that this research will allow a damaged organ to be repaired using compatible tissue where currently a replacement organ would be required.

The BMA welcomed these developments, recognising the potential to benefit vast numbers of people who suffer from disorders that threaten or impede their lives. They could potentially offer a means of overcoming the severe shortage of tissue available for transplantation. In addition, the generation of tissue using the patients' own genetic material would remove the need for them to take the strong immunosuppressive drugs that can be harmful when taken over a long period of time.

In June 2000 an expert group was set up by the Chief Medical Officer to review the potential for developments in stem cell research and cell nuclear replacement to benefit human health. Noting that this work did not fall within any of the categories of research permitted under the Human Fertilisation and Embryology Act, this group nonetheless recommended that embryo research in this area should be permitted. It therefore recommended that the categories of research that could be licensed should be expanded to bring embryonic stem cell research within the scope of the Act.[75] Although it had been suggested that major advances could be made by the use of adult stem cells, the expert group concluded that the use of human embryos was justified. The BMA took the view that, if a similar level of success could be achieved, the use of adult, rather than embryonic, stem cells would be preferable because of the special status of human embryos. Those who were expert in the field, however, believed that there were likely to be limitations to the types of tissue that could be derived from adult stem cells, thus limiting the potential benefits. Until such time as there is clear evidence for the safety and efficacy of the use of adult stem cells, the BMA strongly believes that research using both adult and embryonic stem cells should progress in parallel. By January 2001, both Houses of Parliament had voted to extend the purposes for which embryo research may be undertaken to include this work.[76]

Cell nuclear replacement embryos

The Chief Medical Officer's expert group had concluded that the research use of embryos created by cell nuclear replacement was not prohibited by the Human Fertilisation and Embryology Act, but would be subject to the same restrictions as other embryo research.[77] Shortly after the Regulations were passed, however, the Pro-life Alliance challenged this interpretation and was granted a judicial review, arguing that the definition of "embryo" in the Act did not include an organism created by cell nuclear replacement. It therefore argued that both reproductive cloning and research on embryos created by cell nuclear replacement were completely unregulated in the UK.

The definition of "embryo" in the Human Fertilisation and Embryology Act is: "a live human embryo where fertilisation is complete" and includes "an egg in the process of fertilisation" and "for this purpose, fertilisation is not complete until the appearance of a two cell zygote".[78] The Pro-life Alliance argued that, with cell nuclear replacement, fertilisation does not take place and so the organism created cannot possibly be an "embryo where fertilisation is complete". The Government, although accepting that fertilisation does not take place, argued for a purposive rather than a literal interpretation. On 15 November 2001, Mr Justice Crane accepted "with some reluctance" the Pro-life Alliance's arguments and concluded that to accept the Government's approach would involve "an impermissible rewriting and extension of the definition".[79]

(Continued)

The Government responded quickly by passing the Human Reproductive Cloning Act 2001. Although this put beyond doubt the illegality of reproductive cloning, it did not, as some had anticipated, extend the definition of "embryo" in the Act to incorporate those embryos created by cell nuclear replacement. Instead, the Government launched an appeal against the decision of Mr Justice Crane, arguing that the Act was clearly intended to provide comprehensive control of human reproduction by either prohibiting or licensing particular activities. The Court of Appeal agreed and reversed the earlier decision.[80] The Pro-life Alliance was denied leave to appeal to the House of Lords, but announced that it would submit a petition to the House of Lords. This petition was rejected.

R (on the application of Quintavalle) v Secretary of State for Health[81]

After the Regulations were passed, the House of Lords Select Committee on Stem Cell Research was established. Its report, published in February 2002,[82] concluded that there were strong arguments for research to continue with both embryonic and adult stem cells in order to maximise the chance of medical benefit. The Select Committee also recommended the establishment of an embryonic stem cell bank to ensure their purity and provenance, and to monitor their use. This led directly to the establishment of the UK Stem Cell Bank. The Human Fertilisation and Embryology Authority announced that it would be a condition of the research licence that any cell line derived from human embryos must be deposited in the Stem Cell Bank.

Research and innovation involving fetuses or fetal material

Research involving fetuses is governed by widely accepted guidance rather than legislation. The *Review of the guidance on the research use of fetuses and fetal material* (otherwise known as the Polkinghorne report) was published in 1989.[83] Although there were differing views about the ethical acceptability of using fetal tissue in research, the Polkinghorne Committee unanimously concluded that it should be allowed with certain safeguards.

Safeguards proposed by the Polkinghorne Committee

- There must be clear separation between decisions and actions relating to termination of pregnancy and those relating to the use of fetal material.
- Where the fetal material comes from a terminated pregnancy, consent to the termination of pregnancy must be given before consent is sought to the use of fetal material.

(Continued)

- Written consent from the donor woman should be sought for the use of fetal tissue, but based on general information to avoid the possibility of termination of pregnancy for ulterior motives (such as donation for the treatment of a particular individual).
- No inducements, financial or otherwise, should be proposed to the woman who is donating the material or to other people who may influence her decision.
- There should be no modification to the termination procedure to facilitate research.

All research involving the fetus or fetal tissue must be examined by a research ethics committee, which has a duty to examine the progress of the research or innovative therapy by receiving reports. It should have access to records and be able to examine those of any financial transactions involving fetal tissue. Polkinghorne also said that such projects should continue to be regularly reviewed until the validity of the procedure has been recognised by the Committee as part of routine medical practice. Before permitting the research the research ethics committee must satisfy itself:

- of the validity of the research or use proposed
- that the objectives of the proposed use cannot be achieved in any other way
- that the researchers or clinicians have the necessary facilities and skill.

Clearly, it is essential that a woman's decision to donate fetal tissue is separated from her intentions about her own health care, including her decision to undergo termination of pregnancy. This concept of separation of decisions was central to the Polkinghorne recommendations. The Committee also considered, but rejected, the notion of allowing the donor woman to choose the method and timing of her termination of pregnancy based on factors other than her own health, such as the desire to donate fetal tissue. In 2002 the possible need for re-examining the Polkinghorne guidelines was raised by the Department of Health,[84] which noted that the idea of non-specific consent to the use of the material was increasingly out of step with modern expectations, such that individuals make choices on a properly informed basis.

Genetic research

There is considerable guidance on genetic testing and screening for health care and research. The ethical issues are discussed in detail in Chapter 9. In addition, stored human material is sometimes used in genetic research projects. In 2001 the Medical Research Council published detailed advice on the use in research of samples from both living and dead donors.[85] (The main points in this guidance are summarised on pages 524–5) This includes guidance on genetic research on archived samples. It states that when a genetic test is of known predictive value or gives reliable information about a known heritable condition, samples must be anonymised before testing unless specific consent is obtained. This applies even if the donor has died, because genetic information can have implications for relatives. The Medical Research Council also argues that if the predictive value of the genetic information to be obtained is not known, research on anonymised linked samples is permissible, provided that there is a strong scientific justification for not irreversibly anonymising the samples.[86]

Other research involving retained human material

Samples of human material from living and deceased donors are useful for a range of research projects and for audit. Human material retained after surgery and tissue, such as placentas retained after childbirth, are often described as "surplus" or "discarded", indicating that their retention is not important for the continuing care of the individual. Nevertheless, such material is very valuable for other health goals. In 2001 the Royal College of Pathologists drew attention to the fact that in the past research projects that exclusively used "surplus" material and involved no contact with patients had been perceived as not needing review by research ethics committees.[87] It emphasised that this was no longer acceptable.

Living donors

Living patients undergoing diagnostic or therapeutic procedures for their own health care are the major donors of the human tissue used in research. They should be asked about their willingness to donate surplus tissue for the purposes of research, audit, and education, quite separately to the consent they provide for the surgery or other care. They also need to give specific consent if tissue is taken in excess of what is required for their health care with a view to undertaking research. Hospitals generally have specific consent forms for this purpose, which separate out the patient's consent to the therapeutic procedure and the consent to the use or disposal of surplus tissue. In many cases, however, the person in contact with the patient is not familiar with laboratory procedures, which can obviously impede the provision of accurate information. Although general consent is sufficient for anonymised use, identifiable uses must have express consent. When patients do not wish the material to be used for such purposes after its diagnostic value for themselves is exhausted, their wishes regarding disposal should be respected.

Living donors need to know:

- a summary of the positive and negative consequences of a decision to donate or refuse
- a description as far as is practical of the uses to which tissue may be put
- if known, the likely purpose for which their own tissue will be used
- whether any research will involve the tissue in an identifiable way

- whether it may be used in genetic research
- the fact that, if they agree, it may be stored for future uses yet unforeseen
- an outline of the system for ethical oversight and regulation
- the mechanisms by which their decision will be recorded.

Anonymised surplus material

Human samples, including blood, saliva, or other body fluids that were originally given with appropriate consent for diagnostic purposes, are frequently used in an anonymised way for research once the diagnostic value for the patient has expired. Historical collections of samples obtained in this way continue to be used, subject to appropriate authorisation from a research ethics committee. Current and future patients providing samples should be made aware that surplus materials may be used for research unless they request that their own samples be destroyed. In principle, the BMA has no objection to the use of anonymised data or material as long as projects have appropriate scrutiny by research ethics committees. Obviously, however, consideration needs to be given to the fact that even anonymised samples contain genetic information about the donor.

Deceased donors

There is considerable sensitivity about the notion of retaining samples from deceased people for the purposes of research and, as is discussed in Chapter 12, much of this is due to the general lack of openness about such practices in the past. A consistent message, therefore, in all current published advice[88] is the need for greater transparency and appropriate authorisation from the families of deceased people. Researchers need to be familiar with such guidance as well as with proposed changes in legislation (see pages 523–4).

The forms authorising a postmortem examination and retention of tissue need to be clear and to offer a range of options for which relatives' agreement may separately be granted or withheld. Relatives should be given their own copy of such authorisation. The reports of postmortem examinations should clearly state what, if any, tissue or organs have been retained. Families authorising the use of cadaveric material in research need also to know the purpose for which it is intended, the anticipated time span, and the eventual manner of disposal. Discussing such issues with bereaved relatives is universally acknowledged to be a difficult and challenging task that requires appropriate training. Face to face discussion with families can be usefully augmented with written information. Guidance for relatives has been published by the Royal College of Pathologists[89] and organisations such as the Child Bereavement Trust,[90] which provides support for bereaved families.

Proposals for legal change

From the early 1960s, throughout the UK, legislation made provision for tissue from deceased people to be used for medical education and research in certain circumstances, but this legislation, although "well-intentioned … simply did not contemplate the sorts of issues and concerns" that arose at the end of the century.[91] In March 2000, the Royal College of Pathologists published guidelines on tissue retention[92] and an information leaflet for families[93] explaining what was involved in a postmortem examination and why tissue or organs may need to be kept. These publications sought to introduce greater transparency into an area where it had been significantly lacking. Two months later, in May 2000, the interim report of *The inquiry into the management of care of children receiving complex heart surgery at the Bristol Royal Infirmary 1984–1995* (the Interim Bristol report) was published.[94] This was the first of a series of reports[95] retrospectively examining how the retention of tissue and organs for research and education had been managed in previous decades. It fiercely criticised the fact that parents and relatives of deceased patients had often been unaware of the extent of this practice and lacked any real understanding of what was involved. It was followed in January 2001 by the report of the Royal Liverpool Children's Inquiry, which was also extremely critical of established practice. Similar findings were made in Scotland, where the Independent Review Group on Retention of Organs at Post Mortem considered the retention and use of cadaveric materials.[96] Clinical standards for postmortem retention were subsequently published.[97] The retention of human material was also scrutinised in Northern Ireland.[98] A common conclusion was the urgent need for legislative reform across the UK.

In England in 2001, the Chief Medical Officer published 17 recommendations.[99] Among these, he called for immediate amendment of the Human Tissue Act 1961, a new code of practice, and standardised forms throughout the NHS to obtain families' consent separately for postmortem examinations and for tissue retention. He also recommended the establishment of an independent commission (the Retained Organs Commission) to oversee the return of human material to surviving relatives. The Retained Organs Commission also produced helpful information for families on aspects of return and donation.

In July 2002, the Department of Health consulted widely on proposals for legislative change that would affect the manner in which human tissue or organs could be retained in England and Wales.[100] This covered both living and deceased donors. (Guidance on legislation resulting from the consultation and further developments in Scotland and Northern Ireland will be available on the BMA website.)

Summary – advice on human tissue

This is a summary of some of the main points of the Medical Research Council's guidance.

- Potential benefits must outweigh potential risks.
- Researchers need to be aware of the cultural and religious significance of human material for donors.

- Human biological material should be treated as a gift and the donor's wishes must be respected.
- The host institution receiving donations is responsible for custodianship.
- Human material should not give rise to financial gain.
- Informed consent is needed for new samples from the next of kin of the donor when the donor has died.
- Donors need to know if and how the results of research may impact on their interests.
- Donors need to know and give consent if their material may be used in genetic research.
- Patients should be informed if their surplus tissue may be useful for research.
- Information for donors and families must be understandable to them.
- Particular care must be taken in relation to research involving incapacitated adults and children.
- NHS interpreters or patient advocates should translate when necessary, not relatives.
- Surplus material can be used anonymously without consent.
- Donors need to be aware that their sample, or products derived from it, may be used by commercial companies.
- It may not be possible to go back to donors for new consent when new research is proposed.
- All personal and medical information relating to research participants is confidential.
- Advance thought must be given to the possibility of information being discovered that is relevant to the donor's health or interests.
- When there is a possibility of feeding back information to research participants, their wishes should be sought in advance.

Fraud and misconduct in research and innovative treatment

Independent audits of compliance (or rather the lack of it) with GCP guidelines and regulatory requirements continue to give cause for concern.[101] Misconduct includes ignorance or neglect of accepted standards, failure to obtain proper consent from participants, and attempts to conceal bad practice. Fraudulent research data provide misleading information upon which later treatment options may be decided, putting patients at risk of harm and wasting healthcare resources. When exposed, fraud also undermines public confidence. Within the definition of fraud are also the fabrication of data or cases, the falsification of data, failing to admit when some data are missing, and plagiarism. Traditionally, it was considered acceptable to include as authors senior staff who had not been involved in the actual project and there was no clear obligation to disclose any potential conflicts of interest when publishing. This is no longer the case. Furthermore, because there is immense pressure to publish, redundant publication occurs. Part of the problem concerning fraud and misconduct arises from the inadequate training of researchers.

Measures to improve research practice

- All research should be recorded in log books, which should include details of the research, the achievement of targets, and specified responsibilities of the researchers. The log book should be in the public domain.
- The senior academic or consultant who is conducting the research, or in whose name the research is being conducted, should maintain a personal responsibility for the supervision and management of the project.
- Research projects should be subjected to rigorous scientific evaluation and all but the simplest should undergo external peer review.
- A culture of routine self audit should be developed among research teams.
- There is a need to balance the enthusiasm of researchers with the observance of proper process while avoiding unnecessary obstruction of legitimate research.
- Researchers should receive training in the principles of research practice, including GCP, the full implications of the European Union Directive on Clinical Trials, and UK legislation.
- Consideration should be given to the use of independent third parties to obtain consent to research, particularly where this involves vulnerable groups of patients or especially stressful situations when anxious patients and/or relatives may rely too heavily on medical staff.

In 1996 a highly dramatic and well publicised case of fraud occurred, which increased public and professional unease about the lack of thorough audit and regulation. This case is summarised in the box below. One aspect of the tightening of standards means that senior clinicians who have often been automatically invited to add their name to research papers published by their staff should be aware that it is unacceptable to do so if they have not verified the results for themselves or been closely involved.

Fraudulent research

In August 1996, there was wide media coverage of an important medical advance involving the birth of a baby, after the reimplantation of an ectopic pregnancy by an expert on ultrasonography in obstetrics (the first author). The second author of the case report was the President of the Royal College of Obstetricians and Gynaecologists (RCOG). At the same time, the first author also published an RCT. The two papers were subsequently exposed as being fraudulent when investigation showed that the patient in the first case did not exist and those supposedly involved in the RCT could not be found. Further investigation of previous studies going back to 1989 identified three more fraudulent papers. All of these were retracted. The first author lost his job and was subsequently struck off by the GMC. The President of the RCOG retired or resigned from all his positions, admitting that he had not known that the work was fraudulent, even though his name was on the paper. The concept of "gift authorship", which had been common at the start of his career, was increasingly seen as scandalous by 1996.[102]

Whistleblowing

It is obviously essential that people who become aware of unethical activities in any sphere are able to ask questions and, if unsatisfied by the answer, report them to an appropriate body, such as the GMC. The general issues for whistleblowers are discussed in more detail in Chapter 21 (page 757), but the main point is that they should not be silenced by fear for their own career prospects, or erroneous or misplaced notions of loyalty to colleagues. Speaking out can be immensely difficult, but the GMC has shown itself ready to act against senior clinicians who attempt to threaten or bully potential whistleblowers. On the other hand, if health professionals who are aware of misconduct or fraudulent research fail to take action, they may themselves be considered to be guilty of a culpable omission.

Problems for whistleblowers

In 1997 the GMC heard a case against a doctor who was struck off the register for misleading investigators who were looking at allegations of a cover up in a clinical trial and threatening junior colleagues. He was a professor of respiratory medicine and had previously chaired a research ethics committee. Nevertheless, when his registrar raised concerns about the conduct of the trial of a new asthma drug, the doctor threatened to ruin his career. His threats were taped by the registrar and contributed to the GMC's findings of serious misconduct.[103]

In 2000 a consultant surgeon was found guilty of serious professional misconduct by the GMC for publishing fraudulent research results.[104] He admitted that the results in an abstract he had submitted had been falsified. He had claimed that they were based on urine samples from a dozen healthy adults, whereas, in fact, all the samples were of his own urine. The GMC's Professional Conduct Committee pointed out that this was not only dishonest but also damaging to public confidence, and it was potentially dangerous for patients if a doctor falsified research findings. The misconduct had occurred a decade earlier and, although known about by colleagues, pressure had been brought to bear on them to keep silent. The hospital authorities had selectively shredded the relevant laboratory books. In 2001 the consultant surgeon's research supervisor was also severely reprimanded by the GMC for failing to act over the falsified research.[105]

Committee on Publication Ethics

One of the mechanisms for identifying fraud and misconduct in medical research is the Committee on Publication Ethics (COPE), which was established in 1997 by the editors of several British journals, including the *British Medical Journal* and *The Lancet*. Its establishment reflected a growing anxiety about the integrity of papers submitted to medical journals. Its aims were:

- to advise on cases raised by editors
- to publish an annual report describing those cases

- to produce guidance on good practice
- to encourage research
- to offer teaching and training.

COPE also acts "as an editors' self-help group",[106] providing a forum in which difficult cases can be considered anonymously. It identified over 100 cases of possible misconduct in its first three years and led commentators to believe that existing UK procedures for dealing with misconduct were inadequate.[107] In 2002 it established two subcommittees, one for research in publication ethics and the other to develop educational strategies.

National committees to identify misconduct

Some countries have established national committees to receive and investigate complaints about possible cases of research misconduct and fraud. In 1992, for example, the Danish Medical Research Council initially established a Committee on Scientific Dishonesty composed of a High Court judge as chairman and seven members with health science expertise. Although lacking legal powers, it investigated all manner of scientific misconduct, including deliberate fraud and negligence. This Committee worked until 1998, when new legislation was passed and it was replaced by a series of committees covering fraud in all scientific fields, including research, social science, and agricultural and veterinary science. Most complaints, however, continue to concern medical research.[108] There have been calls in the UK for a similar national panel on research integrity. A consensus conference on misconduct in biomedical research in 1999, for example, recommended the establishment of a national panel to develop models of good practice and investigate alleged misconduct.[109]

Prevalence of misconduct

The real prevalence of fraud and misconduct in research and innovative treatment in the UK is unknown and would obviously depend on the particular definition adopted. In the first 103 cases considered by COPE, 80 contained some evidence of misconduct. The kinds of problems highlighted were:

- undeclared redundant submission or publication (29 cases)
- disputes over authorship (18)
- falsification (15)
- failure to obtain informed consent (11)
- performing unethical research (11)
- failure to gain approval from a research ethics committee (10).

Monitoring of research and innovative treatment

In the past in the UK, in the absence of specific legislation (apart from that governing the use of embryos) research on humans has been conducted according to a vaguely defined common law concept of consent. Safeguards have also been provided by the statutory framework for drug licensing by the Committee on Safety of Medicines. The Human Fertilisation and Embryology Act 1990 brought research on embryos within statutory supervision, but other difficult areas such as research on children, prisoners, and elderly people remained unregulated by law. In 2001 the Independent Review Group on Retention of Organs at Post Mortem that was looking at retained human cadaveric material in Scotland, expressed concern that the framework of research ethics committees was, in some cases, "insufficiently robust to ensure that the ongoing conduct of research is adequately monitored".[110] It recommended, therefore, that consideration be given to placing such committees on a statutory basis, with specific and clear powers to monitor the conduct of projects. As previously mentioned, in 2003 steps were taken to implement the European Directive on the Implementation of Good Clinical Practice in the Conduct of Clinical Trials on Medicinal Products for Human Use. This also had the effect of introducing new regulations and a statutory basis for research ethics committees, with its proposal for a new UKECA. This was intended to establish, recognise, and monitor the work of research ethics committees.

Functions and composition of local research ethics committees

The detailed duties of committee members, the factors they must consider, and other aspects of research governance are set out in detail in the Department of Health framework for research governance (see pages 493-4) and in the regulations implementing the European Directive on Clinical Trials on Medicinal Products.

Factors to be considered are:

- whether the scientific quality of the protocol has been properly assessed – studies that are unscientific are also unethical
- whether the investigator and others involved in the trial are competent and have adequate facilities
- possible hazards to trial participants and precautions taken to deal with them
- measures for providing information and seeking appropriate consent
- whether adequate compensation arrangements are in place in case of any harm arising from the trial
- methods of recruitment and any payments to participants
- payments to investigators
- storage and use of subject identifiable information.

General questions for consideration by research ethics committees

A considerable body of guidance exists for research ethics committees[111] but, in addition to the general factors mentioned above, the main questions include:

- Benefits

    - Can the person consent and how are any risks and benefits to be explained?
    - Is the project intended mainly to benefit the participants or others in the same situation?
    - What, if any, evidence exists for the anticipated benefits?
    - Are there beneficial side effects for the individual (such as enhanced care and attention)?
    - How will the knowledge be used?
    - How severe and common is the problem that it seeks to alleviate?
    - How likely is it to achieve its aims?

- Harms

    - How invasive or intrusive is the project?
    - How severe may the harms associated with it be?
    - How likely are the harms to occur?
    - Are adverse effects likely to be brief or lasting, immediate or delayed?
    - Are a few patients drawn into many projects simply because they are available?
    - Are researchers and clinicians involving patients who already have many problems?

Support structures

- **UKECA:** At the time of writing, a UK Ethics Committee Authority to establish, recognise and monitor research ethics committees is a proposal not yet implemented under draft regulation 4 of the proposed Medicines for Human Use (Clinical Trials) Regulations 2003.
- **COREC:** The Central Office for Research Ethics Committees works on behalf of the Department of Health in England. (COREC works closely with colleagues with similar responsibilities in Scotland, Wales and Northern Ireland.) Its remit is to:

    - coordinate development of operational systems for research ethics committees in the NHS in England
    - manage multicentre research ethics committees in England
    - act as a resource for training for research ethics committee members and administrators

- provide advice on policy and operational matters relating to research ethics committees.

- **AREC:** The Association of Research Ethics Committees is an umbrella group for research ethics committees in the NHS, universities, independent sector, and research establishments, which deals with the ethical review of scientific research involving human participants. It is a charity that holds regular meetings and conferences, as well as providing information about other published guidance and web resources.

As is emphasised throughout this chapter, research and innovative treatment need to be open, accountable, and involve patients and the public. A potential problem for some members of research ethics committees is the vast amount of published ethical guidance of which they are expected to be aware. This is also a sphere of practice that is undergoing change with the enactment of new legislation. The need for support structures such as those mentioned above will be of increased importance.

References

1 World Medical Association. *Declaration of Helsinki.* Ferney-Voltaire: WMA, 1964 (as amended): clause 6.
2 Royal College of Psychiatrists. *Guidelines for researchers and for research ethics committees on psychiatric research involving human subjects. Council report CR82.* London: RCPsych, 2001: sect 3·4.
3 The Bristol Royal Infirmary Inquiry. *Learning from Bristol: the report of the public inquiry into children's heart surgery at the Bristol Royal Infirmary 1984–1995.* London: The Stationery Office, 2001: recommendation 78. (Cm 5207 (II).)
4 Information and guidance are available from the Central Office for Research Ethics Committees (COREC). http://www.corec.org.uk.
5 Directive 2001/20/EC of the European Parliament and of the Council of 4 April 2001 on the approximation of the laws, regulations and administrative provisions of the member states relating to the implementation of good clinical practice in the conduct of clinical trials on medicinal products for human use. *Official Journal of the European Communities* 2001;**L121**:34–44.
6 Department of Health. The Medicines for Human Use (Clinical Trials) Regulations 2003. At the time of writing these are still in draft form.
7 European Agency for the Evaluation of Medicinal Products. *Note for guidance on good clinical practice (CPMP/ICH/95).* London: EMEA, 1996.
8 Department of Health. *Research governance framework for health and social care.* London: DoH, 2001.
9 Scottish Executive Health Department, Chief Scientist's Office. *Research governance framework for health and community care.* Edinburgh: Scottish Executive, 2001.
10 Department of Health. *Research governance framework for health and social care. Op cit:* p. 24.
11 Directive 2001/20/EC of the European Parliament and the Council of 4 April 2001 on the approximation of the laws, regulations and administrative provisions of the member states relating to implementation of good clinical practice in the conduct of clinical trials on medicinal products for human use. *Op cit.*
12 Draft Medicines for Human Use (Clinical Trials) Regulations 2003.
13 Department of Health. *Governance arrangements for NHS research ethics committees.* London: DoH, 2001.
14 Centre of Medical Law and Ethics, King's College London. *Manual for research ethics committees, 6th ed.* Cambridge: Cambridge University Press, 2003. Comprises a collection of helpful articles and guidelines.
15 World Medical Association. *Declaration of Helsinki. Op cit.*
16 See, for example: World Health Organization. *Guidelines for good clinical practice (GCP) for trials on pharmaceutical products.* Geneva: WHO, 1995. World Health Organization. *Operational guidelines for ethics committees that review biomedical research.* Geneva: WHO, 2000.

17 Joint United Nations Programme on HIV/AIDS (UNAIDS). *Ethical considerations in HIV preventive vaccine research*. Geneva: UNAIDS, 2000.

18 *Convention on human rights and biomedicine*. (Oviedo, 4.IV.1997) 1997 (ETS 164).

19 Council for International Organizations of Medical Science (CIOMS), World Health Organization. *International ethical guidelines for biomedical research involving human subjects*. Geneva: CIOMS, 2002.

20 The European Group on Ethics in Science and New Technologies. *The ethical aspects of biomedical research in developing countries*. Brussels: EGE, 2003.

21 Nuffield Council on Bioethics. *The ethics of research related to healthcare in developing countries*. London: Nuffield Council on Bioethics, 2002.

22 General Medical Council. *Research: the role and responsibilities of doctors*. London: GMC, 2002.

23 X v Denmark, European Commission of Human Rights, Application No. 9974/82.

24 See: British Medical Association. *The impact of the Human Rights Act 1998 on medical decision-making*. London: BMA, 2000.

25 Kennedy L, Bates P. Research ethics and the law. In: Centre of Medical Law and Ethics, King's College London. *Manual for research ethics committees, 6th ed. Op cit*: p. 15.

26 Information Commissioner. *Use and disclosure of health data – guidance on the application of the Data Protection Act 1998*. Wilmslow: Information Commissioner, 2002:ch 3.

27 Moore v Regents of the University of California, 793 P 2d 479 (Cal, 1990).

28 Central Office for Research Ethics Committees. *Guidelines for researchers – patient information sheet and consent form*. London: COREC, 2001. This document is under review at the time of writing.

29 Consumers for Ethics in Research. *Medical research and you*. London: CERES.

30 See, for example: Mellor, E, Raynor D, Silcock J. Writing information for potential research participants. In: Centre of Medical Law and Ethics, King's College London. *Manual for research ethics committees, 6th ed. Op cit*: p. 96.

31 Royal College of Paediatrics and Child Health. Guidelines for the ethical conduct of medical research involving children. *Arch Dis Child* 2000;**82**:177–82.

32 Doyal L. Informed consent in medical research. *BMJ* 1997;**314**:1107–11.

33 Hall A. The role of effective communication in obtaining informed consent. In: Doyal L, Tobias JS, eds. *Informed consent in medical research*. London: BMJ Books, 2000: 292.

34 Doyal L. Informed consent in medical research. *Op cit*.

35 The Royal Liverpool Children's Inquiry. *The Royal Liverpool Children's Inquiry report*. London: The Stationery Office, 2001.

36 This case is discussed in detail in: McNeill P, Pfeffer N. Learning from unethical research. In: Doyal L, Tobias JS, eds. *Informed consent in medical research. Op cit*.

37 Nicholson RJ. Final act in the Evelyn Thomas case. *Bull Med Ethics* 1992;**75**:3–4: 3.

38 O'Rourke DM, Slattery J, Staniforth T, Warlow C. Evaluation of a stroke family care worker: results of a randomised control trial. *BMJ* 1997;**314**:1071–6.

39 Bhagwanjee S, Mukart D, Jenna PM, Moodley P. Does HIV status influence outcomes of patients admitted to a surgical intensive care unit? A prospective double blind study. *BMJ* 1997;**314**:1077–81.

40 Wilkie P. Ethical considerations in research. In: Carter Y, Shaw S, Thomas C, eds. *Patient participation and ethical considerations*. London: Royal College of General Practitioners, 2001:9.

41 This is discussed in: Pfeffer N. Informed consent in medical research: the consumer's view. In: Doyal L, Tobias JS, eds. *Informed consent in medical research. Op cit*.

42 West Midlands Regional Office. *Report of a review of the research framework in North Staffordshire Hospital NHS Trust (Griffiths inquiry)*. Birmingham: NHS Executive, 2000: para 10·2.

43 European Agency for the Evaluation of Medicinal Products. *Note for guidance on good clinical practice (CPMP/ICH/95). Op cit*: para 1·61.

44 British Medical Association. *The medical profession and human rights: handbook for a changing agenda*. London: Zed Books, 2000:11–12.

45 Department of Defense. Request for exemption from informed consent. *Federal Register* 1990 Dec 21;(55):52813–17.

46 Annas GJ. Changing the consent rules for desert storm. *N Engl J Med* 1992;**236**:770–3.

47 Simms v Simms, PA v JA (Also known as: A v A, JS v An NHS Trust) [2003] 1 All ER 669

48 General Medical Council. *Seeking patients' consent: the ethical considerations*. London: GMC, 1999: para 37.

49 The Adults with Incapacity (Ethics Committee) (Scotland) Regulations 2002. (SSI 2002 No. 190.)

50 Department of Health. *Consultation on the draft guidance on consent by a legal representative on behalf of a person not able to consent under the Medicines for Human Use (Clinical Trials) Regulations 2003*. London: DoH, 2003.

51 Adults with Incapacity (Scotland) Act 2000.

52 Department of Health, Medicines and Healthcare Products Regulatory Agency. *Consultation on the UK's draft Medicines for Human Use (Clinical Trials) Regulations 2003, implementing EU Directive 2001/20/EC.* London: DoH, 2003.

53 Department of Health, Medicines and Healthcare Products Regulatory Agency. *MLX 287. Consultation letter on the Medicines for Human Use (Clinical Trials) Regulations 2003.* London: MHRA, 2003.

54 This is discussed, for example, in: Meslin, EM. A perspective from the USA and Canada. In: Doyal L, Tobias JS, eds. *Informed consent in medical research. Op cit.*

55 Royal College of Paediatrics and Child Health. *Safeguarding informed parental involvement in clinical research involving newborn babies and infants.* London: RCPCH, 1999.

56 Saugsted OD, Rootwelt T. Resuscitation of asphyxiated newborn infants with room air or oxygen: an international controlled trial: the Resair-2 study. *Pediatrics* 1998;**102**:e5.

57 Royal College of Paediatrics and Child Health. *Safeguarding informed parental involvement in clinical research involving new-born babies and infants. Op cit:* p. 2.

58 The ethical arguments for including children in research are explored in a number of published guidelines. See, for example: Medical Research Council. *The ethical conduct of research on children.* London: MRC, 1991.

59 Royal College of Paediatrics and Child Health. Guidelines for the ethical conduct of medical research involving children. *Op cit:* p. 177.

60 *Ibid.*

61 Draft Medicines for Human Use (Clinical Trials) Regulations 2003.

62 Royal College of Paediatrics and Child Health. Guidelines for the ethical conduct of medical research involving children. *Op cit:* p. 179.

63 Royal College of Psychiatrists. *Guidelines for researchers and for research ethics committees on psychiatric research involving human subjects. Council report CR82. Op cit:* sect 5·6a.

64 West Midlands Regional Office. *Report of a review of the research framework in North Staffordshire Hospital NHS Trust (Griffiths inquiry). Op cit:* para 4·2·2.

65 Royal College of Physicians. *Research on healthy volunteers.* London: RCP, 1986.

66 Cartwright SR. *The report of the committee of inquiry into allegations concerning the treatment of cervical cancer at National Women's Hospital and related matters.* Auckland: Government Printing Office, 1988. Quoted in: McNeill P, *et al.* Learning from unethical research. In: Doyal L, Tobias JS, eds. *Informed consent in medical research. Op cit.*

67 McNeill P, *et al.* Learning from unethical research. In: Doyal L, Tobias JS, eds. *Informed consent in medical research. Op cit.*

68 British Medical Association. *Asylum seekers: meeting their healthcare needs.* London: BMA, 2002.

69 Medical Research Council. *Personal information in medical research.* London: MRC, 2000.

70 General Medical Council. *Research: the role and responsibilities of doctors. Op cit:* para 31.

71 These issues are discussed in: British Medical Association. *Human genetics: choice and responsibility.* Oxford: Oxford University Press, 1998.

72 General Medical Council. *Research: the role and responsibilities of doctors. Op cit:* para 42.

73 For information on the main points in the debate see: Lee RG, Morgan D. *Human fertilisation and embryology: regulating the reproductive revolution.* London: Blackstone Press, 2001.

74 BMA Annual Representative Meeting, 1985.

75 Department of Health. *Stem cell research: medical progress with responsibility. A report from the Chief Medical Officer's expert group reviewing the potential of developments in stem cell research and cell nuclear replacement to benefit human health.* London: DoH, 2000: para 5·10.

76 Human Fertilisation and Embryology (Research Purposes) Regulations 2001. (SI 2001 No. 188.)

77 Department of Health. *Stem cell research: medical progress with responsibility. A report from the Chief Medical Officer's expert group reviewing the potential of developments in stem cell research and cell nuclear replacement to benefit human health. Op cit:* para 3·10.

78 Human Fertilisation and Embryology Act 1990 s1(1).

79 R (on the application of Quintavalle) v Secretary of State for Health [2001] 4 All ER 1013: 1024.

80 R (on the application of Quintavalle) v Secretary of State for Health [2002] 2 All ER 625.

81 R (on the application of Quintavalle) v Secretary of State for Health [2003] 2 All ER 113.

82 House of Lords. *Stem cell research. Report from the Select Committee.* London: The Stationery Office, 2002. (HL Paper 83(I).)

83 Committee to Review the Guidance on the Research Use of Fetuses and Fetal Material. *Review of the guidance on the research use of fetuses and fetal material.* London: HMSO, 1989. (Cmnd 762.)

84 Department of Health, Welsh Assembly Government. *Human bodies, human choices: the law on human organs and tissue in England and Wales. A consultation report.* London: DoH, 2002.

85 Medical Research Council. *Human tissue and biological samples for use in research: operational and ethical guidelines.* London: MRC, 2001.

86 *Ibid:* para 10·2.

87 Royal College of Pathologists. *Transitional guidelines to facilitate changes in procedures for handling "surplus" and archival material from human biological samples.* London: RCPath, 2001: para 65.

88 See, for example: Department of Health. *Consent to organ and tissue retention at postmortem examination and disposal of human materials: report of content analysis of NHS trust policies and protocols on consent to organ and tissue retention at post-mortem examination and disposal of human materials in the Chief Medical Officer's census of NHS pathology services.* London: DoH, 2000.

89 Royal College of Pathologists. *Examination of the body after death: information about post mortem examination for relatives.* London: RCPath, 2000.

90 For example: The Child Bereavement Trust. *Ordinary days and shattered lives.* High Wycombe: The Child Bereavement Trust, 2000. The Child Bereavement Trust. *Supporting parents when their baby dies.* High Wycombe: The Child Bereavement Trust, 1993.

91 Department of Health, *et al. Human bodies, human choices: the law on human organs and tissue in England and Wales. Op cit:* p. 19.

92 Royal College of Pathologists. *Guidelines on the retention of tissues and organs at post mortem examination.* London: RCPath, 2000.

93 Royal College of Pathologists. *Examination of the body after death: information about post mortem examination for relatives. Op cit.*

94 The Bristol Royal Infirmary Inquiry. *The inquiry into the management of care of children receiving complex heart surgery at The Bristol Royal Infirmary. Interim report: removal and retention of human material.* London: The Stationery Office, 2000.

95 The Royal Liverpool Children's Inquiry. *The Royal Liverpool Children's Inquiry report. Op cit.* The Independent Review Group on Retention of Organs at Post Mortem. *Retention of organs at post mortem: final report.* Edinburgh: Scottish Executive, 2001. The Human Organs Inquiry. *The human organs inquiry report.* Belfast: Department of Health, Social Services and Public Safety, 2002.

96 Independent Review Group on Retention of Organs at Post Mortem. *Retention of organs at post mortem: final report. Op cit.*

97 Clinical Standards Board for Scotland. *Clinical standards: post-mortem and organ retention.* Edinburgh: CSBS, 2002.

98 The Human Organs Inquiry. *The human organs inquiry report. Op cit.*

99 Chief Medical Officer. *The removal, retention and use of human organs and tissue from post-mortem examination.* London: Department of Health, Department for Education and Employment, Home Office, 2001.

100 Department of Health, *et al. Human bodies, human choices: the law on human organs and tissue in England and Wales. A consultation report. Op cit.*

101 McNeill P, *et al.* Learning from unethical research. In: Doyal L, Tobias JS, eds. *Informed consent in medical research. Op cit.*

102 Barker A, Powell RA. Authorship [letter]. *BMJ* 1997;**314**:1046.

103 Dyer C. Professor accused of threatening staff. *BMJ* 1999;**319**:938.

104 Ferriman A. Consultant suspended for research fraud. *BMJ* 2000;**321**:1429.

105 Dyer C. Professor reprimanded for failing to act over fraud. *BMJ* 2001;**322**:573.

106 Farthing M. Research misconduct: an editor's view. In: Lock S, Wells F, Farthing M, eds. *Fraud and misconduct in biomedical research.* London: BMJ Books, 2001:254.

107 White C. Plans for tackling research fraud may not go far enough. *BMJ* 2000;**321**:1487.

108 Brydensholt HH. The legal basis for the Danish Committee on Scientific Dishonesty. *Sci Eng Ethics* 2000;**6**:1–14. Quoted in: Lock S, Wells F, Farthing M, eds. *Fraud and misconduct in biomedical research. Op cit.*

109 Farthing M. Research misconduct: an editor's view. In: Lock S, Wells F, Farthing M, eds. *Fraud and misconduct in biomedical research. Op cit:* p. 255.

110 Independent Review Group on Retention of Organs at Post Mortem. *Retention of organs at post mortem: final report. Op cit:* p. 24.

111 In particular, see: Centre of Medical Law and Ethics, King's College London. *Manual for research ethics committees, 6th ed. Op cit.*

15: Emergency care

The questions covered in this chapter include the following.

- Is it ever permissible to withhold lifesaving treatment after an attempted suicide?
- What is the role of advance refusals ("living wills") in emergency care?
- Should health professionals take blood samples from unconscious drivers?
- Should relatives be encouraged or allowed to witness resuscitation attempts?
- Are doctors obliged to provide "Samaritan" care in an emergency?
- Is it reasonable for doctors to exceed their competence to help an injured person?

This chapter considers ethical dilemmas in emergency care, including those that arise in A&E departments and those involving the urgent treatment of inpatients. Also covered briefly are specialised emergency care procedures and urgent impromptu treatment outside hospitals, such as at the site of a disaster, in aircraft, and at road accidents. We aim to show how core ethical principles apply equally in emergency care as in other branches of medicine, but with some differences in emphasis.

General principles

The general principles applicable to emergency care include:

- the duty to promote patient autonomy and patient centred services
- the responsibility to determine incompetent patients' best interests
- the recognition of the abilities of others in the healthcare team to work across traditional boundaries
- the duty of care both for patients and, in some cases, families
- the obligation to act within one's sphere of competence
- the protection of patient confidentiality, privacy and dignity.

Promoting patient autonomy

Dilemmas in any field of medicine are addressed by application of the general ethical principles of maximising benefit and minimising harm. Throughout this book, we discuss how such principles are interpreted in various contexts, concluding that the competent patient's own views of what is beneficial or harmful are key factors in most ethical decision making. This is equally true in emergency care. As in other areas of care, patient autonomy is important and the majority of patients attending hospital emergency departments have time to receive and consider information about treatment options. For them the normal procedures regarding consent and provision of information apply (see Chapters 2 and 4 for general advice on seeking consent from adults and from minors). All competent people, including minors, should have the treatment options explained to them and be asked for their consent. When patients are incompetent, essential treatment should be provided without delay unless the patient is an adult who is carrying clear evidence of a treatment refusal. (Advance directives are discussed briefly below on pages 540–1 and in Chapter 3, pages 113–6.)

In all cases of children and young people, parents or other people with parental responsibility should also be involved whenever possible, but essential treatment cannot be delayed if they are not immediately contactable. Patient consent should be sought either by the doctor providing the specific treatment or by someone with sufficient training to be capable of doing it so that the real issues, potential complications, and alternatives can be explained appropriately.

The duty to provide information

It must not be assumed that patients requiring urgent interventions are incapable of discussing treatment options. In one study, the majority of patients undergoing urgent surgery for acute abdominal conditions felt capable of assimilating information and deciding on options.[1] Over 80% were in pain and 70% had already received analgesia, but many claimed this did not interfere with their decision. Only a minority, however, felt that they had received a proper explanation of the side effects and complications of surgery. Where there were competing options for treatment with differing side effects and complications, the study found that these were discussed differently between urgent and elective patients. Doctors need to use their judgment in differentiating, for example, between penetrating abdominal trauma or acute conditions associated with major blood loss such as a ruptured abdominal aortic aneurysm and the relatively common clinical emergencies arising from acute appendicitis or acute cholecystitis. For the former, there is no opportunity for detailed discussion, but for the latter treatment plans should be formulated with patient input.

Autonomy and refusal of treatment

Patient refusal of treatment is a common ethical and legal problem faced by doctors providing emergency care; it therefore deserves significant attention here. As is discussed in detail in Chapter 2, competent adults cannot be obliged to accept examination, investigation, or treatment even if their refusal results in death. Nevertheless, when patients seem determined to discharge themselves without accepting treatment for a potentially life threatening injury or illness, questions about their competence arise. Adults can be detained in hospital against their will only under the provisions of mental health legislation. If there is any doubt about their ability to make a valid decision, a psychiatric evaluation should be urgently arranged. Competence can be temporarily affected by factors such as shock, fatigue, medication, or loss of blood. If the patient lacks sufficient mental capacity to make the decision in question, treatment can be provided without consent under the common law criteria of necessity to act in the patient's best interests or with the consent of a proxy in Scotland. If, however, an assessment of their competence indicates that adult patients have sufficient ability to make a valid refusal, their decisions should be respected. (Assessment of capacity is discussed in detail in Chapter 3.) Even if they refuse essential treatment, children and young people can be treated if authorisation is given by someone who has parental responsibility or if treatment is urgently required in their best interests. (The situation may differ in Scotland, as is discussed in Chapter 4, and legal advice may need to be sought.)

Some patients refuse even to attend hospital for examination after an accident or injury and a significant number of these actually have a serious diagnosis.[2] Emergency teams in the community are advised to persist in trying to persuade patients to agree to go to hospital if certain clinical criteria are met, such as indications of a history of drug ingestion, head injury, disorientation, or chest pains, but treatment cannot be forced upon competent patients. Even if refusing hospitalisation, patients should be strongly encouraged to allow their GP to be informed and it should be stressed that they should seek medical help immediately if their condition worsens. Efforts should also be made to find a responsible adult to stay with the patient and call for help if necessary.

In hospitals, Jehovah's Witnesses frequently indicate restrictions on the use of blood products. In such cases, urgent advice needs to be sought about options for bloodless surgery and acceptable blood substitutes if the patient is likely to need a transfusion. Advice is available from the Jehovah's Witness hospital liaison committee. Assumptions should not automatically be made, however, that all Jehovah's Witnesses necessarily refuse all blood products. Where possible, the various options must be discussed with the individual, as with any other patient. If that is not possible because, for example, the patient is unconscious, essential treatment should be provided in an emergency unless there is evidence of the individual's wish to refuse it. (Treatment of adult Jehovah's Witnesses is discussed in Chapter 2, pages 87–8, and of children in Chapter 4, pages 141–2.) The courts have generally taken the view that parents can refuse treatment themselves but not on behalf of their children.

Suicide attempts and self harm

Many patients arriving at A&E departments after a suicide attempt are already incapable of making a valid decision about treatment and they must be treated according to the "best interests" criteria (see Chapter 3, pages 108–9). Common methods by which men attempt suicide include hanging and suffocation, poisoning by gases and vapour, poisoning by substance, drowning, and other measures such as the use of firearms, jumping from high places, and lying in front of moving objects.[3] The speed and lethal effect of these methods mean that lifesaving detection is less likely to happen and, if they are brought to hospital alive, these patients' mental capacity is likely to be seriously affected. Such methods by men also contribute to the suicide rate being predominantly male and the attempted suicide rate being predominantly female. When patients arrive in an incapacitated condition, attempts should obviously be made to try to revive them (but see also the discussion of advance directives below).

Some patients presenting after an episode of self harm are conscious and able to communicate, but refuse urgent medical treatment. Attempts at suicide by apparently competent adults challenge ethical analysis because they combine two conflicting principles. Doctors should respect competent individuals' liberty and right of self determination, but they also have an obligation to try to act in patients' interests. Normally, the former trumps other considerations so that a competent patient's refusal of life prolonging treatment is binding. Therefore, if it is absolutely clear that the patient is competent, informed, and determined, the refusal must be respected and the decision not to proceed should be taken by a senior doctor. The patient should still be offered information and support and may agree to calling relatives or friends, who may be persuasive about the acceptance of treatment. If such patients discharge themselves, however, it should be made clear that the hospital health team remains ready to offer treatment if they change their mind. As mentioned above, if the patient is thought to have impaired capacity or is a minor, refusal of treatment is likely to be invalid. In difficult borderline cases, legal advice should be sought and an application may need to be made to the courts.

An estimated 100 000 people, approximately 19% of whom are young, are referred to hospitals in England and Wales each year having suffered some form of deliberate self harm or drug overdose.[4] Suicide among the very young seems particularly tragic and many people who attempt self harm are not necessarily making a competent and valid decision to die. Among the range of factors prompting a suicide attempt are mental illness, drug use, child abuse, family or relationship breakdown, loss of employment, and development of illness or disability. There appears to be a significant link between mental illness and suicide. Schizophrenia and depressive illness are commonly found among young men who commit suicide.[5] This is likely to lead health professionals in most cases to conclude that a suicide attempt should not be regarded as a sustained and competent expression of intention. The presence of a mental illness does not in itself automatically render patients incompetent and there may be various matters upon which they can make valid decisions, but when there is any doubt about the patient's competence to refuse treatment a psychiatric evaluation is needed. Although not inevitable, mental illness often does reduce patients' competence to consent or refuse treatment for a physical injury or condition. In such cases, health professionals should provide treatment acting under the common law principle of best interests (see Chapter 3, pages 108–9).

The need for psychiatric assessment in case of self harm

In 1996 a study was conducted involving 104 doctors in 14 A&E departments, seeking their views on the management of a hypothetical but typical case. The details were as follows.

- A 19-year-old woman says she has taken 20 paracetamol and 30 amitriptyline tablets an hour ago.
- Advice from the local poisons centre is for immediate gastric lavage and charcoal therapy.
- Persuaded by a friend to attend A&E, the patient refuses any investigation or treatment.
- She has no history of self harm, is not intoxicated, and seems fully alert.
- She says she wishes to die.

Over half of the doctors had encountered a similar scenario recently and 80 of them correctly identified the need for an assessment of mental capacity. Nevertheless, 43 doctors would have illegally detained the patient against her will even if she was deemed competent and, of these, 19 would have carried out gastric lavage, which they considered to be in her "best interests". On a competent patient, this could have amounted to a battery.[6]

The case example above demonstrates that many health professionals remain unsure about how to deal with apparent competence in patients who have taken an overdose. A particular problem noted by the study authors was that decisions on how to proceed on such complex issues are often made at short notice by the A&E doctor on duty. It is therefore desirable for hospitals to have clear guidelines in place, drawing attention to the likely need for assessment of capacity or recourse to legal advice in cases of uncertainty. One of the key targets of the Health of the Nation strategy in England in 1992 was suicide reduction.[7] This was echoed in 1999 by *Saving lives: our healthier nation*, which set a target of reducing the suicide rate by at least a fifth by 2010.[8] The mental health national service framework[9] described ways of achieving this in its standard 7. It called for A&E departments to develop and implement protocols for those who present with self harm[10] and also highlighted the role of these departments in ensuring that people with mental health problems are put in touch promptly with local services. The framework notes that many people who subsequently go on to take their lives have been in touch with health services in the period prior to their death. Some have had previous admission to hospital and may have a history of self harm or substance abuse. Many were not fully compliant with treatment when discharged.[11] Similar goals for reducing suicide have been set in other parts of the UK. In Scotland, for example, a Framework for Suicide Prevention was developed in 2001, jointly by the Health Department and Scottish Development Centre for Mental Health Services.[12] Part of the overall aim was to provide better access to early psychological treatments via GPs and to ensure continuing support in the community for people with depressive disorders.

Advance refusals

Some adults want to decide in advance about the treatment they are willing to accept later when they may have lost mental capacity or the ability to communicate. They do this by means of an advance statement or "living will" (see Chapter 3, pages 113–6). This form of decision making can be helpful for people who have a serious or terminal condition that is likely to entail loss of mental capacity in circumstances in which they are sure that they would not want cardiopulmonary resuscitation or other invasive procedures to be attempted. Where the patient's refusal is clear, unambiguous, and obviously applies to the current situation, it should be respected unless there is evidence that the patient's views have changed. Advance refusal of resuscitation could also be potentially binding if suicide were attempted by a clearly rational patient suffering from a serious condition and who fears mental decline.

It seems counter intuitive to suggest that a suicide note could prevent treatment being given later because the common expectation is to assume that such notes are written at a time of crisis, without reflective discussion with other people and without reliable witnesses. Arguably, however, in very exceptional cases a suicide note specifically prohibiting resuscitation could constitute a valid advance directive if there were reliable indicators that the individual was competent and informed at the time of deciding. If such cases could indeed be reliably identified – which is questionable – doctors could be seen as acting illegally and unethically in overriding the patient's intention by attempting resuscitation. Much would depend on the reasonableness of the available evidence in the individual case and whether, for example, the patient had undergone an assessment of capacity when making that particular form of advance directive. Factors such as the method chosen to commit suicide may lead health professionals to believe that the individual was ambivalent or expected to be found in time to be resuscitated. For a suicide note to constitute a form of advance statement and legally to prohibit treatment, there would need to be persuasive evidence that the individual had thought through the options and reached a valid decision to decline treatment, being aware that death would result. Urgent legal advice may be needed by health professionals who discover such a document.

In most cases it would be immensely difficult for a resuscitation team to be confident that a suicide note written by a patient who is now unconscious constitutes a valid and binding advance statement refusing treatment. In emergency care the normal assumption when faced with unconscious people who have self harmed is that death was not their true intention or that their capacity to decide in a valid way is likely to have been impaired at the time of deciding. Prior competence cannot be automatically presumed and, as already mentioned, a significant proportion of people who attempt suicide have a psychiatric illness or are prone to substance abuse, which may impair their capacity. Certainly, when there are reasons to doubt individuals' prior competence or their intention to refuse resuscitation knowing that death will result, treatment should be provided. In some cases, the authenticity of the note may be in question. It is conceivable, for example, that potential heirs could fabricate one. There are, therefore, strong public policy arguments for attempting resuscitation in most cases; in the vast majority, this is the right choice.

Arguably, however, a distinction can be made between cases in which the self harm is associated with a history of psychiatric disturbance or erratic behaviour, and treatment refusals that individuals have clearly thought about for a long time and discussed with other people. If a demonstrably competent person took a lethal dose, having clearly, in advance, refused resuscitation or other emergency care, respect for that person would prohibit any coercive attempts at rescue. The fact that other people, such as an adult patient's family, would be distressed would not be sufficient justification for intervening. In exceptional cases, a deliberate suicide accompanied by a clearly articulated advance treatment refusal by a person whose competence has recently been assessed may constitute a legally binding decision.

Potentially binding refusal of resuscitation

W was a prisoner who refused potentially life prolonging treatment and this was discussed with him on numerous occasions. In April 2002, the High Court ruled that he had the mental capacity to make a valid refusal even if this resulted in death. He had previously attempted suicide, but the court deemed this to have been a facet of his need to command public attention. Nevertheless, W said that he did not wish to be resuscitated in future if he were at the point of death as a result of trying to hang himself, cutting his throat, or inducing blood poisoning. In the light of these comments, the judge was asked to say what should happen if he attempted suicide. She suggested that W draw up a statement clarifying his verbal refusal of resuscitation if he were to attempt suicide by any means. Prison service rules required him to be cut down if he again attempted to hang himself, but not necessarily to attempt resuscitation. The judge made clear that the onus was on W to say precisely whether he was serious in refusing all medical help in that situation. In such cases where there was clear forewarning of the patient's wish, the judge said that authorities could risk litigation against them if they resuscitated a person contrary to an express wish.

Re W[13]

This case is also discussed in Chapter 17 (pages 605–7), where it is noted that W is exceptional in having discussed his intentions with lawyers and other people in advance and having had his mental capacity assessed. In most situations, there is not clear evidence of capacity and informed intention. In an emergency setting, there is also unlikely to be time to make enquiries about the existence of a valid advance refusal of treatment if it is not immediately available. The responsibility for ensuring that it is known about rests with the patient and it is often documented in medical notes. It should also have been discussed with relatives or carers who can inform paramedics, ambulance crew, or the health team. Some patients, such as Jehovah's Witnesses, carry clear and specific evidence of their wish to refuse certain procedures by means of a signed statement.

Proxy refusal

When there is no obvious indication of an adult patient's views, relatives may claim that the incapacitated patient held certain views about refusal of life prolonging treatment and doctors must make a reasoned judgment in the light of the available evidence. If the individual has taken no discernible steps to document an advance refusal, doctors are right to have reservations about withholding treatment that, in their clinical judgment, would be beneficial. In England, Wales, and Northern Ireland, relatives cannot legally decide for an incompetent adult. In Scotland, proxy decision makers may refuse medical treatment, provided that in doing so they are fulfilling their duty of care to the adult and are abiding by the general principles in the Adults with Incapacity (Scotland) Act 2000. When it appears that a proxy's decision is contrary to the patient's interests, however, essential treatment should be given, and then the procedures for resolving disagreement between doctors and proxies must be followed (see pages 111–2). Parents or other people with parental responsibility can make decisions on behalf of a young child or a minor who is unconscious. Such decisions must be in the patient's best interests in order to be determinative and so any treatment choice that seems not to be so should be challenged (see Chapter 4). When competent, children and young people should be asked their own views about treatment options; this is discussed further below.

Improving communication

Hospital emergency departments are often excessively busy and traditionally have dealt with a wide range of patients, many of whom could be more appropriately treated in a different setting. A&E departments, for example, are often the first port of call for mentally disturbed patients and also deal with injured people who are drunk or violent. (Management of violent patients, including their removal from hospital premises, is discussed in Chapter 1, pages 58–60.) In such a stressful atmosphere, making time for effective discussion, even with fully competent people, is difficult. Both patients and health professionals find it hard to have a proper dialogue about options and risks. Hospitals should consider ways of addressing this.[14] Separating out patient groups with very different needs, for example, can promote better communication and help to enable patient autonomy and satisfaction. The lack of accessible translation and interpretation services can also hamper communication in an emergency. Translation is also discussed in Chapter 1 (pages 42–3).

Measures to improve communication

Patients with minor injuries attending Ipswich Hospital A&E department were waiting a long time, particularly between triage and first assessment, and from investigation to diagnosis. They also identified problems with a lack of

(Continued)

information and poor communication. A scheme was developed to stream patients with minor injuries to nurse practitioners who clinically assess and treat patients at the front door. This amalgamated triage and assessment processes, fully utilised the skills of the emergency nurse practitioners, improved communication with waiting patients, and diminished patient hostility.[15]

Listening to children and young people

On a typical day, some 33 000 patients, of whom a quarter are children, attend A&E departments because of a wide range of conditions,[16] but provision of specific care for them has sometimes been poor.[17] Ideally, parents should be involved in decisions of a serious nature about their child, but in an emergency this is not always possible and, where no-one is available to give valid consent, it is lawful to proceed with treatment that is immediately necessary and in the child's interests. Competent children and young people can consent to treatment on their own behalf, as outlined in the general advice given in Chapter 4. If they refuse essential treatment, attempts should be made to ascertain the reason, but ultimately the patient's wishes may have to be overridden if urgent interventions are required. Their views must be considered, but generally health professionals are not bound by a refusal that would result in harm to a child patient. (There may be exceptions, however, in Scotland, where a competent child can refuse treatment in some circumstances and an urgent application may need to be made to the court to clarify individual cases. This is also discussed in more detail in Chapter 4.)

Refusal of blood products

A was aged nearly 16, suffered from leukaemia, and urgently needed a blood transfusion, which both he and his parents refused because the family were Jehovah's Witnesses. The young man knew he would die without a transfusion, but had not been told the details of the prolonged and painful death facing him. The High Court judge adjudicating A's case concluded that A was generally intelligent enough to make his own decisions but, nevertheless, he was insufficiently mature to grasp all of the implications. He was considered to lack competence to refuse the urgent treatment, but the judge made clear that it was important to be aware of A's own wishes when deciding what was in his best interests. The hospital was given permission by the court to carry out any necessary treatment, including blood transfusions. When A reached 18, however, he refused further transfusions and, as an adult, could not be overruled, and eventually he died.

Re E (a minor) (wardship: medical treatment)[18]

Treating detained people in A&E

Communication can be difficult with patients who are brought to an emergency department by prison staff. The BMA receives many queries about the use of handcuffs or shackles in such situations, and the fact that accompanying prison staff can make difficult any confidential discussion with the patient. In brief, risk assessment procedures should have been used by the prison or detention centre prior to transferring the detainee so that hospital staff would have a good idea of whether restraints could safely be removed. Clearly, the medical condition of the detainee is also likely to be a factor in whether violence or escape are risks. A&E doctors occasionally report, however, that their requests to assess in private a patient who very clearly poses no threat are sometimes refused; the position of a junior doctor in being able to insist on the removal of shackles can be difficult. The general rules on these issues are set out in detail in Chapter 17.

Summary – promoting patient autonomy

- The fundamental principles in emergency care are similar to those that govern other areas of treatment.
- Informed consent is desirable. Assumptions should not be automatically made that patients cannot consent in a valid way, even if in pain or having received anaesthesia.
- Emergency settings differ from other healthcare contexts when doctors have only a brief interaction with a patient rather than a continuing relationship.
- In some cases, patients' capacity to participate in decision making is impaired by the effects of an accident or acute illness.
- Nevertheless, any reliable indicators of the patient's own preferences must be taken into account.
- If shown to be valid and informed, advance directives are as binding as in other contexts.

Determining patients' best interests

Incapacitated adults

Wherever possible, patients must be involved in treatment decisions. Nevertheless, the delivery of emergency care frequently involves situations in which immediate and irreversible decisions have to be made without being able to discuss the implications or knowing the patient's preferences. Therefore there are some similarities with the situation in which incapacitated people are treated in line with a medical assessment of their "best interests". The general factors relevant to an assessment of best interests are set out in Chapter 3 (pages 108–9) and include identifying effective options that are least likely to restrict patients' future choices. In normal practice, such assessment is time consuming and involves talking to people who are close to the patient about that person's likely wishes or prior opinions. When the potential benefits and burdens of a particular intervention are finely balanced, for example, the views of people close to the patient can be informative, even though they may have no standing in law. Ultimately, however, the clinician in overall charge must make a decision about what is in the patient's best interests, even if this does not match the views of relatives. In Scotland, if patients have appointed a proxy decision maker, that person's views should be sought if it is reasonable and practicable to do so, but not if this would delay or jeopardise essential care (see Chapter 3, pages 110–2). In an emergency, this type of input into the initial best interests assessment is often unobtainable when the health team must make a quick decision. When patients are unconscious or incapable of communicating, it is reasonable to assume that most would want any intervention likely to save life or prevent disability, or that, if they hold strong objections to particular treatments, they will have taken steps to make that fact known in advance (see pages 540–1 on advance refusals).

Young and incapacitated children

With regard to immature or unconscious children, the health team must act in the child's best interests. Wherever possible, parents should be involved in decision making, but it is clearly important not to delay essential treatment. In the absence of a person with parental responsibility, any person who has care of the child, such as a grandparent or child minder, can do "what is reasonable in all the circumstances of the case for the purpose of safeguarding or promoting the child's welfare".[19] This is likely to include agreeing to treatment on the child's behalf unless the carer is aware that the parents would object. Ultimately, however, in an emergency situation, obtaining consent to proceed with essential treatment is not the most important issue. Even if families oppose treatment, it is lawful and ethically justifiable to administer lifesaving treatment to a child against his or her wishes if the situation is an emergency and any delay would lead to serious harm or even death. If time permits, however, attempts must be made to resolve the matter without overriding the family's wishes. Legal advice should be sought and the courts may need to be involved. Legal advice may also be needed in cases where the benefits and burdens of treatment are finely balanced and the family takes a view different to that of the health team.

Dilemmas in assessing patients' interests

A&E doctors are sometimes faced with very difficult dilemmas in attempting to assess patients' best interests. Withdrawal of futile treatment and decisions not to attempt cardiopulmonary resuscitation, for example, are discussed in Chapter 10.

Other examples of dilemmas include drug smugglers who may be brought to hospital by the police or customs officers. Some of these individuals are suspected of having concealed drugs, which may mean that they are at risk of harm if the packaging is flimsy, while others are likely to have ingested packets of drugs to avoid detection. In the latter case, the risk of toxicity is likely to be even higher. The BMA has well established policy on intimate body searches and says that they should normally be done by doctors only with the person's consent. (This is discussed in Chapter 17, page 640.) Nevertheless, cases may arise where the individual is losing or has lost capacity and doctors feel obliged to intervene to save the person's life or minimise harm.

Interventions not in patients' interests

Forensic testing of unconscious patients

Diagnostic testing in patients' interests is uncontentious, but decisions may also have to be made about whether other forms of testing should be allowed. In general, doctors may legally carry out on incompetent adults only procedures that are in their best interests or are, at least, not in any way contrary to their interests. Touching competent adults without their consent or incapacitated people against their own best interests may constitute a battery or assault (see Chapters 2 and 3). Therefore, wherever feasible, it is best to wait for an unconscious patient to recover consciousness and be able to give consent if this would not prejudice the reliability of tests that are not related to the patient's treatment.

When a fatality or serious crime has occurred and forensic information from an unconscious patient would probably provide vital clues, there may be strong public interest in carrying out such tests. If an unconscious patient has been a victim of crime, such as an assault or rape, it may also be what the patient would want. Although doctors must act in patients' best interests, such interests are not necessarily confined to purely medical matters. If, for example, a patient has been attacked, it could be argued that is it in the unconscious patient's interests (as well as the public interest) to identify the attacker. A common example in A&E departments concerns the taking of a blood sample from the patient prior to any transfusion in assault cases. If the patient was injured by an assailant who has traces of the patient's blood on his or her clothing, this can help to obtain a conviction. In such cases, blood needs to be obtained from the patient prior to transfusion because subsequent blood samples may contain DNA from a blood donor and the comparison with blood found on an alleged attacker may therefore be invalid. In these cases, delay in taking blood until the victim of the assault regains capacity to consent is not possible, but it is assumed that it is in that individual's interest to take steps to obtain evidence about the attacker. Where it is feasible to do so, it would be good practice to wait for the patient to regain consciousness prior to testing the blood, unless this jeopardises the chances of apprehending the assailant. Doctors should obviously object, however, if any proposal to take forensic samples could be harmful to the patient's care and treatment. Patients' clinical needs should be of paramount importance and doctors must err on the side of caution if they feel that any intervention is likely to jeopardise recovery.

The Association of Police Surgeons has issued guidance specifically on consent in relation to complaints of sexual assaults.[20] Regarding patients who lack capacity, it states that the forensic medical examiner should:

- inform the consultant responsible for the patient's care of the proposed examination and ensure that the consultant has no objections
- inform any contactable people close to the patient about the purpose of the proposed examination so that they can say whether the patient previously held strong views about such tests
- document such enquiries clearly in the patient's medical record
- ensure that the patient is informed about what has been done, and why, as soon as the patient has recovered sufficiently to understand.

Testing unconscious patients for blood alcohol levels

Legally, forensic samples cannot be taken from competent people against their will. Competent individuals' refusal to provide a specimen to the police must be respected, but if they are charged with a drink driving offence their refusal results in automatic conviction. Even if the court considers an individual not guilty of the driving offence, disqualification from driving normally follows refusal to provide a sample.

The possibility of taking and testing blood samples that may not be in an unconscious patient's interests, but could be in the public interest, was debated by the BMA for many years. Although in some cases, prompt testing of unconscious drivers who have been in accidents exonerates some of them from any blame, it is still a non-therapeutic act done without consent. In 2002, however, the Police Reform Act made such testing legal without consent in specific circumstances in England, Wales, and Scotland. (At the time of writing, Northern Ireland is also considering introducing such legislation.) The Act allows for a police constable to ask a doctor to take a specimen of blood from an incapacitated person who had been involved in a road traffic accident. Samples should not be taken by any doctor involved in the care of the patient, but rather by a police surgeon.

Taking blood specimens from unconscious drivers

A blood sample may be taken for future testing for alcohol or other drugs from a person who has been involved in an accident and is unable to give consent when:

- a police constable has assessed the person's capacity and found him or her to be incapable of giving valid consent for medical reasons
- the police surgeon taking the specimen is satisfied that the person is not able to give valid consent (for whatever reason)
- the person does not object to or resist the specimen being taken and
- in the view of the doctor in immediate charge of that patient's care, taking the specimen would not be prejudicial to the proper care and treatment of the patient.

The specimen taken must not be tested until the person regains competence and gives valid consent for it to be tested.

The BMA supported legislation to permit this, having adopted a policy in 2001 stating that "police surgeons should be legally empowered to take blood samples for testing for alcohol and drug levels without consent from a driver without capacity after a road traffic accident and that testing should occur later only with the consent of the driver".[21] This policy is based partly on public interest arguments and partly on the belief that patients should not be denied the opportunity for exoneration because they are unable to give valid consent.

Although it would be lawful for a police surgeon to take a blood sample in the circumstances covered by the Act, the police cannot require a doctor to take a specimen. Legally, doctors taking specimens can do so irrespective of the need for consent, as long as they believe that the patient lacks capacity to give valid consent. Clearly, any doctor involved in taking samples specifically for forensic use must be appropriately trained so that the sample is forensically useful. The BMA and the Association of Police Surgeons believe that doctors should not take samples if the patient refuses or resists and consider it ethically unacceptable to use force or restraint. It is also unlikely to be appropriate to take a specimen without consent if the person is expected to recover capacity within a very short period of time. The BMA and the Association of Police Surgeons have joint guidance for those involved in taking blood specimens from incapacitated drivers.[22]

Summary – determining best interests

- When they are mentally competent, patients are most suitably placed to judge their own best interests.
- Parents and proxy decision makers can make only those decisions that appear to promote the best interests of young children and incapacitated adults.
- Exceptionally, it may be possible to take forensic samples without consent when this is likely to be in the interests of justice and is not contrary to the interests of unconscious patients.
- After a road accident, best interests may not come into the discussion since the law allows some taking of samples from unconscious drivers in limited circumstances.

Recognition of the skills of all members of the team

Effective use of resources is an ethical issue and includes using appropriately the skills of all members of the healthcare team. In 2001 the Audit Commission criticised existing practice saying that more nurse practitioners should be treating and discharging patients without the need to involve doctors. Lack of recognition of their ability to treat patients was seen as "a missed opportunity given that 60% of patients attending A&E departments are not classified as urgent".[23] In particular, nurses specially trained to deal with children were seen as an important indicator of quality care. Just as team working has assumed greater importance in other spheres of medicine, similar developments have occurred in emergency care. Nurse practitioners play a growing role in treating patients rather than simply assessing them. Increasingly, they request diagnostic procedures, interpret results, give medication and discharge patients. Although consultants spend more time on the most complex cases, more responsibility is given to physiotherapists, radiographers, and paramedics to deal with straightforward cases. As in all other spheres of medicine, good communication and teamwork are vital. Effective teamwork recognises the skills of various professionals and encourages good communication between them. A&E departments particularly illustrate how beneficial this can be for patient care. More information about teamworking is provided in Chapter 19.

Challenging rigid professional roles

Experienced nurses in one trust were guiding senior house officers in the treatment of minor injuries, but their role expansion had not been formally recognised. Staff could see that there were problems with strict demarcation of roles and restricted boundaries of practice. A need was identified for developing autonomous practice consistent with ensuring patient safety. The minor injury nurse treatment service was established, whereby nurses could work at three levels, developing their skills within a competency framework and moving up the levels as their skills increased.

- Level 1 nurses work under the supervision of a level 2 or 3 practitioner and can initiate certain investigations.
- Level 2 nurses work with minimal supervision and peer support from a level 3 practitioner. They initiate and interpret some investigations, but do not refer or discharge patients.
- Level 3 are senior nurses working without direct supervision. They interpret the results of investigations, assimilate those into the overall clinical picture, and can treat and discharge patients.

The effect was to challenge the traditional role of emergency nurses, develop their skills, and improve patient flow.[24]

Samaritan acts

Emergency situations differ from normal practice, not only because the patient's choices and active involvement may be constrained but so are doctors' options. As a general principle, in an emergency, health professionals do not have the option of non-involvement and they may not have the choice of waiting for someone better qualified to handle the situation. The General Medical Council says that "in an emergency, wherever it may arise, you must offer anyone at risk the assistance you could reasonably be expected to provide".[25] Doctors who have a conscientious objection to abortion, for example, can generally opt out of participating except in an emergency when they must do what they can to assist the pregnant woman (see Chapter 7, pages 248–51).

The BMA is sometimes asked to clarify the duties of ordinary doctors in relation to volunteering help when off duty and outside the healthcare setting. For doctors not specialised in emergency care, there may be a difficult decision about whether to intervene at all in emergencies for which they are ill equipped. On the other hand, very basic but prompt measures taken on the spot can be life saving. Although many European countries have legislation requiring doctors to render emergency assistance, those in the UK do not have this legal obligation unless there is a pre-existing doctor–patient relationship[26] (see page 552). Nevertheless, the BMA's general advice is that doctors should be willing to identify themselves in such cases and offer help in a road traffic accident or aircraft emergency, for example. Doctors frequently worry, however, that they may exceed their competence and incur litigation if they embark upon an intervention outside their normal sphere of practice. Fear of liability has traditionally been cited as the common reason for doctors' reluctance to offer help in an in-flight emergency.[27] Generally, airlines are legally liable for any negligence or misconduct that occurs during an in-flight emergency. As far as can be ascertained, however, there is no evidence that litigation has ever been brought against a doctor who rendered assistance during such an emergency.[28]

When there is clearly likely to be a long delay in obtaining specialised help, immediate non-specialised medical assistance can make the difference between life and death. How much to intervene or whether to risk acting beyond one's competence must be considered within the context of the case. Doctors dealing with an aircraft emergency on a long flight are more likely to need to intervene to the very limits of their competence than a doctor coming across a traffic accident to which an ambulance is on its way. Doctors are normally advised to restrict themselves to interventions well within their competence. In an emergency far from a hospital, however, they may well be justified in going beyond what they would normally attempt as a last resort when no other help is at hand.

Advice from an indemnifying body

The fact that you are not a consultant in emergency medicine, have never been trained in advanced trauma life support (ALTS), and do not have a fully equipped crash trolley should not be a barrier to helping someone to the best of your ability. However, you should remember that whatever you do would be classed as a clinical intervention. You must therefore, record the name of the patient, make a clinical record of what you are doing and give your name and address to a suitable official such as a member of the aircraft cabin crew. Remember to take appropriate precautions with infectious diseases although advance airline permission may be required for doctors to take needles, syringes or other equipment for their use. Remember also the duty of confidentiality to patients, which continues beyond death, especially if there is media interest subsequently.[29]

Nevertheless, doctors seem increasingly reluctant to come forward in such situations. Many airlines have developed a form of telemedicine, whereby expert medical assistance is made continually available by telephone. Several companies provide continuous ground to air medical advice and employ doctors trained in emergency and aviation medicine.[30] Airline staff are trained to use the first aid equipment on board the aeroplane and can also follow instructions provided by the ground-based doctor. In-flight medical events are relatively common on some airlines (an American study,[31] for example, found a rate of 13 such events each day) but most are not serious. Nevertheless, serious cardiac, neurological, and respiratory emergencies do occasionally occur and these account for the majority of instances in which airlines have to make unscheduled landings.[32] There do not appear to be standard international guidelines on the management of in-flight medical events, but each airline has its own policy. The role of medical passengers who volunteer help is not to take sole control but to assist the flight crew, who remain responsible for the patient.

Even within hospital settings, critical situations can arise when doctors have to balance the likely harms and benefits and may need to act to the limits of their capacity and training rather than await a more specialised colleague. For example, career A&E doctors (as opposed to senior house officers) receive training in anaesthesia, but current practice in most A&E departments is for all anaesthetics to be provided by qualified anaesthetists or anaesthetists in training. Nevertheless, urgent situations can arise when an anaesthetist is unavailable and an A&E doctor has to weigh up the comparative risks of proceeding or delaying. There are also some situations in which a trained A&E doctor knows the procedure that is required, but has not actually carried it out previously. For example, if no more experienced practitioner is available, it may be necessary for someone who has never carried out an emergency thoracotomy to attempt it. Many A&E consultants have never done this procedure for penetrating chest trauma with recent cardiac arrest, but all should know the indications requiring it.

In addition, as doctors become more senior, working fewer clinical hours, their exposure to certain clinical techniques may decline, with consequent deskilling, and they need to decide whether to cease attempting a certain procedure at all. Ideally, general advice should be sought in advance of an emergency from colleagues and from trust lawyers. Conceivably, however, there may be rare occasions when they should attempt a procedure they rarely do if the choice is genuinely between that and risking serious harm to the patient through a delay in intervening. In all such cases, judging what is "reasonable" and most likely to preserve life or reduce harm needs to be considered on a case by case basis. Clearly, doctors should be well aware of their own limitations and never act beyond their competence if there is a viable alternative. The need for such emergency interventions should be audited and steps taken to minimise their occurrence. If inadvertent harm is caused to a patient by a doctor acting at the limits of his or her capacity, this should be discussed with the patient at the earliest appropriate opportunity.

In the event of an accident or terrorist act incurring multiple casualties, the medical team has a duty of care not only to the patients undergoing treatment but also to those as yet unassessed. It may well be more ethically correct to maximise the numbers assessed so that certain cases can be appropriately prioritised, rather than provide comprehensive treatment to only limited numbers.

Legal considerations

In some countries, and in some American states, there are "good Samaritan" or "failure to stop" laws obliging any passing health professional to offer assistance in an emergency. There are no parallel legal obligations in the UK, although doctors may be considered to have special obligations to people with whom they already have a therapeutic relationship. One of the anxieties experienced by doctors in such a situation is that they may incur liability if they intervene without improving the patient's situation or if they make it worse. In general terms, the law expects doctors to do what appears most reasonable in the circumstances and the Medical Defence Union says that "if you are trying to do the right thing by using your professional expertise to help a fellow human continue to live . . . the chances of you facing legal action are so low they are almost non-existent".[33] In respect of errors, "judges have recognised that in an emergency responsible professionals may be more prone to errors" and "the fact that a mistake is made should not lead lightly to a finding of negligence".[34] Such situations are said to reflect "battle conditions".[35] The BMA advises doctors who are frequent flyers and who are often asked to intervene to check their indemnity situation with their defence body. Most medical defence organisations offer policies covering good Samaritan acts anywhere in the world.[36]

Reimbursement

Although it is not strictly a matter of medical ethics, some doctors object to volunteering help for airline emergencies without some form of reimbursement because they sometimes feel that advantage has been taken by the airline. If no thorough checks are made prior to embarking sick passengers, the likelihood of an emergency is increased. Doctors can ask for payment, but none of the major airlines has a policy of hourly rates for good Samaritan acts, although some offer upgrades or free flight vouchers as tokens of gratitude. Some airlines have a clear policy not to offer payment in such circumstances.[37]

Summary – the duty to help

- Doctors are expected to give whatever assistance they can in an emergency.
- Doctors should not normally intervene beyond or at the limits of their competence, but in an emergency situation this may be the only alternative to permitting serious harm to occur.
- Such interventions in a hospital setting should only ever be exceptional. Audit and appropriate planning should ensure that they are not repeated.

Duties to families

In the hospital situation, teams working in emergency care often have to help relatives as well as patients. Care of people who have been suddenly bereaved is part of the responsibility of A&E departments, but it has not always received sufficient attention. The Royal College of Nursing and the British Association for Accident and Emergency Medicine conducted a study in 1995, which identified good initiatives in A&E departments to help people to cope with an unexpected bereavement.[38] Nevertheless, they also found that the high standards were not evenly distributed and many departments had no written policy. Detailed recommendations were set out in the report, which included checklists as an aid to audit and advice concerning relationships with parents after the death of a baby. Special arrangements for bereaved children after the sudden death of their parents are also covered.

Principles for bereavement care in A&E departments

The Royal College of Nursing and the British Association for Accident and Emergency Medicine point out that the quality of the initial care has major importance for families' experience of bereavement. Their principles of good practice include the following.

- There should be up to date written policies for bereavement care.
- Appropriately trained individuals should be specifically allocated to relatives to provide consistency and continuity.
- There should be follow up care.
- Staff should have good communication skills and information for relatives should be provided in appropriate languages.
- Relatives should have access to the deceased person as a matter of right. Their needs should be paramount.
- Caring for bereaved people is emotionally demanding. Staff should be trained for this and staff support should also be available.[39]

Asking families about research and education

One of the difficult issues that may have to be raised with the families of incapacitated people in the emergency care setting is that of the possible involvement of their loved one in research initiatives, innovative treatment, or medical education. All doctors have general obligations to maximise useful knowledge and make appropriate efforts to improve care. Treatment should be evidence based, but in emergency and acute care, there are few opportunities to carry out research on potential treatment options with properly informed patient consent. For example, it may be important to research different modes of cardiac compression to ascertain what is most effective in cardiac arrest or to compare different possible ways of attempting to resuscitate babies. To introduce changes in practice without evidence of efficacy and research data is likely to be unethical. These kinds of dilemmas are discussed in Chapter 14 on research and innovative treatment, where the importance is emphasised of involving patients or people close to them, wherever possible, in any discussion of experimental procedures. In particular, the parents of children must be involved in deciding whether they wish the child to be involved in any research or innovative treatment. In 2003 the Government issued its proposals for a system of proxy decision making throughout the UK on behalf of incapacitated people who may be involved in trials of medicinal products.[40] In its consultation document, it emphasised the importance of not unduly hampering the conduct of research in emergency situations, and suggested that research ethics committees could consider schemes for seeking authorisation on the patient's behalf from an appointed "legal representative" if people close to the patient were not contactable when the decision about participation in emergency care research had to be made (see Chapter 14, pages 509–10). Obviously, all research proposals in any context must be scrutinised in advance by an appropriately constituted research ethics committee.

As well as research and innovative treatment, another extremely sensitive issue that may need to be raised in the emergency care setting is the fact that medical education occurs there and needs support from patients and their relatives. Seeking consent for patient involvement in education is discussed in Chapter 18.

Asking families about organ and tissue donations

A difficult issue for relatives can be the question of organ and tissue donation when an unexpected death occurs, although in the long term many families derive comfort from the knowledge that other lives have been saved or transformed. In some cases there are good reasons for not raising the issue because, for example, the organs are likely to be unusable, but whenever donation is an option this should be raised with the family. General issues concerning organ donation and discussion with relatives are covered in Chapter 12 (pages 431–4).

Confidentiality and privacy

All patients are entitled to privacy and confidentiality of their personal health information, although this right is not an absolute one. (This is discussed in detail in Chapter 5.) Nevertheless, in an emergency people who are emotionally close to the patient expect to act as advocates and be consulted about decisions when time permits. Sharing general information with families should be with the patients' permission. In the case of incapacitated people, it is normally seen as in the patients' interest unless previously prohibited by them.

Information sharing in the healthcare team

Effective and prompt sharing of essential information is vital for assessment, diagnosis, and treatment in A&E departments. Good links with primary care services are obviously also important. Information obtained at each stage of the patient's transit through the system should be available to other professionals seeing that person, subject to patient consent and to the introduction of appropriate safeguards to preserve confidentiality. Nevertheless, safeguards to protect confidentiality are sometimes difficult to ensure. In an emergency where paramedics attend a patient who has previously been treated in hospital, they may want to advise the A&E staff to call up the individual's medical record urgently, so that it is available when the person reaches hospital. To do this, however, identifying information generally has to be passed by the insecure medium of the ambulance radio. Emergency frequencies are scanned by many people in the community and sometimes the medical condition of celebrities has been passed to the press in this way.[41] Clearly, however, the context of each case should be weighed up and a decision made about which would be likely to be the more serious harm. Avoidable delay in accessing vital information about the patient's past treatment and medication may be a more serious problem than the risks of a breach of confidentiality.

Confidentiality and disclosure to the police

A&E health teams are also often approached by the police and other authorities, such as the courts, about patients who have been treated after an assault or other violent incident, where there may be a strong public interest in ensuring that perpetrators are identified. Such requests should be directed to the consultant in charge of the patient's care, who should ascertain what kind of information is sought and why. Wherever possible consent should be sought prior to disclosure. When consent is refused, or it proves impossible to contact the patient concerned, doctors should consider their duty of confidentiality and disclose information only if there is an overriding public interest. If the injured person is a suspect hurt in the course of a serious crime, the public interest is likely to override the medical duty of confidentiality owed to that person. Further guidance on confidentiality and disclosure in the public interest is provided in Chapter 5 (pages 189–92).

In 2003 the Association of Chief Police Officers proposed a system whereby any patient admitted to hospital with a gunshot injury should be notified to the police in a non-identifiable way. The police would then visit the hospital and, if the injured person agreed, discuss the details of what had occurred. Both the BMA and the General Medical Council supported the proposal for automatic reporting of the fact of such an injury, but considered that the identity of the patient should be disclosed only when there is a public interest justification. An obvious example would be when a serious crime is suspected.

It is also likely that some patients attending A&E departments are illegal immigrants, who are seldom registered with primary care services. The BMA has firmly rejected any role of doctors in denouncing such patients to the authorities, while recognising that information about any patient should be shared when that person represents a clear threat of harm to other people.

Domestic violence

In 1998 the BMA issued advice concerning the management of the sequelae of domestic violence.[42] This noted that, in the UK, one in four women experience domestic violence at some stage in adult life and they are highly represented among A&E patients. There are also strong links between domestic violence and child protection issues. Traditionally, A&E staff believed that the high turnover of such patients and difficulties with follow up meant that any intervention with the patient would be unlikely to effect any change in the abusive situation. Nevertheless, studies have shown that the process of empowerment for many women is a gradual one, and over time health professionals can play an important role in reinforcing basic messages.[43] A vital first step is systematically to question patients who are likely to be in this category, including attempting to discover whether other people are at risk of harm. The fact that an adult may refuse to allow disclosure of information about an abuser does not mean that health professionals do not continue to have some duty to other vulnerable persons, such as children or elderly people, who may be caught up in an abusive situation.

Guidelines about domestic violence issued to UK A&E departments

- Examine injuries thoroughly, remembering that the presenting complaint may be only one part of the overall picture.
- Document injuries meticulously.
- Treat the injuries and ask the patient direct questions about them.
- Encourage the patient's own decision making.
- Discuss the next steps for the patient and offer contact numbers and written information about where further help is available.[44]

In many cases, it is counterproductive to attempt to force a patient to agree to disclosure of information about domestic violence to the police, a GP, or others who are in a position to help. Successful protocols to deal with such cases in A&E are being developed, however, which often involve a dedicated domestic violence team member to act as the patient's advocate and link to community and health services. Such protocols require advance planning and must be backed by an educational programme for health professionals, who must be encouraged to believe in the utility of their interventions.

Suspected child abuse or neglect

When children come into emergency care in situations in which non-accidental injury, other abuse, or neglect is suspected, a meticulous record must be made and as thorough an explanation as possible sought from carers. Competent children should be sensitively encouraged to talk through what has happened without the involvement or presence of accompanying persons. Specialist staff need to be involved at an early stage with a view to possibly initiating child protection procedures and interagency cooperation. Where any doubt exists about the safety of a child who is due to be discharged back to family care, specialist advice should be taken. Wherever possible, keeping families together is an important goal, but the safety of the child must be the paramount consideration. Child protection issues are discussed in more detail in Chapter 4 (pages 156–62).

Disclosure of information about patients

The general rules about disclosure are discussed in Chapter 5. Some categories of patients give rise to particular concern. For example, emergency staff often come into contact with patients who feign pain to obtain prescription medicine or narcotics under false pretences. They also see patients who suffer from Munchausen's disease and may embark on lengthy and expensive diagnostic and treatment initiatives for them. Once identified by one emergency team, the question sometimes arises about whether identifying information can be passed to other hospitals in the locality where the same patient is likely to present. Arguably, it is in the public interest that abuse or fraudulent use of the system be addressed, even at the cost of the individual's confidentiality. As a general principle, the BMA has recommended that patients be told in advance of disclosure. In addition, general notices about such information sharing should be displayed in hospital facilities, so that everyone is aware that attempts to obtain drugs or unnecessary treatment will be made known to other medical facilities in the area.

Privacy and witnessed resuscitation

This section considers patients' rights to privacy and the wishes of other people to be present when resuscitation is attempted. We focus primarily on people who are emotionally close to the patient, but health professionals in training may also want to observe the process as part of their own education. When they are part of the team that is attempting to assist the patient, they have a right to be present, but if people are in attendance simply to observe and learn, patients or their families need to be aware of this and have an opportunity to say if they have any objections.

The BMA is sometimes asked about its views on whether people who are emotionally close to the patient should be invited to remain in the room when resuscitation is attempted in hospitals. This is not an issue upon which the Association has a firm policy, neither does there seem to be a consensus within the profession, but some general factors for consideration can be set out.

Privacy and witnessed resuscitation

The following factors should be considered:

- whether additional people in the vicinity would hamper the resuscitation efforts
- whether their presence would be what the patient would have wanted
- whether witnessing a resuscitation attempt is likely to have a bad effect on the witnesses or leave them with very disturbing memories
- whether being present would reassure them that everything possible has been attempted
- whether the family needs to express emotions physically or vocally at such a time and, if so, whether this can be accommodated in a manner that does not distract the resuscitation team
- whether there are appropriately trained staff available to concentrate just on looking after relatives
- whether there is time to provide a proper explanation and choice for those who may want to be present.

If having additional people present would hamper the patient's treatment, or would be contrary to the patient's known wishes, then clearly families should be excluded.

In cases of terminal illness, it is common for family members to stay with their loved one at the end of that person's life, but this has not generally been the case when patients die in A&E departments during attempted cardiopulmonary resuscitation. A 1995 study found that, in a sample of A&E departments, less than a quarter allowed families unrestricted access to the room during attempted resuscitation, and 60% allowed relatives in once the resuscitation attempts had ceased.[45] Generally, health professionals seem to have little objection to bringing in people who are close to the patient once resuscitation efforts are being scaled down, either because the process has been unsuccessful or when the patient appears to have survived the worst. Health professionals have concerns, however, if family members are exposed, without appropriate preparation and support, to the team's efforts to revive a patient.

A report by the UK Resuscitation Council, however, found that the majority of relatives or friends of deceased people who had been present during attempts to resuscitate their loved one preferred to be there and believed that it helped in coping with their bereavement when the patient died.[46] Some saw it as a last opportunity to communicate and be heard by the dying person, and thought that it was important both for the patient and themselves to be together in the final moments. The Council also cited anecdotal evidence that the presence of a loved one could be beneficial to some patients with fleeting consciousness, increasing their will to live. It noted that patients undergoing resuscitation after cardiac arrest may retain some awareness. The report concluded that attitudes about the presence of families were changing and that "for many relatives it is more distressing to be separated from their loved one during these critical moments than to witness attempts at resuscitation".[47] The positive benefits were especially felt by younger adults (under the age of 40).

The BMA has had concerns about relatives *automatically* being invited to witness resuscitation or, indeed, allowed to attend other medical procedures, such as surgery. Part of its concern is that, unless thorough preparations have been made in advance, the presence of relatives could jeopardise the chances of successful resuscitation. Relatives' distress could distract or hinder the health professionals providing resuscitation and make the situation more stressful for the healthcare team. Clinicians occasionally cite examples of large groups of family members crowding into the room, or very emotional relatives throwing themselves on to patients and inadvertently hampering efforts at defibrillation.[48] There is also concern that the presence of relatives could have an influence on the decision to stop resuscitation at times when the health team believe it to be in the patient's interest to continue. Conversely, the family may try to insist on resuscitation being continued beyond the point at which it has become futile. On the other hand, many of these concerns could be addressed by thorough preplanning, appropriate safeguards, and prior explanation to the family members if time and staffing levels permit. Where known, the patient's own wishes are important factors to consider. It may be completely appropriate, for example, for parents to be with an injured child and they may experience feelings of guilt or of having failed their child if they are excluded. If families are invited to witness resuscitation, however, appropriate support and supervision to prevent interference with the procedure are needed. They should be given information about what to expect and also have an opportunity to leave with dignity if they feel that they cannot cope. Staff also need appropriate training and additional support themselves because witnessed resuscitation is likely to impose additional stress for them, at least initially. Guidance should make clear to the health staff what relatives must be told in advance.

Summary of Resuscitation Council guidance

- Acknowledge the difficulty of the situation. Ensure that relatives understand that they do not have to be present and should not feel guilty about declining.
- Relatives should be accompanied by staff to care specifically for them and should know who these staff are. They should be introduced and know each other's names.
- Relatives should be given a clear explanation of what to expect to see, the nature of the illness or injury, and the procedures they will witness.
- They should know that they can leave the room and will be accompanied.
- Relatives should be aware that they cannot intervene or touch the patient until they are told this is safe. They should be given opportunities to touch the patient when it is safe to do so.

(Continued)

- Procedures should be explained to relatives as they occur. This includes telling them when resuscitation is not succeeding and will be abandoned, and when the patient has died.
- They should be advised that, when the person has died, there may be an interval during which the equipment is removed, after which they can have time alone with the deceased person. They need to know if the coroner is likely to require certain tubes to be left in place.
- Relatives should be offered time to think about the situation and ask questions.[49]

In addition to providing general guidance for witnessed resuscitation in the hospital setting, the Resuscitation Council's report also gives brief guidelines on the presence of relatives when resuscitation is attempted in the field by paramedics.

Although the Resuscitation Council took a very positive approach to witnessed resuscitation and felt that professional reservations were diminishing, it also noted that many health professionals still had anxieties about it. A subsequent pilot study at Addenbrooke's Hospital in 1997 found significant support from relatives, no reported adverse psychological effects among those who witnessed a relative's resuscitation, and strong support from staff.[50] In fact, the trial had to be terminated early as the clinical team became so convinced of the benefits of allowing relatives to be present that there was no point in continuing the experiment. Subsequently, nurses have argued that relatives should be allowed to choose whether or not they want to watch the resuscitation process. The issue was debated at the 2000 Congress of the Royal College of Nursing, where there was overwhelming support for relatives being present. The College published detailed guidance on the subject in 2002, which also included a model hospital policy for witnessed resuscitation.[51] The College thought that, among other benefits, witnessed resuscitation was likely to reduce complaints from relatives and lawsuits because families would see for themselves that all reasonable steps had been taken.

Privacy after death

The medical duty of confidentiality extends beyond the death of the patient, but this must be balanced with other moral imperatives. Relatives and people who are close to the deceased patient want information and reassurance about what has occurred, and need to be consulted about procedures such as postmortem examinations. These issues are discussed in detail in Chapter 12.

Summary – confidentiality and privacy

- As in other spheres of treatment, patients have a right of confidentiality but this is not absolute.
- People close to the patient expect to be involved in receiving information as long as the patient has not expressed an objection.

- The interests of justice may require disclosure contrary to the patient's wishes.
- Disclosures without consent should be within an agreed framework.
- Decisions about disclosures to the police without patient consent should be discussed by senior doctors and senior police officers.

General issues in immediate and prehospital care

In this final section, the focus is on issues likely to arise outside the hospital setting. Prehospital emergency care in the UK developed after a major rail disaster at Harrow station in the early 1950s drew attention to the field hospital techniques used by American military medical units. Such units based nearby attended the crash and provided stabilising care *in situ* to crash victims. Immediate and prehospital care then developed significantly as a specialist area of medicine from the 1970s. The British Association for Intermediate Care (BASICS), established in 1977, continues as a voluntary organisation, providing volunteer medical help. BASICS doctors often work with prehospital paramedic teams and can make critical on the spot decisions to assist paramedics who have to work strictly to protocols. In the past, perceived role divisions sometimes hampered cooperative work between doctors and paramedic teams, or between volunteers and professionals. Part of the important contribution of BASICS has been to foster good teamwork across such barriers.

Triage

Triage is essential when there are multiple casualties and may occur both at the scene of a disaster and in the A&E department. Medical assessment and pain relief are vital for all the injured, but most attention has to be centred on those with the best chance of survival and recovery. Therefore, in disasters, the commonsense rule of triage is to attend to people whose condition does not appear to be fatal but requires immediate attention, without which they will deteriorate seriously. The most severely injured people may simply be made as comfortable as possible but left untreated if their care would mean that people with better chances of recovery are left to deteriorate. Utilitarian considerations about saving the greatest number tend to come to the fore rather than focusing on doing the best for a particular individual.

Teamwork

Mobile specialist care is delivered in various ways, ranging from a motorcycle paramedic to a mobile coronary unit or helicopter emergency team. It can be provided by a single emergency expert or a team including appropriately trained technicians. Paramedics play an ever growing role in emergency care and are increasingly developing their own codes of ethics that reflect changing practice. In the past, paramedics and ambulance staff were expected to work to fairly inflexible guidelines in which all decision making was left with doctors. In the 1980s and 1990s, the BMA received queries, for example, from ambulance staff who had been instructed always to attempt resuscitation unless directly instructed to the contrary by a doctor, generally a GP. This caused dilemmas when they were faced by patients who collapsed at home having clearly made an advance refusal of such treatment, but when the GP was not immediately contactable. In such cases, a lack of preparation for such eventualities meant that emergency workers were caught in the middle between relatives supporting non-resuscitation on the basis of an advance directive and rules requiring a doctor to make a judgment. Gradually, however, more attention has been given to the need for emergency workers, like all other health professionals, to take account of patient autonomy and abide by evidence of patients' refusals of treatment. Although bound by certain widely agreed protocols, emergency healthcare workers are independently responsible for decision making within their sphere of competence.

Ambulance paramedics have extended training in advanced life support skills. Despite this, there are some procedures and emergency decisions that protocols decree should be undertaken only by doctors. Dilemmas can arise, however, if no doctor is immediately available and another health professional is faced with the choice of breaching protocols and attempting a procedure normally outside his or her competence or risking the patient's death. Paramedics' training should prepare them for such dilemmas before they arise.

Dealing with stress and trauma

A difference between emergency medicine and most other spheres of treatment concerns the impact on the health professionals involved. All medicine requires health staff to deal with tragedy and grief in some form, but emergency care at a disaster site, such as a major crash or bombing, can be particularly dangerous and traumatic. The risks of post-traumatic stress disorder for health staff after major disasters have to be taken into account and plans devised. Emergency care can involve exposure to sudden large numbers of deaths, horrific injuries, and mutilation, the effects of which can be extremely stressful for health professionals. Immediate care doctors and hospital emergency departments also have a duty to deal with the suddenly bereaved relatives of patients who do not survive. The option for health staff to obtain support and counselling without adverse career implications is essential. Some of the effects of persistent stress on doctors are discussed further in Chapter 21.

Summary – care at disaster sites

- In emergency settings, doctors may have to make difficult decisions about which patients to treat first.
- They have duties to those awaiting assessment as well as those for whom treatment has begun.

- Effective teamwork is essential.
- Health professionals also need to bear in mind their own need for support in order to continue providing care effectively.

References

1 Kay R, Siriwardena AK. The process of informed consent for urgent abdominal surgery. *J Med Ethics* 2001;**27**:157–61.
2 Cooke MW. *Churchill's pocket book of pre-hospital care.* Edinburgh: Churchill Livingstone, 1999.
3 Lloyd T. *Men's Health Forum briefing paper: young men and suicide.* London: Men's Health Forum, 2000.
4 Hawton K, Fagg J. Deliberate self-poisoning and self-injury in adolescents: a study of characteristics and trends in Oxford, 1976–1990. *Br J Psychiatry* 1992;**161**:816–23.
5 Lloyd T. *Men's Health Forum briefing paper: young men and suicide. Op cit:* p. 5.
6 Hassan TB, MacNamara AF, Davy A, Bing A, Bodiwala GG. Managing patients with deliberate self harm who refuse treatment in accident and emergency departments. *BMJ* 1999;**319**:107–9.
7 Department of Health. *The health of the nation: a strategy for health in England.* London: HMSO, 1992.
8 Department of Health. *Saving lives: our healthier nation.* London: DoH, 1999.
9 Department of Health. *Mental health – national service frameworks.* London: Department of Health, 1999.
10 *Ibid:* p. 80.
11 *Ibid:* p. 78.
12 Scottish Executive. *Health in Scotland 2001.* Edinburgh: SE, 2001:45.
13 Re W (adult: refusal of treatment) [2002] EWHC 901 (Fam).
14 See, for example: Emergency Services Collaborative. *Improvement in emergency care: case studies.* London: NHS Modernisation Agency, 2002.
15 *Ibid.*
16 Department of Health. *Reforming emergency care: practical steps.* London: DoH, 2001.
17 Audit Commission. *Accident and emergency: review of national findings.* London: Audit Commission, 2001.
18 Re E (a minor) (wardship: medical treatment) [1993] 1 FLR 386.
19 Children Act 1989 s3(5). The Children (Northern Ireland) Order 1995 art 5(8). Children (Scotland) Act 1995 s5(1).
20 Association of Police Surgeons. *Consent in relation to complainants of sexual assault.* Harrogate: Association of Police Surgeons, 2001:2–3.
21 British Medical Association Annual Representative Meeting, 2001.
22 British Medical Association, Association of Police Surgeons. *Taking blood specimens from incapacitated drivers: guidance for doctors on the provisions of the Police Reform Act 2002 from the British Medical Association and Association of Police Surgeons.* London: BMA, 2002.
23 Audit Commission. *Accident and emergency: review of national findings. Op cit:* p. 12.
24 Emergency Services Collaborative. *Improvement in emergency care: case studies. Op cit:* case study 1c.
25 General Medical Council. *Good medical practice.* London: GMC, 2001: para 9.
26 Genreau MA, DeJohn C. Responding to medical events during commercial airline flights. *N Engl J Med* 2003;**346**:1067–73.
27 Rayman RB. Inflight medical kits. *Aviat Space Environ Med* 1998;**69**:1007–10.
28 Genreau MA, *et al.* Responding to medical events during commercial airline flights. *Op cit:* p. 1070.
29 Kirkpatrick A. Good Samaritan acts. *BMJ* 2002;**324**:S29.
30 Genreau MA, *et al.* Responding to medical events during commercial airline flights. *Op cit.*
31 DeJohn CA, Véronneau SJ, Wolbrink AM, Larcher JG, Smith DW, Garrett J. *The evaluation of in-flight medical care aboard selected US air carriers: 1996 to 1997.* Washington DC: Federal Aviation Administration, Office of Aviation Medicine, 2000. (Technical report DOT/FAA/AM-0013.)
32 Genreau MA, *et al.* Responding to medical events during commercial airline flights. *Op cit:* p. 1067.
33 Kirkpatrick A. Good Samaritan acts. *Op cit:* p. S29.
34 Montgomery J. *Health care law, 2nd ed.* New York: Oxford University Press, 2002:179–80.
35 Wilsher v Essex AHA [1986] 3 All ER 801: 812.
36 Kirkpatrick A. Good Samaritan acts. *Op cit.*
37 Dyer C. Doctor demands payment for helping airline passenger. *BMJ* 1998;**317**:701.
38 British Association for Accident and Emergency Medicine, Royal College of Nursing. *Bereavement care in A&E departments.* London: RCN, 1995.
39 *Ibid:* p. 1.

40 Department of Health. *Consultation on the draft guidance on consent by a legal representative on behalf of a person not able to consent under the Medicines for Human Use (Clinical Trials) Regulations 2003.* London: DoH, 2003.

41 Gorovitz S. Suicide. In: Iserson K, Sanders A, Matthieu D, eds. *Ethics in emergency medicine.* Tucson, AZ: Galen Press, 1995.

42 British Medical Association. *Domestic violence: a health care issue?* London: BMA, 1998.

43 Stevens KLH. The role of the accident and emergency department. In: Bewley S, Friend J, Mezey G, eds. *Violence against women.* London: RCOG Press, 1997.

44 British Association of Accident and Emergency Medicine. *Domestic violence: recognition and management in accident and emergency.* London: Royal College of Surgeons, 1994.

45 British Association for Accident and Emergency Medicine, Royal College of Nursing. *Bereavement care in A & E departments. Op cit.*

46 Resuscitation Council (UK). *Should relatives witness resuscitation?* London: Resuscitation Council (UK), 1996:5.

47 *Ibid:* p. 6.

48 Womersley T. Let families view resuscitation, say casualty nurses. *Daily Telegraph*, 2000 Apr 7.

49 Resuscitation Council (UK). *Should relatives witness resuscitation? Op cit:* p. 9.

50 Robinson SM, Mackenzie-Ross S, Campbell Hewson GL, Egleston CV, Prevost AT. Psychological effect of witnessed resuscitation on bereaved relatives. *Lancet* 1998;**352**:614–17.

51 Royal College of Nursing. *Witnessing resuscitation: guidance for nursing staff.* London: RCN, 2002.

16: Doctors with dual obligations

The questions covered in this chapter include the following.

- How does the nature of the doctor–patient relationship change when doctors have contractual obligations to third parties?
- What rights of confidentiality do patients have when reports are being written about them by independent medical examiners?
- Should doctors act as referees for firearms licences?
- Can information about genetic tests be put into medical reports for third parties?
- How do occupational physicians balance their duty of confidentiality to their patients with their obligations to management?
- What duties of confidentiality do sports doctors owe to players and athletes?

When do dual obligations arise?

Much of medical practice is concerned with the direct relationship between doctors and patients (see Chapter 1) and, although the impact of decisions on others is important, there are only two main parties to the relationship. This chapter concerns situations in which there is a third party, which may be an insurer or employer to whom the doctor has contractual responsibilities, or a court for which a doctor is acting as a witness. Obligations to third parties may be express or implied, real or perceived. The common factor is that the doctor–patient relationship cannot be reduced to the usual model of a therapeutic partnership and this has implications for both the doctor and the patient. (Doctors who have dual obligations as a result of working in custodial settings are dealt with separately in Chapter 17.)

Implications of having dual obligations

Traditionally, codes of medical ethics have centred on the notion that a doctor's primary loyalty is to the welfare of the patient. International codes such as the World Medical Association's Declaration of Geneva (the modern restatement of the Hippocratic Oath) emphasise that the health of the patient must be a doctor's first consideration.[1] Whereas all doctors have multiple professional loyalties, such as those to colleagues, health service employers, and society at large, these are generally in the background. The duties at the forefront of doctors' concern are normally those owed to individual patients. When loyalties conflict, doctors have to be prepared to support their patients by, for example, reporting poor practice by colleagues or employers that has put their patients at risk (see Chapter 21).

In the doctor–patient relationship, decision making is usually a joint process, with the patient's health and wellbeing as the primary concern. In the situations covered in this chapter, however, the welfare of individual patients may not be the main focus, although all doctors have some responsibility for the people they see or advise professionally. Dual obligations are a live issue in any debate about civil and political rights since it is generally assumed that doctors with pronounced dual obligations are at risk of subordinating the rights of patients to other interests. Although this is particularly true for doctors working in custodial settings (see Chapter 17), it is also true of occupational health physicians whose responsibilities are divided between protecting the health of workers and advising management on all aspects of occupational health.[2]

Many of the issues covered in this chapter are drawn from the cases that doctors bring to the BMA for advice. Although doctors in these situations recognise that they may have some therapeutic role, they also acknowledge that they have a strong obligation to another party or a wider population, such as an employer, insurer, or court of law. In many cases, this duty to another may appear to come into conflict with the patient's usual rights, particularly the right to confidentiality. In these circumstances, doctors often feel that their responsibilities towards the patient are vague and unspecified, while their duties to their employer or the body paying for the medical report are more clearly defined. There is also a risk that they will assimilate the norms and values of the third party rather than acting in accordance with their professional standards. A central argument in this chapter is that, although doctors may be acting outside the normal therapeutic relationship, the usual ethical standards still apply. In particular, they have a duty to inform their patients of the nature of their obligations to any third party and the impact of those obligations on the patient.

Circumstances in which dual obligations arise

This chapter focuses on three areas. Within each there are a number of different examples:

- **Doctors providing medical reports for third parties:** Doctors write medical reports for the immigration service, employers, insurers, the courts, and others. A common factor is that the medical report serves a purpose other than facilitating treatment. Reports for third parties are often carried out by a patient's own GP, although sometimes an independent expert is commissioned to examine a patient and write a report.
- **Doctors who are employed by third parties:** This includes occupational physicians, doctors in the armed forces, and sports doctors employed by, for example, professional football clubs.
- **Doctors whose job does not focus on individual patients:** In this final category we consider the work of doctors in the media and those with business interests.

Public health physicians are covered separately in Chapter 20. Doctors working in custodial settings are the subject of Chapter 17.

General principles

The following principles should inform doctors' actions where they have dual obligations.

- Doctors acting for a third party must ensure that the patient understands that fact, and its implications.
- Doctors appointed and paid by a third party still have a duty of care to the patient whom they advise, examine or treat, and must abide by professional guidelines on ethics and law.
- Medical reports must be objective and impartial.
- Consent is as important as it is in other areas of medical practice.
- Doctors have a duty of confidentiality, and information should not normally be disclosed without the patient's knowledge and consent.
- Doctors have a duty to monitor and speak out when services with which they are concerned are inadequate, hazardous, or otherwise pose a potential threat to health.

Providing reports for third parties

This section outlines some general points that are common to all situations in which doctors write reports for non-medical purposes. Specific advice about the most common areas can be found on pages 570–86.

When doctors are called upon to write medical reports, they should ensure that they are factual, detailed, and carefully worded, avoiding assertions that cannot be defended. They should also bear in mind who will be reading the report. Responsibility for assessing medical reports for insurance rests with the insurance company's chief medical officer. In contrast, medicolegal reports are mainly read by non-medical officials, so abstruse medical terms should be avoided or, if they must be used, they should be defined.

Confidentiality

All the health information that doctors obtain about identifiable individuals and which they learn in a professional capacity is subject to the duty of confidentiality. It follows that all doctors who write reports about patients need consent for the report to be released. They should be prepared to discuss the contents of reports with patients, and be aware of patients' statutory rights of access to reports (see Chapter 6, pages 216–22).

General Medical Council (GMC) advice on confidentiality and medical reports

"If you are asked to write a report about and/or examine a patient, or to disclose information from existing records for a third party to whom you have contractual obligations, you must:

a. Be satisfied that the patient has been told at the earliest opportunity about the purpose of the examination and/or disclosure, the extent of the information to be disclosed and the fact that relevant information cannot be concealed or withheld. You might wish to show the form to the patient before you complete it to ensure the patient understands the scope of the information requested.
b. Obtain, or have seen, written consent to the disclosure from the patient or a person properly authorised to act on the patient's behalf. You may, however, accept written assurances from an officer of a government department that the patient's written consent has been given.
c. Disclose only information relevant to the request for disclosure: accordingly, you should not usually disclose the whole record. The full record may be relevant to some benefits paid by government departments.
d. Include only factual information you can substantiate, presented in an unbiased manner.
e. The Access to Medical Reports Act 1988 entitles patients to see reports written about them before they are disclosed, in some circumstances. In all circumstances you should check whether patients wish to see their report, unless patients have clearly and specifically stated that they do not wish to do so.

Disclosures without consent to employers, insurance companies, or any other third party, can be justified only in exceptional circumstances, for example, when they are necessary to protect others from risk of death or serious harm".[3]

Doctors who are writing independent reports sometimes think that the very fact that a patient has cooperated with an examination, and volunteered information about health, means that the patient gives consent for the disclosure of information. This does not automatically follow, and doctors should ensure that they have written consent to disclosure once the examination is completed.

Breach of confidentiality for disclosure of a report

Pamela Cornelius was a schoolteacher who felt that her mental health was being affected by difficulties that the school was suffering, which she blamed on the head teacher. She was considering resigning and bringing a claim for constructive dismissal, and therefore approached a solicitor.

Her solicitor advised that they should seek a report from a consultant psychiatrist to ascertain whether Mrs Cornelius's health problems could

(Continued)

properly be attributed to her conditions of employment. Dr Taranto was commissioned to write a report.

Mrs Cornelius was seen by Dr Taranto, and a report prepared. Dr Taranto wanted to refer Mrs Cornelius to a consultant psychiatrist, and claimed in court that she had consented to do so. As part of the referral, she sent a copy of the report to a psychiatrist and Mrs Cornelius's GP.

Mrs Cornelius claimed that she had neither given consent for the referral to be made, nor for the report to be sent to a psychiatrist or her GP. As such, her confidentiality had been breached. Dr Taranto, on the other hand, argued that Mrs Cornelius had agreed to being referred for treatment and that sending the report to the other doctors was a consequence of that. The medical records showed no note of a discussion about consent for the referral or disclosure of the report.

The judge in the Court of Appeal upheld Mrs Cornelius's claim and said that her express consent for the report's transmission to a third party was necessary, even if she had agreed to the referral.

Pamela Cornelius v Dr Nicola de Taranto[4]

Access to reports

The BMA strongly supports openness between doctors and patients, and encourages doctors to share the reports they write with patients whenever possible. Reports written for insurance or employment purposes by a doctor with whom the patient already has a therapeutic relationship are covered by the Access to Medical Reports Act 1988 and Access to Medical Reports (Northern Ireland) Order 1991. The legislation gives specific rights to be informed when a report is sought, to be offered the opportunity to see the report before it is sent, and to have any inaccuracies amended. Detailed advice is given in Chapter 6 (page 221).

In addition, all health records, including, in the BMA's view, reports written by independent medical examiners, are covered by the subject access provisions of data protection legislation. Detailed advice is given in Chapter 6 (page 221).

Impartiality

Doctors must do their best to avoid being influenced by the requirements of a third party who is commissioning a report or by sympathies they may have for the individual being examined. They should not be drawn into speculation if asked, for example, to offer an expert opinion on insufficient or flawed evidence, or on something outside their area of expertise. In such cases, it is important to state clearly either the limits of what can be deduced or the extent of the doctor's expertise.

Impartiality can be a particular issue for doctors, such as GPs, who have developed a professional relationship with a patient over a period of time, and who see their role as the patient's advocate. It is important therefore that doctors who have a prior relationship with a patient and are called upon to provide a report relating to that patient should ensure that the nature of the relationship and of the doctor's interest is explained to all relevant parties.

Patients, or the person commissioning the report, sometimes try to persuade doctors to change a report to make it more favourable from their perspective. Although factual errors can, and should, be corrected, this pressure must obviously be resisted.

GMC advice on report writing

"You must be honest and trustworthy when writing reports, completing or signing forms, or providing evidence in litigation or other formal inquiries. This means that you must take reasonable steps to verify any statement before you sign a document. You must not write or sign documents which are false or misleading because they omit relevant information. If you have agreed to prepare a report, complete or sign a document or provide evidence, you must do so without unreasonable delay".[5]

Medical reports for insurance

One of the most common situations in which doctors have a duty to another party is when they are completing medical reports about patients who want to buy insurance cover. Patients are under no obligation to accept either an examination or the release of personal medical information, although financial constraints do put pressure on patients to agree to examination and disclosure. There is, however, little that doctors can do in such situations after impartially counselling the patient. Ultimately it is for the patient to decide whether or not to accept the terms laid down by the insurance company or to consider other alternatives. Detailed advice about the use of medical information in insurance can be found in joint guidance from the BMA and the Association of British Insurers (ABI).[6] The release of information about deceased patients to insurance companies is covered on pages 220–1.

How is medical information for insurance collected?

Insurance companies gain information about their applicants' health in a number of ways. The most common is direct from the applicant. Applicants have a legal duty to reveal all information that is material to the insurer's actuarial decisions, whether or not it is specifically requested. Failure to do so could invalidate a policy.

Where more detailed information is needed, insurers sometimes seek a report from the applicant's GP (see page 571) or an independent medical examiner (see pages 571–2). Occasionally, applicants are asked to have specific tests, for example for HIV. Doctors' responsibilities in all these situations are to ensure that they have consent from the applicant and to respond truthfully to the questions they are asked. Their role is to provide factual information about the applicant's health. Doctors should not express opinions about whether an applicant's condition merits the application of a "normal" or "increased" rate of insurance. If they are asked questions that are inappropriate for them to answer, they should indicate this on the form.

General practitioner reports

Insurance companies generally prefer to ask the applicant's GP to write a report based on the medical notes rather than arrange an independent examination. A GP is likely to be able to provide an overall picture of the applicant's health instead of just the snapshot seen by an independent examiner. A GP's report (GPR) can, for example, validate the information that the applicant has provided or clarify whether an applicant's condition is being controlled. Some applicants also prefer this option as it may be more convenient than having an independent examination.

Some GPs have expressed concerns about this process as they believe that it endangers the open, trusting nature of the doctor–patient relationship. There is anecdotal evidence to suggest that some patients do not share information with their GP or avoid going to their GP for advice or treatment because they think the information will not be kept confidential. They may believe that it will jeopardise their chances of obtaining insurance at standard rates or of obtaining insurance cover at all. The BMA is concerned about the effects on the health of individuals and the public of information being withheld from doctors who are providing care. The scale of this problem is not known, but the BMA believes that it is an issue that must be addressed, and that it would be helpful if insurance companies offered applicants a choice between GPR and an independent examination.

BMA policy states that doctors should refuse to complete insurance reports about their patients unless a copy of the applicant's written consent has been provided for the doctor's retention. The consent form should make it clear that the applicant understands the nature and purpose of the report and any examination, and to whom information will be disclosed. Doctors should rely on an electronic copy of the applicant's signed consent form only if they are satisfied that the company has in place robust mechanisms for verifying that the document has not been altered in any way.

At the time of writing, an electronic GPR was being developed, the "e-GPR", which would compile and send medical reports from the doctor's existing electronic medical records without revealing information that is not relevant to the insurance application. Exactly as with the paper system, doctors must check the report and edit it, and give patients the opportunity to see it before it is sent.

Legal rules governing the sending of medical reports to insurers give patients rights of access to them. These are covered in detail in Chapter 6 (page 221).

Independent medical reports

Instead of seeking a GPR, or sometimes as well as, insurance companies may ask applicants to be seen and examined by an independent doctor. Doctors undertaking these examinations must be satisfied that the company has explained the nature and purpose of the examination, together with the necessary practical details. The examining doctor also has responsibilities to ensure that the applicant gives valid consent to the examination, and understands the nature and implications of any tests involved. Consent is also needed before information about the applicant may be disclosed to the insurance company.

Occasions arise where the examining doctor detects some significant abnormality or other feature of the applicant's health that requires investigation or treatment, and of which the applicant may not be aware. In such cases, the examining doctor has an ethical responsibility to ensure that either the applicant or, with the applicant's consent, his or her GP, is informed. The examining doctor should undertake this task. Examining doctors may find it helpful to ascertain the applicant's views on disclosure to the GP before the examination, and to obtain permission to liaise with the GP, should the need arise.

Rights of access to independent medical reports are discussed in Chapter 6 (page 221).

Consent for disclosure

Doctors' professional, ethical, and legal duties require them not to disclose information about patients without their consent. This is true in all but the most exceptional of circumstances (see Chapter 5).

When seeking a medical report, the insurance company or agent is responsible for ensuring that the consent is competently given and is based on a full understanding of the request. There is anecdotal evidence that, in the past, the subjects of GPRs have not always been aware of the extent of the information that is requested. At the time of writing, the BMA and the ABI are working on ways to improve the consent process. A useful step would be to provide applicants with a copy of the questions the doctor will be asked, with time allowed for the information to be read and understood before consent is given.

If doctors are in any doubt about whether valid consent has been given, they should check with the applicant. The GMC requires doctors to:

> Be satisfied that the patient has been told at the earliest opportunity about the purpose of the examination and/or disclosure, the extent of the information to be disclosed and the fact that relevant information cannot be concealed or withheld. You might wish to show the form to the patient before you complete it to ensure the patient understands the scope of the information requested. [7]

Content of reports

There are some restrictions on the use of medical information in insurance. Data protection legislation prohibits insurers from having more information about applicants than is relevant for the insurance product being sought. The doctor therefore needs to be aware of what the product is, and what information is relevant to it, before completing a report. A brief explanation of different insurance products, and the information insurers need in relation to each, is given in joint guidance from the BMA and ABI.[8]

The sections that follow highlight some specific areas where special rules apply.

Sexually transmitted infections

The possibility that information about sexually transmitted infections (STIs) will be revealed to another party, such as an insurance company, discourages some people from approaching their GP about this aspect of their health. The problem of information being withheld from the GP is particularly pronounced in this area because genitourinary medicine is a field of specialist medical care that patients can access without a referral from their GP. Anecdotal evidence suggests that patients sometimes seek services direct from genitourinary medicine clinics because they prefer to retain their anonymity, or in order to conceal from their GP information that they believe may affect their chance of obtaining insurance at the standard rate, or of obtaining it at all. Some doctors clearly believe that the insurance issue puts people off seeking advice about and testing for HIV.[9]

The BMA is concerned about the health implications of patients not seeking advice and testing for HIV and other STIs, and of patients' refusal to allow their GPs to be kept informed about certain aspects of their health care. In 2002 the BMA and the ABI agreed that insurers should not request, and doctors should not reveal, information about an isolated incident of an STI that has no long term health implications, or even multiple episodes of non-serious STIs, again where there are no long term health implications. The fact that this is likely to have only a negligible impact on insurance companies, coupled with the potential to overcome some patients' disincentive to seek advice and testing regarding STIs, makes a strong medical and public health argument for this information being excluded from insurance reports.

HIV, and hepatitis B and C

Insurance companies should not ask whether an applicant has had an HIV or a hepatitis B or C test, received counselling in connection with such a test, or received a negative test result. Doctors should not reveal this information when writing reports and insurance companies do not expect it to be provided. Insurers may ask only whether someone has had a positive test result, or is receiving treatment for HIV/AIDS, or for hepatitis B or C.

For high value policies or when there is a need to clarify the level of risk, insurers may send applicants a supplementary questionnaire and/or request that they are tested for HIV, or for hepatitis B or C. A test must be administered only after the applicant has:

- been notified of the test procedure
- given valid consent in writing
- nominated a doctor or clinic to receive the results if the test is positive
- received appropriate counselling before the test is undertaken.

Existing life insurance policies are not affected in any way by undergoing an HIV test, even if the result is positive. Providing that the applicant did not withhold any material facts when the life policy was taken out, life insurers will meet all valid claims whatever the cause of death, including AIDS related diseases. Material facts that the applicant may need to reveal include information about activities that increase the risk of HIV infection.

Lifestyle questions

Doctors are expert in clinical matters and can give professional advice only about issues in which they have expertise. They should refuse to answer questions that invite speculation about a patient's lifestyle. Although doctors often do hold some information about certain "lifestyle" issues, such as smoking, alcohol intake, eating habits, or sexual behaviour, it is, of course, only the individual himself or herself who has accurate, up to date information about these things.

At the time of writing, it is common for insurance companies to ask doctors to include in medical reports what the health records said about lifestyle issues. The BMA would prefer insurance companies to seek this information only from the applicant, and it is hoped that this will be the case in the future. Meanwhile, doctors need to be careful to avoid becoming involved in speculation about lifestyle issues and should restrict their responses to factually verifiable and clinically relevant information.

Of course, medical conditions that have arisen as a result of a patient's lifestyle choice are legitimate areas for doctors to comment on, with appropriate consent.

Genetic information

The use of the results of genetic tests by insurers is tightly controlled, and doctors must ensure that they work to the latest rules. Those in force at the time of writing are set out below; information about any changes will be put on the BMA's website.

In October 2001 the Government and the ABI reached the following agreement, covering the whole of the UK.

- There would be a 5 year moratorium on the use of predictive genetic test results by insurers.
- This would apply to life insurance policies up to a total value of £500 000 and to critical illness, long term care, and income protection policies up to a total value of £300 000.
- Over these limits, the insurance industry may use genetic test results only where the tests have been approved by the Government's Genetics and Insurance Committee (GAIC).
- A review of the financial limits would take place in 2004.
- Individual companies would decide on their policy regarding the use of favourable results.

Doctors should not, therefore, disclose unfavourable genetic test results in insurance reports for policies up to the limits set out above, and insurance companies should make it clear that such information is not required. Information about a family history of a genetic disease is not covered by the moratorium, and is discussed further below. Doctors with concerns about whether a particular test falls within the scope of the moratorium may seek advice from the ABI.

In some circumstances, patients may wish to opt to disclose a genetic test result, however. When an individual has had a favourable predictive genetic test that would avoid the need for additional premiums, this information may be provided with the explicit consent of the patient.

Monitoring compliance with the moratorium falls to both the Association of British Insurers and GAIC. The ABI also monitors compliance with its own voluntary code of practice on genetic testing,[10] the main points of which are listed below.

- Applicants will not be asked to undergo a genetic test in order to obtain insurance.
- Insurers will take account of existing genetic test results for policies that fall outside the terms of the moratorium (for example policies that exceed the financial ceilings) only when their reliability and relevance to the insurance product has been established by GAIC.
- There will be no effect on the premium or on the terms offered unless a relevant and reliable genetic test result indicates an increased risk. An increase in the risk will not necessarily justify an increase in premium.
- If underwriters wish to take account of a genetic test result (that falls outside the terms of the moratorium), they will always consult a medical practitioner, normally the company's chief medical officer, who will consult a genetics specialist if necessary.
- Mechanisms are in place to deal with complaints.
- Standards for security and confidentiality are set out.

Further discussion of the use of genetic information by insurance companies can be found in Chapter 9 (pages 335–6).

Family history information

As mentioned above, information about a patient's family history of disease is not covered by the moratorium on the use of genetic information in insurance. It is usual for insurance companies to ask doctors to include in their reports information about a patient's family history when this is recorded in the health records and it is clear that the information originated from the patient himself or herself. If there is information in a patient's record about family history that is recorded only because of the doctor's independent knowledge of the family member, it must not be revealed. Essentially, insurance companies are asking doctors to confirm that the information in health records matches the patient's disclosure of information. The BMA has concerns about this process, and would prefer insurers not to ask doctors to report on information that is merely "hearsay". The insurance industry is, however, keen to preserve this "check" on patients' declarations.

Explanations

Insurance companies must provide written reasons for any higher than standard premium or rejection of an application to applicants, on request. They must not ask applicants' doctors to explain their actuarial and underwriting decisions. If the company is concerned that the applicant is not aware of a health condition that has influenced the underwriting, or, if it believes that further care or treatment may be beneficial, a medical officer of the company should discuss the best way to proceed with the applicant's GP. Any health concerns that the insurance company has brought to the attention of the GP should be discussed, if the GP feels it to be necessary, in a normal NHS consultation.

Summary – insurance reports

- GPs must see the patient's written consent before writing insurance reports.
- Insurers and their agents have responsibility for ensuring that applicants give valid consent, although, if there is any doubt, doctors should check with the patient.
- Patients should be encouraged to access reports before they are sent.
- Doctors need to be aware of the type of information that is relevant to the insurance report, and of any rules that apply to special categories of information, for example, genetic test results.

Expert witnesses

Ordinary witnesses in court are asked to report what they have seen or heard. Experts, on the other hand, are invited to say not only what they have seen and heard, but also to express an opinion. When doctors are employed as expert witnesses, their primary duty is to assist the court and, it follows, to remain independent of the parties, regardless of who called the doctor to court. Detached objectivity is required of medical experts at all times and it is not the role of doctors to plead the case of the side paying the fee. Expert witnesses are not advocates and should not have, or be seen to have, an interest in the outcome of the case. The weight of a doctor's opinion is clearly likely to be diminished if it appears biased. Doctors should bear in mind that their opinion may be challenged in court, and that their evidence and their reasoning may be subject to intensive and searching cross examination.

Experts may be asked to prepare a report outlining what, if any, injury has been sustained, the role of pre-existing or coincidental factors, the likely causation, and prognosis. Since solicitors must represent their client's best interests, they are concerned to present such evidence as will assist in advancing the client's case. Solicitors are under no obligation to inform doctors from whom they are commissioning a report of any facts adverse to the case. Doctors cannot, therefore, assume that they have been given all the material facts. In such a situation, the onus is upon doctors to seek all relevant information such as any pleadings, witness statements, investigation reports, incident or accident reports, and previous medical records, and to report upon any material features whether they consider these may be adverse to the case of the party instructing them or not.

Submission of an expert report in the context of litigation

Unless instructed otherwise, a report to a court should be addressed to the court and it should:

- give details of the expert's qualifications
- where there is a range of opinion on the matters dealt with in the report, summarise the range of opinion and give reasons for the conclusion the expert reached
- give details of any literature or other material that the expert has relied on in making the report; it should also contain a statement setting out the substance of all (written and oral) material instructions to the expert
- contain a statement that the expert understands his or her duty to the court
- be verified by a "statement of truth" which confirms that the expert believes that the facts he or she has stated are true, and that the opinions expressed are correct.[11]

If individuals are medically examined for a report, doctors need to check that the solicitor has properly communicated to the client the exact reason for the medicolegal appointment. Doctors may need to reiterate the fact that it is not a therapeutic exchange and information will be disclosed in the doctor's subsequent report. Consent should of course be sought. When writing reports, it is important that doctors restrict comments to relevant clinical issues and do not ask questions that lead the report towards unnecessary or inappropriate assumptions of potential liability. Nor should doctors get drawn into commenting on the standard of care the patient has received unless specifically invited to do so. When writing reports, doctors should bear in mind that they will be read by all parties involved in the action, as well as the presiding officer of the court.

As a general principle, an expert should not accept instructions in any matter in which there is an actual or potential conflict of interest. If doctors are acquainted with the person, or if they stand to benefit, they need to consider seriously whether it is appropriate to give evidence as an expert. In exceptional cases, if full disclosure of the nature of the conflict is made by the medical expert and acknowledged by those commissioning the report, it may be acceptable to take instructions. If an actual or potential conflict of interest arises only in the course of preparing the report, the doctor must notify all concerned of this and, if appropriate, return the instructions and resign from the case.

In order to provide constructive feedback for medical experts, some judges arrange for their judgments to be provided to the experts at the end of the case, and recommend that they are given debriefing letters from the instructing solicitors. This can clearly assist experts in their practice, and doctors offering expert witness services should consider requesting such feedback as a routine part of their work. Many courts also provide witness training days, which offer an opportunity to develop the skills necessary to become a good expert witness.

The BMA's Medico-legal Committee publishes detailed advice on acting as an expert witness.[12] It is likely that new standards and guidance will arise from the Home Office review of forensic pathology services.[13] In 2003 it announced measures for training expert witnesses and setting standards for their competence.[14]

Summary – expert witnesses

- The primary duty of the expert witness is to assist the court.
- Impartiality is essential.
- If individuals are medically examined for a report, doctors need to check that the solicitor has properly communicated to the client the exact reason for the medicolegal appointment, and consent should of course be sought.

Refereeing firearms licences

Doctors are sometimes asked to act as referees for people wanting to own firearms. Applications for a firearm or shotgun licence require a signature from two people of "good character" who are resident in the UK.[15] Referees have to sign a declaration that they know of no reason why the applicant should not be permitted to possess a firearm. Although responsibility for deciding whether or not to issue a licence rests with the chief constable, considerable weight is given to the endorsement of the referee.[16] The form expressly states that the referee is not guaranteeing the future good behaviour or conduct of the applicant, but doctors asked to sign these forms feel that their opinion will be decisive and that they are being asked to comment on a patient's likely "future dangerousness".

The form asks whether the referee has knowledge of any medical or emotional problems, alcohol, drugs or medication related abuse, or mental or physical disability suffered by the applicant. Doctors have pointed out that they will seldom have sufficient knowledge of a patient to certify that he or she has not suffered from *any* mental disorder, and in such cases should decline to act as a referee. Doctors should countersign application forms only if they believe they have a sufficiently detailed knowledge of the patient to be confident that the individual can safely possess a firearm. The BMA expects that very few doctors will feel this confident about their knowledge of a patient.

Doctors are not alone in being seen as people of good standing for the purposes of this form. Lawyers and magistrates, for example, can also be asked to act as referees. When the applicant is not a patient, the relationship is arguably clearer because it is personal not professional. There is nothing to prevent doctors from countersigning forms in this situation, although they should bear in mind that the law regards doctors as *de facto* experts on mental capacity and as such their signature may carry more weight than that of a non-medically qualified person.

If doctors have reason to believe that individuals have access to firearms and are a danger to themselves or to society, they should be prepared to breach confidence and inform the appropriate authorities, in this case the chief constable or other senior police officer. (For further information on breaching confidentiality, see Chapter 5.) If in doubt, doctors should seek further advice from their professional, regulatory, or indemnifying body.

Summary – refereeing firearms licences

- Any person of good standing may act as a referee on firearms licence applications.
- Doctors often feel that they are being asked to comment on an applicant's "future dangerousness".
- Doctors should not act as referees unless they are confident that the individual can safely possess a firearm.

Doctors examining asylum seekers

The intensification of political instability in several parts of the world during the 1990s led to a significant increase in the number of people applying for political asylum. Those who arrive in the UK claiming that they had suffered torture or maltreatment in their country of origin are offered an examination by medical officers employed by the Department of Health. Some of these new arrivals will apply for asylum. The BMA recognises that the identification of torture sequelae requires particular expertise and training, and cannot be done quickly. Nevertheless, brief but adequate notes and, where possible, photographs, of abnormalities taken by port medical officers could be crucial in the later assessment of the validity of an asylum seeker's case. It is helpful if any record made by port of entry medical officers is made available, with the patient's consent, to other doctors who examine the same individual later in connection with an asylum application. In the past, independent doctors providing reports at a later date have been unable to gain access to medical records made at the time of entry to the country.

As with all medical reports, doctors must be impartial and should indicate where there is more than one possible cause of an asylum seeker's symptoms. Doctors who undertake this form of work invariably build up expertise in the patterns of maltreatment or torture common to the region of the applicant's origin. They may offer an opinion about the most likely aetiology of the asylum applicant's condition, based upon observed facts, but should not speculate more widely.

People who have suffered torture, maltreatment, and psychological trauma in their country of origin rely partly upon medical documentation of the detectable sequelae to substantiate their claim for asylum. This can be an emotive area, and doctors asked to provide a medical report for asylum seekers must ensure both the impartiality of their report and that each application is subject to careful and disinterested scrutiny. The doctor's role is to discover and report on any material features that he or she considers relevant, even if they may adversely affect the case of the instructing party.

Expert assessment

Asylum seekers may be housed in the community pending adjudication, or they may be detained in custody. (For more detailed information on the ethical implications of doctors treating detained asylum seekers, see Chapter 17, pages 634–7.) They do not form a homogeneous group, but some common health problems have been identified by experienced doctors working with torture survivors' rehabilitation organisations.[17] These draw attention to the fact that the full effects of any maltreatment that the applicant may have suffered are unlikely to be immediately evident upon initial examination. Although conclusive physical signs are apparent in only a minority of cases, predictable patterns of psychological sequelae are nevertheless common. It should be noted, however, that medical opinion varies concerning the extent to which such sequelae may be categorised as exclusive to survivors of certain types of trauma.[18]

Many of the psychological sequelae of torture take a long time to emerge, which can be problematic given the time limits imposed upon asylum applications. Discussing past physical abuse, particularly if it involved cultural taboos such as sexual humiliation, is likely to be extremely difficult for the applicant. Doctors must also recognise that there are often cultural differences in the way in which patients present medical symptoms and the importance they accord to different types of injury. Doctors should bear in mind when examining asylum seekers that it is not part of their function to give an opinion on whether asylum should be granted.

The London-based Medical Foundation for the Care of Victims of Torture provides volunteer doctors experienced in documenting evidence of torture, who can give a medical assessment. The Foundation and the BMA have joint guidelines on the examination of asylum seekers who make Home Office applications.[19] The BMA also publishes a separate guide to the health needs of asylum seekers.[20]

Translation services

Finding appropriate interpretation services for asylum seekers can sometimes present a problem. In some cases, other members of the patient's family or cultural group offer to interpret. This can cause grave problems with confidentiality and should be avoided unless there is an emergency and no other interpreter can be found. Confidentiality issues can be particularly acute if patients want to discuss sensitive information or need to access services such as family planning, abortion, or HIV testing. Some UK commissioners of health services, including most of those in London, have interpretation services, although paying for them can present problems. Wherever possible, sensitivity should be exercised in selecting interpreters, with regard to factors such as gender and political or cultural background. This is particularly important in cases where patients need to discuss very personal issues such as sexual health. It is essential that health services do not rely on embassies or official agencies of the patient's home country if the patient claims to have been persecuted or tortured because information may be collected that puts patients at risk and may jeopardise the safety of their relatives. For further information on translators and interpreters, see Chapter 17 (page 609).

Summary – doctors examining asylum seekers

- Impartiality is essential.
- Identifying the sequelae of torture requires specialist knowledge and sensitive interaction with patients.
- Where translators are used, doctors need to give particular consideration to issues of confidentiality.

Pre-employment reports and testing

Employers sometimes need to confirm prospective employees' medical fitness for the job. They often have duties to third parties that require them to assess whether their employees pose any threat to others. NHS trusts, for example, owe a clear duty of care to their patients and, if they fail to undertake suitable vetting procedures for prospective employees, they may be failing in this duty. This was highlighted by the 1994 Clothier Report, which examined the deaths and injuries caused by nurse Beverly Allitt and put forward recommendations for the screening of people entering the nursing profession.[21]

The case of Beverly Allitt

Between February and April 1991, three children died suddenly on the children's ward at Grantham and Kesteven General Hospital. Another baby died at home shortly after discharge, and nine other children and babies collapsed unexpectedly, some more than once. On 30 April, police were called in to investigate and in November of the same year nurse Beverly Allitt was charged with four murders, nine attempted murders, and nine counts of causing grievous bodily harm.

The independent inquiry into the case of Beverly Allitt made the following recommendations in relation to pre-employment checks.[22]

- For all those seeking entry into nursing, in addition to routine references, the most recent employer or place of study should be asked to provide at least a record of sick leave.
- Nurses should undergo formal health screening when they obtain their first posts after qualifying.
- The possibility should be reviewed of making available to occupational health departments any records of absence through sickness from any institution that an applicant for a nursing post has attended or where he or she has been employed.
- Consideration may be given to how GPs could, with the consent of candidates, be asked to certify that there is nothing in the medical history of candidates for employment in the NHS that would make them unsuitable for their chosen occupation.

Like insurance companies, employers may obtain information about the suitability of potential employees by commissioning GP reports or independent examinations. Consent is always needed in these cases. Those applying for jobs may effectively bar themselves from that particular post if they do not agree to information being disclosed, but the BMA does not believe that pressure of that nature necessarily invalidates their consent, provided that they are properly informed and only relevant information is sought.

If potential employees prohibit doctors from disclosing information to the employer, doctors must respect their decision. The fact of refusal must be made clear to the employer, taking care to avoid revealing any details, although there may be exceptional circumstances in which confidentiality may be breached, and information disclosed to a potential employer.

Patients have statutory rights of access to reports written about them for employment purposes. Detailed advice is given in Chapter 6 (page 221).

When doctors are involved in designing pre-employment medical questionnaires, they should encourage employers to limit the information requested to that which is directly relevant to an individual's fitness for the particular work concerned. The doctor involved should obviously be familiar with both the workplace and the types of employment involved. Wherever possible, specific information should be requested and "catch all" type questions should be avoided. Doctors need to be aware that claims of racial, sexual, or disability discrimination could arise from the collection of irrelevant medical data. It could also breach the third data protection principle that information "shall be adequate, relevant and not excessive in relation to the purpose or purposes for which they are processed".[23]

Pre-employment testing for HIV, drugs and alcohol

When any pre-employment testing is carried out, it must be done to the highest clinical and ethical standards, and the consent of the individual must be obtained. This involves informing the person of the precise nature of the tests and to whom the results may be disclosed. The Faculty of Occupational Medicine publishes guidance on the ethics of drug testing in the workplace, which sets out good practice for testing both job applicants and current employees for illicit substances.[24] When employers wish to use pre-employment testing, a clear explanation must be given to potential employees so that they can make an informed choice about whether or not to undergo that test.

Consent for pre-employment testing

When applying for a temporary position with the European Commission as a typist, Mr X had a medical examination but refused to be screened for HIV antibodies. During the examination, a blood sample was taken and the medical officer ordered blood tests in order to determine the T4 and T8 lymphocyte counts. When these were below the normal ratio, the medical officer concluded that Mr X was suffering from a significant immunodeficiency constituting a case of full-blown AIDS. He was thus rejected on the grounds of his physical condition. Mr X brought a legal case on the grounds that he had been effectively subjected to an AIDS screening test without his consent.

Although the Court of first instance supported the employer's decision, the European Court of Justice held that the manner in which Mr X had been medically examined and declared physically unfit constituted an infringement of his right to respect for his private life as guaranteed by Article 8 of the European Convention on Human Rights. The court said that:

> The right to respect for private life, embodied in Article 8 and deriving from the common constitutional traditions of the Member States is one of the fundamental rights protected by the legal order of the Community. It includes in particular a person's right to keep his state of health secret.[25]

It went on to say that:

> although the pre-employment medical examination serves a legitimate interest of the Community institutions, which must be in a position to fulfil the tasks required of them, that interest does not justify the carrying out of a test against the will of the person concerned ... If the person concerned, after being properly informed, withholds his consent to a test which the medical officer considers necessary in order to evaluate his suitability for the post for which he has applied, the institutions cannot be obliged to take the risk of recruiting him.[26]

X v The European Commission[25]

GP involvement in pre-employment assessments

Some of the same concerns that arise with reports for insurance are evident in queries from BMA members about pre-employment reports. GPs sometimes question the extent of medical information that potential employers seek. They point out that, although the patient gives consent, in areas of high unemployment, for example, the individual has little free choice in the matter. There are also concerns that patients may decline to inform their doctors of certain episodes of illness if they believe that they may need a pre-employment report at a later date.

Some argue that this pressure on patients to agree means that any consent cannot be valid. The BMA is concerned about anecdotal evidence that patients do withhold information, but considers that it would be incorrect for doctors to pre-empt patient choice and to assume it is necessarily contrary to the patient's interest to provide information. The decision about whether to authorise disclosure must ultimately rest with the patient. Patients should be encouraged to see the report before it is sent if GPs believe that there is information that may affect their chances of getting the job, so that patients are forewarned. Although at this stage patients may choose to withdraw their consent for the report to be sent, they cannot, of course, demand that information is withheld selectively. If asked to do this, doctors should explain that they cannot write a misleading report.

In a similar vein, patients may give consent for the release of information to a potential employer because if it is withheld the employer will draw adverse conclusions. The BMA believes that it is not for the doctor to enquire into the motives that underlie a consent freely given in full knowledge of the implications. Therefore, provided the statutory requirements relating to consent for reports have been met (see Chapter 6, page 221), doctors should accept the consent given. As with insurance reports, doctors should retain a copy of the letter of consent, and, if they have any concerns about its validity, they should check with the patient.

In their reports, GPs should limit themselves to statements of fact. Commenting on whether they are aware of any health reason why a patient would be unsuitable for a job is acceptable, but they should be wary of making more general judgments about suitability for employment or to make value judgments about previous periods of absence through sickness. It is not the role of the GP to predict future actions by patients, or to try to judge the likelihood of future health problems. GPs should limit themselves to certifying whether there is anything in the medical record that raises concerns about the suitability of the person for the job or activity in question. It is then for the prospective employer to make a judgment about suitability for employment. It goes without saying that the GP should have sufficient relevant knowledge of the nature and context of the job for which the person has applied before making any assessment about fitness for work or related matters.

Genetic screening for employment purposes

As genetic predisposition to disease is increasingly identified, it is expected that employers may wish to introduce screening of employees and prospective employees in order to identify those most at risk of developing adverse reactions to hazards in the workplace.

In the early years of the twenty-first century, there was no evidence that any employer was asking potential or existing employees to undergo a genetic test to predict for future disease or general health, as a condition of employment. If there were to be such proposals, the potential benefits to the employer would need to be balanced against the potential harms both to the individual and to society in general. In the BMA's view, the individual's right to make a free and informed decision about whether to seek genetic testing is likely to outweigh any theoretical advantages to the company. The BMA would strongly object to individuals being required to take a predictive genetic test as a condition of employment unless this was directly linked to their ability to carry out their work safely.

Although there is no evidence of employers asking specific questions about existing genetic test results,[27] doctors sometimes ask the BMA about their responsibility to disclose such information in response to general health questions. General questions may enquire whether there is anything in the medical record that raises concerns about the individual's current or future health or ability to meet the requirements of the job, or about recent referrals to specialists. Clearly, a positive predictive genetic test result, or a referral to a geneticist because of a family history of a late onset genetic disorder, falls into that category and doctors may be obliged to release the information in order to answer the question truthfully. There are a number of difficulties with this information being requested in this indirect manner. First, the patient may not be aware that the information will be provided if there is no specific question about genetic tests, so the consent obtained may not be valid. Secondly, the employer or occupational health department receiving the information may not have the necessary expertise to interpret it accurately. There is therefore a risk that all people who have had a positive genetic test, or those with a family history of a genetic disorder, may be excluded from employment even though they may not be affected by the disorder for many years, or possibly at all. Although people with disabilities have some protection under the Disability Discrimination Act 1995,[28] those who have had an unfavourable genetic test do not if they are asymptomatic because they would not fall within the definition of a person with a "disability". A further problem with such indirect requests is that the true extent to which employers are using genetic information is hidden. This presents difficulties for those who are responsible for monitoring the situation and deciding whether additional safeguards are needed.

If sensitive information is required to answer questions on the report accurately, doctors must ensure that the patient is aware of any such information that may be revealed, and has given consent on that basis. Even when patients have chosen not to see the report before it is sent, it would be a sensible precaution for the doctor to discuss its content with the patient in these circumstances. Doctors presenting genetic information in reports also have a responsibility to see that it is both accurate and fair, and provides sufficient detail to put it in context. This could include providing information about the meaning of a particular genetic test and possibly to suggest that additional specialist advice should be sought. Occupational health doctors receiving such information, in turn, have a responsibility to respond fairly and, where necessary, to seek more specialist advice.

The Department of Health has accepted, in principle, that pre-employment medical reports should focus on the individual's current ability to carry out the work in question.[29] Until such time as this policy is acted upon by the Government, however, doctors should continue to provide information, on request, with patient consent along the lines set out above. (Up to date information may be obtained from the BMA, the Human Genetics Commission, and the Faculty of Occupational Medicine at the Royal College of Physicians.)

Information about occupational hazards

Genetic testing may also be suggested as a way of identifying those who are more susceptible to the occupational hazards of a particular type of employment. In theory, this information could help people to make informed decisions about their choice of employment, although it needs to be recognised that, in some areas of high unemployment, such choices may be constrained. Employers could use screening to help them to fulfil their duties under health and safety legislation to provide a safe working environment without making themselves liable under current antidiscrimination legislation. A common concern, however, is that, rather than improving the working environment, employers could simply exclude from employment anyone who represents a higher than the average risk. This would save the employer the cost of making improvements to the working environment and may also save them from paying out compensation for work related injuries at a later stage.

At the time of writing, there is no evidence that such screening is being used, although this is largely due to the current lack of certainty about the genetics of susceptibility to hazardous substances in the workplace.[30] It is possible, however, that such screening could be developed in the future, particularly with advances in pharmacogenetics (see Chapter 13, pages 484–6). The BMA is keeping this matter under review.

Summary – pre-employment reports and testing

- Pre-employment medical reports should be restricted to information that is relevant to the job.
- Patients must be properly informed about the nature and purpose of any disclosure to a potential employer.
- Patients have a right of access to reports.
- Consent for disclosure of reports is essential, and doctors should not assume that simply because patients are under pressure to give consent that this is necessarily invalid.

Occupational health physicians

Occupational medicine deals with the effects of work on health and the impact of the employee's health on his or her performance and that of others in the workforce.

The objectives of an occupational health service can be summarised in five points:

- to promote and maintain the health and safety of employees
- to provide emergency treatment for sick and injured employees
- to advise on rehabilitation and suitable placement of employees who are temporarily or permanently disabled by illness or injury
- to promote safe and healthy conditions by informed assessment of the working environment and by providing advice or educative material
- to promote research into causes of occupational diseases and the means of their prevention.[31]

Occupational physicians must act as impartial professional advisers, concerned with the health of all those employed in the organisation. Such responsibilities can, however, lead to very real dilemmas such as when the doctor believes that the working environment may exacerbate health problems for certain employees or applicants for employment. Statutory and other periodic medical examinations may also affect continued employment. Pilots, workers in the atomic energy industry, and medical staff who develop allergies to drugs are examples of difficult cases. Here, occupational physicians must be careful not to take over the role of the line manager in deciding whether such an individual should be offered employment or dismissed. The patient must be reminded that the doctor's role, as the agent of a third party in such cases, is to advise the employer, with the individual's consent, of possible health problems that could arise.

Pre-employment assessment

When occupational health physicians undertake pre-employment assessments, their primary responsibility is to the employer, although there is still a duty of care owed to the applicant to conduct a clinically sound examination that is appropriate for the job in question. Generally speaking, a medical examination is normally justified only when the job involves working in hazardous environments, requires high standards of fitness, is required by law, or when the safety of other workers or of the public is concerned. Usually, a health assessment by questionnaire should suffice, and occupational health physicians have an important role in advising about what standards of mental and physical health are necessary for a particular job.

Confidentiality

Although paid by the management, the occupational physician's duties concern the health and welfare of the whole workforce, both individually and collectively. They have the same duties of confidentiality as other doctors. The fact that a doctor is a salaried employee gives no other employee of that company any right of access to medical records or to the details of examination findings. With the employee's consent, the employer may be advised of any relevant information relating to a specific matter on a strictly need to know basis, the significance of which the employee clearly understands. If an employer explicitly or implicitly invites an employee to consult the occupational physician, the latter must still regard such consultations as strictly confidential.

The occupational health physician and nurse are responsible for ensuring the confidentiality of clinical records. The arrangements for custody of the records should be defined in the occupational physician's contract of employment. Under the supervision of the occupational health team, clerical support staff may see clinical records in the same way as staff in a GP's surgery, that is, when they have a legitimate "need to know" the information for the purposes of providing support to the occupational health clinician. The occupational physician must ensure that such staff understand the need for confidentiality and have a contractual obligation to preserve it.

Although individual clinical findings are confidential, their significance may be made known to an appropriate third party, such as the employer or health and safety representatives. Thus, while the reading of a laboratory result is confidential to the individual tested, it is nonetheless proper to disclose to those with a responsibility for overseeing safety that a group, or an individual, shows, for example, a significant degree of exposure to a potentially toxic hazard. Similarly, although a report of being "fit" or "unfit" for work can be made known to the employer, the clinical details cannot be disclosed unless the individual gives consent.

Where occupational physicians believe that a process or product in the workplace constitutes a risk to health, they should try to persuade the employer to take action. Even when there are issues of commercial secrecy, the doctor's responsibility for the health of workers exposed to the hazard takes precedence over the obligations to management. If employers fail to take necessary action, doctors should take urgent advice from their professional, regulatory, or indemnifying bodies. Alternatively, the Health and Safety Executive is also able to offer impartial and, if necessary, anonymous advice.

Consent to examination

In some companies, employees are required by statute or their contracts to undergo medical examinations. Examples of examinations of fitness required by statute include drivers of heavy goods or public service vehicles and airline pilots. Industries that involve food handling frequently impose contractual obligations on employees to undergo examination after sickness absence or where they have been in contact with anyone with a gastrointestinal infection or virus. Examinations are also required under legislation regulating hazardous substances. Doctors working in this field will be aware of these requirements, and advice is given by the BMA's Occupational Health Committee.[32]

It is important not to infer from an employee's attendance at a contractually imposed health assessment that the person agrees both to the examination and to the disclosure of the result. Doctors should ensure that employees understand the context in which the examination takes place, the nature of the examination, the need for disclosure of the significance of the findings, and what, if any, clinical information is to be disclosed. Employees should be informed of these things in their contract of employment or corresponding reference documents, and consent forms should be signed by the employee on each occasion that a medical examination is required by the employer. One-off or "blanket" consent for examination or subsequent disclosure at the start of the contract is not sufficient.

Random drug testing

The Association is sometimes asked to comment on schemes for doctors to conduct random drug or other testing among both applicants for employment and current employees. Such testing, which, at the time of writing, is not widespread in the UK, is sometimes justified by the argument that the employee or applicant may endanger the lives of others if impaired by drugs or alcohol.

The BMA believes that job applicants and employees should be informed in advance, for example, via clauses in the contract of employment, that testing is required on a regular or random basis. General advice about drug misuse should also be provided.

When employees provide samples to be tested for other purposes, it is not acceptable for them to be tested for drugs without these individuals being told of this possibility and giving consent. Seeking to use samples for other purposes could breach employees' rights to privacy as enshrined in Article 8 of the European Convention on Human Rights and given effect in UK domestic law by the Human Rights Act 1998.

Clinical tests for alcohol or drugs are subject to the same degree of confidentiality as any other medical examination. Where, however, the results indicate that the person is affected by drugs or alcohol and is, as a result, putting others at risk, doctors may need to consider whether or not it is appropriate for information to be passed to management. A line may need to be drawn between intoxication at work, for which there should be appropriate disciplinary procedures, and the health effects of chronic misuse. In some cases it may be sufficient for the doctor to declare that the individual is unfit for work without specifying the reasons. When disclosure is necessary, voluntary disclosure should be the aim. Circumstances in which it may be necessary to override confidentiality in the public interest are discussed in Chapter 5 (pages 189–92). Advice about what to do if doctors are abusing drugs is given in Chapter 21 (pages 760–5).

The involvement of health staff in the "policing" of employment procedures should be avoided. It is not a legitimate role for them to adopt and it may also undermine their status as confidential medical advisers.[33]

Sickness absence

Occupational physicians do not usually become involved in confirming or refuting that an individual employee's absence from work is due to sickness or injury, but can sometimes assist in the management and analysis of sickness absence. In such cases, it is crucial to separate out the roles and responsibilities of managers and occupational physicians, and for employees to be aware of these different roles.

On an employee's return to work, the occupational physician is responsible for advising management on the worker's fitness for the job and may be asked to assess whether temporary or permanent modifications to the work are necessary. Doctors should inform employees of the advice they intend to give management and seek the employee's consent to discuss with the employer any important changes required by the employee's present health.

In order for occupational physicians to be able to give informed advice to an employer about a member of staff who has had long or frequent sick leave, they need to be able to see and examine the employee and, if necessary, to contact the relevant GP or hospital consultant, with the written consent of the employee. The importance of good communication between the occupational physician and the GP or hospital consultant cannot be overstated. This is vital in helping the occupational physician to give informed advice to both employer and employee. If the occupational physician examines a worker who is or has been absent for health reasons, the GP should, with the patient's consent, be informed of any conclusion reached.

If an employee's record of sickness absence is very prolonged, the occupational physician may be asked to advise both employee and employer about future employability. Although the employer has no right to clinical details of sickness or injury, it is reasonable for employers to expect the doctor to give an opinion about the anticipated date of the employee's return to work, the employee's work capacity, the likely degree and duration of any disability, and the likelihood of future absences. If employees request that doctors do not release this information to their employers, doctors should take advice from their professional, regulatory or indemnifying body. It is the prerogative of management to take action against an employee who has been sick long term or is too frequently absent from work. In any case where the dismissal is challenged by the individual as unfair or discriminatory under the Disability Discrimination Act, the occupational physician may be called upon by either party to give expert evidence to the employment tribunal.

Occupational health records

Occupational health records provide a factual record of employees' health status for the purposes of workplace risk management and safety. In addition, they can be a very powerful tool in research into work related diseases. The usual rules about patient consent for the use of records in research apply, and any research using occupational health records should have the approval of an appropriately constituted research ethics committee (see Chapter 14). Access to occupational health records is governed by the Data Protection Act 1998 (see Chapter 6, pages 216–8).

If an employee has incurred injury or illness at work and is taking legal action against the employer, the occupational physician may, with the individual's written informed consent, provide the legal advisers of both sides with factual information about attendance at medical departments, first aid, and other treatment. In all questions of litigation, clinical records or abstracts from them should not be released without the individual's written consent. A court or employment tribunal may, however, order disclosure. It is also important that written consent is obtained for records to be released to trade union representatives.

If a particular document or set of documents is ordered to be disclosed, then the doctor or nurse has a duty to disclose them or to challenge the disclosure in the court or tribunal. However, if the nurse or doctor is to challenge the disclosure, then he or she must bring the originals to court in case the order is upheld.

Transfer of records

Arrangements must be made for the proper transfer of health records to another doctor or occupational health nurse when the occupational physician leaves the company. In some cases, where the doctor does not have a clear contract or agreement, supervision of the records is left in doubt when the doctor moves on. In some cases, doctors have attempted to take records with them in the belief that they own them, but the position in law is not clear. The BMA believes that if no other doctor or nurse has been appointed to succeed the occupational physician, the latter retains responsibility for the custody of those records. If an occupational health department closes, the medical records should be transferred to the care of medical staff on another site in that organisation. Alternatively, the records may be offered to a part-time doctor if there is one, or to a suitably qualified nurse who has responsibility for workers. In the absence of occupational health staff, it is acceptable for medical records to be kept securely locked, within the organisation, as long as they can be accessed only by a registered medical practitioner. If the employer's business closes down, the clinician who was in charge of occupational health should take advice from the regional Health and Safety Executive officer about appropriate retention or disposal. Doctors may also contact the BMA's Occupational Health Committee for advice. When the continued security of medical records cannot be guaranteed, the records may be offered to the patients or, if the patients decline or cannot be traced, destruction of the records may be considered.

Occupational health records should normally be retained for at least 10 years after the termination of an employee's service. Records of significant exposures, episodes, or accidents should, however, be retained for at least 30 years. There are also statutory requirements relating to the retention of records that relate to exposure to ionising radiation and other substances that may be hazardous to health. Detailed advice on the requirements is available from the BMA's Occupational Health Committee, the Faculty of Occupational Medicine, and the Society of

Occupational Medicine. In order to save space or to improve clerical efficiency, old records may be stored on microfiche or computer. If external contractors are used to assist in the archiving process, their contract must contain a confidentiality clause. It may be necessary to "weed out" old records if they go back many years, but this should be a matter of last resort.

Liaison with colleagues

Doctors may delegate clinical duties either to specially trained nurses or to nurses who have demonstrated competence in the appropriate tasks. Generally speaking, it is for the doctor to determine the range of clinical duties that nursing staff may undertake. Doctors should bear in mind that they may be liable to prosecution for negligence if they are shown to have delegated a task to a nurse that was outside the scope of the duties that he or she would normally be expected to perform.

Relationships with occupational health nurses

Miss Woodroffe took up employment as a nurse with British Gas. Her original job description made no reference to taking blood samples or to giving talks on health matters. Shortly after she was employed, a new occupational health physician was appointed and he thought that Miss Woodroffe should take blood samples and give talks to employees. Miss Woodroffe explained that she was not trained to perform these tasks, so the occupational health physician offered her additional training. Initially she refused, but after some time she reluctantly agreed to take on the extra responsibilities, although she did not undergo any training. After some time the company became dissatisfied with her work, particularly her record keeping and, in the end, dismissed her. The dismissal was held to be fair by the Court of Appeal. It is interesting, however, that the Employment Appeal Tribunal held that, had she refused to carry out the additional tasks, she could not have been criticised, for they were not tasks for which she had originally been employed. They added that, had she accepted the specialist training, the problems with her work may well have been resolved.

Woodroffe v British Gas[34]

The occupational health practitioner deals constantly with the patients of other doctors and, in order to ensure the best management of these patients, should generally provide treatment only in cooperation with the patients' own doctors, except in an emergency. Similarly, in an emergency, the occupational physician may refer a patient to a hospital or to a specialist, but thereafter they should inform the patient's usual doctor of the action taken. Patient consent must be obtained for liaison between the occupational physician and the GP. In a non-emergency situation, the occupational physician should urge employees to consult their GPs if a referral is necessary, or arrange referral in agreement with the GP.

Summary – occupational health

- Occupational health physicians must act as impartial professional advisers.
- Occupational health physicians have the same duty of confidentiality as other doctors.
- Rarely, it may be necessary to reveal information without consent, but employees should be informed and clinical details kept to a minimum.
- The involvement of health staff in the "policing" of employment procedures should be avoided.
- Patients must be reminded of doctors' obligations to third parties and the impact of such obligations on the patient.
- Consent is required every time an employee undergoes an examination or tests.

Doctors in the armed forces

Constraints on serving doctors

All members of the armed forces are subject to both civil and military law. A doctor in the armed forces must obey any lawful command; disobedience is punishable by means of various sanctions including those determined by court martial. In addition, however, like all doctors, those serving in the forces must behave in accordance with professional ethics.

Doctors working in the armed forces are responsible for their professional actions to the same extent as any other doctor, and are expected to work to the same ethical standards. It follows therefore that it would be unethical for a medical officer to be required to treat a patient under the constraint of non-medical orders when the doctor believes that treatment is not in the individual's best interests.

One matter that has been raised with the BMA on several occasions concerns armed forces doctors who object to boxing matches. These doctors, who do not agree with boxing as a sport, have been required to carry out pre-bout medical examinations. The BMA has advised that a full explanation of the doctor's objections to boxing as a sport should be given to the commanding officer and that the matter should be handled through the recognised appeals procedure. Doctors may also wish to refer to the BMA's objections to boxing.[35] Some doctors who feel strongly on the matter have considered resigning from the forces, rather than having anything to do with boxing matches. Some doctors have also complained that they had insufficient examination time and facilities to assess adequately the potential risk to each participant. Where doctors believe that the examination facilities or the way in which the sport is practised do not minimise the risk of severe injury, they should report these dangers to the commanding officer, making clear the distinction between these concerns and any conscientious objection they may have.

Another ethical issue sometimes facing doctors serving in the armed forces relates to soldiers asking to be declared unfit for active service after receiving notification that they are to be sent to a war zone, or upon learning that war has been declared. Here, doctors must not be influenced either by the soldiers or their commanding officer, but must make a dispassionate and independent evaluation of the individuals concerned on the basis of sound medical principles.

When doctors in the armed forces believe that the medical resources available to them are substandard, it is important that they discuss this with their commanding officers. If this fails to remedy the situation, doctors need to consider whether the best interests of their patients would be served by "blowing the whistle". Advice can be sought from the BMA's Armed Forces Committee.

Confidentiality

When people join the armed forces they relinquish some rights and freedoms. One of these is the right to strict confidentiality. Doctors may at times need to balance the interests of the individual patient's confidentiality and the interests of the unit of which he or she is a part. It follows therefore that there will be occasions when a medical officer is required to discuss the personal health information of patients with a commanding officer. Wherever possible, they should do this with consent. Doctors working in the armed forces have the same duty of confidentiality as other doctors, although the extreme situations in which they work means that information needs to be shared much more often than in civilian life. Ill health of service personnel can put the lives of others at risk and jeopardise military goals, so circumstances are likely to arise where, even if the patient refuses, the "public interest" in disclosure overrides confidentiality (see Chapter 5, pages 189–92). When a doctor in the armed forces feels that it is appropriate that information is disclosed to a commanding officer, he or she should notify the patient of the information that is to be released and the reasons for its disclosure. Doctors should ensure that only information that is necessary to the issue at hand is released. Additional details that do not have a bearing on the health of the individual patient and are not relevant to the issue for which disclosure is required (such as his or her sexual orientation) should not be released.

In many cases, the liberties that people in the armed forces have given up are also lost to other members of their families, who may find that, in practice, they have no choice of medical practitioner and have reduced rights of confidentiality, because it is assumed that the health of the families may affect the servicemen and the unit. This raises some very difficult issues for families of serving personnel. If, for example, a child is suspected of having suffered abuse, it would be customary for the officer in charge of welfare to attend the case conference. In effect, this is involving a representative of the employer, and would be unacceptable in other situations.

Consent

To a certain extent, individuals who join the armed forces freely revoke some of their autonomy for the duration of their term of service. They are expected to follow orders issued for the benefit of the unit, platoon, ship, or squadron of which they are part and to the interests of which they subject their own. Discipline is an essential part of the effective functioning of the services, which must inevitably set limits to the exercise of autonomy. This extends to some degree to consent for certain medical procedures. When there may be a doubt, for example, about a soldier's fitness for combat, or if it is believed that his or her mental or physical health presents a threat to others, the soldier may be ordered to submit to appropriate medical testing, or, exceptionally, to certain forms of treatment such as vaccination. A refusal to obey a direct order in this context may well be dealt with by means of the ordinary disciplinary procedures that would apply to any refusal to obey an order.

Summary – doctors in the armed forces

- Doctors in the armed forces must work to the same ethical standards as other doctors.
- Doctors should raise concerns about standards with the commanding officer, in the first instance.
- Although there are likely to be more circumstances in which confidential health information should be disclosed than in civilian life, this should be with the patient's cooperation and consent whenever possible.

Sports doctors

Doctors who are employed by sports teams and by sports clubs may find themselves subject to the tension of conflicting loyalties. On the one hand they are agents of the team or club with the contractual obligations of an employee, and, on the other, as doctors, they are advocates for the individual athletes or players who are their patients.

The most obvious area in which problems may arise is in relation to confidentiality. This can be particularly true in the case of high profile teams or clubs, such as in professional football, where considerable pressure from officials, from the media, or even from sponsors, can be exerted on doctors to release confidential information.[36] Players may also have contractual obligations to pass relevant information on to their managers. There is no commonly held code of ethics governing the way in which English football clubs handle confidential information, and there is considerable variation in both the type, and the amount, of information about players that doctors release to managers.[37]

The British Olympic Association, on the other hand, has a position statement on athlete confidentiality.

> ## The British Olympic Association's position statement on athlete confidentiality – a summary
>
> - All members of medical support staff are bound by professional codes of conduct. They must ensure confidentiality of information.
> - Where information about athletes is to be exchanged within multidisciplinary support staff meetings, the athlete must be told who will be present, and consent should be obtained in advance.
> - Athletes need to give consent before coaches are informed of their problems.
> - If athletes feel that their medical support team will not respect their confidentiality, they can seek advice elsewhere.
> - Athletes who have signed a consent form may still withhold consent for any specific consultation, test, or treatment.
> - A refusal to consent to disclosure must be respected even in the event of an athlete taking a prohibited substance.[38]

Ethically, sports doctors need to be aware that their chief loyalty is to their patients, and that, contractual issues notwithstanding, the duty of medical confidentiality remains unchanged (see Chapter 5). Unless expressly indicated in the terms of the player's or athlete's contract, confidential information can be released only with the express consent of the patient, and breaches of confidentiality can be justified only when there is a risk of serious self harm or harm to a third party.

Individuals who have sustained injuries may come under pressure from managers to continue to play, particularly in team sports where the outcome of a match is crucial for the team's long term success. This may be the case even when continuing to play may exacerbate injuries or incur risks of long term damage. Furthermore, there is evidence to suggest that, in professional football, there is a presumption that players will continue to play with pain and injury.[39] Here, the doctor's chief obligation must be to the long term health and wellbeing of individual players. In such a situation, doctors must inform both player and manager of the risks involved so that both parties can make an informed decision about whether play should continue. A note of any such discussion should be recorded in the relevant health record.

Doctors may from time to time be asked by players or athletes to provide performance enhancing drugs such as anabolic steroids. Not only must doctors clearly operate, and be seen to operate, within the law, but also the long term health interests of the patients must be their primary concern. Although, as the box above indicates, the British Olympic Association recommends that patient confidentiality must be respected even when participants are taking banned substances, it may be necessary to breach such confidentiality in exceptional circumstances, where, for example, the drug taking could lead to serious harm for the player or his or her team mates.

In a statement issued in 2000 on prescribing performance enhancing drugs, the GMC stated that: "doctors who prescribe or collude in the provision of drugs or treatment with the intention of improperly enhancing an individual's performance in sport would be contravening the GMC's guidance, and such actions would usually raise a question of a doctor's continued registration."

This does not preclude the provision of any care or treatment when the doctor's intention is to protect or improve the patient's health.[40]

Both the World Medical Association's *Declaration on principles of health care for sports medicine*[41] and the BMA's *Doctors' assistance to sports clubs and sporting events*[42] have further advice on these issues.

Summary – sports doctors

- Sports doctors have contractual obligations to the employing team or club, as well as the usual ethical obligations to the sports men and women who are their patients.
- Consent is needed for the disclosure of information to coaches or managers.
- Doctors must not be involved with providing drugs or treatment aimed at improperly enhancing a sports person's performance.

Media doctors

Some doctors choose to work partly or exclusively in the media, for example by editing medical journals or commenting on health issues for newspapers and television. Their role is often to provide general medical advice or background commentary on medical issues in a form that lay people find accessible. When providing commentary about specific cases or individuals, doctors must distinguish between the legitimate provision of background information – commenting, for example, in a general way on the ordinary nature and prognosis of a disease – and the far more questionable practice of speculative diagnosis. Doctors should also resist any temptation to comment on information that they think may have been improperly released into the public domain.

The issues of confidentiality that arise when doctors working in clinical practice are asked to release information about patients to the media are discussed in Chapter 5 (pages 187–8).

Many areas of the media offer discussion with doctors about health issues. This may be in the form of a "helpline", where callers discuss problems with a health professional either by telephone or email. The GMC warns of the dangers that may arise if a doctor offers advice to a patient whom the doctor has not seen or examined.[43] The Council does not take exception to recorded messages or to internet databases giving standard advice on health matters by doctors or others. Nor does it object to helplines giving general information. Nevertheless phone-in programmes and helplines that attempt to provide individual advice may create problems. To supply detailed and specific medical advice of the nature usually provided by the patient's own GP is not appropriate in these circumstances. It must be made clear that the information provided by the telephone advice line or website is designed to support, not replace, the relationship between patients and their GPs.

Where websites or advice lines are supported by commercial organisations, this support must be clearly identified. If advertising is a source of funding, this must also be stated and any advertising or promotional material must be presented in a manner that makes it easily distinguishable from the advice on offer. Any claims relating to the benefits of particular treatments or services, particularly those in which the individual or group running the service has a financial interest, must be supported by appropriate, balanced clinical evidence, and the nature of the financial interest must be clearly acknowledged. As with advertisements published in practice leaflets (see Chapter 19, page 700), the BMA recommends that doctors do not advertise health related products and services. It is also inappropriate for sites to carry advertisements for products that clearly affect health adversely.

Summary – media doctors

- Doctors who comment to the press must not make speculative diagnoses.
- Doctors should not comment on information they think may have been improperly released into the public domain.
- Helplines must not provide specific medical advice to callers.
- When websites or advice lines are supported by commercial organisations, this support must be clearly identified.

Doctors with business interests

For doctors who either direct or hold a financial interest in medical or non-medical enterprises, the main ethical considerations include the function of the enterprise, the manner in which it may generally be promoted, and whether the doctor can refer patients to the organisation, where, for example, it offers medical or nursing services. It is important that doctors do not seek to use their reputation and standing as medically qualified people to influence the potential customers of companies in which they have business interests.

Doctors invest in a wide range of medical and non-medical schemes. It is clear, however, that doctors treating patients in an institution in which they, or members of their immediate family, have a financial interest can lead to serious conflicts of interest. The BMA regards with almost equal gravity situations in which patients believe erroneously that the doctor's judgment is influenced by such financial holdings and circumstances in which this belief is well founded. In this situation, patient confidence in the doctor may be compromised just as surely as if the doctor were indeed putting personal financial interests first. Financial investment in pharmaceutical companies is covered in Chapter 13 (pages 469–70).

Although it may be acceptable for doctors to refer their patients to facilities in which they have a financial interest, both the BMA and the GMC[44] advise that in such cases they must declare their interest to patients. When treating NHS patients, doctors must also inform the healthcare purchaser. When doctors offer specialist services, they must not accept patients unless they have been referred by another doctor who will have overall responsibility for managing patient care.

Where GPs have a financial interest in a residential or nursing home, it is inappropriate for them to provide primary care services to patients in that home, unless patients ask them to do so or there are no alternatives. It is important in such instances that the patients or, if appropriate, their relatives, are informed of the nature of the financial interest. The GMC points out that in such instances doctors may be called upon to justify their decision.[45]

One area about which the BMA receives enquiries is in relation to doctors selling, or endorsing the selling of, vitamin supplements or other health related products. In such cases the BMA advises that when doctors have a commercial interest in such products, they should not be involved in promoting, endorsing, or otherwise selling them. Furthermore, GPs' terms of service prohibit them from selling a wide range of health products and services, including any drugs or appliances needed for treatment.[46] When acting as medical practitioners, doctors' recommendations of products must be based solely on clinical effectiveness and on the individual patient's best interests.

Summary – doctors with business interests

- It is essential that doctors' financial interests neither affect, nor are perceived to affect, the way they treat, refer, or prescribe for their patients.
- Doctors must disclose any relevant financial interests to patients and, if working in the NHS, to the NHS purchaser.
- When acting as medical practitioners, doctors' recommendations of products must be based solely on clinical effectiveness.

References

1 World Medical Association. *International code of medical ethics (Declaration of Geneva)*. Geneva: WMA, 1983.
2 International Dual Loyalty Working Group. *Dual loyalty and human rights in health professional practice: proposed guidelines and institutional mechanisms*. Boston, MA: Physicians for Human Rights, School of Public Health and Primary Health Care, University of Capetown Health Sciences Faculty, 2002.
3 General Medical Council. *Confidentiality: protecting and providing information*. London: GMC, 2000: paras 34–35.
4 Pamela Cornelius v Dr Nicola de Taranto [2002] 68 BMLR 62.
5 General Medical Council. *Good medical practice*. London: GMC, 2001: para 51.
6 British Medical Association, Association of British Insurers. *Medical information and insurance: joint guidelines from the British Medical Association and the Association of British Insurers*. London: BMA/ABI, 2002.
7 General Medical Council. *Confidentiality: protecting and providing information. Op cit:* para 34.

8   British Medical Association, *et al. Medical information and insurance: joint guidelines from the British Medical Association and the Association of British Insurers. Op cit.*

9   Department of Health. *AIDS and life insurance.* London: HMSO, 1991. Report prepared for the Department of Health and the Association of British Insurers by British Market Research Bureau Limited.

10   Association of British Insurers. *Genetic testing – ABI code of practice.* London: ABI, 1999.

11   In England and Wales, the rules for submission of an expert report are contained in: Lord Chancellor's Department. *Civil procedure rules. Practice direction. Part 35: experts and assessors.* London: LCD, 2002: 1–2. In Northern Ireland, the submission of medical evidence is regulated by Order 25 of the High Court Rules of Northern Ireland. Information regarding expert witnesses and the submission of medical evidence in Scotland can be found in: Henderson H, Thomson JM, Miller K, eds. *The laws of Scotland: Stair memorial encyclopaedia.* London: Butterworths, 1988: paras 650–1.

12   British Medical Association. *The expert witness: a guidance note for BMA members.* London: BMA, 2002. For further information on acting as an expert witness, see: Mr Justice Wall, Hamilton I. *Handbook for expert witnesses in Children Act cases.* Bristol: Jordan Publishing, 2000. Expert Witness Institute. *The law and you: code of guidance for expert witnesses.* London: EWI, 2002. Information is also available from the Council for the Registration of Forensic Practitioners.

13   Home Office. *Review of forensic pathology services in England and Wales.* London: Home Office, 2003.

14   Home Office press release. *Delivering a first-class forensic pathology service: better regulation, improved performance.* 2003 Mar 17.

15   The law relating to certification for firearms and shotguns in England and Wales is contained in the Firearms Act 1968 and the Firearms Rules 1998 s3–10. In Scotland the law is contained in the Firearms (Scotland) Rules 1989 s 3–10. (SI 1989 No. 889.) In Northern Ireland, certification for firearms and shotguns is contained in the Firearms (Northern Ireland) Order 1981 part 3 (as amended).

16   British Medical Association. *Interim firearms guidance note.* London: BMA, 1996.

17   See, for example: Forrest D, Hinshelwood G, Peel M. The physical and psychological findings following the late examination of victims of torture. *Torture* 2000;**10**(1):12–15.

18   See, for example: Bracken P, Giller J, Summerfield D. Psychological responses to war and atrocity: the limitations of current concepts. *Soc Sci Med* 1995;**40**:1073–82.

19   British Medical Association, Medical Foundation for the Care of Victims of Torture. *Asylum applicants – medical reports: guidelines for examining doctors.* London: BMA, 1993.

20   British Medical Association. *Asylum seekers: meeting their health care needs.* London: BMA, 2002.

21   Clothier C, Macdonald CA, Shaw DA. *The Allitt inquiry: independent inquiry relating to deaths and injuries on the children's ward at Grantham and Kesteven General Hospital during the period February to April 1991.* London: HMSO, 1994. For further information on pre-employment checks on NHS staff in England, see: NHS Employment Policy Branch. *Pre-employment checks for NHS staff [extract taken from HSG 98/064].* Leeds: NHS Employment Policy Branch, 2001 (under review at the time of writing). For advice in Wales, see: National Assembly for Wales. *Pre and post-employment checks for all persons working in the NHS in Wales.* Cardiff: National Assembly for Wales, 2003. (WHC (2003) 007.) In Scotland and Northern Ireland, at the time of writing, the need for guidance for pre-employment checks is under review.

22   Clothier C, *et al. The Allitt inquiry: independent inquiry relating to deaths and injuries on the children's ward at Grantham and Kesteven General Hospital during the period February to April 1991. Op cit:* pp. 128–9.

23   Data Protection Act 1998 s1.

24   Faculty of Occupational Medicine. *Guidance on the ethics of drug testing in the workplace.* London: Faculty of Occupational Medicine of the Royal College of Physicians, 1999.

25   X v The European Commission [1995] IRLR 320: 321.

26   *Ibid.*

27   Human Genetics Commission. *Inside information: balancing interests in the use of personal genetic data.* London: Department of Health, 2002:138.

28   The Disability Discrimination Act 1995 applies to England, Scotland, and Wales. Although the Act also extends to Northern Ireland, in their application to Northern Ireland the provisions of the Act in Schedule 8 have effect subject to the modifications set out in that Schedule.

29   *Government response to HGAC report on genetic testing and employment.* Letter from Lord Sainsbury and Yvette Cooper to Baroness Helena Kennedy, Chair, Human Genetics Commission. London: Department of Health, 2000.

30   Human Genetics Commission. *Inside information. Op cit:* pp. 140–2.

31   For further advice for occupational health physicians, see: Faculty of Occupational Health. *Guidance on ethics for occupational physicians.* London: Faculty of Occupational Health of the Royal College of Physicians, 1999.

32   British Medical Association. *The occupational physician.* London: BMA, 2001.
33   See: Faculty of Occupational Medicine. *Guidance on the ethics of drug testing in the workplace. Op cit.*
34   Woodroffe v British Gas [1985] unreported. The case is written up in: Kloss D. *Occupational health law.* Oxford: Blackwell Science, 1998:54.
35   British Medical Association. *Boxing packs a punch.* London: BMA, 1999.
36   Waddington I, Roderick M. Management of medical confidentiality in English professional football clubs: some ethical problems and issues. *Br J Sports Med* 2002;**36**:118–23.
37   *Ibid:* 119.
38   British Olympic Association. The British Olympic Association's position statement on athlete confidentiality. *Br J Sports Med* 2000;**34**:71–2.
39   Waddington I. Management of medical confidentiality in English professional football clubs: some ethical problems and issues. *Op cit:* p. 122.
40   General Medical Council Standards Committee, personal communication, 13 January 2000.
41   World Medical Association. *Declaration on principles of health care for sports medicine.* Geneva: WMA, 1999.
42   British Medical Association. *Doctors' assistance to sports clubs and sporting events.* London: BMA, 2001.
43   General Medical Council. *Providing advice and medical services on-line or by telephone.* London: GMC, 1998. See also Health on the Net Foundation. *Code of conduct for medical and health websites.* http://www.hon.ch/HONcode (accessed 4 May 2003).
44   General Medical Council. *Good medical practice. Op cit:* para 58.
45   *Ibid.*
46   National Health Service (General Medical Services) Regulations 1992 (SI 1992 No. 635): schedule 2, para 38.

17: Doctors working in custodial settings

The questions covered in this chapter include the following.

- Do doctors' ethical obligations differ significantly in custodial settings?
- Can detainees refuse essential medical treatment?
- Can detainees make advance refusals, including when on hunger strike?
- What rights to confidentiality do detainees have?
- Do different rules about consent apply if the detainee is a minor or has a history of mental illness?
- Is it acceptable for health professionals to be involved in sedating asylum seekers to facilitate deportation?

Duties in custodial settings

Chapter 16 discussed fundamental aspects of dual loyalties and this chapter considers how divided loyalties can be problematic in custodial settings. There are six sections, the first two of which look at the principles and problems common to any form of custodial setting. We then discuss the specific ethical issues that arise in four categories of custodial setting: prisons, young offender institutions, detention centres for asylum seekers, and police stations. Attention is also given briefly to alternatives to custody.

In all of these situations, doctors have a normal therapeutic role and ethical obligations to the people they see. They also have some obligations to other parties, including employers, non-medical colleagues, and the public. The institutions in which they work are concerned with public security, law enforcement, and the containment of inmates, although they also have clear responsibilities for detainees' welfare. For many of the practical problems raised in this chapter, guidance has already been developed and we point out where guidelines designed for one specific setting have wider utility.

General principles

In custodial settings, the following principles are important. All health professionals must:

- remember their duty of care for individuals even when health assessments occur for other purposes than the provision of treatment (such as for forensic purposes)
- do their best to ensure that health care is of a comparable standard to that provided in the community

- ensure that they are able to act with clinical independence in their referral and prescribing decisions
- facilitate good cooperation and communication between all members of the health team and try to ensure continuity of care
- observe the duty to provide information to patients about treatment options
- be continually aware of the obligation to respect detainees' human rights and sensitive to the ways in which those rights can be compromised
- seek informed consent, even if the law does not oblige consent to be provided (such as intimate body searches)
- observe the ethical duty of confidentiality – patients should be aware at the time they provide information if it will be used other than for their care and they should know what those purposes are likely to be
- preplan the appropriate use of restraint – restraint should be the minimum necessary to ensure the safety of all, including the patient; staff should have training in conflict avoidance and safe methods of restraint
- monitor and speak out when services are inadequate or pose a potential threat to health
- audit their own expertise and know their limitations.

General issues of consent, confidentiality, and choice

There should be no need for separate codes of medical ethics specifically for use in custodial institutions since the general principles that apply in custodial settings are the same as those underpinning all other situations. In all interventions, doctors should seek consent if the patient is competent. All patients are owed a duty of confidentiality, but this is never an absolute duty. It is particularly limited in relation to forensic examinations (see the discussion of confidentiality in relation to police surgeons on pages 641–2). Situations arise in all healthcare settings in which other considerations override the individual patient's rights, but this should be discussed with patients in advance of any disclosure. Good communication with patients and with colleagues is clearly also a key requisite in all healthcare settings. All health professionals have duties to draw attention to inadequacies in the service that pose a hazard to health and so need to be wary of employment contracts that seek to limit their ability to do so. (BMA members can obtain advice on this from BMA regional offices.) Doctors working in institutions have a duty to ensure that treatment guidelines are observed and any signs of neglect or maltreatment are properly investigated. Normally, these issues can be raised through a monitoring and complaints system. Internal procedures for reporting suspicions should be followed, but if health professionals are unable to obtain a satisfactory answer through such mechanisms, they need to consider other action. This is often a very difficult and isolating decision in which health professionals can expect support from professional bodies such as the BMA.

Some practical differences exist between the provision of health care in the community and custodial health care. In the latter situation, patients are more vulnerable because they have fewer choices and it may be difficult for them to complain effectively. They are more marginalised. The media and the public are often uninterested in their treatment or unsympathetic to their plight. Aspects of their autonomy are lost. In the past, health services for this population have been significantly underresourced, which has also often affected the efficacy and morale of treatment providers.

In 2003, helpful guidance on best practice was published by the Department of Health.[1] Although designed to cover the provision of primary care services in prison, much of this guidance is equally applicable to doctors working in other places of detention. One of its key points is that normal ethical standards apply to doctors working in such settings and practical examples of good practice are provided.

Seeking consent

In terms of consenting to treatment or refusing it, the same general rules apply as in the community. Adult detainees can accept or refuse as long as they are competent and informed of the implications (unless compulsory treatment is required under mental health legislation; see Chapter 3, pages 123–6). Minors can also consent if they are competent and informed. If aged over 16, they are assumed to be competent to decide unless there is evidence to the contrary. Alternatively, consent can be provided on their behalf by someone with parental responsibility. In relation to young people who are detained, a local authority, court appointed proxy or authorised person with an emergency protection order may have been awarded parental responsibility, in addition to parents. The fact of detention in custody does not in itself remove the ability of parents to consent to treatment on behalf of their children (see Chapter 4 for the general rules for treatment of minors). In 2002, detailed guidance was issued on consent in custody, the main points of which are summarised below.[2]

Summary of guidance on patient consent

- Respecting people's rights to determine what happens to their own bodies is a fundamental part of good practice.
- Valid consent requires the individual to be competent, informed and not under duress.
- Adults should be assumed to be competent unless the opposite is proved. Special effort may be needed to explain treatment decisions to people with learning disabilities.
- Competent minors can consent to treatment, but may have less option to refuse it.
- Seeking consent is a process. Detainees must be aware that they can change their minds.
- Verbal consent is as valid as written consent, but it is good practice to have consent forms for treatments that are complex or involve significant risk or side effects.
- Competent adults can refuse any treatment and cannot be treated against their will unless they fall within the remit of compulsory mental health treatment.

In prisons, all inmates, including those held on remand, are routinely asked to undergo a medical examination on reception into custody. International guidelines emphasise the importance of undertaking this examination within 24 hours of the prisoner's arrival.[3] This is intended primarily to identify symptoms of physical illness, communicable conditions, mental illness, or suicide risk, and to ensure that prisoners continue to receive medication previously prescribed. The fact that this has generally been an automatic and routine procedure does not mean that properly informed consent can be forgone. If detainees refuse to be examined, their refusal is respected and recorded unless it is judged that the patient is likely to have a mental illness. When this is the case, assessment under mental health legislation can be carried out (see Chapter 3, pages 123–6).

Respecting refusal

Individuals who are informed and able to understand the implications of their choice cannot be treated against their will (except under mental health legislation). They can refuse contemporaneously or in advance of losing their mental capacity.

It follows from what has been said above that prisoners can refuse medication if they are competent and understand the implications. The Department of Health consent guidance emphasises that prisoners should not be pressured into accepting treatment by, for example, implying that a refusal could affect their privileges or remission of sentence.[4] As in other areas of medical practice, seeking consent and explaining the implications of medication in an unbiased way are important. Wherever possible, patients should be given opportunities to be cooperatively involved in treatment. Occasionally, doctors have expressed concern to the BMA that the prevailing culture in certain prisons results in some prisoners not receiving an appropriate explanation that they can refuse referral, examination, or treatment in situations in which it is not a question of treatment under mental health legislation. In particular, paedophiles, other sex offenders, and prisoners with a history of violent behaviour need to be as aware as other patients when they have a choice about being referred for treatment. This can be difficult for doctors because obviously some patients prefer to avoid confronting their past behaviour, but are under some unavoidable pressure to accept treatment for it because parole is considered only on the basis of the patient being perceived as no longer a risk to others. Implicitly, therefore, there is pressure on patients to accept treatment in order to be eligible for early release. Generally, prisoners are well aware of this, but it is important that doctors do not contribute to the pressure by directly or indirectly implying that referral does not require patient consent.

Scope and limits of prisoners' choice

W was a high security prisoner, convicted of murder in 2000. He was judged to have a psychopathic disorder and was initially sent to Broadmoor Special Hospital, where doctors found him impossible to treat because of his aggressive behaviour. After being transferred to a prison segregation unit,

(Continued)

however, he began to mutilate his right leg in protest as he believed he was denied his rights to be treated in a special hospital. He said that he wished to receive mental health care, but not treatment for his leg and that he was willing to die if kept in the prison unit. He was told that continuing to mutilate his leg would result in blood poisoning, septicaemia, and death. In April 2002, the High Court ruled that W had the mental capacity to decide whether or not to accept medical treatment for his leg. The judge was satisfied that W understood he would die if he continued his protest and refused medical help for the leg. She upheld his right to refuse and also made clear that transfer to a mental health unit would be dependent upon his doctors' recommendation, rather than his own choice or that of the Prison Service. The judge also drew comparisons with prisoners' suicide attempts by hanging when they had made a clear advance refusal of resuscitation. In such cases, the judge said that prison authorities could risk litigation against them if they resuscitated a prisoner against his or her express wish.

Re W (adult: refusal of treatment)[5]

Advance refusal and suicide attempts

In the legal case described above, attention was drawn by the judge to the theoretical possibility of a person attempting suicide after having made a clear and informed advance refusal of resuscitation. The dilemmas arising in such a circumstance are discussed in detail in Chapter 15 (page 541), but they are also particularly pertinent to the custodial setting. Enormous efforts have been made to reduce the level of self harm and suicide in custody and so health professionals find it counterintuitive and contrary to their training to refrain from all lifesaving efforts when suicide is attempted. In the BMA's opinion, a distinction can be drawn between a demonstrably well reasoned, sustained, informed, and documented advance refusal of treatment made by a fully competent person and a refusal for which there is no clear evidence of such validity. In the case of W, there were opportunities to discuss with him the implications of his choice and assess his ability to make it. This is not the case with most attempted suicides, where doctors lack firm evidence of whether or not the individual was in a disturbed or a reasonable frame of mind when initiating the attempt. In any case of doubt and when there is a possibility of reviving the person, the BMA strongly recommends that resuscitation be attempted.

Assessment of capacity

In order to make a valid refusal contemporaneously or to cover future treatment, prisoners must be mentally competent. Doctors may need to carry out an assessment.

- When prisoners are highly disturbed or violent, it may be impossible to assess their capacity. If there are some indicators of incapacity, doctors should assume incapacity until such time as a proper assessment can be carried out.

- Doctors are accountable for their decisions and so must be able to justify the evidence for these decisions.
- Most people, including those with a learning disability, can make some decisions validly.
- When prisoners have a serious mental disorder warranting compulsory treatment under mental health legislation, they must be transferred out of prison as soon as possible.
- Prisoners who lack capacity can be treated according to the "best interests" criteria, which is a broad term that includes their own likely wishes. They cannot be given treatment for which they have made a valid advance refusal, unless it is compulsory treatment under mental health legislation.
- In order to assess the patient's best interests, doctors should review the patient's history and seek views from colleagues who know the person, including prison officers, other healthcare staff, and probation officers, but they should also bear in mind the duty of confidentiality to the patient.
- People who are close to the patient may also have helpful views and, in Scotland, any proxy appointed for an incapacitated person should be consulted (see Chapter 3, pages 110–3).
- Monitoring is required so that, if the patient regains capacity at any point in the treatment, consent to continue it can be discussed.[6]

The BMA and the Law Society have issued detailed guidance on assessing mental capacity.[7]

Respecting confidentiality

All detainees have rights of confidentiality, but in some cases these are limited and disclosure without consent may be required by statute or by a court. The general principles concerning confidentiality and disclosure in the public interest, as well as the relevant legislation, are discussed in detail in Chapter 5. Individuals should be made aware of the foreseeable use of their information when they provide it. Helpful general information that is relevant to custodial settings is available.[8] Although primarily designed for use in the prison system in England and Wales, the guidance could be helpful in other similar contexts. In particular, it stresses the importance of appropriate interagency information sharing with the individual's consent and according to locally agreed protocols. The prison services in Scotland, England, Wales, and Northern Ireland have moved towards a system of keeping multidisciplinary healthcare records, which are accessible to all members of the healthcare team. This facilitates good communication between professional groups. Detainees have rights of access to their own medical records so that they can see what information may be shared among those who are treating them. Ensuring continuity of care after release is emphasised in the guidance and this is particularly important for people with mental health problems.

Achieving a good balance between detainees' confidentiality and the legitimate security interests of the institution can sometimes be problematic. The fundamental presumption, however, should be that detainees see health personnel out of earshot and sight of other people. In some cases, however, the risk assessment process indicates the advisability of using a chaperone or arranging other supervision (see also page 639). All non-medical staff should have contractual obligations to maintain confidentiality. Nevertheless, when detainees attend hospital appointments outside the detention centre or prison, wherever possible accompanying staff should not be in a position to overhear the consultation. Details of treatment can be passed between the hospital and prison medical team via the accompanying staff, but must be in sealed envelopes.

One of the issues raised by doctors with the BMA and with the medical defence bodies is the question of confidentiality in cases where a patient apparently confesses to previous crimes or denounces other people during counselling or therapy sessions. Ideally, patients should be aware in advance that absolute confidentiality cannot be guaranteed in all circumstances, and that doctors have a duty to consider the public interest and the interests of justice as well as the confidentiality owed to patients. Where information could prevent serious harm or injustice or solve a serious crime, it is clearly important to bring it to the attention of the police or other professionals able to act upon it. More difficult to assess are cases where the information is unverifiable or likely to be unreliable. Professional judgment is required to assess such statements. In some cases, the individual may be deluded or deliberately seeking to mislead or wrongly incriminate others. It is helpful to collect details and clarify inconsistencies. Nevertheless, doctors are not able to investigate such claims and need to bring allegations of substance to the attention of the relevant authorities. This, and general issues of disclosure in the public interest, are discussed in Chapter 5.

Doctors who work in custodial facilities are sometimes faced with a conflict between maintaining patients' confidentiality and the obligation to assist in ensuring the safe and proper management of the institution. When governors or managers need information in order to protect the security or safety of inmates, doctors have an obligation to divulge it. Nevertheless, disclosure of personal health information should be made only on the strictest "need to know" basis unless, for example, the patient requests disclosure to a solicitor or other advocate. Doctors working in prisons must be able to keep independent confidential records. In the course of their duties doctors may make written or verbal reports to courts, adjudication boards, prison governors, or other authorities. Prisoners should be told when there is an obligation to pass medical information to other people and its purpose. On transfer from police to prison custody, patient information provided by a police surgeon should be made available only to the prison health team and transferred immediately to the prison medical record. It is not acceptable for medical details to be included in the prisoner's main prison record, with the exception of opinions about the prisoner's fitness for work or matters directly affecting a prisoner's management by prison staff.

Translation and interpretation

Detainees are a diverse population and some immigration detainees are held in the mainstream prison system (although this is not generally an appropriate setting for them and they are increasingly being transferred to immigration detention centres). The need for competent and independent interpretation and translation in custodial settings is well recognised. In 1997 an agreement was drawn up by a wide range of organisations forming the Trials Issues Group, on arrangements for interpreters within the criminal justice system in England and Wales.[9] The agreement has subsequently been revised and provides minimum measurable standards for interpreters in this context. It recommends the use of interpreters from the National Register of Public Service Interpreters. In Scotland, there is no national register, but proficiency standards have been set for interpreters working in courts and guidance about interpreters is available from the Crown Office and Procurator Fiscal Service.[10] In addition, the Association of Chief Police Officers has published guidance for the police, emphasising, for example, that the interpreter attending a court appearance should not be the same interpreter who previously assisted police enquiries in that case. In all cases, contractors must make the confidentiality requirements clear to all employees, including interpreters and translators of medical records. Other detainees should not be asked to act as translators; to do so would completely undermine the notion of medical confidentiality and could give other detainees information that could be misused about the particular vulnerabilities or anxieties of the patient.

Choice of doctor

People who are detained in police stations have the right to request examination by their own doctor, at their own expense. The BMA's General Practitioners Committee advises that, if the patient has a routine complaint and the station is within the area of the GP's practice, the GP should attend. If the police initiate a medical assessment or if the patient has been injured, or claims to have been injured, while in custody, then the examination should be carried out by a police surgeon.

Individuals held on remand also have a right to consult a doctor or dentist of their own choice, although this appears to be rarely exercised. Consultations should be arranged through the individual's solicitor and with the assistance of the prison doctor. Although the doctor or dentist of the individual's choice can make recommendations regarding treatment, the final decision about the treatment offered rests with the prison doctor or dentist. A frequent question to the BMA on this issue concerns whether GPs who have no connection with prisons are obliged to attend remand prisoners who are on their list and who request a visit. Obviously much depends on the location, which may be far from the practice. Also, opinions differ about the extent of the legal and ethical obligations in such cases and so the situation remains unclear. GPs need to look at the factors in the individual case and if, for example, the circumstances are such that the doctor would normally carry out a home visit and the remand centre is within the practice area, there are grounds for arguing that either the GP or the GP's out of hours service should respond to such a request. Legally, convicted prisoners have no freedom of choice regarding the doctor they see, but in practice if a request is made for a consultation with a prisoner's own doctor, and the doctor is willing to attend, it would be very unusual for this to be refused.

Practical problems common to various detention settings

Although all doctors have to juggle their various responsibilities to patients, patients' relatives, and the community, particular dilemmas arise when dual loyalties are in sharp focus and are an integral feature of daily work. In custodial settings, doctors can find that their ethical duties towards their patients involve a different mindset to that of colleagues whose main focus is on the management and control of detained people. All staff need to work cooperatively to promote an orderly environment, but doctors must also ensure that their patients' rights are respected with regard to confidentiality and self determination on questions of medical treatment.

Doctors working in various custodial settings are often dealing with a transient population of patients who have pre-existing health problems. People detained under the criminal justice system are not generally a healthy population prior to their detention. Many are not registered with a doctor or dentist and a high proportion come from socially excluded sections of the community. Some detainees do not live in one place long enough for all their health problems to be effectively addressed, and ensuring aftercare can be difficult. Health professionals also need to be highly aware of cultural diversity in their patient population and to be knowledgeable about any special laws applicable to the health care of detainees.

In custodial situations, health teams can come under exceptional stress. They can face a particularly difficult task in maintaining trust with patients owing to tensions resulting from reduced patient autonomy. They may also need greater peer support than other doctors because of the complexity of their case load. In places of detention, they may be faced with fatalities resulting from suicide, hunger strike, or other deaths in custody. Despite having followed good practice guidance, health professionals cannot always predict and forestall distressing cases of self harm.

Suicides in prison

In March 2002, fatal accident inquiries were held concerning two deaths at Corton Vale Prison in Scotland.[11] There was considerable discussion of the efficacy of the suicide risk management strategy in the prison because, between April 1995 and October 2001, 10 women at Corton Vale had taken their own lives by hanging. These included Michelle McElver and Frances Carvill.

(Continued)

In respect of the most recent deaths, however, the sheriff concluded that the risk assessments had been carried out appropriately and society had to accept that not all suicides were preventable. One of these prisoners, Michelle McElver, had been admitted to jail late on 23 October 2001 and assessed as not a suicide risk. She was experiencing heroin withdrawal symptoms and was given medication for these as well as being assessed independently by a doctor and a nurse. By 5 p.m. on 24 October, however, she was found dead, hanging by her shoelaces on a hook in the bathroom after a visit to the nurse. The sheriff was satisfied that the assessments of risk had been carried out appropriately and there was no obvious way in which the death could have been avoided. In the same prison, two days later, another woman, Frances Carvill, who had a history of self harm, hanged herself from the bars at the bathroom window and died in hospital on 29 October. In these troubling cases, there was no criticism of the health professionals but rather a recognition by the sheriff that such cases raised hugely difficult issues of patient management, in which it would always be difficult to strike the right balance.[12]

While seeking to promote a good doctor–patient relationship, doctors have here a challenging patient group, some of whom regard them with suspicion (although this is by no means inevitable). Some asylum seekers, for example, have had little previous interaction with health professionals or may associate doctors with previous bad experiences at the hands of the authorities in their country of origin. Health teams looking after them may have to deal with distressing accounts of torture or other trauma and need to be aware of their own need for support.

Ensuring good communication with patients

Good communication depends on trust, but also on health professionals having sufficient time to explain about patients' rights to confidentiality and choice. Lack of time in some institutions is one of the problems doctors raise with the BMA; this has also been noted by the Chief Inspector of Prisons.[13] Guidance on maintaining trust is included in *Good medical practice for doctors providing primary care services in prison.*[14] This draws attention to the risks of detainees becoming institutionalised in their approach to life and seeing doctors as another authority figure. The additional tension in the relationship resulting from this, and from the patient's reduced autonomy, is something doctors need to consider.

Ensuring good communication with other health professionals

It is important that health professionals working in custodial settings should maintain good contact with colleagues in the community and keep aware of any changes in best practice in the community, so as to avoid professional isolation and to facilitate continuity of care of individuals. A severe problem faced by doctors working in custodial settings, however, concerns that of contacting previous treatment providers and obtaining accurate medical information about an individual's previous history. The health team often has to rely initially upon information provided by patients when they come into detention, which may be inaccurate or incomplete. Transfer of health records between prisons has also been problematic at times and hampers continuity of care. Detainees have a right to withhold medical details but often problems arise from confusion. Some do not know details of their medical history, having not had regular contact with the health service. Some detainees are suspicious of the purposes for which information is required or are not convinced that it will be kept confidential. When they have been registered with a GP, prisoners should be asked to provide details and to allow the health team to contact that doctor to obtain confirmation of the medical history. If they have been previously assessed by a police surgeon, that assessment should be made available to the prison health team. The importance of such liaison cannot be overemphasised.

The importance of good communication

At a fatal accident inquiry in Glasgow in 1999, the sheriff drew particular attention to the need for any report made by a police surgeon while an individual is in police custody to be made promptly available to those subsequently responsible for the individual's care. In this case, a 21-year-old man who had previously been assessed by a police surgeon later died by hanging in Barlinnie Prison. In Scotland, the legislation requires the sheriff to consider whether such deaths could have been avoided and whether any defects in the system of working contributed to the death.[15] As part of his duty to identify defects in the system, the sheriff highlighted the importance of good communication in respect of individuals going through the custodial system. He recommended that "if a police surgeon's report is prepared when an accused is in police custody, a copy of that report should accompany the accused if he/she is committed to prison".[16]

In Northern Ireland, the 2002 review of prison health care identified difficulties in ensuring access to past GP records, partly due to problems in obtaining informed patient consent. Prisoners were sometimes either "deliberately or unintentionally vague about their present state of health other than to insist that they have been prescribed high dosages of various drugs".[17] The BMA agreed that promoting exchange of health information in both directions – from GPs on prisoners' admission to detention and back to GPs on prisoners' release – was the single most important recommendation of the prison review.[18] Subsequently, the Northern Ireland Prison Service Management Board agreed to set in place arrangements to ensure a better two-way flow of information.[19] Clearly, in such cases detainees need to be made aware that liaison with their past doctor is essential in determining currently appropriate medication.

In the past in England and Wales, prison health care did not come under the auspices of the NHS and some GPs requested fees before agreeing to supply a report about a patient's past health to the doctor providing prison medical care. Negotiation about fees sometimes delayed the delivery of reports. Some doctors working in prisons said that they were also being asked to pay a fee simply to have access to information in a prisoner's GP medical record, although this did not involve preparing a report. As a general point, however, NHS bodies should not normally charge each other and certainly information needed for the purposes of continuing patient care should not be delayed. Therefore, although there was some uncertainty initially about whether a fee could legally be charged, as the provision of health care started to come directly under the umbrella of the NHS, the BMA's advice was that demanding a fee was inadvisable. Doctors working in the prison health service were increasingly employed directly by primary care trusts, which meant that a community GP requiring a fee would effectively be creating a situation whereby one NHS practitioner was asking another for a fee as part of patient care. When a special report is needed for non-clinical reasons, such as for a parole meeting, however, some delay may be unavoidable for a full review to be carried out of the patient's notes. This may involve a fee.

GPs also reported delays in receiving medical information from the prison health team after the prisoner's release. The BMA believes that there is an ethical duty for doctors promptly to provide clinical information, such as a disease and drug summary, with the patient's consent. In emergencies, information should be provided by telephone. Prompt liaison is particularly significant when a detainee suffers from a psychiatric illness and information about past medication needs to be available to current health staff.

Ensuring access to appropriate care

All detainees are entitled to a standard of medical and nursing care commensurate with what is available in the community at large. This includes prompt access not only to primary care services but also to psychiatric services, physiotherapy, rehabilitation services, and appropriate diets.

Right to a range of medical care

All detainees, regardless of the reason for their detention, should have a clear right to a medical examination and access to a doctor when necessary. In 2003 the European Committee for the Prevention of Torture and Inhuman or Degrading Treatment or Punishment (CPT) pointed out that the UK's Anti-Terrorism, Crime and Security Act 2001 made no mention of the right of access to a doctor or lawyer.[20] In the aftermath of the terrorist attacks of 11 September 2001 in the USA, the UK had enacted this legislation to allow the indefinite detention of

(Continued)

foreigners believed to pose a risk to national security. Such detainees need not be charged with any criminal offence, nor is it a requirement that they even be suspected of a specific offence. At the time of the CPT visit to the UK in February 2002, eight people were detained under this legislation and they had indeed been promptly screened by health staff and medically examined after admission to prison. Therefore, despite what the CPT saw as a deficit in the legislation regarding prompt examination, it judged that, in practice, access to a doctor on admission for this group of detainees was satisfactory. Nevertheless, the CPT reported that the detainees had complained about subsequent delays in being able to see a doctor and that the treatment they had been receiving prior to their arrest was discontinued in prison. The CPT noted that some of the detainees had previously been tortured in other countries and two of them had been diagnosed as suffering from post-traumatic stress disorder. One prisoner had a psychiatric history that included inpatient treatment and suicide attempts. The CPT stressed the importance of psychological and possibly psychiatric support being routinely available for such detainees. In its response, the Government refuted the allegation that access to a doctor had been delayed in these cases and emphasised the availability of a wide range of multidisciplinary skills.[21] It agreed that the special needs of any prisoner should always be taken into account by prison health teams.

All healthcare resources are rationed in some way, but detainees should not be subjected to lower levels of care. Health professionals have an obligation to draw attention to poor quality care. Under the Human Rights Act 1998,[22] everyone has the same rights set out in the European Convention on Human Rights, such as the right to life (Article 2). The state is under a positive obligation to take adequate measures to protect life and thus Article 2 may be engaged if medical treatment were so deficient as to put detainees' lives at risk. Similarly, Article 3 (prohibition of torture and of inhuman or degrading treatment or punishment) could be invoked if there is a failure to provide proper treatment. Also, Article 14 (freedom from discrimination in respect of Convention rights) could be relevant if detainees receive treatment that is inferior to that provided to other sectors of society and Articles 2 or 3 are invoked. In some cases, it is possible that detainees who may otherwise be deported but need continuing medical care can claim this under human rights legislation.

Claim to treatment under human rights legislation

D was born and spent most of his life in St Kitts. On arrival in the UK in 1993, seeking permission to enter for two weeks, he was found to be in possession of a substantial quantity of cocaine and was sentenced to six years' imprisonment. While in prison D was found to be HIV positive and developed AIDS for which he was receiving medical treatment. On his release on licence, D applied to remain in the UK on compassionate grounds, so that he could continue to receive the level of medical care he needed. This request was turned down and he took his case to the European Court of Human Rights.

(Continued)

> D's solicitor argued that D's removal to St Kitts would entail the loss of the medical treatment he was currently receiving, thereby shortening his life expectancy. Furthermore, such action would condemn him to spend the rest of his remaining days in pain and suffering in conditions of isolation, squalor, and destitution. The court held that, although it could not be said that the conditions that would confront him in the receiving country were themselves a breach of the standards of Article 3, D's removal to St Kitts would expose him to a real risk of dying under most distressing circumstances and would thus amount to inhuman treatment in violation of Article 3.
>
> *D v United Kingdom*[23]

Limited resources can result in pressure on doctors not to refer patients outside the institution for treatment owing to the cost of accompanying guards. In the 1980s and 1990s, the BMA saw an increase in enquiries and complaints from doctors working with prisoners and asylum detainees who were worried about the impact of this on patients. Another similar problem has involved last minute cancellation of outpatient appointments because of a lack of escorts. This disadvantages detained patients, wastes NHS resources, and is preventable. Some cases reported by doctors to the BMA involved conflicts with prison governors who were looking at measures to cut costs. Recruitment of prison managers with an NHS background should help to deal with disputes about the use of resources in relation to health care. In the meantime, doctors cannot ignore the cost implications of their recommendations but, by measures such as regular audit of their own referral and prescribing practice, should be able to demonstrate that their practice reflects the standards applied in the community. Their referral rates should be comparable with those in society at large for similar medical conditions.

The fact that detainees are entitled to a similar standard of care as is available in the community does not mean that they have a right to every possible medical intervention. Clearly, it would be inappropriate for prisoners to have special access to interventions that are unavailable or very scarce for others in society. An unusual example of this was the legal judgment in the case of convicted murderer Gavin Mellor, who requested assisted reproduction as part of his claimed right to have a family under Article 12 of the European Convention on Human Rights.[24] Mellor's imprisonment made it impossible for his wife to conceive his child naturally, but his application for fertility treatment was refused. The judge made clear that it was for the Secretary of State to formulate a policy for dealing with such requests by prisoners and to decide particular cases. The case is discussed in detail in Chapter 8 (pages 270–1).

Minimising harm

Assessment of potential for self harm

Assessing each detainee's risk of suicide or other self harm is a key part of the role of health professionals. In England, in 1999, the NHS national service framework for mental health set strategies for reducing suicide rates in the community by one fifth by 2010 and also called on local health and social care organisations to support prison staff in preventing suicides in prisons.[25] Screening procedures during reception are intended to identify potentially self harming prisoners and meet their individual needs. In the case of prisons, data show that people serving life sentences are at high risk of suicide during detention,[26] but the Howard League for Penal Reform has also drawn particular attention to the risk of suicide and self harm after the release of people who have served only short sentences. The League claims that over 50 people each year kill themselves shortly after release from prison, due in part to the lack of preparation for release and post-release support that is provided for those who serve long sentences.[27] In 2003, after carrying out a 6 month study, the Howard League also reported that the level of self harm in jail was substantially higher than had been previously thought.[28] The report claimed that 1 in 10 women, 1 in 20 minors, and roughly 1 in 40 male prisoners harmed themselves by cutting, burning, biting, or strangulation. It recommended more training for prison staff, wider use of materials published by the National Self-Harm Network, and more effort to involve inmates' families. In its response, the Home Office agreed with the figures put forward by the Howard League, but said that the apparent increase in self harm was due to more rigorous reporting of such incidents.[29]

In 2001, the Prison Service in England and Wales had piloted a number of schemes as part of a suicide prevention strategy that involved trained suicide prevention coordinators and risk assessment tools.[30] In 2002, standards for suicide and self harm prevention were issued, emphasising the provision of special training for all staff, support activities to be offered, and case conferences.[31] In Northern Ireland, too, the need for enhanced psychology services as part of suicide prevention strategies and to address the needs of sex offenders has been well recognised,[32] but the service has had recruitment problems. As with the recruitment of other healthcare personnel into the Northern Ireland prison service, lack of career opportunities, professional isolation, and dissatisfaction with remuneration has hampered the provision of appropriate services. This also meant that, to the concern of doctors and psychiatrists, group therapy replaced any option for individual counselling sessions. A shortage of multidisciplinary teams, and poor coordination and information sharing between professional disciplines have also posed problems.

Measures to provide emergency attention

A crisis card scheme was introduced at Moorland Prison whereby inmates with mental health problems could have access to a mental health professional within 30 minutes, day or night. Prisoners who have been assessed as likely to benefit from the reassurance provided by immediate access are issued with a card, which, if they feel they are in crisis, they can show to prison officers, who will call the health team. Prison officers know which inmates have a card but no other details of prisoners' health status.[33]

(Continued)

Prisoners trained by the Samaritans to act as listeners and to support other prisoners who are at risk of self harm are perceived to be an extremely valuable resource, highly appreciated by both staff and detainees. They provide essential human contact and a sounding board for fellow prisoners. According to the Howard League for Penal Reform, trained listeners are one of the best defences against suicide and self injury, especially when there is also provision of special rooms for use by listeners where efforts are made to create a more relaxed atmosphere than in normal cells.[34]

Prompt assistance should be available in advance, both during and after a crisis. Healthcare teams need to have training in recognising and dealing with self harming behaviour. Very detailed strategies have been developed in institutions around the UK to reduce the occurrence of self harm. Comprehensive guidance is available from a range of organisations, including the Howard League for Penal Reform; some very basic steps were outlined in 2002 by the Chief Inspector of Prisons.

Summary of steps for the prevention of self harm outlined by the Chief Inspector of Prisons

- All reasonable steps must be taken to establish an environment to protect against self harm.
- While bearing in mind detainees' right to confidentiality and respect for their dignity, essential information about prisoners who are at risk of self harm should be effectively communicated by those who hold it to those who need it and integrated into a support plan.
- Prisoners should be enabled to access help promptly in times of crisis.
- Raising detainees' self esteem should be part of the establishment's culture.[35]

Auditing and monitoring medication

Prescribing practice has been very variable in institutions. A study in 1997, for example, found that while one prison had two thirds of its population on benzodiazepine tranquillisers or hypnotics, others operated policies of non-provision of such drugs except for withdrawal and were successful in reducing patient dependence.[36] Obviously, medication should not be used simply as a means of control, nor should prescriptions be routinely renewed without proper assessment. Within institutions, medication that is not directly administered or supervised by health professionals can become a valuable commodity to be traded among detainees. In 2001, for example, the Chief Inspector of Prisons emphasised the importance of separating detainees who are undergoing detoxification from the general population of the institution because they were likely to be subject to bullying or pressure to surrender their medication to other inmates.[37] In Northern Ireland and Scotland, regional drugs and therapeutics committees have a lead role in introducing and implementing policies regarding the use of prescribed medicines that are liable to be abused.[38] Part of the prison health work programme outlined in England and Wales in 2003 was an analysis of the provision of pharmacy services to identify good models of future delivery and provide pharmaceutical advice.[39]

Communicable diseases

Healthcare services in custodial settings should ensure that information about transmittable diseases (hepatitis and dermatological infections, as well as HIV) is available to detainees, who need to be aware of preventive strategies as part of general information to improve their health. In England and Wales, the *Prison health handbook* contains details of key contacts for the national control of communicable diseases and the development of harm minimisation measures. One aim of such measures is to reduce the risks to prisoners, their families, and the wider community from bloodborne diseases such as hepatitis B and C, and HIV.[40] The handbook also gives advice on vaccination in prison for certain communicable diseases, including influenza, and on the diagnosis and treatment of tuberculosis.

The provision of condoms in prison to reduce the transmission of sexually transmitted infections has long been a matter of debate. Since 1988, the BMA's policy has been that condoms and health education, including information about HIV infection, should be freely available in prisons. In 1993 the World Health Organization recommended that "since penetrative intercourse occurs in prisons, even when prohibited, condoms should be made available to prisoners throughout their period of detention".[41] Subsequently, the Director of Prison Health Care in England and Wales wrote to doctors working in prisons, encouraging them to prescribe condoms and lubricants to individual prisoners who were thought to be at risk of HIV infection through sexual behaviour. The letter drew attention to the possibility of doctors being seen as in breach of their duty of care if condoms were not provided when appropriate, and also emphasised that homosexual acts between consenting adult prisoners were not necessarily unlawful. In 1997, however, the BMA Foundation for AIDS finalised a survey which indicated that, although there was general awareness among doctors about the option of prescribing condoms, informing prisoners at risk was sometimes problematic.[42] Some establishments, for example, did not publicise condom availability but relied on prisoners disclosing their risky behaviour to the health team. The survey also reflected the continuing stigma attached to homosexual activity within the macho culture of prisons, which meant that condoms were often routinely provided only to prisoners who were going home. Some doctors said that they did not know of any inmate at risk and so did not see a need to prescribe condoms, or they believed that such prescribing would be seen as "condoning homosexuality", although the Director's letter had made clear that sexual behaviour involving adult prisoners was not automatically unlawful. Some prison staff appeared to regard condoms as contraband that prisoners were not allowed to possess. In some cases, prison management agreed to condom provision in principle, but refused to meet the cost. In young offender institutions, some doctors thought that the fact that inmates were aged under 18 meant that condom provision would be inappropriate. The main conclusions of the survey were that most doctors working in English and Welsh prisons had taken some steps to implement the Director's guidance on condom provision, but there was still great variation in how it was interpreted.

The BMA has also long argued for effective measures to minimise risky needle sharing among detained individuals, given that illegal drug use appears impossible to eliminate completely.[43] Common arguments against the provision of needle exchange are that it may appear to endorse illegal activity, encourages drug use, or increases the risk of needles being used as weapons. In the BMA's view, however, such fears are not necessarily borne out in practice. Therefore, while recognising the drawbacks of needle exchange programmes, the Association has supported the concept of pilot schemes as part of broader strategies of education and risk reduction. At the time of writing in 2003, needle exchange is not available in UK prisons, although the policy is under review. The BMA also considers it important to make available to detainees guidance about decontaminating injection equipment. Sterilising or cleansing tablets to clean injecting equipment and information about how to use them are available in many prisons. They have been freely available in all Scottish prisons, for example, since 1993 and should eventually be accessible in all prisons, although there is no definite date for this to be achieved.

Clearly, HIV positive prisoners and young people in detention need not only appropriate medication but also living conditions that allow them to benefit from it. They need to be able to take their medication at the correct time, for example, regardless of normal prison timetables and any associated dietary requirements need to be met. Interruptions to treatment need to be avoided by means of good liaison when they are transferred between prisons. Guidance for health professionals working in custodial settings generally emphasises the opportunities that detention can bring, not just to tackle existing health problems and addiction but also to engage prisoners in health promotion. Primary care providers are reminded, for example, that:

> the lifestyle of some patients and their lack of previous interaction with health care services may mean that there is an opportunity whilst they are in prison for them to be advised about and possibly engage in health promotion activity. A doctor working in prison should be aware of the opportunities to influence their patients' life style.[44]

Solitary confinement

The term "solitary confinement" implies no contact with others, although prisoners who are in individual cells should be able to socialise with others at appropriate times. The CPT has published guidance on the use of solitary confinement.[45] This states that the principle of proportionality requires that a balance be struck between the requirements of the case and the use of solitary confinement. This type of regime can have harmful consequences for the individual and, according to the CPT, can, in certain circumstances, amount to inhuman and degrading treatment. The CPT has been "particularly concerned about the placement of juveniles in conditions resembling solitary confinement" and stresses that, if they are held separately from others, they should be guaranteed appropriate opportunities for contact and outdoor exercise, as well as having access to books and other materials.[46] Yet, in the UK, young people have been routinely placed in solitary confinement. An estimated 3776 young people were placed in segregation cells between April 2000 and January 2002, of whom 976 were segregated for more than a week.[47] On the other hand, lack of privacy in a shared cell can also put pressure on detainees who may be at risk of self harm. The BMA considers that therapy or counselling should be an integral part of the care and treatment pattern for "at risk" offenders and supports the move away from solitary confinement for prisoners who are perceived to be potentially suicidal.

The medical role in restraint and control

When restraint is essential in dealing with detainees' health needs, health professionals need to be involved. If, however, restraint or control measures are invoked for the purposes of maintaining order or discipline, this should not involve health staff. The BMA has published advice on the use of restraint in institutional settings.[48] It makes clear that it should only ever be used as an act of care and control, not as punishment or a convenience. The use of restraint can result in psychological morbidity, demoralisation, and feelings of humiliation. Advice specifically to police surgeons emphasises that rapid tranquillisation should be performed only where equipment for cardiopulmonary resuscitation is present and there are trained staff to use it.[49] In prisons, the security rules set out the appropriate conditions in which restraint may be used and international guidance is available from the CPT.[50]

Summary of CPT guidelines

- The use of physical restraint against violent prisoners requires safeguards.
- Prisoners who are subjected to physical restraint should be kept under constant supervision, and the restraint should be removed at the earliest opportunity.
- Restraint should never be prolonged or applied as a punishment.
- A record should be kept of every use of restraint or force against prisoners.
- Prisoners who have been subjected to force should be examined and, if necessary, treated by a doctor as soon as possible.
- If possible, medical examination should be conducted out of sight and hearing of non-medical personnel; a note should be made of findings and this should be available to the prisoner.
- Effective inspection and complaints procedures must be in place. Prisoners should be aware of the avenues of complaint open to them.

Restraint of detainees in NHS facilities

Detainees may need treatment in NHS hospitals and other healthcare facilities. From the perspective of prison staff, hospitals are sometimes seen as the weak link in the chain of secure custody where detainees may try to give a false impression of their medical condition in order to attempt to escape. Health professionals are often unsure about whether they are entitled to ask for handcuffs to be removed during assessment and treatment, and if they can ask accompanying guards to leave the room. They should certainly do so if the method of restraint interferes with treatment or if the detained person is clearly too incapacitated either to threaten others or to abscond. The general advice given to prison staff around the UK is to comply where feasible with such requests. (Advance risk assessment procedures should have already clarified the potential threat of escape or violence.) In England and Wales, the *Prison security manual* makes it plain that physical restraints should normally be removed if health professionals request it.[51] Sometimes terminally ill patients have been handcuffed to a hospital bed when clearly unfit to escape although, again, the *Prison security manual* stipulates that restraints must not be used to attach any prisoner to furniture, fixtures, or fittings.[52] Whether or not restraint is advisable should be discussed between health professionals and the detaining authorities, and judgments made on a case by case basis. In some cases, it is unnecessary and humiliating for the detainee to be shackled and closely attended by guards. For example, restraints should be removed from pregnant women attending hospital for antenatal care and those in labour. Where there is a risk of escape or violence to others, the safeguards employed should be commensurate with the risk. Some hospitals located near to prisons have special secure areas for the treatment of detainees. The *Prison security manual*[53] sets out the rules that should be observed by all prison staff and the BMA also has very similar guidance on restraint specifically in NHS facilities.[54]

Prison Service rules on restraint in NHS facilities

The *Prison security manual* includes the following rules.[55]

- Risk assessment must be carried out prior to a prisoner going to hospital.
- Assessment determines the degree of supervision.
- Assessment includes the prisoner's condition, any medical objection to the use of restraints, nature of the prisoner's offence, security of the consulting room, and the risk of violence or hostage taking.
- When escape is unlikely, escort and bedwatch by one officer is sufficient, without restraints.
- Prison governors must establish good working relations with hospitals and agree the arrangements under which prisoners will be seen.
- Prisoners should have a single room with bathroom to avoid disruption to other patients.
- Hospitals should be informed in advance about the levels of escort and restraint envisaged, and hospital staff should have an opportunity to discuss when the use of restraint is clinically unacceptable. In those cases, prison management should consider alternative security arrangements.

(Continued)

621

In addition, Prison Service Order 1600 emphasises the following.[56]

- Force is a measure of last resort when alternatives (persuasion or negotiation) are ineffective.
- Only minimum force for the minimum amount of time to ensure safety can be used.
- There should be safe and supervised use of control and restraint techniques and equipment.
- The use of force or restraint should be justified and records kept.
- There is a requirement to seek immediate advice from health professionals when restraint is used.

Restraint in transit

Any means of restraint can be dangerous if improperly applied. Methods whose level of risk has not been thoroughly investigated should not be used. In 1998 the BMA objected to the use of CS spray in confined spaces such as police vans. It argued that there was a lack of data about the full effects of the interaction of the CS and the carrier spray, especially on people who were already taking medication. In March 2000, a report by the Police Complaints Authority noted that a third of public complaints about CS resulted from police officers squirting the spray at near pointblank range in breach of guidelines.[57] Health professionals need to speak out if they are aware of any such breaches of established guidance.

An issue raised with the BMA concerns the role of in-flight nurses and doctors who are escorting asylum seekers who have been refused residence in the UK and are deported either to the first country they passed through or their country of origin. Concerns were raised about the use of both physical and chemical restraints in situations in which a doctor and a nurse were accompanying 50–100 people at a time, with a private security organisation managing the process. In the BMA's view "the involvement of doctors in the forcible removal of refugees or illegal immigrants constitutes an inappropriate use of medical skills".[58] It supports the World Medical Association's view that health professionals should not become involved in providing medication that cannot be medically justified. In 1998 the World Medical Association resolved that doctors "cannot be compelled to participate in any punitive or judicial action involving refugees or to administer any non-medically justified diagnostic measure or treatment, such as sedatives to facilitate easy deportation from the country".[59] The BMA makes a distinction between health professionals being available to provide necessary medical attention to the passengers and being there as part of an "enforcement" procedure. It recognises that people whose appeals have been heard fairly should be returned to their first port of entry, but the BMA would be greatly concerned if it were seen to be the role of doctors to keep deportees passive.

Health professionals need to make sure that their presence is primarily to deal with complications that may arise during repatriation of deportees. Nevertheless, it can be difficult to separate necessary medical attention from the enforcement procedures. Their conditions of employment and the circumstances in which they are expected to use their skills should be made clear at the outset. They should act with the deportees' health needs foremost in their minds and keep a focus on treatment and care. The BMA also recommends that agencies involved in deportations should be informed that this is the only appropriate role of health professionals.

Management of hunger strikes

Hunger strikes are a form of protest in prisons, remand centres, and holding centres for people facing deportation. Principles for their management remain the same in each setting and involve ascertaining as far as possible the individual's wishes and intention. A broad distinction can be drawn between the protesting food refuser who wants to protest or gain some concession, but intends to survive, and the person determined to fast to death. A psychiatric assessment may be required in order to clarify a detainee's ability to make a valid refusal. Patients who appear to be suffering from depression or mental impairment should be promptly referred for appropriate treatment.

Forcible feeding

In March 2000, the High Court decided that convicted murderer, Ian Brady, could not make a valid and binding decision to starve himself to death. Brady's lawyers argued that Ashworth Hospital had exceeded its powers in tube feeding Brady against his will and attempted to obtain the court's authority to prevent further artificial feeding. Despite the fact that Brady claimed not to be suffering a mental illness and a forensic psychiatrist said his decision was a rational one, the judge was swayed by medical arguments that Brady was psychopathic and prone to need to control others. His attempts to prevent feeding were seen as part of this condition because Brady had previously employed hunger strikes as a tactic, which he claimed gave him a "massive psychological boost" in what he perceived as a battle of wills with the prison authorities.

R v (1) Dr James Donald Collins (2) Ashworth Hospital Authority, ex parte Ian Stewart Brady[60]

Doctor–patient discussion

At the start of a hunger strike, detainees should be offered a medical examination and accurate clinical information about the foreseeable effects of fasting. They need to be aware that underlying health problems are likely to come to the fore and should indicate whether they accept treatment or pain relief for these. Doctors should discuss what the patient intends and whether health staff are expected to intervene before permanent damage occurs. They must make their policy about resuscitation clear and explain the difficulties involved. Patients need to be aware that resuscitation attempts, particularly at a late stage, may not be successful and that, even when they are, residual neurological problems may persist. In the absence of such detailed advance discussion, it is likely to be difficult for health staff to judge later what the individual would want if concessions are achieved after the patient has lost mental capacity. If a significant concession is made, doctors may feel justified in intervening on the grounds that the current situation differs substantially from that envisaged by the patient when the treatment refusal was made. Where mass hunger strikes occur, detainees are often under considerable peer pressure to participate. Even when solitary hunger strikes are begun, this can be the result of certain individuals being chosen by the peer group. Medical staff must have opportunities to speak to patients privately about their decision and, if it is clear that the fast is non-voluntary, efforts should be made to remove the pressures on the detainee.

Hunger strikes and advance directives

In the 1980s, a system of advance decision making developed in Northern Ireland, enabling prisoners to make their intentions unequivocally clear at the start of a hunger strike.[61] After being told the implications of their hunger strike, prisoners completed a form specifying their intention, which could include refusal of both medical intervention and all forms of medical monitoring. Even when patients lost mental awareness, health professionals were then bound to follow these instructions. Some doctors found this documented approach useful because it appeared to clarify the patient's intention and exonerated the medical team from blame. Others saw it as a hazard for prisoners who could be inadvertently pressured to decide formally in advance before their own views of the hunger strike were clear. As with any form of advance directive, there is a risk that patients want to change their mind later, which, of course, they are entitled to do while they retain competence. In most situations in the community, a change of heart is unproblematic. In a custodial setting, a documented advance refusal can effectively deprive patients of an opportunity to retract without losing face. In private discussion with prisoners, doctors found that some were willing to cease their strike if even a minor concession allowed this without loss of peer respect. If freely made by a competent and informed person, however, advance refusals are as binding in detention as in other settings (see Chapter 3, pages 113–6).

Advance refusal of nutrition

In November 2001, Barry Horne died in hospital of liver failure resulting from a hunger strike in Long Lartin High Security Prison in Worcestershire. He was an animal rights activist serving an 18 year sentence who had carried out many hunger strikes, previously narrowly avoiding death on a 68 day strike in 1998. In his last hunger strike, he signed an advance directive, refusing medical intervention, at a time when he was declared to be of sound mind. The prison and hospital authorities were therefore bound to abide by his refusal.[62]

Respecting treatment refusal

Respecting the voluntary refusal of competent and informed patients accords with the principles set out in the World Medical Association's Declaration of Tokyo.[63] This affirms that, when competent prisoners refuse nourishment in full knowledge of the consequences, they should not be fed artificially. Doctors sometime take over care only when it is too late to be certain about the individual's real intention. If there is good reason to believe that death was not intended, resuscitation should be attempted. Patients should be transferred to appropriate hospital care, either within the custodial setting or to an NHS hospital. If resuscitation is likely, the hospital or medical room needs to be suitably equipped. When it is clear that detainees intend to continue the strike until death, they must be allowed to die with dignity. It should be decided at a relatively early stage whether they will die in the prison or detention centre hospital, where the staff know them, or be transferred to an NHS hospital. Transfer to an NHS hospital may be easier for the family, but should be arranged in time for some rapport to develop between the patient and staff before the patient becomes incompetent.

Summary – problems common to various custodial settings

Strategies need to be in place to deal with:

- differences in approach of health professionals and other staff
- the opportunities to introduce patients to good disease prevention habits
- the time needed to ensure good communication with both patients and colleagues
- difficulties in ensuring prompt patient access to care in detention and continuity of care after release
- the potential for misuse of medication
- the identification and prevention of opportunities for self harm
- the appropriate use of restraint
- the medical role in management of hunger strikes
- the stress on health professionals and the complexity of their caseload.

Health care in prisons

Prison health reform

Across the UK, prison health services were under considerable pressure in the late 1990s. The general problems that have already been noted as applicable to any custodial setting were often acute in prisons. In 1999, for example, 91 suicides were recorded in English prisons, when the suicide rate reached 140 per 100 000 inmates compared with 12 per 100 000 in the general population.[64] Cases such as that of Paul Wright (see box below) also attracted much criticism. All around the UK, the recruitment and retention of suitable doctors posed problems and the service was criticised for providing inferior health care.[65] Reports focused on the lack of adequate training and the fact that some doctors worked beyond the limits of their ability.[66] The BMA noted that doctors working in prisons were struggling to cope.[67]

In some areas, overseas doctors had to be recruited to cover the staffing shortage. A welcome development, however, has been the growing role of appropriately trained nurses, although they are sometimes inhibited by rigid work profiles from undertaking tasks suited to their competence. It has been suggested that prison rules should be changed to allow nurses greater autonomy, for example, in assessing detainees.[68]

Past inadequate care in prison

Paul Wright died in Leeds prison from an asthma attack in 1996. His death was the subject of the first public inquiry into a death in custody ordered by a judge under the Human Rights Act. In July 2002, the inquiry report found that Wright died after substandard medical treatment at the prison where he was serving three and a half years for fraud, drugs, and driving offences. The GP who treated him had been prohibited from practising independently by the General Medical Council (GMC) and should not have had unsupervised responsibility for prisoners' health care. The inquiry chairman said that in the months before his death the medical service provided for Mr Wright was inadequate and he lacked the medication that might have saved him. The same doctor was later criticised at an inquest into the suicide of another Leeds prisoner, when the doctor stopped resuscitation after the prisoner hung himself in his cell. The doctor was removed from the medical register.[69]

Considerable analysis and change were generated around the turn of the new century. In England and Wales, the Prison Health Policy Unit and Task Force was established jointly by the Home Office and the Department of Health in 2000 to modernise prison health care. In December 2001, a report was published with many recommendations about normalising prison care and bringing it into line with NHS care.[70] It recommended, for example, that all doctors should work at least part of the time in the NHS. Among improvements made were the transfer of commissioning of prison health care, the introduction of NHS mental health in-reach teams, improved detoxification programmes, and more training for prison health teams. The BMA had long called for the prison health service to be brought within the aegis of the NHS and, in 2001, the Chief Inspector of Prisons for England and Wales also recommended that the NHS should assume responsibility for prison health care.[71] In September 2002, the Government announced that funding responsibility for health services in English prisons would be transferred from the Home Office to the Department of Health in 2003/2004.[72] Similar proposals were put forward for the four prisons in Wales. This was envisaged as the first step in a five year process during which prison health care in England would become part of the NHS, attracting extra funding and hopefully dealing with many of the longstanding problems.

The Scottish Prison Service carried out a review of medical services in 1999.[73] In November 2000, medical care was outsourced and the contract awarded to a private provider, Medacs. Nevertheless, the Scottish Prison Service Head of Health Care continued to advise on policy issues and deal with complaints.

The Northern Ireland review of prison health care (see below) looked at the previous reviews that had been undertaken in Scotland, England, and Wales, and considered following the Scottish model of contracting out primary medical services. However, it could not identify an appropriate service provider within the country. It suggested, however, that contracting out prison health services to suppliers in other parts of the UK, Ireland, or western Europe could be considered in future. Its general thrust was to support greater integration between prison health care and the NHS in Northern Ireland. Although the funding for most of the health care provision is to be supplied by the Northern Ireland Prison Service, the overall responsibility for the provision of health care remains with the Department of Health, Social Services and Public Safety.

Improvements have undoubtedly been made, but providing health care in prisons will always be a complex task. From a health perspective, detention represents an opportunity to tackle neglected health problems and doctors working in such settings are generally aware of the possibility to influence patients' attitudes positively.[74] Many patients, however, have behavioural disorders, a history of violence or a history of self harm. The majority of prisoners are said to have a diagnosable mental illness, substance abuse problem, or both.[75] The patient group is far from static because the prison population has increased steadily, but turnover is high in some prisons.[76] Patient demand for care can be very high; in 2002, for example, 20% of women in prison requested access to a doctor or nurse every day.[77] Although services around Britain developed new strategies and training for health professionals in risk management,[78] and despite considerable efforts made to tackle prisoner suicide rates, these remain problematic. In 2002 the Director General of the Prison Service expressed concern that jail suicides were reaching record levels and overcrowding was driving up the number of deaths.[79]

Changes to the prison health service in Northern Ireland

Prison services around Great Britain generally function in similar ways, but Northern Ireland has been noticeably different and this has had an impact on the provision of health care. In 1974, in contrast with arrangements in the rest of the UK, the Northern Ireland Prison Medical Service became the direct responsibility of the Department of Health and Social Services (now the Department of Health, Social Services and Public Safety). The political situation in Northern Ireland gave rise to a rapid increase in the numbers of people in custody in the early 1970s, when the average detained population, including internees, reached 2517.[80] Doctors were professionally responsible to the Government's chief medical officer, although operationally accountable to the prison governor. This separation of duties made medical staff very clearly distinct from the prison management at a time when the service was under intense scrutiny from human rights organisations. Prison rules were derived from the same Home Office rules operational elsewhere in the UK but reflected the differing responsibilities of doctors in Northern Ireland. The moral dilemmas facing doctors there were highlighted in 1981 when a high profile series of prison hunger strikes resulted in 10 deaths. Doctors provided advice and medical supervision for the duration of the strikes while respecting prisoners' refusal of nutrition. Although clearly an extreme example of the stresses and moral tensions, it demonstrates how health professionals working in prisons have a very ethically demanding job.

The signing of the Belfast Agreement in April 1998 triggered a significant reduction in the prison population, which fell to an average of 934 by April 2001. This impacted on the range of services, including health care, as the health needs of the prison population changed, becoming more reflective of underlying socioeconomic deprivation. Increasing problems were identified with drug and alcohol abuse, communicable diseases, and mentally disordered offenders.[81] An expert review group was established in April 2001 to look at the structure and management of healthcare provision. Its report published in April 2002 carried 60 recommendations emphasising, for example, the need for sufficient time to be available in prisons for healthcare assessment, more autonomy for nurses, formal arrangements to allow female prisoners to see female doctors, and demanding that specific training in prison health care be provided and funded.[82] It also drew attention to the problems of professional isolation that could arise if there was insufficient contact with doctors working in the community and which could also reduce the influence of health service initiatives such as clinical governance and clinical audit.

Mental health services

A frequent problem for doctors has been the difficulty in transferring mentally ill prisoners who need specialised care to a suitable mental health establishment. The unacceptability of prolonged waiting periods was highlighted in 2001 by the CPT, which called on the Government to ensure that immediate steps were taken to address this.[83] Prison doctors have frequently faced reluctance from hospitals to accept such patients, although the standards set out in the national service framework for mental health[84] and the NHS plan for England, and the equivalents in Wales and Scotland, apply to prisoners as to other patients.[85] In 2002 the Government acknowledged that the volume, range, and quality of mental health services in English and Welsh prisons were not meeting prisoners' needs.[86] At its annual meetings, the BMA consistently called upon Government to ensure that prison health services matched care provided in the community. It particularly identified a need for improved psychiatric services for prisoners. Expert studies reinforced the view that the quality of services for mentally ill prisoners had often fallen below NHS standards.[87] In 2001 the Government published a new strategy for improving mental health services in prisons in England and Wales.[88] This drew attention to the particular mental health needs of women, young prisoners, and people from ethnic minority groups, and pointed out that effective care could benefit society by reducing reoffending rates. It set out a series of goals to be attained over five years, emphasising early diagnosis and rapid transfer to the NHS where necessary. However, it acknowledged that there were also problems in ensuring sufficient mental health training and appropriate skill mix in prisons. Balancing patient confidentiality with efforts to improve information flow between prisons, social services, probation officers, police, and courts was seen as potentially problematic, and the establishment of information-sharing protocols was recommended so that everyone would be clear about what information could be shared and how.

In Scotland, it was recommended in 1999 that prisons should contract with their local primary care trust for the provision of mental health services for prisoners.[89] In practice, however, this has proved problematic despite the efforts of the Scottish Prison Service because of a lack of sufficient psychiatrists able to take on additional work with prisoners.

In Northern Ireland, the prison health care review recommended a fundamental assessment of mental health services in prisons to be carried out under the implementation process. In addition, an independent review of mental health services and legislation was initiated. The prison service is a partner in this review, which is expected to report in 2005.

Management of pregnancy and child care

The number of pregnant women held in prisons is not routinely collated, but in 2002 a survey of prisons in England and Wales identified 75 pregnant women prisoners.[90] An important issue is the ability of women to attend routine antenatal care sessions and give birth without invariably being handcuffed or constantly monitored by accompanying prison personnel. In the 1990s, the Howard League for Penal Reform publicised a number of cases of women who were allegedly handcuffed while being given an antenatal examination, while giving birth, and while trying to breastfeed.[91]

Management of pregnancy and health care: advice from the *Prison security manual*

- For antenatal visits, pregnant women should have restraints removed unless there is a high risk of escape.
- Escorting staff should not be present for intimate examinations or labour unless the woman requests that.
- Birthing partners should be allowed as long as there is no risk to safety or security of other people.[92]

In 1995 the BMA was one of a number of organisations that lobbied the Home Office about inadequate provision of places where babies and toddlers could be with their mothers in prison in England. At that time, more than twice as many babies were eligible to stay in prison with their mothers than the actual places available for them. In 1998 the director of the prison service promised a full review of the system and of the allocation of places.[93] In 2002 standards for mother and baby units were published.[94] These emphasised the importance of an open and equitable system of allocating places and stressed the interests of the child as the basis for decision making. A full range of health services for babies and toddlers must be available, equivalent to what is provided in the community. Separation plans must be drawn up and discussed with the mother when her application for a child place is refused and aftercare support should be offered to women who are not permitted to keep their babies with them. Alternative carers need to be identified for babies when this is judged to be in their best interests. For women who keep their children with them, childcare plans still need to include potential arrangements for separation as part of the child's development needs.

In addition to the women who give birth while imprisoned, many women in jail have dependent children at home. Although data are not routinely collected, a study carried out in 2000 found that 66% of the female prison population had dependent children.[95] Nevertheless, childcare arrangements are not necessarily taken into consideration when women are allocated to a prison, with the result that women can be serving their sentence hundreds of miles away from their children, making visits impossible. Clearly, when their families are a source of anxiety, there needs to be appropriate liaison between the relevant agencies.

Independence of health professionals

Health professionals should not have a disciplinary or punitive role in any institution, although they must be aware of the need for order and discipline to be maintained. They are primarily responsible for the physical and mental health of inmates and should not be expected to fulfil both clinical and disciplinary roles. Some confusion about role identity can exist. In Northern Ireland, for example, the review group welcomed the contribution of nurses, but thought that the speed of change had uncovered "a potential for conflict between the delivery of healthcare and security requirements" that impinged on nursing standards.[96]

Doctors must be able to make independent clinical and ethical judgments concerning patients' health care. A problem in the past, however, was the wide variation in prescribing practice in prisons.[97] Clearly, clinical decisions in any context should be evidence based and all health professionals should have regard to equitable use of resources. For example, in prisons, doctors may be asked to prescribe from a limited drug list, with medicines not on the list requiring special justification. As this is intended to reduce costs in an equitable manner without damaging the health of individual patients, the principle of using prescribing protocols is ethically acceptable and such protocols are also common outside custodial settings. Doctors sometimes object, however, that they cannot prescribe what they judge to be the most appropriate product for individuals and feel that patient trust can be undermined as a result. Doctors are accountable to the GMC for their standard of care, including the medications they prescribe, but they also have to work within the financial constraints of prison budgets. In particular, they must "only prescribe treatments which make an effective contribution to the patient's overall management" and "take resources into account when choosing between treatments of similar effectiveness".[98] Pharmacy protocols should contribute to better standardisation. Prescribing issues are discussed in depth in Chapter 13.

Independence and the duty to speak out

Doctors working in UK prisons have traditionally been bound by the Official Secrets Act 1989 but this is rarely a problem in practice.[99] Nevertheless, the BMA has received a steady trickle of enquiries from doctors who assume that this duty of secrecy prohibits them from speaking out about poor conditions or evidence of abuse. The Association's advice is that health professionals cannot be impeded from taking appropriate action when detainees appear to be subject to abuse or brutality by prison staff or other inmates. Suspicions should be reported to the governor of the institution and, if this appears to have no effect, advice should be sought from the relevant area manager and medical director of prison health via the BMA's Civil Service Committee. Senior BMA doctors experienced in prison medicine can also provide further advice if necessary. In this situation, doctors need to obtain objective clinical evidence and keep a firm grip on reality to ensure that they have not been manipulated by their patients. There must be accurate clinical recording of findings and it may be prudent to ensure that copies of such records are kept in a secure place in addition to the medical file.

Diversion from prison: drug treatment and testing orders

Strategies to divert some categories of offender away from custodial care can raise dilemmas for health professionals because medical treatment in the community could then be seen as part of the criminal justice system. Conflict has arisen in the past in relation to drug treatment and testing orders (DTTOs), whereby patients are "sentenced" to take part in a specified treatment regimen as an alternative to a prison sentence. DTTOs can be imposed only if the court is satisfied that the offender is dependent on drugs or has a propensity to misuse them. The dependency or propensity must not only require treatment, but also be treatable.[100] The patient must be willing to give consent. The orders include both a treatment and a testing requirement, and specify whether treatment should be on a residential or non-residential basis.

An inherent problem with such orders is the different perspectives, aims, and objectives of the various parties involved. One key concern is that "ethical codes of conduct governing the treatment provider's relationship with such patients do not fit neatly with the responsibilities which they have to the criminal justice system if their services have been purchased in order to effect a DTTO".[101] These tensions can manifest themselves in a number of ways. Some health professionals have concerns about providing treatment when the patient has effectively been coerced to consent. As mentioned throughout this book, however, there are other circumstances in which there are pressures on consent, but where the consent is nonetheless considered to be valid. Although patient choice is restricted, ultimately the decision of whether to accept the treatment regimen that is offered as an alternative to prison rests with individual patients. They must understand their options and the implications of their choices in order to give valid consent but, provided this information has been given, it is for each individual to decide whether treatment is the best option for them. This must include an awareness and acceptance that the usual rules of confidentiality do not apply and that information must be provided to other agencies.

Although the treatment provider is involved with drawing up the treatment schedule, this must be within the general framework set out in the national standards for DTTOs.[102] This includes stipulations such as that contact, including treatment, should be over 5 days a week, with a minimum of 15 hours a week, for the first 13 weeks. If progress is satisfactory, the minimum period reduces to 9 hours per week for the remainder of the order (which could be up to 3 years). Conflicts can arise when the treatment provider does not believe that the requirements set out in the national standards are in the individual patient's best interests. In the final report of the pilot scheme, for example, some of the offenders themselves reported that it had been difficult coming into contact with other users during the contact periods.[103]

Some doctors report that they do not believe that a treatment order, along the lines of the national standards, is in the best interests of a particular patient, but they are concerned that changing the programme could lead to difficulties for that patient. There have also been cases in the past where doctors have complained to the BMA about the requirement in the national standards for urine samples to be produced under direct observation. They considered that, despite the punitive aspect to such treatment orders, patients should be entitled to the maximum amount of dignity and privacy consistent with the aims of the testing. This problem is likely to diminish in the future because the testing of urine samples has largely been replaced by the testing of oral fluid.

When doctors have concerns, they should discuss them with the named treatment provider and others involved with enforcing the treatment orders with a view to maximising the likelihood of the patient succeeding in the programme. If appropriate, such issues could be raised at one of the scheduled review hearings. Although only the court has the power to amend any of the order's specific requirements or provisions, in practice the court is likely to depend on advice from the treatment provider or supervising officer about any necessary amendments.[104] The aim should be to find a balance between the treatment needs of the patient and the aims of the court to enforce the terms of the order and to prevent the patient from reoffending.

As with other cases in which doctors are prescribing, it is important, with the patient's consent, to keep the GP informed of any medication prescribed and of the progress of treatment.

Young offenders' facilities

Many reports have criticised youth detention facilities and drawn particular attention to the problems of self harm and bullying.[105] As many as one in four people known to be involved in crime are children or young people. Drug dependency, alcohol abuse, and mental health problems lie behind much of this. Clearly, many of the same issues arise with young offenders as with the care of adult detainees, with the additional vulnerability that is likely to be experienced by a young person in custody. As with adult prisoners, an important factor directly affecting the quality of care for young detainees has been the lack over many years of appropriately trained doctors who are willing to work in custodial settings. In 2001, for example, the CPT drew particular attention to the lack of sufficient doctors and nurses at Feltham Young Offender Institution and Woodhill Prison, which resulted in prisoners facing long delays in accessing a health professional.[106]

Young people's consent and refusal of care

The general rules on consent relating to young people are set out in Chapter 4 and summarised on page 604. Legally, competent young people are able to consent on their own behalf, but may not always be able to refuse an intervention that is deemed to be in their best interest if people with parental responsibility consent on their behalf. Where the relationship between parents and the young person is strained, as is often the case for detainees, parents still have a legal right to consent, but this does not necessarily mean that doctors are obliged to carry out their wishes. It is always important to listen to the views of young people and try to understand why they object. Health professionals are very reluctant to impose a medication or treatment that a competent young person refuses since this is likely to undermine their relationship with that patient. Chapter 4 provides advice on the action to be taken when a young person refuses a procedure that has been validly authorised by parents.

Child protection in detention

In a High Court ruling in 2002,[107] the judge held that the Children Act 1989 applies to people under the age of 18 held in custody. Mr Justice Munby noted that "bullying, self-harm and suicide remain serious and in some instances untackled problems"[108] for this group. His judgment means that local authorities in England and Wales have a legal duty for the welfare of detained minors. Some experts believe that this is likely to result in more child protection investigations involving young detainees and greater involvement of social services in assessing the needs of the most vulnerable young people.[109] Local authorities have to undertake a needs assessment if the young person falls within the statutory criteria set out in the Children Act and develop a care plan that meets those needs. This obviously has huge resource and staffing implications for services that are already stretched.

Research by the Howard League for Penal Reform has indicated that, in the decade ending in 2003, 18 young people killed themselves while in detention. From April 2000 to November 2001, 554 incidents of self harm by juveniles were recorded.[110]

Self harm and assessing suicide risk

It is particularly important that training in assessment of detainees takes account of the differing needs between young people and adult prisoners. In 2002, in an inspection of an establishment for young offenders in Northern Ireland, the Chief Inspector of Prisons drew attention to the need for prisons to have a comprehensive vulnerability assessment procedure rather than relying upon evidence of previous attempts to self harm.[111] In relation to the detention of adolescents, she noted that staff generally had had inadequate training in the particular problems of young people. The report made it clear that this was not unique to Northern Ireland since the Chief Inspector had previously highlighted similar problems in England and Wales.[112] The Northern Ireland Prison Service had already recognised that its suicide and self harm policy was inadequate and had commissioned research into best practice in this area. A working group was also established to produce guidance and local policies for the prevention of suicide and self harm in institutions in Northern Ireland.[113]

Tackling bullying

At the young offenders facility at Wetherby it was found that those individuals who failed to meet their set targets or refused to become involved in activities such as physical education were also at risk of self injury or being bullied. In March 2001, the departments of psychology and physical education worked together to design a new programme entitled the "access course", involving classroom sessions and physical exercise. New skills such as problem solving, assertiveness, communication, and emotion management were acquired and then put into practice through physical exercise or acting as a referee in games. A preliminary analysis of results appears to demonstrate a reduced risk of self injury and victimisation by bullies.[114]

Detention centres for asylum seekers

In the BMA's view, the detention of people who are not convicted of a criminal offence should be a measure of last resort, used only in exceptional circumstances. In such cases, the detainees should be informed, in a language they understand, of their rights and the procedures applicable to them, in line with the 1998 guidance from the CPT.[115] The lack of understandable information about the reasons and likely duration of detention can obviously contribute to anxiety and depression in this patient group. Detainees should also receive accessible information relating to the provision of health care.

Duty of care for detainees held in immigration detention

From the mid-1980s, the Home Office has increasingly used powers available under the Immigration Act 1971 to detain thousands of asylum seekers who are awaiting decisions. The Asylum and Immigration Appeals Act 1993 further increased the use of detention. Subsequently, in 2002 the Government proposed to establish a system of induction and accommodation centres, including the Oakington Reception Centre for fast tracking some asylum seekers' claims.[116] In April 2003, however, the Chief Inspector of Prisons strongly criticised detention centres for asylum seekers in England.[117] Among the problems she noted were the lack of respect shown to inmates and the superfluous use of random strip searches in some facilities. Poor translation services were criticised, as was the general lack of information for detainees about what would happen to them. She expressed fears that immigration detainees in a number of centres were targeted by unscrupulous advisers who charged them large sums of money with promises of sorting out their applications to remain in the country. A general complaint about the detention centres visited by the Chief Inspector was the lack of support for detainees with mental health problems, especially those who had suffered trauma.

All detainees are entitled to the same range and quality of services as are received by the general public. In addition, immigration detainees and asylum seekers may need extra services to address their own specific health problems. The BMA has analysed some of the health problems that are common among asylum seekers.[118] For example, many women and female children from countries such as Eritrea, Ethiopia, and Somalia have undergone female genital mutilation, which can affect their health. Access to second opinion and out of hours care should be available according to the same criteria used by GPs in the community, rather than decided solely on management priorities. The BMA has particular concerns about the potentially pejorative mental health impact of detention on asylum seekers, some of whom are likely to have previously been the victims of abuse or violence. A study published in 1996 found that many detained asylum seekers have suffered multiple traumatic experiences.[119] Typically, although the majority of this group could cope with the initial month or two of detention, they deteriorated after three to four months. In many cases they had been inadequately assessed prior to detention, which meant that their health problems were not monitored while they were detained. In the past, they received little information about the reasons for detention or its likely duration.

If detainees are to have timely access to hospital services on the same basis as patients in the community, it is obviously important that such referrals are not delayed merely for administrative convenience. As with prison inmates, the BMA has received reports of access to hospital being denied or postponed because of the costs of providing escorts.

The provision of medication should be in line with that for comparable conditions in the community and take into account recommendations from bodies such as the National Institute for Clinical Excellence (see Chapter 13, page 464). Policies on the provision and recording of all medication in this setting need to be developed by, for example, a drug and therapeutic committee that includes a pharmacist.

Health care for detainees in immigration detention centres

The BMA supports the principles of good practice documented in sections 33–37 of The Detention Centre Rules 2001 (Statutory Instrument 2001 No. 238), which deal with the provision of health care to detainees in immigration detention centres. These set out the following rules for every detention centre.

- A fully registered GP shall be available.
- A healthcare team is responsible for detainees' physical and mental health.
- Team members should recognise medical conditions in a diverse population and be culturally sensitive.
- Professional guidelines on confidentiality will be observed.
- Requests to see the doctor will be recorded and passed on.
- The doctor has discretion to consult other doctors.
- Detainees can request a doctor and dentist of their own choice if:

  - they pay the costs incurred
  - the request is reasonable
  - attendance is in consultation with the detention centre doctor.

- As far as possible, the doctor will obtain detainees' previous medical record.
- Medical records will be passed on appropriately when the detainee leaves.
- Doctors must ensure that detainees know they can request a doctor of their own sex.
- Any doctor chosen by a detainee facing legal proceedings must have reasonable access to examine the detainee in connection with the proceedings.

The Operating Standards accompanying these rules draw attention to the need for health professionals to have access to training on aspects of health care that are likely to be particularly relevant for this patient group.

Consent in immigration detention centres

Detainees must be offered a physical and a mental examination within 24 hours of admission. This cannot proceed if the detainee refuses. In such cases, the detainee is entitled to an examination upon request. Under Schedule 12 of the Immigration and Asylum Act 1999, however, the manager of the centre can require that a detainee be medically examined in the interests of other people in order to ascertain if he or she has a transmissible disease. In such cases, doctors must still seek consent, explain the nature of the suspected disease, and tell the patient that refusal, without reasonable excuse, is an offence.

Examination for the purposes of providing an independent report for the immigration services or courts is discussed in Chapter 16 (pages 579–81).

Confidentiality in immigration detention centres

Interpretation and translation are particularly important in the care of this population. The BMA has been concerned about the alleged use of fellow detainees as interpreters or of other people who happen to speak the same language as the patient. Family members are also not appropriate because people who have survived torture are often unwilling to disclose the details in front of people they know. Asylum seekers can also be greatly concerned if the interpreters appear to represent officialdom or are recommended by embassies that they fear will filter back information to the authorities in their own country or carry out reprisals on relatives.

Rule 35 of the Detention Centre Rules requires the doctor to report to the manager any detainee whose health is likely to be pejoratively affected by continued detention and any person at risk of suicide. The same general advice discussed previously about providing a supportive environment for people who are likely to harm themselves is equally valid here. Rule 35 also requires the reporting to managers of detainees believed to be torture survivors. This is usually in the detainee's interests. Most torture survivors want that information known as it is likely to support their case and they also may need treatment. The fact that doctors believe an individual to have been subjected to abuse should be noted appropriately, although managers do not necessarily need any detail. Patients should be aware of how their information will be used and their agreement to any disclosure should be sought, as would be common practice in any other sphere. Doctors working with immigration detainees and asylum seekers have sometimes expressed concern to the BMA that, although such information is passed on to the Home Office, it is not acted upon. It is important, therefore, that detainees or their authorised representative can access their own health record to see (and, if appropriate, challenge) what has been written and passed on in reports about their health. Access to health records by patients and their representatives is discussed in Chapter 6 (pages 216–18).

Detainees have also alleged that medical reports made on them by independent experts have sometimes been improperly transcribed by detention staff. In October 2001, the BMA expressed some concerns to the Home Office about such allegations by detainees that the recommendations for release or specialist treatment submitted by community psychiatrists had been toned down. The BMA strongly emphasises the importance of accuracy and transparency in passing on the recommendations made by consultants in such cases. One option is for detainees to access their records under the provisions of the Data Protection Act 1998 in order to address the problem of improper transcription or inadvertent error. Clearly, medical reports and assessments should not be altered unless shown to be inaccurate in some way and then the alteration should be clearly marked and the reasons for it given. As in all other cases, health professionals are accountable for what they write and should be able to show proper justification for their decisions, including a decision not to act upon views provided by specialists.

> ### Summary – care in prisons, young offender institutions and asylum centres
>
> - Specific training for health professionals should be available and properly resourced.
> - Professional isolation is a risk. Good contact with community services needs to be preserved.
> - Independence and a clear sense of the medical role need to be maintained.
> - Doctors should not be involved in disciplinary issues.
> - Strategies are needed to ensure prompt access to care, including mental health care.
> - All detainees should be aware of their rights regarding consent to or refusal of treatment.
> - The need for appropriate liaison and prevention of self harm needs to be balanced with prisoners' rights to confidentiality.

Police surgeons

Police surgeons (increasingly known as forensic physicians) have both forensic and therapeutic roles. They examine, on behalf of the police, victims and suspected perpetrators of crime, as well as examining and treating people who are taken ill while in custody. They see detained people to determine their fitness for custody or interview, and may examine people, detained or otherwise, for forensic purposes or to obtain forensic samples. In all cases, police surgeons should identify themselves to the person to be examined and tell that person how their role differs from that in the usual doctor–patient relationship. Although complicated by the fact that the examinations they carry out have both a therapeutic and a forensic content, police surgeons still have obligations to respect patient consent and confidentiality. In general terms, therapeutic information is subject to the same degree of confidentiality accorded to other patients (bearing in mind that no patient's right to confidentiality is absolute). Forensic information, however, is likely to have greater implications for the public interest and the need to ensure justice.

Police surgeons and consent

Consent for examination of victims of crime

Evidential examination is different in aim, and in procedure, from clinical examination. Its purpose is to elicit material evidence regarding a possible criminal charge. Although the police sometimes ask GPs or hospital doctors to provide a report of injuries sustained in an alleged criminal act, documenting those injuries for forensic purposes is a specialised task requiring a trained police surgeon. When a serious crime, such as rape or assault, has occurred there is inevitable pressure to act quickly to protect others. The time limits for obtaining supporting evidence and full information on the alleged crime dictate that examinations be carried out promptly. This has to be explained to the victim. The police have done much admirable work to address sensitive issues surrounding sexual crimes and generally have specially trained officers to provide counselling and support. Nevertheless, the doctor cannot assume that the person's presence implies consent. In order to consent validly, the individual needs to know what is entailed by the examination and understand that forensic information will be passed to the police. Everyone involved should be sensitive to patients' preferences regarding the gender of the examining doctor. It is also important, in cases of suspected child sexual abuse, that children are not subjected to repeated examination. It is good practice for one examination to be carried out jointly by a police surgeon and a paediatrician. Discussion of children's consent to examination and treatment is discussed in Chapter 4 and more detail is provided in the BMA's book *Consent, rights and choices in health care for children and young people.*[120]

Consent for examination of a person held in custody

If detainees are conscious and competent, their consent for medical examination must be sought. The purpose may be to look for evidence of involvement in a crime or to deal with any illness or injury. In either case, the individual has the right to refuse to be examined or treated, or to provide specimens. (It is lawful for an intimate body search to be undertaken without consent, although the BMA and Association of Police Surgeons consider that doctors should participate only with the individual's consent; see page 640.) In order for consent to be valid, the detainee should be competent, informed of the purpose of the examination or specimens, and not subjected to coercion. The ability of detainees to give consent can obviously be compromised by factors such as illness, distress, or the effects of alcohol or drugs, and their very situation is likely to make them feel somewhat pressured. Nevertheless, most people can make valid choices even in difficult situations.

Consent should be written or, if verbal, witnessed and recorded in the medical notes. A police officer may be present for the examination but, if possible, should be out of immediate earshot. This is not always attainable and depends on the circumstances. Assaults on police surgeons are not uncommon and unfounded allegations are also sometimes made against them. The Association of Police Surgeons strongly recommends the presence of a chaperone when doctors examine a detainee of the opposite sex. If detainees agree, their solicitor can attend the examination. An informed refusal to be examined or treated must be respected. If consent for examination is unobtainable because the detainee is incapacitated at the time, information should not generally be passed to the police until the person can consent.

Problems can arise when the examination begins with one purpose, which is explained to the individual, but the information obtained is later wanted for another purpose, which has not been mentioned. Patients with minor injuries, for example, are examined to ascertain their fitness for custody, but their injuries may be the result of assaulting another person. Therefore detainees should be made aware that information obtained from the examination may be requested by the police or by lawyers.

Consent by minors

When the detainee is a minor, relatives may be present at the examination if the young person agrees. For people aged under 16, no forensic examination or samples should be undertaken without the consent of the young person *and* someone with parental responsibility. In addition to ensuring that valid consent has been obtained, the police surgeon also needs to ensure that any legal considerations are met regarding the admissibility in court of any forensic evidence obtained.[121]

Incapacitated detainees

As with any other patients, when detainees lack the capacity to consent, treatment should be provided in their best interests (see Chapter 3, pages 108–9). Specimens can be taken for diagnostic purposes. They should not be taken or used for forensic tests except where a blood sample is taken from an incompetent driver under the terms of the Police Reform Act 2002 (see Chapter 15, pages 546–8).

Acting without consent

Intimate body searches   Intimate body searches without consent are lawful, provided that appropriate authorisation has been received.[122] Nevertheless, the ethical obligation to seek consent applies. The BMA and the Association of Police Surgeons have a joint guidance note setting out their policy that doctors should not carry out intimate body searches without consent.[123] (The principles have also been supported by the GMC's Standards Committee.) Detainees faced with the prospect of an intimate search often request that a doctor does it rather than a police or prison officer. Doctors working in an environment in which intimate searches are likely should seek agreement that they are always called when an intimate search is proposed. This does not commit them to carrying out searches, but allows doctors to ascertain the detainee's wishes and establish whether consent has been given. When detainees refuse to be searched, this should be recorded in the notes. The BMA and the Association of Police Surgeons advise doctors not to participate, although in rare circumstances an intimate search may be justified in order to save the individual's life when, for example, a toxic substance is being concealed.

Taking blood samples to test for alcohol and drugs   Police surgeons may be asked by the police to take a blood sample from an incapacitated driver to test for alcohol or drugs. In the limited circumstances set out in the Police Reform Act 2002 this would be lawful in England, Scotland, and Wales, and, in the BMA's view, would also be ethically acceptable. (Similar proposals are under consideration in Northern Ireland at the time of writing.) The BMA and the Association of Police Surgeons have produced joint guidance for those involved in taking blood specimens from incapacitated drivers (see also Chapter 15, pages 546–8).[124]

Confidentiality and police surgeons

The primary purpose of most examinations conducted by police surgeons is to obtain evidence for a possible prosecution. Confidentiality is a difficult issue and people who are examined – both victims and suspects – should be clear about the use that will be made of their information. Police surgeons should say explicitly at the outset that part of their job is to collect evidence for the police and so no assurances about confidentiality can be given. They should also explain that they are required to disclose information obtained during the examination that might affect the outcome of the case.

In the mid-1990s some confusion arose about the conflict between police surgeons' duty to disclose information to the police and their duty of confidentiality. On one side, it was argued that police surgeons are part of the "prosecution team" and are obliged to provide the police with all notes of their examinations, including medical history and any purely therapeutic (as opposed to forensic) information. On the other, a distinction was drawn between the two categories of information. The situation was clarified for England, Wales, and Northern Ireland in parliamentary debate on the Criminal Procedure and Investigations Act 1996. It was made clear that the reports police surgeons prepare for criminal proceedings must be given to the police, but any information obtained for therapeutic purposes would be subject to the usual rules of confidentiality.[125] In order to do this, however, police surgeons need to separate out the forensic evidence (and any other information obtained that is likely to affect the outcome of the case) from information that is not germane to the case and was provided solely in a therapeutic context. Only forensic information and other information likely to affect the case should be included in the statement prepared for the police. If the police or the Crown Prosecution Service requests access to the therapeutic information, the individual's written consent should be sought. If the individual refuses or consents only to partial disclosure, that decision must be respected unless a judge orders full disclosure. In court, police surgeons should state why the information should not be disclosed or why they think it would not affect the outcome of the case. If, however, a court order is issued, the patient should be told of this and the information must be disclosed. The BMA and the Association of Police Surgeons have issued joint guidance on confidentiality for police surgeons in England, Wales, and Northern Ireland.[126] Doctors in Scotland should take advice from their defence body. (In addition, see Chapter 5 on general issues of confidentiality.)

Patient confidentiality in the police station setting

- Careful attention must be given to ensuring that people who are being examined understand the role of the forensic doctor.
- Before any information is volunteered, doctors should state explicitly that part of their role is to collect evidence for the prosecution. They should make clear that any information given may be so used and that

(Continued)

confidentiality cannot be guaranteed. The patient should understand and agree to this prior to examination or to the collection of the information.

- Doctors should explain that, in addition to forensic evidence, they are required to provide to the police any information obtained during the examination that may affect the outcome of the case.
- Before an examination takes place, doctors should ensure that the patient has consented to the forensic examination, the provision of medical care, and the disclosure of forensic evidence and any other information likely to affect the outcome of the case.
- While carrying out the examination, doctors should consciously attempt to separate out forensic evidence, other information obtained that is likely to affect the outcome of the case, and information that is not germane to the case but is given solely in the therapeutic context.
- A statement should be provided for the police, giving all the forensic evidence and any other information obtained that is likely to affect the outcome of the case.
- If the police request further information about the medical examination that was not included in the report, the specific consent of the patient should be sought before this is disclosed.
- If the patient refuses to consent, or consents to only partial disclosure, the doctor should abide by that decision unless, exceptionally, disclosure can be justified by the potential for serious harm to others or a likely miscarriage of justice, or a court order.

Information to be included in police station records

Full notes of any examination should always be kept. Any notes made in station records should be relevant to the care of the prisoner, or briefly describe the relevant injuries in the case of a victim. Doctors must be aware that, as such records are widely accessed, they should contain a minimum of clinical information. As far as the person's health is concerned, only the information necessary to enable the police to take proper care of the individual should be disclosed. In the case of serious illness in a person in custody, information relevant to supervision may be given to the police. Worries are sometimes expressed that police surgeons document details such as the HIV status of detainees in police records without the person's consent. Unless this information is necessary for the provision of appropriate care, this would be a breach of confidentiality.

A confidential record of any medical treatment provided or requested by the police surgeon while the individual is in police custody should accompany the person when transferred elsewhere. It should accompany detainees when they first appear in court, in a sealed envelope marked "confidential". This information may be relevant to the granting or refusal of bail and may be used by court forensic psychiatrists or other doctors who later become responsible for the care of the prisoner. When the care of a patient is passed over from one police surgeon to another, all relevant information must be provided to ensure continuity of care.

Summary – police surgeons

- Doctors should seek consent from competent individuals, even if that is not a legal requirement.
- People who are examined in custody may want their lawyer to be present.
- People who are examined for forensic purposes need to be aware that any information obtained may be used as evidence in court.
- Confidentiality cannot be guaranteed, but a distinction should be made between information obtained for therapeutic and forensic purposes.
- Police surgeons should make every effort to ensure continuity by passing on medical information to health professionals who subsequently provide care.

References

1 Department of Health, Welsh Assembly, HM Prison Service, General Practitioners Committee, Royal College of General Practitioners. *Good medical practice for doctors providing primary care services in prison.* London: DoH, 2003.
2 Department of Health, Welsh Assembly, HM Prison Service. *Seeking consent: working with people in prison.* London: DoH, 2002.
3 European Committee for the Prevention of Torture and Inhuman or Degrading Treatment or Punishment. *The CPT standards.* Strasbourg: Council of Europe, 2002:31. (CPT/Inf/E (2002) 1.)
4 Department of Health, *et al. Seeking consent: working with people in prison. Op cit.*
5 Re W (adult: refusal of treatment) [2002] EWHC 901 (Fam).
6 Summary of guidance in: Department of Health, *et al. Seeking consent: working with people in prison. Op cit.*
7 British Medical Association, The Law Society. *Assessment of mental capacity: guidance for doctors and lawyers, 2nd ed.* London: BMJ Books, in press. This book covers the law in England and Wales.
8 Department of Health, Welsh Assembly, HM Prison Service. *Guidance on the protection and use of confidential health information in prisons and inter-agency information sharing.* London: DoH, 2002. (PSI 25/2002.)
9 Lord Chancellor's Department Trials Issues Group. *Agreement on the arrangements for the attendance of interpreters in investigations and proceedings within the criminal justice system.* London: Lord Chancellor's Department Trials Issues Group, 2001. Available from the signatory groups, which include the Association of Chief Police Officers, Bar Council, Crown Prosecution Service, Home Office, Law Society, Lord Chancellor's Department, Magistrates Association, Victim Support, and National Probation Service.
10 Crown Office and Procurator Fiscal Service. *Review of arrangements for instruction of interpreters by procurators fiscal: guidance on policy and best practice.* Edinburgh: COPFS, 2001. (Crown Office Circular 17/2001.)
11 Determination by Robert Alastair Dunlop, QC, Sheriff Principal of the Sheriffdom of Tayside Central and Fife following an Inquiry held at Stirling on 4, 5, 6, 7 March 2002 into the death of Michelle McElver. Determination following an Inquiry held at Stirling on 8, 12 and 13 March 2002 into the death of Frances Carvill.
12 Determination by Robert Alastair Dunlop QC, following an Inquiry held at Stirling on 8, 12 and 13 March 2002 into the death of Frances Carvill: 6.
13 HM Chief Inspector of Prisons. *Report on an unannounced follow-up inspection of HM Prison Bristol, 3–5 September 2001.* London: Home Office, 2001: para 1·170.
14 Department of Health, *et al. Good medical practice for doctors providing primary care services in prison. Op cit.*
15 Fatal Accidents and Sudden Deaths Inquiry (Scotland) Act 1976. Section 6(1)(c) requires the sheriff to determine whether reasonable precautions were taken that might have avoided the death, and section 6(1)(d) requires the sheriff to determine whether any defect in the system of working contributed to the death.

16 Determination by TA Kevin Drummond, Sheriff of the Sheriffdom of Glasgow and Strathkelvin after an inquiry held at Glasgow on 17 February 1999 into the death of Daniel Lynch: 1. Documentation provided by the Medical and Dental Defence Union of Scotland.

17 Northern Ireland Review Group. *Review of prison healthcare services.* London: Home Office, 2002:7.

18 Response of the British Medical Association Northern Ireland Consultants and Specialists Committee to the *Review of the provision of healthcare services to prisoners.* Belfast: BMA, 2002.

19 The Northern Ireland Prison Service Management Board and the Associate Director of Health Care have drawn up an implementation plan. Northern Ireland Prison Service Management Board, personal communication, 21 Mar 2003.

20 European Committee for the Prevention of Torture and Inhuman or Degrading Treatment or Punishment. *Report to the Government of the United Kingdom on the visit to the United Kingdom by the CPT from 17 to 21 February 2002.* Strasbourg: Council of Europe, 2003: 10. (CPT/Inf 2003 18.)

21 Lord Chancellor's Department. *Response of the UK Government to the report of the European Committee for the Prevention of Torture and Inhuman or Degrading Treatment or Punishment on its visit to the UK from 17 to 21 February 2002.* Strasbourg: Council of Europe, 2003:21–3.

22 For further information and advice about the Act see: British Medical Association. *The impact of the Human Rights Act 1998 on medical decision making.* London: BMA, 2000.

23 D v United Kingdom [1997] 24 EHRR 423.

24 R v Secretary of State for the Home Department, ex parte Mellor [2001] 2 FLR 1158.

25 Department of Health. *Our healthier nation, mental health national service frameworks.* London: DoH, 1999:76.

26 Secretary of State for Home Affairs. *House of Commons official report (Hansard).* 2002 Apr 26: col 481W.

27 The Howard League for Penal Reform. *Suicide and self-harm prevention: following release from prison.* London: The Howard League, 2003.

28 The Howard League for Penal Reform. *Suicide and self-harm prevention: the management of self-injury in prisons.* London: The Howard League, 2003.

29 Anonymous. Self-harm in prison "triples". *BBC Online,* 2003 Mar 3. http://news.bbc.co.uk (accessed 4 May 2003).

30 Secretary of State for Home Affairs. *House of Commons official report (Hansard). Op cit.*

31 HM Prisons Library. *Prison service standards.* London: HM Prison Service, 2002. http://www.hmprisons.gov.uk/library (accessed 4 May 2003).

32 Northern Ireland Review Group. *Review of prison healthcare services. Op cit:* pp. 23–4.

33 Department of Health. *Changing the outlook: a strategy for developing and modernising mental health services in prisons.* London: DoH, 2001:18.

34 The Howard League for Penal Reform. *Suicide and self-harm prevention: the management of self-injury in prisons. Op cit:* p. 18.

35 Based on: HM Chief Inspector of Prisons. *Report on a full announced inspection of HM YOC Hydebank Wood, 4–8 February 2002.* London: HM Chief Inspector of Prisons, 2002.

36 Reed J, Lyne M. The quality of health care in prison: results of a year's programme of semi-structured inspections. *BMJ* 1997;**315**:1420–4.

37 HM Chief Inspector of Prisons. *Report on an unannounced follow-up inspection of HM Prison Bristol 3–5 September 2001. Op cit:* para 1·74.

38 Northern Ireland Review Group. *Review of prison healthcare services. Op cit:* p. 21. Former Head of Health Care, Scottish Prison Service, personal communication, 13 March 2003.

39 Department of Health, Welsh Assembly, HM Prison Service. *Prison health handbook.* London: DoH, 2003.

40 *Ibid.*

41 World Health Organization. *WHO guidelines on HIV infection and AIDS in prisons.* Geneva: WHO, 1993:5.

42 BMA Foundation for AIDS. *Prescribing of condoms in prisons: survey report.* London: BMA Foundation for AIDS, 1997. This survey was carried out jointly by the BMA Foundation for AIDS (now the Medical Foundation for Aids and Sexual Health) and the National AIDS and Prisons Forum.

43 British Medical Association. *The medical profession and human rights: handbook for a changing agenda.* London: Zed Books, 2001:113.

44 Department of Health, *et al. Good medical practice for doctors providing primary care services in prison. Op cit:* p. 15.

45 European Committee for the Prevention of Torture and Inhuman or Degrading Treatment or Punishment. *The CPT standards. Op cit:* p. 20.

46 *Ibid:* p. 60.

47 Davies R. Children locked away from human rights in the UK. *Lancet* 2003;**361**:873.

48 British Medical Association. *The medical profession and human rights: handbook for a changing agenda. Op cit:* pp. 304–5.

49 Police Complaints Authority. *Policing acute behavioural disturbance.* London: PCA, 2001:8. See also: Herring J. Fitness to be detained. In: Stark MM, Rogers DJ, Norfolk GA, eds. *Good practice guidelines for forensic medical examiners.* London: Metropolitan Police, 2001.

50 European Committee for the Prevention of Torture and Inhuman or Degrading Treatment or Punishment. *The CPT standards. Op cit:* pp. 19–20.

51 HM Prison Service. *Prison security manual. Prison Service Order 1000.* London: HM Prison Service, 1998:37·92 (v) (updated 9/99); 37·133 and 37·144 (both updated 12/2000).

52 *Ibid:* 37·135.

53 *Ibid.*

54 British Medical Association. *Guidance for doctors providing medical care and treatment to those detained in prison.* London: BMA, 1996.

55 HM Prison Service. *Prison security manual. Prison Service Order 1000. Op cit:* ch 37. This chapter of the manual is publicly accessible and not restricted, although others are.

56 HM Prison Service. *Use of force. Prison Service Order 1600.* London: HM Prison Service, 1999. (PSI 38/1999.) This Order applies only in England and Wales.

57 Hopkins N. Police warned over point-blank use of CS spray. *The Guardian* 2000 Mar 27.

58 British Medical Association. *The medical profession and human rights: handbook for a changing agenda. Op cit:* pp. 407–8.

59 World Medical Association. *World Medical Association resolution on medical care for refugees.* Ferney-Voltaire: WMA, 1998.

60 R v (1) Dr James Donald Collins (2) Ashworth Hospital Authority, ex parte Ian Stewart Brady [2001] 58 BMLR 173.

61 Northern Ireland prison doctor at BMA meeting on hunger strikes. BMA House, personal communication, 12 Sep 2001.

62 Anonymous. Animal activist dies on hunger strike. *BBC Online* 2001 Nov 5. http://news.bbc.co.uk (accessed 4 May 2003).

63 World Medical Association. *Guidelines for medical doctors concerning torture and other cruel, inhuman or degrading treatment or punishment in relation to detention and imprisonment.* Ferney-Voltaire: WMA, 1975.

64 Howard League for Penal Reform. *Desperate measures: prison suicides and their prevention.* London: The Howard League, 1999:8.

65 Smith R. Prisoners: an end to second class care? *BMJ* 1999;**318**:954–5.

66 Royal College of Physicians, Royal College of General Practitioners, Royal College of Psychiatrists. *Report of the working party of three medical royal colleges on the education and training of doctors in the health care service for prisoners.* London: Home Office, 1992.

67 British Medical Association. *Prison medicine: a crisis waiting to break.* London: BMA, 2001.

68 Northern Ireland Review Group. *Review of prison healthcare services. Op cit:* p. 11.

69 Wainwright M. Jail attacked by inquiry into death of prisoner. *The Guardian* 2002 Jul 12.

70 Department of Health, HM Prison Service, National Assembly for Wales. *Report of the working group on doctors working in prisons.* London: DoH, 2001.

71 Her Majesty's Inspectorate of Prisons for England and Wales. *Report of Her Majesty's Chief Inspector of Prisons.* London: The Stationery Office, 2001.

72 Home Office press release. *Prison health transferred to Department of Health.* 25 Sep 2002. 64 N/02.

73 The results of the Scottish Prison Service's review of medical services have not been published.

74 See, for example: Department of Health. *Health promoting prisons: a shared approach. A strategy for promoting health in prisons in England and Wales.* London: DoH, 2002.

75 Department of Health. *Changing the outlook: a strategy for developing and modernising mental health services in prisons. Op cit.*

76 In England and Wales, 13% of sentenced prisoners were serving less than 1 year and more than half of these were sentenced to less than 6 months; a further 38% were serving between 1 and 4 years. Home Office. *Prison population brief for England and Wales.* London: Home Office, 2002:7.

77 Home Office press release. *Prison health transferred to Department of Health. Op cit.*

78 For example, the Scottish Prison Service adopted a suicide risk management strategy in 1998. The Northern Ireland Prison Service commissioned a research report into best practice in order to develop new policies.

79 Burrell I. Prisoners who refused medical help near death. *Independent* 2002 May 20.

80 Northern Ireland Review Group. *Review of prison healthcare services. Op cit:* p. 4.

81 *Ibid:* p. 7.

82 *Ibid.*

83 European Committee for the Prevention of Torture and Inhuman or Degrading Treatment or Punishment. *Report to the Government of the UK on the visit to the UK carried out by the European Committee for the Prevention of Torture and Inhuman or Degrading Treatment or Punishment (CPT) from 4–16 February 2001.* Strasbourg: Council of Europe, 2002:31.

84 Department of Health. *A national service framework for mental health.* London: DoH, 1999.

85 Department of Health. *Our healthier nation, mental health national service frameworks. Op cit.* Department of Health. *The NHS plan.* London: The Stationery Office, 2000. NHS Wales. *Improving health in Wales. A plan for the NHS with its partners.* Cardiff: National Assembly for Wales, 2001. NHS Scotland. *Our national health. A plan for action, a plan for change.* Edinburgh: Scottish Executive, 2000.

86 Department of Health, *et al. Changing the outlook: a strategy for developing and modernising mental health services in prisons. Op cit:* p. 5.

87 Reed J, *et al.* Inpatient care of mentally ill people in prison: results of a year's programme of semi-structured inspections. *Op cit.*

88 Department of Health, *et al. Changing the outlook: a strategy for developing and modernising mental health services in prisons. Op cit.*

89 The Scottish Office. *Health, social work and related services for mentally disordered offenders in Scotland.* Edinburgh: The Scottish Office, 1999.

90 Benn H. *House of Commons official report (Hansard).* 2003 Feb 24: col 122W.

91 Howard League for Penal Reform. *Prison mother and baby units.* London: The Howard League, 1995.

92 HM Prison Service. *Prison security manual. Prison Service Order 1000. Op cit.*

93 The Howard League for Penal Reform. *Prison mother and baby units. Op cit.* This is discussed in: British Medical Association. *The medical profession and human rights: handbook for a changing agenda. Op cit:* p. 100.

94 HM Prisons Library. *Prison service standards. Op cit.*

95 Benn H. *House of Commons official report (Hansard).* 2003 Feb 24: col 119W.

96 Northern Ireland Review Group. *Review of prison healthcare services. Op cit:* p. 13.

97 Reed J, *et al.* The quality of health care in prison: results of a year's programme of semi-structured inspections. *Op cit.*

98 Department of Health, *et al. Good medical practice for doctors providing primary care services in prison. Op cit:* p. 24.

99 In Scotland, for example, prison doctors, as civil servants, have traditionally been bound by the Official Secrets Act, although they are not actually required to sign it.

100 Crime and Disorder Act 1998 s61–64. Act of Adjournal (Criminal Procedure Rules Amendment No. 4) (Drug Treatment and Testing Orders), SSI 1999 No. 191. The Criminal Justice (Northern Ireland) Order 1998, SI 1998 No. 2839 (NI 20).

101 Walsh C. Sentenced to treatment. *Web Journal of Current Legal Issues* 1999;**5**:5. http://www.webjcli.ncl.ac.uk/1999/issue5/walsh5.html (accessed 4 May 2003).

102 Home Office. *National standards for the supervision of offenders in the community.* London: Home Office, 2002: Annex D.

103 Turnbull PJ, McSweeney T, Webster R, Edmunds M, Hough M. *Home Office research study 212. Drug treatment and testing orders: final evaluation report.* London: Home Office Research, Development and Statistics Directorate, 2000:62.

104 Home Office. *Guidance for practitioners involved in drug treatment and testing order pilots.* London: Home Office, 2000.

105 See, for example: Davies R. Children locked away from human rights in the UK. *Op cit.*

106 European Committee for the Prevention of Torture and Inhuman or Degrading Treatment or Punishment. *Report to the Government of the UK on the visit to the UK carried out by the European Committee for the Prevention of Torture and Inhuman or Degrading Treatment or Punishment (CPT) from 4–16 February 2001. Op cit:* p. 29.

107 R (on the application of the Howard League for Penal Reform) v the Secretary of State for the Home Department and Department of Health [2003] 1 FLR 484.

108 *Ibid*: 526.

109 Epstein R, Wise I. Children behind bars. *New Law J* 2003;**153**(7068):263–4.

110 The Howard League for Penal Reform. *Suicide and self-harm prevention: the management of self-injury in prisons. Op cit:* p. 17.

111 HM Chief Inspector of Prisons. *Report on a full announced inspection of HM YOC Hydebank Wood, 4–8 February 2002. Op cit.*

112 *Ibid:* p. 13.

113 Northern Ireland Prison Service, personal communication, 21 Mar 2003.

114 The Howard League for Penal Reform. *Suicide and self-harm prevention: the management of self-injury in prisons. Op cit:* p. 17.

115 European Committee for the Prevention of Torture and Inhuman or Degrading Treatment or Punishment. *Foreign nationals detained under aliens legislation.* Strasbourg: Council of Europe, 1998.

116 Home Office. *Secure borders, safe haven: integration with diversity in modern Britain.* London: The Stationery Office, 2002.

117 HM Chief Inspector of Prisons. *Report on an inspection of Campsfield House, Haslar, Lindholme, Oakington Reception Centre and Tinsley House, carried out during February and March 2002.* London: HM Chief Inspector of Prisons, 2003.

118 British Medical Association. *Asylum seekers: meeting their healthcare needs.* London: BMA, 2002:5–10.

119 Pourgourides CK, Sashidharan SP, Bracken PJ. *A second exile: the mental health implications of detention of asylum seekers in the United Kingdom.* Birmingham: North Birmingham Mental Health NHS Trust, 1995.

120 British Medical Association. *Consent, rights and choices in health care for children and young people.* London: BMJ Books, 2001.

121 Association of Police Surgeons. *Consent from children and young people in police custody.* Ipswich: APS, 2002.

122 Police and Criminal Evidence Act 1984 as amended by the Criminal Justice and Public Order Act 1994 s55 (England and Wales). Police and Criminal Evidence (Northern Ireland) Order 1989 art 56 (Northern Ireland). In Scotland, "proper authorisation" is the authority of a sheriff's warrant.

123 British Medical Association, Association of Police Surgeons. *Guidelines for doctors asked to perform intimate body searches.* London: BMA, 1999.

124 British Medical Association, Association of Police Surgeons. *Taking blood specimens from incapacitated drivers. Guidance for doctors on the provisions of the Police Reform Act 2002 from the British Medical Association and Association of Police Surgeons.* London: BMA, 2002.

125 Blatch B. *House of Lords official report (Hansard).* 1996 Feb 5: col 50.

126 British Medical Association, Association of Police Surgeons. *Revised interim guidelines on confidentiality for police surgeons in England, Wales and Northern Ireland.* London: BMA, 1998.

18: Education and training

The questions covered in this chapter include the following.

- Why and how should medical students learn about medical ethics and law?
- Is patient consent needed for the presence of medical students during consultations?
- Should patients be told if a medical student is to carry out part of their treatment?
- What is the "hidden curriculum"?
- Are there ethical dilemmas that are particular to medical students?
- What should medical students do if they witness unethical practice?

The ethical practice of medicine

The aim of Medical education is to provide doctors with the knowledge and skills needed to practise medicine within an ethical and legal framework. As discussed in the introductory chapter, doctors are confronted by ethical issues every day of their working lives; the medical training they receive must equip them with the skills and confidence needed to deal with these situations in an appropriate manner. This chapter examines the contribution that the teaching of medical ethics and law makes to medical education. This is a contribution that extends well beyond the provision of a body of knowledge about ethics and law, to the teaching of analytical and communication skills, and appropriate attitudes and behaviour towards patients. As the object of medicine is to maximise the health and wellbeing of patients, however technically proficient or knowledgeable doctors may be, if their practice is unethical they are failing to meet their objective. An understanding of ethics, and of the ethical practice of medicine, is therefore essential to being a good doctor.

This chapter considers three related but distinct areas. It begins by considering the way in which medical education has changed, introducing a greater emphasis on medical ethics as a core part of the medical curriculum. This part of the chapter focuses primarily on the teaching of law and ethics in the medical undergraduate curriculum, but recognises the increasing role of continuing professional development throughout a doctor's career. The chapter goes on to look at the related matter of the ethical issues that arise in medical education, focusing on the ethics of teaching and ways of ensuring that medical students can gain the experience they need without risk to patients, either physically or through undermining their autonomy. The final section considers whether there are particular ethical issues that arise for medical students.

General principles

The following general principles apply in education and training.

- An understanding of medical ethics and the ethical practice of medicine is essential to being a good doctor.
- In addition to knowledge of medical ethics and law, teaching should aim to provide medical students with the skills and confidence necessary to address difficult ethical dilemmas.
- Education and training is an ongoing process throughout a doctor's career.
- Tutors must ensure that teaching, both formal and informal, complies with good ethical practice; careful attention should be paid to consent and confidentiality when medical students are present during consultations.
- Medical students who witness unethical practice have a responsibility to make their concerns known.
- Teaching institutions have a responsibility to establish mechanisms for students to raise ethical concerns about aspects of their training without fear of repercussions.

Medical education: the changing landscape

The General Medical Council (GMC) has statutory responsibilities for undergraduate medical education, in terms of determining the knowledge and skills to be taught and the standard of proficiency required at qualifying examinations. In 1993 the GMC published the results of a comprehensive review of undergraduate medical education, which deplored the "gross overcrowding of most undergraduate curricula". It described the education of medical students as a process that "taxed the memory but not the intellect" while sacrificing the "truly educational" aspects of the course in favour of rote learning and cramming.[1] In future, the report suggested, medical education should provide "the graduate about to embark on a professional career with the capacity and the incentive to acquire and apply new knowledge and with the ability to adapt to changing circumstances, many as yet unforeseen".[2] One feature of this as yet unseen landscape was considered to be the appearance of new ethical dilemmas driven by changes in technology and medical practice, so the GMC concluded that any new curriculum would need to contain teaching in medical ethics and law at its core. The GMC published a series of recommendations, setting out the knowledge, understanding, skills, and attitudes that students must acquire from their undergraduate medical education and worked with medical schools to ensure that the necessary modifications were made to the curricula. In 1999 the GMC reported that, of its 13 recommendations, three had been implemented in most medical schools, eight had been substantially implemented in most medical schools, and only two were still awaiting implementation.[3] In 2002 its guidance was revised to take account of progress towards meeting the requirements and changing expectations.[4]

In the mid-1990s the BMA had also turned its attention to the perceived shortcomings in medical education and its findings echoed the GMC's recommendations.[5] The Association established a Medical Education Working Party in response to a number of resolutions passed at its Annual Representative Meetings, calling for complete reform of the undergraduate curriculum. It concluded that medical education had become overloaded with fact acquisition to the detriment of learning, ignoring established principles of education and insights from the psychology of learning. As discussed in Chapter 1, too much emphasis had been placed on the science of medicine and too little on the art of medicine.

BMA recommendations for all professional training

- It should recognise that students are capable of being (and should be encouraged to become) self directed learners.
- Learning should focus on making connections rather than the acquisition of isolated facts.
- Theoretical principles must be related to practical (preferably first hand) experiences.
- Constructive feedback should be provided by teachers to students on their progress.
- A positive social and emotional learning environment should be created to encourage cooperation and collaboration rather than competitiveness.
- Self assessment of performance should be encouraged alongside effective external assessment.[6]

The BMA emphasised that, although educational structures may be formal, teachers should be seen as facilitators of learning rather than providers of information. They should help students to see their own role as an active one and encourage them to revisit earlier work to see its relevance.

In its detailed recommendations, the BMA stressed that medical undergraduates should:

- have well developed skills of thinking and reasoning
- have skills for personal development and self criticism
- be taught and understand the ethical principles underpinning medical practice
- know their limitations and when to call for help
- have good communication skills
- develop attitudes appropriate to the practice of medicine
- be given support at all levels
- have interactive teaching to encourage them to reflect on, and critically evaluate, their own work
- be encouraged to define educational objectives to meet their personal learning needs
- have teachers who are kind and thoughtful towards them
- have access to a confidential counselling service separate from the appraisal system.

Selection for medical schools

The traditional prioritisation, within the medical curriculum, of technical and rational skills above capacities such as compassion and intuition has inevitably been reflected in the type of students selected for medical school. In 1999 the BMA considered the appropriateness of the selection techniques used by medical schools and, in order to develop a more diverse student body, concluded that:

- there should be greater emphasis on graduate entry
- the social basis of medicine needs to be widened
- information about the variety of non-standard entry requirements should be distributed more widely.[7]

> ### Selection for medical school
>
> In February 1999 the Council of Heads of Medical Schools and Deans of UK Faculties of Medicine published some guiding principles for the admission of medical students. The principles recognised the interplay of academic and non-academic qualities that go together to make up a successful doctor. Among these was
>
> > the recognition that patient care is the prime duty of a doctor. Honesty, integrity and an ability to recognise one's own limitations and those of others are central to the practice of medicine. In addition, medical students should be expected to have good communication and listening skills, an understanding of professional issues such as teamwork and respect for the contribution of other professions. Curiosity, creativity, initiative, flexibility, and leadership are all desirable characteristics for the aspiring doctor.[8]

The BMA is opposed to all forms of inappropriate discrimination in the selection of candidates to study medicine. This opposition is formally expressed in a wide range of policy statements drawn up at the BMA's Annual Representative Meetings, including the statement, drawn up in 2000, that "racism and discrimination in any form must be eliminated in the NHS".

The teaching of medical ethics and law

Although the introduction of medical ethics as a core part of the undergraduate medical curriculum is a relatively recent development, the notion that practical expertise should be accompanied by an awareness of certain moral standards goes back to the beginning of medicine. A surprisingly consistent set of values and standards is reflected in all codes of medical ethics, regardless of their cultural, geographical, or historical context. The teaching of medical ethics was traditionally intended to pass on these professional values to future generations of practising doctors, but in the past such teaching was often skimpy and formulaic. In many medical schools, medical ethics was either barely mentioned or was chiefly taught as a measure to protect medical staff against potential litigation.

As the teaching of ethics has become more formal, both in the UK and elsewhere, its aims, methodology, and content have changed. Various events prompted this change, including the publication in 1987 of the Pond Report,[9] which was the first major survey of UK medical schools focusing on the scope, aims, and methods of their teaching, and the GMC's report, *Tomorrow's doctors*,[10] which required changes to the medical curriculum. Despite the subsequent improvements identified by the GMC,[11] a 1997 survey of medical schools indicated that there remained considerable variation in the quality and quantity of undergraduate ethics teaching.[12] Among the problems highlighted by the authors were a lack of teachers and a paucity of appropriate teaching materials. A further study in 1998, carried out by the BMA, sought to assess how ethical issues were being presented to undergraduates and also to question whether there was a demand for human rights teaching as part of ethics courses (see pages 658–9).[13] The responses confirmed the continuing variations in both the time allocated to the subject and the depth in which ethical issues were explored. They also indicated that various methods were being used to develop questioning attitudes and skills in moral reasoning. However, promisingly, it was clear that an increasing amount of very detailed and sophisticated educational material was being produced for undergraduate use.

At the time of writing there is increasing recognition of the need for an updated version of the Pond Report and for a thorough assessment of the ethics and law component of postgraduate medical education.

Educational goals of teaching ethics and law

The teaching of medical ethics is sometimes criticised for being impractical. There is no place, it is argued, for philosophical abstractions amidst the messy contingencies of day to day medical practice, and cumbersome philosophical theories are more of a hindrance than a help to busy doctors. As discussed in the introductory chapter, however, a practical approach to resolving ethical dilemmas does not demand a detailed understanding of the philosophy underpinning discussion about medical ethics. In some cases, reaching a reasoned decision may demand little more than attentiveness to the dignity and autonomy of patients, together with knowledge of the relevant laws and guidance. Inevitably, however, difficult dilemmas arise that involve a more formal critical analysis of, for example, the conflicting duties owed to different people; training in and understanding of medical ethics equips doctors to deal with these situations. Furthermore the BMA, and other bodies, have come increasingly to recognise the absolute centrality of good communication skills to medical practice.[14] It sometimes becomes clear that certain complaints of unethical practice would never have arisen but for a breakdown in dialogue between doctors and patients. Good communication, recognising as it does the subjectivity of patients, is therefore critical to ethical practice, and is an area of education in which a small amount of attention could reap considerable benefit.

Objectives of teaching medical ethics and law

Teaching should ensure that students develop:

- an ability to identify the morally relevant principles at stake in particular dilemmas
- the skills to analyse these in order to reach a balanced and morally satisfactory answer
- an awareness of their legal and professional obligations to patients, employers, and the community
- the competence to communicate well with patients and professional colleagues
- an understanding of the generally complementary nature of ethics and law
- an overview of the implications for medical practice of ethical principles and law
- skills in communicating ethical concepts in a professional environment
- an attitude of respect for patient rights as an integral part of medical ethics and law.

In the UK, the last decades of the twentieth century saw a rapid development in legal aspects of medical practice, both through new statutes and developments in case law (see introductory chapter). Although some study of law has always been advisable for medical students, and is particularly relevant to certain medical specialties such as forensic medicine, it was often seen as a precautionary measure to help doctors to avoid litigation and raise their awareness of potential liability. Increasingly, however, the courts have become involved in deciding about the legal scope within which doctors may decide to give or withhold treatment. In some cases, sophisticated, imaginative, and complex ethical debates have taken place in the courts about the purpose of medical treatment and definitions of life and death. It is important that doctors should understand the key principles of law that affect medical practice and have knowledge of their legal obligations and duties. Students also need to be introduced to the nature of legal reasoning and exposed to the reality that definitive answers to some questions may not be available.

GMC recommendations on medicolegal and ethical issues for students

Graduates must know about and understand the main ethical and legal issues they will come across. For example, they must:

- make sure that patients' rights are protected
- maintain confidentiality
- deal with issues such as withholding or withdrawing life prolonging treatment
- provide appropriate care for vulnerable patients
- respond to patients' complaints about their care
- deal appropriately, effectively, and in patients' interests, with problems in the performance, conduct, or health of colleagues
- consider the practice of medicine within the context of limited financial resources
- understand the principles of law and good practice when seeking consent.[15]

Academic misconduct

Patterns and habits of conduct learnt at medical school can clearly set the basis for ethical practice throughout a doctor's career. As it is vital that doctors are honest and trustworthy, the ethical conduct of students during the academic parts of their training, when they will have no direct contact with patients, is also of the first importance. Reported problems with the academic conduct of medical students include plagiarism and fraud.[16] It is clear that students need to be aware that the ethical practice of medicine extends beyond the doctor–patient relationship and incorporates all aspects of their working lives. Furthermore, as medicine is widely seen as a career that entails lifelong learning, the need for scrupulous academic honesty throughout both undergraduate and postgraduate training is essential.

A core curriculum for teaching ethics and law

In 1998 the *Journal of Medical Ethics* published a consensus statement by teachers of medical ethics and law in the UK.[17] This outlined a model core curriculum for the UK (see below) with the aim of responding to the GMC's two objectives for the teaching of ethics and law, as outlined in its 1993 report[18]:

- to ensure that students acquire a knowledge and understanding of ethical and legal issues relevant to the practice of medicine and
- to ensure that students develop an ability to understand and analyse ethical problems so as to enable patients, their families, society, and doctors to have proper regard to such problems in reaching decisions.

A core curriculum for medical ethics and law

- **Informed consent and refusal of treatment:** why respect for autonomy is so important; adequate information; treatment without consent; competence; battery and negligence
- **The clinical relationship – truthfulness, trust and good communication:** ethical limits of paternalism; building trust; honesty, courage and other virtues in clinical practice; narrative and the importance of communication skills
- **Confidentiality:** clinical importance of privacy; compulsory and discretionary disclosure; public versus private interests
- **Medical research:** ethical and legal tensions in doing medical research on patients, human volunteers, and animals; the need for effective regulation
- **Human reproduction:** ethical and legal status of the embryo/fetus; assisted conception; abortion, including prenatal screening
- **The new genetics:** treating the abnormal versus improving the normal; debates about the ethical boundaries of and the need to regulate genetic therapy and research

(Continued)

- **Children:** ethical and clinical significance of age to consent to treatment; dealing with parental/child/clinician conflicts
- **Mental disorders and disabilities:** ethical and legal justifications for detention and treatment without consent; conflicts of interests between patient, family and community
- **Life, death, dying and killing:** the duty of care and ethical and legal justification for the non-provision of life prolonging treatment and the provision of potentially life shortening palliatives; transplantation; death certification; and the coroner's court
- **Vulnerabilities created by the duties of doctors and medical students:** public expectations of medicine; the need for teamwork; the health of doctors and students in relation to professional performance; the GMC and professional regulation; responding appropriately to clinical mistakes; whistleblowing
- **Resource allocation:** ethical debates about "rationing" and the fair and just distribution of scarce health care; the relevance of needs, rights, utility, efficiency, merit, and autonomy to theories of equitable health care; boundaries of responsibility of individuals for their own health
- **Rights:** what rights are, and their links with moral and professional duties; the importance of the concept of rights, including human rights, for good medical practice.

The consensus group concluded that medical ethics and law should be introduced systematically throughout the entire clinical curriculum, including the house officer year, and that each clinical discipline should address the ethical and legal issues of particular relevance within it. Students and teachers should be formally assessed with the same rigour as for other core subjects, and successful completion of the course should be a prerequisite for graduation. Although not wishing to produce rigid guidelines about how medical ethics should be taught, the group was convinced that adequate teaching of medical ethics and law required at least one full time senior academic in ethics and law with relevant professional and academic expertise. It could no longer "be taught by well-disposed clinicians without some consistent interaction with, and support from, specialists".[19]

Graduation oaths

Studies show that about half of all UK medical schools and almost all medical schools in the USA administer an oath of some kind either on graduation, or at the beginning of medical studies, in order to acknowledge formally the student's or graduate's commitment to medicine.[20] Texts vary. Some use a version of the Hippocratic Oath (see appendix A), while others use the World Medical Association's Declaration of Geneva (see appendix B), or an oath formulated by the institution itself. Some are applicable only to doctors; others reflect the reality of current multidisciplinary practice.

One of the strengths of the "Hippocratic tradition" of asking that doctors pledge themselves to demanding ethical standards has been its contribution to the understanding of the unique position, and the unique powers and responsibilities, of members of the medical profession; the ethical standards are demanding in proportion to doctors' potential to act for good or bad in their patients' lives. Views differ about the benefits and drawbacks of such ceremonies.[21] Those who support them draw attention to their perceived benefits, including the development of ethical sensitivity, the promotion of professional bonding, and the recognition by students of the gravity of their undertaking. Those who oppose their use focus on the potential drawbacks, including their promotion of cultural and professional isolation, the confusing number of oaths available and reservations about whether medical students are yet sufficiently experienced to understand the ramifications of the oath they take.

The BMA supports the practice of health professionals making some formal commitment to ethical standards as an awareness raising act at the beginning of their careers.

Postgraduate training in ethics

Although most of this chapter focuses on the training of undergraduate medical students, medical education generally and training in medical ethics specifically are ongoing processes throughout a doctor's career. In addition to their own educational needs, doctors are also involved in teaching more junior colleagues, both formally and informally. In order to fulfil this role adequately, all doctors need to keep their knowledge and skills up to date and ensure that their practice complies with current expectations of good practice (see pages 665–7). Continuing education and professional development is not an optional extra; they are part of the professional obligations of all doctors, the assessment of which forms part of the revalidation process (see Chapter 21, page 760). The GMC advises doctors: "you must keep your knowledge and skills up to date throughout your working life. In particular, you should take part regularly in educational activities which maintain and further develop your competence and performance".[22]

From theory to practice

One of the consistent problems raised by junior doctors with the BMA has been that, although as students they learn the importance of medical ethics and medical law, once graduated they are often expected by other professionals to conform to accepted custom and practice. The force of tradition is hard to resist and is compounded by younger doctors' anxieties that their career prospects can easily be jeopardised by questioning or objecting to the instructions of senior health professionals.

One of the most important issues in medical ethics is that of communicating effectively with patients in order to enable them to consent to or refuse particular treatment options. Seeking consent, however, has traditionally been a task passed to the most junior member of the healthcare team, who is often unable to answer all the patients' questions or does not have the experience properly to convey information that may be potentially distressing. In 1998 a resolution was passed at the BMA's annual meeting noting that "the current practice of obtaining informed consent is inadequate and fails to serve patients or doctors". It was clear that the primary concern of doctors lay not with any lack of guidance as to what constitutes ethical practice, but with the implementation of that guidance. A BMA working party was established to consider the problem, in consultation with the royal colleges of medicine and nursing, patient groups, and lawyers. After a wide consultation exercise it was found that, despite the proliferation of legal and ethical guidance, general awareness of the main principles relating to consent remained inadequate. Nevertheless, there was felt to be little point in merely reiterating those principles, and efforts were made to find ways of ensuring that information reached the appropriate people in a way that would ensure its implementation.

Implementing best practice on consent

The BMA took the following steps in its attempts to implement best practice on consent.

- It produced a report outlining the problems and made 17 recommendations for action, which emphasised the importance of senior clinicians becoming involved in both the formal teaching of consent issues and leading by example.
- It sent copies of the report to all UK medical schools and 4000 copies were sent to clinical and medical directors of trusts throughout the UK, together with the recommendation that trusts develop their own internal guidelines and policy statements on how consent should be sought and by whom.
- It produced a pocket sized "consent tool kit", comprising a series of "reminder" cards containing frequently asked questions.
- It distributed more than 70 000 copies of the tool kit to practising doctors by, for example, inclusion as a supplement in *BMA News*.
- It sent copies of the tool kit to all new doctors on their graduation and, on request, to teachers, students, and others.
- It made the report and the tool kit freely available through the ethics department's website, with no copyright restriction.
- It drew attention to the practical obstacles that stand in the way of good practice and called for change.
- It was represented on the Department of Health's good practice in consent initiative, which resulted in the publication of guidance, patient information leaflets, model policy, and model consent forms (see Chapter 2, page 73).

Developing trends in teaching medical ethics

In addition to changes in what is taught, the way in which ethics is taught has also been undergoing change, with increasing involvement from other disciplines.

Multidisciplinary teaching

Medical ethics is increasingly taught on a multidisciplinary basis. One of the aims of this is to try to avoid professional compartmentalisation, to create a better understanding of the complementary roles of different professionals in the team, and to engender mutual respect between all healthcare professions. In the past, for example, nurses and doctors saw their ethical obligations to patients in rather different terms, with nurses often seeing themselves as the patient's advocate. In this context, *The report of the public inquiry into children's heart surgery at the Bristol Royal Infirmary 1984–1995* (the Bristol report) makes several recommendations about strengthening links between medical schools and schools of nursing "with a view to providing more joint education between medical and nursing students".[23]

Reinforcing this process, the development of patient centred care is increasingly leading to a softening of traditional boundaries between the various healthcare professions, and the professional status and range of responsibilities of nurses and other non-doctors in the medical team is also increasing. Awareness of the role of other healthcare professionals is also becoming a core activity in the training of doctors. Furthermore, given the general applicability of core ethical issues such as consent and confidentiality to all healthcare professionals, it is likely that joint teaching in this area is something that will continue to develop.

Although multidisciplinary teaching presents administrative and logistical problems, and its effectiveness needs to be assessed, the BMA nevertheless strongly supports the principle of exploring multidisciplinary education. Further information in this area can be obtained from the BMA's Board of Medical Education.

Human rights

The integration of human rights into medical ethics teaching is symptomatic of a growing recognition that human rights are not only of concern in a few specific countries, but that they increasingly coincide with the ordinary ethical dilemmas with which health professionals are faced. Policy making in terms of health care, for example, frequently raises questions about the rights (and duties) of the individual versus those of society at large, thus echoing one of the central concerns of human rights.[24] In addition, since the Human Rights Act 1998 came into force in the UK, lawyers and ethicists have begun specifically to consider traditional ethical issues, such as the allocation of healthcare resources and the marginalisation of some patient groups, through the prism of human rights discourse. The relationship between medical ethics and human rights is discussed further in the introductory chapter.

In 1994 Amnesty International undertook a survey to assess the level and nature of human rights teaching in UK medical schools.[25] Of the 22 schools responding, 14 said that their ethics courses included, or would in future include, a human rights component, covering issues such as abuse in psychiatry and general failure to obtain informed consent. The BMA conducted a further study of medical schools in 1998–1999, which found that the extent of human rights teaching had not significantly increased, but that the teaching of medical ethics generally had become more formalised, detailed, and comprehensive, particularly on issues such as informed consent.[26] Human rights issues, such as prison medicine or treatment of asylum seekers, however, were absent. In 1999 the annual meeting of the World Medical Association passed a resolution calling for the inclusion of medical ethics and human rights in the curricula of all medical schools worldwide.[27]

Although an awareness of ethical and legal principles is essential for all health professionals, a knowledge of the connections between law, ethics, and human rights assumes a particular importance for those working in environments that are most likely to generate human rights violations or to bring health workers into contact with the evidence of abuse. Forensic doctors, prison doctors, police surgeons, and those employed by the armed services should have training that focuses on their particular dilemmas. Similarly, doctors visiting or working in otherwise "closed" institutions, such as psychiatric hospitals or children's homes, many need additional training. These doctors work in specialties in which it is easy to become isolated from mainstream practice and to absorb the mind set of other workers, whose dominant concern may be for the maintenance of order rather than the maximisation of welfare. Their dilemmas are also the ones least addressed in ethical guidelines or training.

Humanitarian and global issues

There is increased recognition that the views of medical students themselves should be sought about the components to be included in undergraduate teaching. Medical students' organisations are very conscious of the number of subjects that already have to be compressed into the curriculum. One student organisation active in this sphere is the Medical Students' International Network (MedSIN), which campaigns for the curriculum to be extended to include humanitarian and global health issues. In the UK, MedSIN works closely on education issues with another organisation, Medact, which has produced an undergraduate teaching pack with a public health focus, covering:

- social and economic development
- environmental change and pollution
- the health implications of conflict
- the interconnections between poverty, environmental pollution, and conflict.[28]

These teaching materials can be used flexibly to suit local needs, either as a complete course or as separate modules. Some UK medical schools have been very responsive to the inclusion of these materials as special study modules in global health. Among the key topics that MedSIN recommends as appropriate for inclusion in the curriculum are: human rights generally; social inequality; migration and refugees; conflict and trauma; and ethics and reproductive health. In addition to its projects on the curriculum, MedSIN undertakes a range of practical community and public health activities to encourage medical student involvement in community and intersectorial work. Such projects complement the theoretical and academic teaching in human rights and may produce a more enduring impact on future doctors' views and attitudes.

Medical humanities

In *Tomorrow's doctors* the GMC stresses the importance of developing the cultural sensitivities, imagination, and interpretive skills of medical students.[29] The medical humanities have been portrayed as one means of achieving this, by relating issues in medicine to those portrayed in art, literature, popular culture, film, and theatre. The integration of medical humanities into the teaching of medical ethics has the key aims of helping students to:

- think of themselves as embryonic doctors and promote an understanding of professional identity by reference to cultural images of the profession
- understand the disparity between the reality of medicine and public expectations
- develop analytical and interpretive skills and
- come to terms with their own mortality.

Concerned as they are with imagination and insight, the medical humanities fit closely with a great deal of core ethical discourse. Literature, art, and poetry share with medical ethics a preoccupation with the most troubling human questions relating to death, illness, suffering, and disability. Some see the subject as a counterbalance to a potentially excessive focus on scientific knowledge alone. Goodwin argues

> Science can tell us nothing about an individual. Science speaks in terms of probabilities, of means and standard deviations, the behaviour of groups of electrons or proteins or people, not of individual entities. Everything that makes an individual an individual, everything that importantly defines an individual's life, is outside the realm of science. The practice of medicine involves only individuals.[30]

Ideally, of course, doctors and other health professionals should be exposed to a wide range of influences that can contribute positively to their personal and professional development and to the manner in which they approach patients.

Distance learning materials

The BMA has long been aware of an international need for teaching packs consisting of basic learning materials in ethics and relevant law. Such packs could either be used as self teaching tools or as a means of training medical students and others where access to such material is impossible. It has urged that high quality teaching materials be made available via media such as the internet, so that they can be accessed by doctors and medical students who have no easy means of increasing their knowledge about medical ethics. Most BMA ethics and law materials are freely available on its website. Clearly, however, in a competitive market, it may be difficult for academic institutions to disseminate material without charge.

Summary – the teaching of medical law and ethics

- In its 1993 report the GMC advised that medical ethics and law should form part of the core curriculum for medical undergraduates.
- Medical ethics teaching has the two main objectives of ensuring that medical students acquire:

  - a knowledge and understanding of ethical and legal issues relevant to medicine and
  - an ability to understand and analyse ethical problems.

- Good communication skills are essential to the ethical practice of medicine.
- The BMA supports the practice of health professionals making a formal commitment to ethical standards at the beginning of their careers.
- Education and training are continuing processes throughout a doctor's career.
- The teaching of medical ethics has increasingly adopted methods and principles from other disciplines, such as human rights and medical humanities.

Ethical issues raised in teaching medical students

In addition to teaching medical ethics, tutors, supervisors, and other doctors also need to ensure that the practice of teaching medical students is undertaken in an ethical manner. Inevitably, during their training, medical students come into contact with patients and, in some cases, they undertake examinations or procedures. The general ethical principles that guide all medical practice are also central to any contact between patients and medical students. This section considers the issues raised by such encounters and also other aspects of the ethical teaching of medicine.

Consent in the context of teaching

It is essential that medical students develop their clinical skills through steadily increasing involvement with patients, but this should be done only with the knowledge and consent of the patients concerned. In order for this consent to be valid, patients need to be aware of:

- who will be present
- why they will be present
- what, if any, involvement they will have with the procedure being undertaken.

All patients must also be given the opportunity of refusing to have students present and should be reassured that this will not, in any way, affect the care they receive.

When the patient is a young child, the consent of someone with parental responsibility should be sought. Older children and young people may themselves be capable of giving consent to being examined by a student, but may also wish to involve their parents. Extreme care needs to be taken before including incapacitated people in teaching processes, whether they are temporarily incapacitated, as a result of an accident or trauma for example, or have long term incapacity. When considering whether to include an adult who is lacking capacity in teaching, it is important to consider whether the intervention could cause any physical or emotional harm. If it can be shown to be neutral or beneficial in its effects, then there are no obvious reasons for not involving incapacitated adults, although it would be good practice to discuss the matter with those close to these patients and with any appointed health care proxies in Scotland. Additional information about consent can be found in Chapters 2, 3 and 4.

These basic principles about consent apply whether training is undertaken in a teaching hospital or in any other clinical setting. All healthcare establishments involved in education and training may find it helpful to draw up protocols about the extent to which medical students and other doctors in training will be present during, and involved with, examination and treatment.

Introducing students

The BMA is sometimes asked how students should be introduced to patients, whether as "medical students" or "student doctors", for example. The most important factor is that the patient must be left in no doubt about whether the individual is a qualified doctor who is learning new skills or is an undergraduate undergoing his or her initial training. The BMA believes that the phrase "medical student" is the most appropriate and unambiguous term for those who are undergoing their undergraduate training.

Presence of medical students

Even when medical students will not be involved in the consultation and are simply observing the practice of the treating doctor, consent is needed for them to be present; this includes where large numbers of students are present during ward rounds. The doctor who is carrying out the consultation should explain to the patient that one or more observers would like to be present during the consultation, examination, or procedure, who they are, and why they wish to observe. Patients should be given the opportunity to refuse the presence of medical students or, if they prefer, to limit the number who will be present. Patients should be reassured that their decision will not affect their treatment. In most circumstances, it is possible and good practice to give patients the option of considering this request prior to the arrival of the students.

Examining patients

Learning to carry out examinations with the necessary degree of technical expertise and appropriate communication skills is an essential part of medical training. As with doctors, any touching of patients by medical students needs consent. When patients are conscious and competent, the nature and the purpose of the examination should be described, and they should be asked for permission for one or more students to examine them. It should be made clear whether the procedure is being undertaken as part of their own treatment, or for the educational benefit of the examining students. Where procedures or examinations are solely for the purpose of educating students, it is essential that the patient understands this, and gives explicit consent for it to take place. If the patient does not give consent, students should not take part in the examination.

Whenever possible, students should learn their technical skills by working with competent patients who have given consent. Inevitably, however, they also need to learn to examine and interact with people who lack capacity. Care must be taken, however, to ensure that incapacitated people are not subjected to repeated examinations simply because they do not appear to object. If patients are distressed, the examination should stop.

Students who are present while patients are anaesthetised are sometimes asked to examine the patient or simply to "have a feel" of the surgeon's findings. In the past, it was common to conduct rectal or vaginal examinations on patients under anaesthesia, often without their consent.[31] Such practice is entirely unacceptable. Doctors must not ask students to be involved in any physical touching or exploration unless the patient has given consent in advance, and students should refuse to participate if they are not satisfied that proper permission has been obtained. In addition to the ethical problems that can arise, the Royal College of Obstetricians and Gynaecologists has questioned the value of pelvic examination under anaesthesia because it does not teach students the "combination of communication and expert examination that characterise sensitive pelvic examination".[32] Instead, it recommends that students should learn how to don gloves and handle a vaginal speculum in a classroom, and practise using a mannequin in a clinical skills laboratory. Observation of an awake patient in an outpatient clinic is the next step, before ultimately the student performs pelvic and speculum examination of an awake and competent patient under supervision and with the patient's consent. This model of acquiring technical expertise and observing good practice is important throughout medical training. Whether students are performing the examination or merely observing, explicit consent is required from patients. When consent cannot be obtained, intimate investigations by or in the presence of students should not be undertaken.

Failure to obtain consent for teaching

At the beginning of 2003 the results of an exploratory survey into the quality of the consent sought for intimate examination of anaesthetised patients by students was published.[33] The survey found that up to a quarter of intimate examinations on these patients did not have adequate consent. This survey echoes an earlier and more detailed exploration of the ethical dilemmas facing medical students undertaken at the University of Toronto in 2001.[34]

Carrying out procedures as part of the patient's care

Medical students and doctors in training often carry out procedures that patients need as part of their care, such as taking blood samples. The Department of Health advises that

> assuming the student is appropriately trained in the procedure, the fact that it is carried out by a student does not alter the nature and purpose of the procedure. It is therefore not a legal requirement to tell the patient that the clinician is a student, although it would always be good practice to do so.[35]

The BMA supports the view that patients should be told if a student is to undertake the procedure, but they should be reassured that the student has had the necessary training and will be given an appropriate level of supervision. A similar view was expressed in the Bristol report, which said that "surgeons or other clinicians who undertake invasive clinical procedures for the first time must be properly trained and directly supervised ... Patients are entitled to know what experience the surgeon or clinician has before giving consent".[36] Openness and honesty with patients is the key if their consent to the procedure is to be valid.

Responsibility for seeking consent rests with the doctor recommending the procedure, who should tell the patient what the procedure involves, including a discussion of the various treatment options, the alternatives available, the prognosis, and the risks associated with the intervention. Although the process of seeking consent may be delegated in certain circumstances (see Chapter 2, pages 74–6), the person seeking consent must always be suitably trained and have sufficient knowledge and understanding of the proposed procedure and the risks involved.

As with qualified doctors, if students are asked during their training to carry out procedures they do not feel competent to do, they should make their concerns known and ask for additional guidance and supervision.

Confidentiality in the context of teaching

Patients who are involved in teaching do not relinquish their rights to, or their interests in, confidentiality. In the process of seeking consent to the presence or involvement of medical students during consultations (see above), patients should be advised that necessary information will be shared with students as part of that process. Patients should be reassured that medical students have a duty to keep the information confidential.

The amount of information that medical students are given should be judged on the same basis as deciding whether information should be shared within healthcare teams. Information should, therefore, be limited to those who have a demonstrable "need to know" it as a part of their role in providing care (this is discussed further in Chapter 5). When medical students, or doctors in training, are providing care to a patient, they should be provided with as much information as they need in order to carry out the procedure safely and effectively. When, however, they require information solely for their own education, it is essential that patients are made aware of this and give explicit consent to the sharing of information for that purpose. If patients refuse consent to this information being released, this must be respected. When patients give consent, the information disclosed should be the minimum necessary to achieve the purpose. If student involvement is limited to teaching on the basis of patient notes, or if students are using the case studies of particular patients for a dissertation, anonymised information should be used wherever possible. If identifiable information is required, patient consent must be sought, ideally by the responsible tutor, and either a written statement of consent or a record of verbal consent placed in the notes.[37] The involvement of children who lack the capacity to consent to projects of this kind requires consent from someone with parental responsibility.

Work observation and experience

Young people who are reaching the end of their secondary education and are considering applying to medical school, sometimes ask doctors if they can observe their work (shadowing) in order to gain a clearer picture of the reality of medical practice. When considering such requests, doctors must emphasise the importance of patient confidentiality, and must be satisfied that the observer is mature and responsible enough to understand the principles of confidentiality. As with the presence of medical students, observers should be present only during consultations if patients have given their consent. Patients should be given time to consider such requests without the observer present and it must be made clear that a refusal will not in any way influence their treatment. Further guidelines for doctors on work observation are available from the BMA.[38] Prospective medical students sometimes also ask to observe postmortem examinations; this is discussed in Chapter 12 (page 443).

Young people also sometimes seek work experience or part-time positions in healthcare settings, in the process of which they may have access to some confidential medical information. As with all employees, it is the doctor's responsibility to advise them about the importance of confidentiality and the employer retains overall responsibility for any breaches that might occur.

The "hidden curriculum"

It has long been recognised that students learn not only from their formal teaching but also from their experiences of observing and working with practising doctors. This aspect of teaching has been referred to as the "hidden curriculum".[39] Many doctors provide excellent role models and reinforce the lessons and principles that students have learnt throughout their studies. It has been argued, however, that it is in the corridors and cafeteria, and in the methods and manners of their teachers, that medical students absorb a distinctive "medical morality", a "morality" that is sometimes at odds with the interests of their patients.[40] The example of how their tutors practise can be a far more powerful influence in the development of ethical, or unethical, practice than the edicts of formal ethics teaching.

This conflict between formal and informal learning underlies the tensions that many medical students, motivated as they are to be "good doctors", articulate in their response to the teaching of ethics. On the one hand they have strong moral instincts and express considerable interest in ethics, but on the other they aspire to the professionalism and confidence of their senior colleagues, some of whom may seem to pay scant attention to medical ethics in their actual practice. In fact, their senior colleagues may unwittingly give the impression that medical ethics gets in the way of good practice. Anecdotal support for the existence of this tension has been reported to the BMA by its student members, who describe how they learn about ethics in the classrooms of medical school but sometimes find that some of their senior colleagues appear to ignore ethical and legal precepts.

One possible effect of this tension is the growth of cynicism and the erosion of ethical beliefs and conduct.[41] "When there is a discrepancy between what students are taught about good ethico-legal practice and what they experience on clinical firms, anger, disillusionment and cynicism may follow".[42] Feudtner and colleagues have studied a range of ethical dilemmas faced by medical students in their clinical practice, all of which displayed this tension between the formal and the hidden curricula.[43] When asked why they did not respond when they witnessed unethical behaviour by other, frequently senior, members of medical teams, medical students gave the following responses:

- wanting to be seen as "team players" and
- concern that if they did not "toe the line" they would receive negative evaluations from other team members.

The way in which medical students can begin to address this type of situation, given the inevitable imbalance of power, is discussed on pages 670–2. It is essential, however, that all doctors are conscious of the impact of their words and behaviour on those who are learning. In terms of their own practice, as well as their informal role as teachers, doctors should ensure that they always act in accordance with good ethical practice and that they are willing to respond to questions and challenges about their methods and decisions.

The ethical doctor: teaching skills or inculcating virtues?

It has been suggested that part of the response to the problems caused by the "hidden curriculum" lies in the recognition that ethical principles need to be fully integrated into doctors' professional identities before they can begin to resist unethical practice.[44] Essentially, medical ethics cannot be taught in the same way as science or technical skills, but requires an understanding of the virtues that make a good doctor. Virtue ethics, which is discussed further in the introductory chapter, focuses discussion of medical ethics on the inner moral development of doctors and asks questions about what values doctors have absorbed rather than what rules or duties they should respect. In drawing attention to the centrality of virtues such as caring, concern for others, appreciation of their predicament, a proper sense of humility, and the ability to communicate clearly and compassionately with a person while he or she is under a great deal of stress, virtue ethics points to qualities that are "the heart and soul of good clinical judgment".[45]

Creating the necessary distance: professionalism or dehumanisation?

The training and practice of medicine is intellectually and emotionally demanding. An important part of medical training is to help medical students to develop the skills required to assist people during some of the most difficult times of their lives, without themselves ceasing to function either as professionals or as human beings.[46] The relative youth and inexperience of the majority of medical students mean that they are frequently unprepared for the experiences of suffering and death they will inevitably encounter.[47] In order to deal with this "a kind of emotional hardening has to take place ... the student must quickly learn ways of coping not only with cadavers, but with the pain, distress, and mutilation associated with serious disease and injury".[48] A delicate balance is required, however. If the process of "hardening" is too complete, if too great an emotional distance is established, those who become clinically competent may not, in the end, be the best (or even good) doctors. It is during the period of their training, when medical students begin the process of "detachment", that some of the most important ethical lessons are learnt, and habits of feeling towards patients are developed that can persist for a professional lifetime. It is also at this stage that "the informal curriculum reigns",[49] and the scope for ethical teaching to encourage sensitivity towards patients is at its greatest. Those who teach medical students have a responsibility to show by their words and example that this process of detachment can be achieved without diminishing the respect and dignity of those who are suffering or who have died. Reports, such as that below, of cadavers being treated merely as objects, reflect outdated attitudes and practices that have no place in the teaching of medical students.

Encountering death

"The reality of death is thrust at us as medical students. From the moment we swung through the doors of the dissection room in the first year, we were faced with the immensity of what we will have to cope with during our studies and professional lives. Because we did not and still do not understand death and what it involves, we did not know how to react to the bodies, or deal with the horrific thought that we were cutting up human flesh. During our first session, the anatomy demonstrator casually threw a pile of books down on our group's cadaver, making us flinch: this was the first time that the body was treated as an object in our presence."[50]

Students' experiences of the dissecting room inevitably alter their perceptions of human beings and instil in them the importance of emotional distance. They have been described as the "first bridge leading us away from the lay public towards the medical world" where patients come to be seen less as people than as "cases of disease".[51]

One of the clear and essential contributions that the teaching of ethics and law can have at this point is to demonstrate that the process of detachment is not a straight line, but rather a loop. Medical students move away from lay responses – from squeamishness and fear – in order to return, but to return not to see their patients as elaborate machines that require tinkering with, but as suffering human beings whom, through their professionalism, they can assist.

The healing ethos combines this necessary detachment with a genuine concern for the individual patient, an attitude requiring a degree of empathy and emotional closeness. Only when the medical ethos includes a profound respect for the individuality of each patient will it serve the true purpose of medicine – the health of the patient.[52]

Summary – ethical issues raised in teaching medical students

- Tutors, supervisors and other doctors must ensure that the practice of teaching medical students is undertaken in an ethical manner.
- Medical students should be present during, or involved with, consultations only where the appropriate consent has been obtained.
- Medical students should never touch or examine a patient, including those under anaesthetic, without the necessary consent.
- Information should be shared with medical students only with the patient's consent.
- All doctors must be aware of students' informal methods of learning by experience and observation; they must always ensure that their behaviour complies with good ethical practice.
- Doctors should always be willing to respond to questions and challenges from medical students about their methods and decisions.

Particular dilemmas of medical students

The question is often raised of whether there are ethical dilemmas that are peculiar to medical students. In order to ensure that this publication addressed the particular needs of medical students, the Medical Ethics Committee asked the BMA's Medical Students Committee to draw up a list of common ethical dilemmas faced by medical students. These are listed in the box below, which also indicates where in this book the issues are discussed.

Ethical dilemmas faced by students

- the proper form by which students should be introduced to patients (see page 662)
- patients' consent to student involvement in consultations and treatments (see pages 661–4)
- the sharing of confidential information with clinical firms (see pages 664–5)
- inexperience in carrying out procedures (see page 664)
- carrying out intimate examinations on patients while under anaesthetic (see pages 662–3)
- conflicts between medical education and patient care (see pages 662–3)
- witnessing poor practice (see pages 665–6 and pages 670–2)
- how to respond when senior colleagues have impaired judgment (see Chapter 21, pages 754–8)
- physical or verbal assault from patients (see Chapter 1, pages 58–60)
- disclosure from patients that they have been subjected to abuse (see Chapter 5, pages 195–6)
- concealment of mistakes by senior colleagues (see Chapter 21, pages 754–8)
- responding to admissions of criminal behaviour from patients (see Chapter 5, page 194)
- providing medical treatment to family and friends (Chapter 1, pages 53–4, and Chapter 13, page 478)
- when questions arise about the competence or behaviour of fellow students (Chapter 21, pages 754–8)
- students being recruited to take part in the research projects of their teachers (see Chapter 14, pages 503–4).

Although many of the issues highlighted are similar to those encountered by fully qualified doctors, what is different for medical students is their relationship to those dilemmas. Students do not need to take full responsibility for decision making and should seek the advice of clinical tutors if confronted by some of the situations outlined above. If, for example, patients disclose to a student that they have been subjected to abuse or if they disclose past criminal activity, students should seek advice from a senior colleague or member of the teaching staff who can take the matter forward if necessary.

More difficult are cases where students' concerns relate to the behaviour or performance of a senior colleague or teacher. They often feel unable to speak out, even though they recognise unethical practice, because of the power imbalance in the relationship. Medical students are dependent on their senior colleagues and teachers in order to progress in their medical career; criticising them for practising unethically may seem like a certain path to failure. One medical student, commenting on this power imbalance, said:

Clinical students walk this ethical tightrope every day – to refuse or object when placed in an unethical situation you have to be brave and tread carefully. It is often the arrogant clinician, with little interest in ethics, who puts the student in this difficult position, and too often it is the same arrogant clinician who grades the student.[53]

Furthermore, the power difference is based on more than just status. There are inevitably and properly very real differences in knowledge and experience, and a respect for this may lead students to question their own perception of poor practice.

Students and tutors: managing inequalities in power

In a profession as complex, demanding, and technically refined as medicine, students will always begin their training entirely dependent on the expertise and instruction of tutors and senior colleagues, and it is appropriate that they should defer to them. An inability to take instruction or recognise legitimate authority can be as much of an impediment to becoming a good doctor as obsequiousness and a suppression of critical faculties. Lives may be at stake and the overwhelming majority of senior doctors have arrived at their positions because of their professional excellence, and most students recognise this. Frequently, what is at issue is little more than a disagreement over which of several legitimate approaches is the best. In such cases, it is appropriate that the doctor with the most experience and overall responsibility for the patient should have the final word, after discussing and considering the views of other members of the team. Students who disobey instructions whenever they feel they have a better idea are likely to harm their patients;[54] but when students have serious concerns that carrying out orders will significantly compromise patient care, or where the practice they see is seriously at odds with the principles they have been taught, they have a duty to make their concerns known. Initial concerns may be overcome simply by questioning why a particular decision was made, or why one option was chosen over another, and asking the doctor to explain the reasoning behind it. When a satisfactory answer is not received, however, or where there are remaining concerns, further steps may need to be taken despite the huge burden that this can place on the students concerned.

As discussed above, a primary aim of the teaching of medical ethics is to develop within students a questioning, enquiring, and analytical mind; this needs to be backed up by a mechanism for students to exercise these qualities without fear of repercussions. It is therefore incumbent upon teaching institutions to devise safe methods for students and staff to discuss such problems as and when they arise, in ways that enhance rather than jeopardise the students' progress. An important part of addressing such problems is to ensure that teaching in medical ethics and law is not reserved only for students. Those involved with teaching students, both in the classroom and on the wards, need to be aware of the impact of their practice on others, and to recognise that, when students raise legitimate concerns or questions, they have a duty to respond.

Questions students should consider if they believe they have witnessed unethical practice

- Is it possible to raise questions about the episode in an enquiring and non-confrontational manner?
- If not, or if this has proved unsatisfactory:

  - Are there local protocols for managing problems of this nature?
  - Are there personal tutors, mentors or pastoral carers who may be able to advise?
  - Are there other senior colleagues who may be able to give advice?
  - Would it be useful to discuss the concerns with fellow students to see if they agree?
  - If advice on the general ethical issues the dilemma raises is required, would it be helpful to seek advice from the BMA?

BMA members can seek advice on these questions from their regional office.

These problems are not easily resolved, and speaking out can require courage. Singer argues that what is required is a systematic change in the procedures for accountability.[55] Medical schools, he argues, need to develop formal guidelines for ethics in clinical teaching that:

- highlight the responsibility of clinical teaching staff to serve as appropriate role models to medical students and to provide them with an opportunity to discuss ethical challenges
- require university and teaching hospitals to develop processes for reporting ethical concerns
- ensure that medical students and their tutors have access to individuals they can approach with ethical problems
- ensure that when medical students express concern about ethical issues or decline to take part in certain activities for ethical reasons, this will not have any repercussions for them.

Finally, Singer argues that the reporting of ethical problems should model itself upon the "medical error movement", which seeks to promote a blame free environment in which errors and difficulties are openly reported and discussed. Instead of apportioning blame, which can lead to evasion and coverup, systematic solutions should be found for the ethical challenges of medical education.

Rights of patients asked to participate in medical education

In 1996 students at one medical school developed a policy to underline the rights of competent patients who were asked to participate in educational activities that were separate from their clinical care. They argued that, in addition to reminding teachers of their duties as medical educators, such a policy would also help students to question activities they perceived to be unacceptable. The policy included the following.

- Patients must understand that medical students are not qualified doctors.
- Clinical teachers and students must obtain explicit consent from patients before students take their case histories or physically examine them.
- Clinical teachers and students should never perform physical examinations or present cases without the patient's consent.
- Students should never perform any physical examination on patients who are under general anaesthesia without the patients' prior written consent.
- Clinical teachers should obtain patients' consent for students to participate in treatment.
- Students must respect the confidentiality of all information communicated by patients in the course of their treatment or educational activity.
- Patients should understand that students may be obliged to inform a responsible clinician about information relevant to their clinical care.
- Clinical teachers are responsible for ensuring that these guidelines are followed.
- If students are asked by anyone to act contrary to this policy, they must politely refuse, referring to these guidelines.[56]

Summary – particular dilemmas of medical students

- Many of the dilemmas that arise for medical students are the same as those that fully qualified doctors experience, although their relationship to the dilemma is different.
- Students do not need to take full responsibility for decision making and should seek the advice of clinical tutors if confronted by ethical dilemmas involving patients or patient care.
- Difficulties can arise when medical students have concerns about the behaviour or performance of a senior colleague or tutor; this is exacerbated by the imbalance of power within the relationship.
- Medical students who have concerns that carrying out instructions will compromise patient care, or who witness practice that is seriously at odds with the principles they have been taught, have a duty to make their concerns known.
- Those involved with teaching students, both in the classroom and on the wards, need to be aware of the impact of their practice on others and to recognise that, when students raise legitimate concerns or questions, they have a duty to respond.
- Teaching institutions have a responsibility to establish mechanisms for students to raise ethical concerns about aspects of their training without fear of repercussions.

The teaching of ethics and the ethics of teaching

Ethics and law training provide a framework that can help doctors to maintain intellectual independence and to keep sight of accepted moral norms in the face of pressure to compromise. The point of training in ethics is to assist doctors to look beyond the immediate system within which they work and, through analytical reasoning, help them to assess whether the treatment of the patients they see corresponds with public expectations and widely accepted standards. Raising awareness about duties and rights can make a significant difference only if this is accompanied by other practical measures that allow theory to be implemented in daily practice.

Doctors and tutors have a responsibility not only to teach medical ethics but also to teach medicine in an ethical manner. This involves, for example, ensuring that patients have given consent to the presence of, or examination by, students and showing, by example, the respect and dignity owed to patients both during and after their life. Medical students and junior doctors, however, sometimes report discrepancies between the ethical standards they are taught formally and the practices of senior colleagues and teachers. This "hidden curriculum" needs to be recognised and used to emphasise the role of all qualified doctors in the teaching of tomorrow's doctors. Students are being taught to have enquiring minds and to challenge unethical practices; those who are responsible for teaching them have a duty to allow them to do so without jeopardising their future careers.

References

1 General Medical Council. *Tomorrow's doctors: recommendations on undergraduate medical education.* London: GMC, 1993:4.
2 *Ibid:* p. 6.
3 General Medical Council. *Implementing "Tomorrow's doctors". Report of the Education Committee's informal visits to UK medical schools between spring 1995 and spring 1998.* London: GMC, 1999.
4 General Medical Council. *Tomorrow's doctors: recommendations on undergraduate medical education.* London: GMC, 2002.
5 British Medical Association Board of Medical Education. *Report of the working party on medical education.* London: BMA, 1995.
6 *Ibid:* p. 1.
7 British Medical Association Board of Medical Education. *Report of a BMA conference on selection for medical school.* London: BMA, 1999:2.
8 Council of Heads of Medical Schools and Deans of UK Faculties of Medicine. *Guiding principles for the admission of medical students.* London: CHMS, 1999: para 3.
9 Pond D. *Report of a working party on the teaching of medical ethics.* London: Institute of Medical Ethics Publications, 1987.
10 General Medical Council. *Tomorrow's doctors: recommendations on undergraduate medical education.* 1993. *Op cit.*
11 General Medical Council. *Implementing "Tomorrow's doctors". Report of the Education Committee's informal visits to UK medical schools between spring 1995 and spring 1998. Op cit.*
12 Fulford KWM, Yates A, Hope T. Ethics and the GMC core curriculum: a survey of resources in UK medical schools. *J Med Ethics* 1997;**23**:82–7.
13 British Medical Association. *The Medical profession and human rights: handbook for a changing agenda.* London: Zed Books, 2001:480.
14 For further discussion of the importance of communication skills, see: British Medical Association Board of Medical Education. *Communication skills education for doctors: a discussion paper.* London: BMA, 2003.

15 General Medical Council. *Tomorrow's doctors: recommendations on undergraduate medical education.* 2002. *Op cit:* para 29.

16 Rennie S, Rudland J. Differences in medical students' attitudes to academic misconduct and reported behaviour across the years – a questionnaire study. *J Med Ethics* 2003;**29**:97–102.

17 Ashcroft R, Baron D, Benetar S, *et al.* Teaching medical ethics and law within medical education: a model of the UK core curriculum. Consensus statement by teachers of medical ethics and law in UK medical schools. *J Med Ethics* 1998;**24**:188–92.

18 General Medical Council. *Tomorrow's doctors: recommendations on undergraduate medical education.* 1993. *Op cit:* p. 26.

19 Doyal L, Gillon R. Medical ethics and law as a core subject in medical education. *BMJ* 1998;**316**:1623–4.

20 Veatch RM. Medical codes and oaths. In: Reich W, ed. *Encyclopedia of bioethics, 2nd ed.* New York: Simon and Schuster Macmillan, 1995:1419–35.

21 See, for example: Gillon R. A personal view: white coat ceremonies for new medical students. *J Med Ethics* 2000;**26**:83–4. Veatch RM. White coat ceremonies: a second opinion. *J Med Ethics* 2002;**28**:5–6. Veatch RM. Medical codes and oaths. In: Reich W, ed. *Encyclopedia of bioethics. Op cit.*

22 General Medical Council. *Good medical practice.* London: GMC, 2001: para 10.

23 The Bristol Royal Infirmary Inquiry. *Learning from Bristol: the report of the public inquiry into children's heart surgery at the Bristol Royal Infirmary 1984–1995.* London: The Stationery Office, 2001: recommendation 78. (Cm 5207 (I).)

24 This is discussed in several chapters of: British Medical Association. *The medical profession and human rights: handbook for a changing agenda.* London: Zed Books, 2001.

25 Vincent A, Forrest D, Ferguson S. Human rights and medical education. *Lancet.* 1994;**343**:1435.

26 British Medical Association. *The medical profession and human rights: handbook for a changing agenda. Op cit:* p. 480.

27 World Medical Association. *Resolution on the inclusion of medical ethics and human rights in the curriculum of medical schools world-wide. Adopted by the 51st World Medical Assembly, Tel Aviv, Israel 1999.* Ferney-Voltaire: WMA, 1999.

28 Medact. *Global health studies teaching pack.* London: Medact, 2001.

29 General Medical Council. *Tomorrow's doctors: recommendations on undergraduate medical education.* 2002. *Op cit.*

30 Goodwin J. Chaos and the limits of modern medicine. *JAMA* 1997;**278**:1399–400: 1399.

31 Coldicott Y, Pope C, Roberts C. The ethics of intimate examinations – teaching tomorrow's doctors. *BMJ* 2003;**326**:97–101.

32 Royal College of Obstetricians and Gynaecologists. *Gynaecological examinations: guidelines for specialist practice.* London: RCOG, 2002:18–19.

33 Coldicott Y, *et al.* The ethics of intimate examinations – teaching tomorrow's doctors. *Op cit.*

34 Hicks LK, Lin Y, Robertson DW, Robinson DL, Woodrow SI. Understanding the clinical dilemmas that shape medical students' ethical development: questionnaire survey and focus group study. *BMJ* 2001;**322**:709–10.

35 Department of Health. *Reference guide to consent for examination or treatment.* London: DoH, 2001: para 4·1. Welsh Assembly Government. *Reference guide for consent to examination or treatment.* Cardiff: Welsh Assembly Government, 2002: para 4·1. Department of Health, Social Services and Public Safety. *Reference guide to consent for examination, treatment or care.* Belfast: DHSSPS, 2003: para 4·2. At the time of writing, Scotland was looking into producing guidelines in this area.

36 The Bristol Royal Infirmary Inquiry. *Learning from Bristol: the report of the public inquiry into children's heart surgery at the Bristol Royal Infirmary 1984–1995. Summary and recommendations.* London: The Stationery Office, 2001: para 78. (Cm 5207 (II).)

37 Medical Protection Society. *Consent: a complete guide for students.* Leeds: MPS, 2002.

38 British Medical Association. *Work observation guidelines.* London: BMA, 1999.

39 Hafferty FW, Franks R. The hidden curriculum, ethics teaching, and the structure of medical education. *Acad Med* 1994;**69**:861–71: 862.

40 *Ibid.*

41 Roach JO, Yamey G. Witnessing unethical conduct: the effects. *Student BMJ* 2001;**9**:2–3.

42 Doyal L. Closing the gap between professional teaching and practice. *BMJ* 2001;**322**:685–6.

43 Feudtner C, Christakis DA, Christakis NA. Do clinical clerks suffer ethical erosion? Students' perceptions of their ethical environment and personal development. *Acad Med* 1994;**69**:670–9.

44 Hafferty FW, *et al.* The hidden curriculum, ethics teaching, and the structure of medical education. *Op cit.*

45 Campbell A, Gillett G, Jones G. *Medical ethics, 3rd ed.* Oxford: Oxford University Press, 2001:9.

46 *Ibid:* p. 20.
47 Doyal L. Closing the gap between professional teaching and practice. *Op cit.*
48 Campbell A, *et al. Medical ethics. Op cit:* p. 20.
49 Singer PA. Intimate examinations and other ethical challenges in medical education: medical schools should develop effective guidelines and implement them. *BMJ* 2003;**326**:62–3.
50 Finlay SE, Fawzy M. Becoming a doctor. *J Med Ethics: Med Humanities* 2001;**27**:90–2.
51 *Ibid.*
52 Campbell A, *et al. Medical ethics. Op cit:* p. 20.
53 Woodall A. Should I do what they say to secure that grade A? *Student BMJ* 2001;**9**:169.
54 Trotter G. Hierarchy and the dynamics of rank: commentary. In: Kushner TK, Thomasma DC. *Ward ethics: dilemmas for medical students and doctors in training.* Cambridge: Cambridge University Press, 2001:191.
55 Singer PA. Intimate examinations and other ethical challenges in medical education: medical schools should develop effective guidelines and implement them. *Op cit.*
56 Based on: Doyal L. Closing the gap between professional teaching and practice. *Op cit:* p. 685.

19: Multidisciplinary teams and relationships with colleagues

The questions covered in this chapter include the following.

- What are the responsibilities of doctors who lead multidisciplinary teams?
- How should personal health data be made available within teams and to other professionals?
- Is there a different degree of accountability for doctors who refer or delegate treatments to a non-regulated therapist?
- Can patients switch between the care of NHS and private practitioners?
- How can doctors advertise their services?

Good clinical care

Changes in the provision of health care in the UK have demonstrated that the way forward is for increased team working, with recognition and maximum utilisation of the range of skills available in order to improve patient care. The emphasis nowadays is firmly on patient choice in health care and liaison between professionals for the good of the patient. *The report of the public inquiry into children's heart surgery at the Bristol Royal Infirmary 1984–1995* (the Bristol report) summed this up, saying that the "culture of the future must be a culture of safety and of quality; a culture of openness and of accountability; a culture in which collaborative teamwork is prized; and a culture of flexibility in which innovation can flourish in response to patients' needs".[1] The General Medical Council (GMC) highlights the importance of team working, emphasising that, in providing a good standard of care, doctors must recognise their own limitations, and be willing to consult colleagues and keep them well informed when sharing the care of patients.[2] It also advises doctors that they must work cooperatively with colleagues to monitor the general quality of care provided and be willing to deal openly and supportively with problems that arise.

This very strong and positive emphasis on joint working, cooperation, and shared decision making can leave doctors somewhat unsure of the boundaries of their own legal liability and moral accountability. Also, as the UK moves towards developing more public–private partnerships in health care, there is a growing likelihood that patient care will need to be coordinated not only across the traditional professional boundaries but increasingly between public and private healthcare providers. The interaction that takes place within the healthcare setting is discussed in this chapter, including issues such as who should be ultimately responsible for different facets of care, how responsibility is transferred, and how the various professions interact. There is discussion of doctors' relationships with their medical and healthcare colleagues, including professionals such as nurses, midwives, health visitors, pharmacists, and complementary therapy practitioners. Consideration is also given to doctors' relationships with other professionals whose work overlaps with the health sphere, such as social workers.

General principles

The general principles are familiar ones that are stressed in many chapters of this book. Here, however, the main focus is on applying concepts such as the duty to communicate effectively and respect others' views to doctors' relationships with colleagues as well as to their relationships with patients. The principles for working effectively with colleagues include the following.

- The interests and safety of patients are the primary concerns.
- Good communication is needed with medical colleagues and other health and social care professionals and agencies.
- All team members must understand the team's shared objectives.
- All those working together should respect the autonomy, skills, and qualifications of colleagues.
- There is a need to make the best use of the range of skills and expertise available.
- All team members must recognise the need continually to assess their own performance and to work within the limits of their competence.
- Patients need continuity and consistency of care.
- All team members have a responsibility for ensuring the team's competence and functioning.

Working in multidisciplinary teams

Although considerable strides have been made towards the goal of effective multidisciplinary working, it needs to be acknowledged that the legacies of past hierarchies and historical professional rivalries have not entirely disappeared, and further work is needed in this area. When the BMA was established in the nineteenth century, three groups of medical practitioners were recognised: physicians, surgeons, and apothecaries. There was friction not only between these groups but also between the groups and people working outside them. The management of pregnancy and childbirth, for example, was prone to rivalry between medical men and midwives. The early ethicist, Thomas Percival, sought in his code of ethics to encourage cooperation between physicians and apothecaries, claiming it was not only in patients' interests but also a moral duty "when health or life are at stake".[3] Traces of past battles can still sometimes be seen in uneasy aspects of the relationships within, as well as between, the professions. The undercurrent of tension that is sometimes still evident between doctors and nurses has been blamed on "nurses' readiness to be slighted and doctors' reluctance to be challenged".[4] The inevitable and timely shift in the traditional relationship between the professions has, and will continue to, take time to translate from rhetoric into action.

Nurses, more assertive, educated, and competent than ever before, resent what they see as continuing put downs by a profession holding all the cards. Doctors, puzzled and unaccustomed to being challenged, are themselves resentful at the apparent undervaluing of their competence, knowledge and skill by nurses, the public and policymakers.[5]

Teamwork can be frustrated by rivalry and bad communication or can become a mutual experience through which each profession understands better what the other can contribute in a spirit of trust and mutual support. With the increasing multidisciplinary teaching of medical ethics (see Chapter 18, page 658), with emphasis on the common duties and goals of different health professionals, it is hoped that such tensions will become less common.

Many of the types of disagreement that arise, both between different doctors and between doctors and other professionals, would be more accurately described as matters of etiquette than of ethics, but the two are related because ethical behaviour involves truth telling, and good relationships are based on respect for others. However they are categorised, if such disagreements are not handled in a satisfactory way they can give rise to serious disputes; it is in the interests of both doctors and patients that such potential disputes are foreseen and avoided wherever possible. Many disputes can be avoided by effective communication, by sharing of information (with due regard to confidentiality, see Chapter 5), through constructive discussion about areas of disagreement, and through respect for the skills, expertise, and opinions of other professionals.

Nurses, midwives, and health visitors are personally accountable for their practice and are subject to statutory regulation by the Nursing and Midwifery Council. The *Code of professional conduct*[6] by which these professionals are bound is very similar in content to the *Duties of a doctor*,[7] issued by the GMC. As with doctors, professionals such as nurses, midwives, and health visitors have a duty to acknowledge any limitations in their knowledge and to decline to undertake any duties or responsibilities they consider to be beyond their competence or to be inappropriate in the particular circumstances. They are specifically advised not simply to follow directions, with the reminder that "you are personally accountable for your practice. This means that you are answerable for your actions and omissions, regardless of advice or directions from another professional".[8] All members of the team have duties to ensure the avoidance of any inadequacies or errors that could put patients at risk, audit their own professional practice, raise problems for discussion, and draw attention to bad practice. Team members who have concerns over the professional practice of a colleague from another profession should bring these to the attention of the leader of that professional group.

A key commitment in England's 2000 *NHS plan* was to extend the role of nurses and other staff throughout the NHS, with clear messages to employers and managers to make change happen. "The new approach will shatter the old demarcations which have held back staff and slowed down care. NHS employers will be required to empower appropriately qualified nurses, midwives and therapists to undertake a wider range of clinical tasks".[9] Similar commitments were made to expand the role of nurses in Scotland[10] and Wales.[11] These changes are not only relevant in mainstream NHS services but also in contexts such as prison health care (see Chapter 17). Team working, however, does not automatically follow from groups of professionals working together. It involves mutual respect, shared objectives, and joint working towards a common goal to ensure that the professions are working "together" rather than simply "alongside" each other[12]. The World Health Organization defined teamwork as:

> coordinated action, carried out by two or more individuals jointly, concurrently or sequentially. It implies commonly agreed goals; a clear awareness of, and respect for, others' roles and functions on the part of each member of the team; adequate human and material resources; supportive cooperative relationships and mutual trust; effective leadership; open, honest and sensitive communications; and provision for evaluation.[13]

Effective team working also depends upon valuing what each profession brings to collaborative practice while setting aside negative stereotypes. Both the GMC[14] and the Nursing and Midwifery Council[15] emphasise the professional obligation to work effectively and cooperatively within teams.

Flawed team working

A GP was providing care for his 85-year-old patient, Mrs X, in a nursing home. Mrs X had suffered a series of strokes and was unable to swallow. She was fed by food supplements being placed into her mouth by syringe. In June 1995 the doctor gave instructions to the nursing staff that the food supplements should be stopped. The nursing staff disagreed with these instructions and continued to feed Mrs X secretly until the supplements ran out. Mrs X died on 26 August 1995.

The doctor was reported to the GMC, which found him guilty of serious professional misconduct for failing to follow proper procedures in reaching the decision to withdraw the food supplements. In particular, it was found that he had failed to seek a second opinion when he should have done, and failed adequately to seek or heed the views of the nursing staff.[16]

The example given above is an extreme one of a breakdown of teamwork but, on a more frequent basis, patients and families can suffer if different messages are given, or contradictory actions proposed, by different team members. This is discussed, in relation to dying patients, in Chapter 10 (pages 371–2).

Although much of the argument in support of multidisciplinary working has focused on the economic reasons for breaking down professional barriers and making the best use of the range of skills available, there are also good arguments in terms of the quality of care provided and increasing patient satisfaction. Various studies carried out since the 1980s have indicated clear benefits for patient satisfaction and outcomes when professionals cooperate positively.[17]

Multidisciplinary geriatric care

A randomised controlled trial was undertaken to evaluate the effectiveness of an interdisciplinary geriatric evaluation unit compared with the usual treatment (acute care followed by discharge to either home or long term care facilities). Patients who fitted the eligibility criteria – over 64 years old who had a persistent medical, functional, or psychosocial problem – were randomly allocated to the evaluation unit or the control group.

The evaluation unit had among its stated goals: increasing the patient's level of functioning, improving diagnosis and treatment, achieving more appropriate placement, reducing the use of institutional services, and generally increasing the overall quality of care delivered to elderly patients. A multidisciplinary team involving doctors, specialist geriatric nurses, care assistants, and a social worker ran the unit. There was also part-time input from a clinical psychologist, a dietician, a geriatric dentist, an audiologist, occupational and physiotherapists, and a public health nurse. The ratio of doctors and nurses to patients was equivalent to that on other intermediate care wards.

During the first year of follow up there was a great difference in mortality between the two groups: 23·8% of those in the evaluation unit had died compared with 48·3% of the control group. A higher percentage of unit patients (73%) than controls (53·3%) were discharged to their homes as opposed to nursing homes. The unit patients also had better morale, showed more improvement in functioning, spent less time in hospital acute care, and had fewer readmissions to acute care.[18]

Sharing information

The importance of effective communication with patients and other people caring for them is emphasised throughout this book. Written records, assessments, and medical reports need to be understandable not only for the professionals providing care (for whom they are primarily intended) but also for patients who may wish to access what is written about them (see Chapter 6, pages 216–8). It is clearly vital that the exchange of information is prompt, effective, and relevant between primary care practitioners, hospitals, and other facilities where patients may receive care, including psychiatric facilities, prison health services, and centres for asylum seekers. Other community-based services such as palliative care outreach teams and community psychiatric nurses also need to have well coordinated contact with the primary care team. The team providing care in a hospital setting needs to have access to the information necessary to provide care safely and appropriately. Nevertheless, doctors clearly need to be discriminating about what information they release for specific purposes; the fact that an individual is a health professional does not mean that he or she is entitled to access to patients' records. Access to confidential medical information should be on a clear "need to know" basis in connection with the care of the patient (see Chapter 5, page 180).

Leading teams

Within multidisciplinary teams, all professionals have responsibility for ensuring the proper functioning of the team, but one person must be ultimately accountable for making certain that the patient's care is properly coordinated and managed. The team leader is often, but not always, a doctor, and could be a social worker, a community psychiatric nurse, or a health visitor if care is carried out primarily in the community, with the GP as one member of the broader team that may include specialists in palliative care, mental health, and optical and dental services among its members. In hospitals the consultant in charge of the patient's care is assumed to be the team leader unless otherwise agreed and designated. The GMC offers guidance to doctors who lead teams about their responsibilities, which include ensuring that:

- the doctors in the team comply with the standards set out by the GMC
- any problem that may prevent other professionals from complying with the standards for their profession are identified and addressed
- all team members understand their personal and collective responsibility for the safety of patients, and for openly and honestly recording and discussing problems
- each patient's care is properly coordinated and managed and the patient knows who to contact if he or she has any questions
- cover is provided at all times
- regular reviews and audit of the standards and performance of the team are undertaken and any deficiencies are addressed
- systems are in place for dealing supportively with problems in the performance, conduct, or health of team members.[19]

Junior doctors have sometimes expressed concern about the perceived lack of support from their senior colleagues when they are faced with ethical dilemmas. Those who lead teams should ensure that adequate and appropriate support is available so that, in difficult ethical situations, junior doctors are not expected to make critical decisions without formal and comprehensive input from a senior colleague.[20]

Doctors as managers

Many, if not most, doctors take on some management responsibilities either in terms of leading a team (see above), employing staff, or adopting a management role within the NHS. This section focuses primarily on the last category. These doctors have responsibilities to patients, the wider community, the organisation in which they work, and their colleagues; these responsibilities can sometimes come into conflict. In 2002 the Department of Health produced a *Code of conduct for NHS managers,* listing the following principles that NHS managers in England are expected to observe:

- making the care and safety of patients their first concern and acting to protect them from risk
- respecting the public, patients, relatives, carers, NHS staff, and partners in other agencies
- being honest and acting with integrity
- accepting responsibility for their own work and the proper performance of the people they manage
- showing their commitment to working as a team member by working with all their colleagues in the NHS and the wider community
- taking responsibility for their own learning and development.[21]

This is supplemented by *Managing for excellence in the NHS*,[22] which draws specific attention to health service mangers' role in contributing to the modernisation of the NHS and the delivery of the *NHS plan*.

The GMC also reminds doctors who take on management roles that they remain professionally accountable to the GMC for their clinical decisions and professional conduct.[23] In their role as managers, doctors may receive information about individuals, certain forms of practice, or resource failings that put patients at risk. When such information comes to the attention of managers, they have a duty to investigate and, if the concerns are substantiated, to take whatever action is considered appropriate. (For further information on reporting poor performance, whatever its origin, see Chapter 21.) Doctors who receive reports of possible risks to patients must also be alert to the possibility that the complaints may not be well founded and should seek to establish the facts as soon as possible.

Failure of management

The chief executive of the United Bristol Healthcare (NHS) Trust was informed by senior medical colleagues of serious concerns about the excessive mortality of patients undergoing paediatric cardiac surgery. He ignored these concerns and took no steps to establish the truth or to obtain impartial advice from appropriate specialists. In respect of one patient, he was approached and asked not to let the operation go ahead, but took no steps to prevent the operation from proceeding.

In 1998 the chief executive was found guilty of serious professional misconduct by the GMC.[24] It found that, as a registered medical practitioner, he had a duty to put patients' safety and needs first. As such he should have made enquiries in response to the concerns brought to his attention and intervened to ensure the safety of patients. In view of the gravity of the case his name was erased from the medical register.

The chief executive appealed against the decision. One of the grounds for his appeal was that, as he was not practising as a doctor, his name should not have been removed from the register. The appeal was dismissed. It was held

(Continued)

that, as a registered medical practitioner, he was required to take action to protect patients from harm. Although he was entitled to leave routine day to day clinical decisions to the professional staff, there could be circumstances in which more would be expected of him. Even though he had no specialised expertise in that particular aspect of medicine, his general medical knowledge would have been relevant and applicable. As such, the GMC had been entitled to find that his failures constituted serious professional misconduct and to erase his name from the register.[25]

Although responsible for their personal conduct, doctors who take part in corporate decision making, for example by serving on the board of a commissioning body, are not accountable to the GMC for those decisions. If doctors become concerned that decisions made by the board would put patients at risk of harm, however, they have a duty to make their concerns known through the appropriate channels and should ensure that they are noted and recorded by the board. If their concerns are not addressed, they may need to consider taking their concerns further. Doctors who are in this position should contact their defence body or BMA regional office for advice.

Pressure to meet waiting list targets

A common area of conflict for doctors who act as managers is in the allocation of resources, where the needs of individual patients and the needs of a population frequently come into conflict. Resource allocation is an inevitable part of health service management and difficult decisions must be made. Doctors should ensure that their decisions are equitable, supported by sound evidence from research and clinical audit, and can be justified. They should also take account of the priorities set by the Government and the NHS, but any pressure, whether explicit or implied, to adjust NHS waiting lists inappropriately to meet waiting list targets must be resisted. Similarly, managers must not unduly persuade others to manipulate waiting lists and clinicians should protest if they feel under pressure to comply with target setting that does not reflect the urgency of the case. Patients should always be prioritised in the first instance according to clinical need, not in order to meet externally imposed targets.

The National Audit Office reported on waiting list initiatives in 2001 and restated the Department of Health's view that "it is a fundamental principle of the NHS that the order in which patients should be operated on by a particular consultant should be determined by their clinical priority so that those in greatest need are treated first".[26] It went on to say that waiting times should be taken into account only when deciding priority for treatment when two patients have the same clinical urgency and that it would be "inappropriate to operate on routine patients in preference to, and to the detriment of, those who require urgent treatment solely to meet waiting list targets".[27] A further report from the National Audit Office in 2001 identified a number of cases in which managers had inappropriately adjusted NHS waiting lists in order to meet waiting list targets. The report made it clear that such action was entirely inappropriate.[28] Despite this emphasis on honesty in relation to waiting lists, during "spot checks" of NHS hospitals in England in 2003 the Audit Commission found evidence of deliberate misreporting of waiting list information in three trusts.[29]

Summary – working in multidisciplinary teams

- Disagreement within teams can often be avoided by effective communication, sharing of information (with due regard to confidentiality), constructive discussion about areas of disagreement, and respect for the skills, expertise, and opinions of other professionals.
- Team working involves mutual respect, shared objectives and joint working towards a common goal.
- Both the GMC and the Nursing and Midwifery Council emphasise the professional obligation to work effectively and cooperatively within teams.
- There is evidence of clear benefits in terms of patient satisfaction and clinical outcomes when professionals cooperate positively.
- Within multidisciplinary teams all professionals have responsibility for ensuring the competence and proper functioning of the team.
- Access to confidential medical information should be on a clear "need to know" basis in connection with the care of the patient.
- The team leader must accept ultimate responsibility for ensuring that the patient's care is properly coordinated and managed.
- The first consideration of all managers should be the interest and safety of patients.
- Registered medical practitioners acting as managers remain professionally accountable to the GMC for their clinical decisions and professional conduct, although not for corporate or board decisions.

Working with others in primary care

At the heart of patients' contact with health services are GPs and the primary care team. Those working in primary care hold the main responsibility for maintaining patient records, arranging referrals, and keeping an overview of care arrangements. They also coordinate health measures such as screening programmes and recruitment of patients into relevant research. However, as discussed in Chapter 1, they are also drawn into many non-health related tasks, such as providing reports for employers, insurers, and housing and benefits agencies, and certifying fitness to drive, travel abroad, to adopt children, or act as child minders (general issues around dual obligations, and some of these specific issues, are discussed further in Chapter 16). The scope of such tasks means that GPs often have a detailed and intimate knowledge of individuals and their families. They also have contact with a very wide range of other professionals, some as part of the primary care team and others outside the team who are responsible for specific aspects of their patients' care, either in hospitals or in the community.

The primary care team

Primary care is increasingly provided by a specialised, multidisciplinary team with each member having particular areas of expertise and responsibility. Some members of the team are based within the GP practice while others work in the community but liaise closely with the patient's GP. In addition to GPs, the primary care team frequently includes other health professionals such as nurses, health visitors, physiotherapists, and others such as counsellors, complementary therapists, practice managers, receptionists, and secretaries. Midwives also work closely with the primary care team. Nurses, health visitors, midwives, and some other therapists are professionally accountable for their own actions. Nevertheless, GPs retain liability for any acts and omissions of all the staff they employ under the doctrine of vicarious liability.

In the past, professionals such as nurses, midwives, and health visitors have often felt that their role and independence were not adequately recognised, and this has undoubtedly been the case. As part of the general effort to push back professional boundaries, however, and to make the best possible use of the range of expertise available, the nurse's role in the primary care team has expanded, with the development of the independent professional roles of the practice nurse and nurse practitioner. For some patients, the practice nurse is the first point of contact, providing referral to a GP only if that is considered necessary and appropriate. In addition, as nurse prescribing continues to increase (see Chapter 13, page 475), the independent role of the nurse practitioner will continue to expand. Increasing the role of nurses not only makes effective use of the resources available but, from the patients' perspective, high levels of satisfaction have been found with nurse consultations in general practice, and evaluation of the clinical outcomes shows them to be comparable with those of doctors.[30]

Nurse consultations for minor illnesses

A multicentre, randomised controlled trial was undertaken to assess the acceptability and effectiveness of a practice-based minor illness service led by practice nurses compared with routine care offered by GPs.[31] The nurses took the history, performed a physical examination, offered advice and treatment, issued prescriptions (which required a doctor's signature), and referred the patient to a GP when appropriate. Consultations with the nurse took around 10 minutes (compared with 8 minutes for consultations with the GP).

(Continued)

The key outcome variable was patient satisfaction, measured by questionnaire. Information was collected from the doctors and nurses, including the nature of the complaint, the number of prescriptions written, and the number of patients referred by the nurses to the doctors. Two weeks after the appointment with the nurse a further questionnaire was sent to patients asking about their health status, their compliance with drug treatment, their rating of the information provided, and whether they had returned to the surgery.

Of the 790 patients seen by the nurses, 73% were managed without referral to a doctor, 19% had to be seen by a doctor, and 8% involved the nurse having a discussion with the doctor. Nurses and doctors wrote prescriptions for a similar proportion of patients, although nurses reported giving more advice on self medication and general self management than doctors. Patients generally expressed greater satisfaction with the nurses, although both groups reported that they were very satisfied with the general advice and explanation they had been given. Those who were referred by the nurse to the doctor were less satisfied with the service they had received. There was no difference between the groups in the patients' ratings of clinical improvement in their health status after two weeks.

Both hospital- and community-based nurse practitioners aim to offer a holistic approach to patient care. They are often particularly aware of the range of patient needs because of the regular contact they have with patients and their families. Specialised nurses such as Macmillan nurses, and others who work in the community, may have opportunities to develop an insight into the overall situation and problems of both patients and their families. GPs may have a different perspective, having often been responsible for the family's treatment over a prolonged period. Both are important to providing appropriate care to patients, and good communication is essential to enable nurses and doctors to respect each other's area of expertise and to benefit from their particular respective insights in order to develop the most appropriate management plan for the patient.

Liaison between GPs and pharmacists

As discussed in Chapter 13, the role of pharmacists within the NHS is also changing to make maximum use of their skills and expertise. Increasingly, pharmacists are working alongside GPs and some GPs employ them as prescribing advisers. Proposals for a more integrated care system require closer liaison and shared responsibility for patient care. A number of initiatives have demonstrated that the role of pharmacists can be usefully developed to improve patient care and manage demand. Strategies include:

- recognising the benefits of patients consulting pharmacists rather than their GP for self limiting illnesses
- supporting patients to implement self care through advice on over the counter medication, thereby reducing demand for GP appointments

- repeat dispensing of long term medication through instalments reviewed by the pharmacist rather than by repeat GP visits
- medication reviews and advice from pharmacists for patients with complex conditions requiring a number of different medications.[32]

GPs employing other practitioners

The shape of primary care has changed and many practices now offer a wide range of health services within the surgery. This sometimes includes physiotherapists, chiropodists, dieticians, counsellors, and acupuncturists. When these practitioners are employed by NHS GPs, patients may not be charged for the use of their service because this is deemed to be part of the service patients are entitled to receive within the NHS. GPs also need to be aware that they retain liability for any acts or omissions of these staff when delegating any aspect of patient care.

Sharing premises with non-medical practitioners

In some cases other non-medical practitioners share premises with an NHS general practice, but operate independently. Although this may be convenient for patients, it is important that their status in relation to the practice is unambiguously clear. If the practitioners are operating on a private basis and patients will be charged for a consultation and treatment, they need to be made aware of this at an early stage. There should also be no pressure on patients to seek private treatment. When the treatment is necessary and is available within the NHS, an NHS referral should be provided unless the patient asks to be referred for private treatment. Where the practice is renting rooms to the practitioner, and therefore arguably has a financial interest in the success of the venture, GPs need to be careful when referring patients to, or advising them about, the service, so that they are not seen to have a conflict of interest. Any financial relationship with the practitioner should be explained to the patient, who should also be made aware of other practitioners in the area.

Referral and delegation in primary care

The level of responsibility retained by GPs when they ask another person to undertake part of a patient's care depends, primarily, upon whether a particular task is being delegated to another person or the patient is being referred for more specialist care.

Delegation occurs when doctors ask other people to carry out procedures or provide care on their behalf. This may involve a GP asking a practice nurse to take a blood sample from a patient, for example. When tasks are delegated, the doctor retains clinical responsibility for the care provided to the patient. The person to whom care is delegated need not be medically qualified or subject to a statutory regulatory body, but the doctor must ensure that tasks are delegated only to those who are competent to fulfil them.

Referral takes place when responsibility for the patient is transferred, usually temporarily, to someone with more specialised knowledge to carry out specific procedures, tests, or treatment that fall outside the sphere of competence of the referring doctor. An example is the referral of a patient to an oncologist, cardiologist, or physiotherapist. Referrals are usually made to another registered health professional. If this is not the case, the referring doctor must "be satisfied that any healthcare professional to whom [a patient is referred] … is accountable to a statutory regulatory body, and that a registered medical practitioner, usually a GP, retains overall responsibility for the management of the patient".[33]

Traditionally, referrals have been made to registered medical practitioners who may then, in turn, delegate care to other members of the team. This process has been challenged, however, as not making the most effective use of the resources available and not representing the best option for patients. The *NHS plan*, for example, says that employers must empower nurses, midwives, and therapists by giving them the right to make and receive referrals, admit and discharge patients, order investigations and diagnostic tests, run clinics, and prescribe drugs.[34] The BMA welcomes the greater use of the range of specialist skills within the health service, but has some concerns about the implications for GPs, in terms of legal liability, if patients are to be referred to non-medically qualified practitioners. Clear guidelines and standards of practice would need to be established to determine whether, in a particular case, referral to a consultant or other health professional was appropriate. In obstetric care, for example, the BMA would expect clear guidance to be provided to GPs about the factors that would categorise a pregnancy as "low risk" such that a direct referral to a midwife, rather than to an obstetrician, would be appropriate.

Referral to practitioners of complementary and alternative medicine

A common enquiry to the BMA concerns requests from patients for referral to complementary and alternative medicine (CAM) practitioners. A study published in 2000 estimated that up to 5 million people may have consulted a practitioner specialising in CAM in the previous year and that many more have consulted a statutory health professional practising CAM.[35] This reflects growing public awareness of and interest in complementary therapy, as well as changing attitudes within the medical profession. As a result, CAM is increasingly being integrated into treatment programmes offered by the NHS, as illustrated by the fact that in 1999 acupuncture was reported to be available in 86% of NHS chronic pain services.[36] The BMA also undertook a random survey of GPs, which showed that 58% had arranged CAM for their patients.[37] The BMA's Board of Science and Education has undertaken some work on the safety, efficacy, and regulation of CAM, focusing primarily on the discrete clinical disciplines of homeopathy, osteopathy, chiropractic, acupuncture, and herbal medicine.[38] These are distinguished from other therapies in a number of ways, but primarily because they are not only increasingly the therapies of choice for the UK public but they also have the greatest potential to do harm.

There is no problem with GPs referring patients to CAM therapists who are subject to a statutory regulatory body as with chiropractors or osteopaths, or if the person carrying out the therapy is a registered doctor or nurse. For other therapists, the GP is considered to have delegated care and so retains responsibility for the overall management of the patient. When GPs employ CAM therapists who are not subject to a statutory regulatory body, they need to be satisfied that the individual is suitably qualified and experienced to undertake the role. GPs should also be aware that, in such circumstances, they may be held liable for any harm arising to their patients.

Information sharing within primary care teams

One of the problems that frequently arises from GPs' intimate knowledge of patients' lives is the question of how much individual members of the practice team should be able to access patients' personal health information. The BMA's general advice is that essential information should be shared on a "need to know" basis, which means that not all members of the primary healthcare team need to have access to all of a patient's notes. Some members of the team, such as health visitors or counsellors, may make their own records of aspects of care that they feel should not be integrated into the general GP health record. The counselling of people experiencing distress after bereavement, violence, or abuse is likely to elicit very sensitive information that should not be shared with others without the patient's express consent. Nevertheless, the BMA sometimes receives complaints from patients who have consented to a very generally worded authorisation of disclosure of information in their GP record to third parties, such as insurers or pension schemes, not knowing that notes of very personal conversations with counsellors would be included. Although there may be some advantages to having shared records, varying levels of access must be integrated into the system to follow the general rule that people providing care to patients should have access only to the information they need to know in order to provide that care. Issues concerning security of data, access, record keeping, and informed consent to disclosure are discussed in detail in Chapters 5 and 6.

The BMA occasionally receives reports of residential care homes for elderly people requesting the transfer from the patient's GP of entire patient records for residents who remain on the GP's list. Clearly, pertinent information can be shared, with appropriate patient consent, but entire records should not be automatically passed on unless the home retains a fulltime doctor and the patient wishes to transfer to that practitioner's care completely, in which case the appropriate procedures for transferring records between GPs should be followed.

Information sharing outside the team

Liaison with researchers

GPs are often approached by researchers seeking to recruit patients for specific projects. The BMA believes that patient data, including name and address, should not be disclosed without the patient's agreement. Consent for disclosure to a researcher is usually a legal requirement, although in some circumstances disclosure may be legally permitted under section 60 of the Health and Social Care Act 2001 (see pages 182–3). Initial invitations to participate in research projects should usually be sent out from the GP's surgery and patients should be given the opportunity to decide whether or not they wish to participate. Research is discussed in detail in Chapter 14.

Liaison with social workers

Primary care services often liaise with social workers, particularly in relation to the management of suspected cases of abuse or neglect of children, elderly people, or physically or mentally incapacitated people, both in the community and in residential facilities. All published guidance on this subject emphasises the vital need for well coordinated interagency liaison between professionals caring for such client groups. Nevertheless, the need to support and protect such patients must be balanced with their rights to confidentiality, especially in relation to very sensitive information. Whenever feasible, patients should be actively involved in deciding how their information should be shared, although in some cases the overriding need to ensure the protection of vulnerable individuals precludes this. When families are dysfunctional and exhibit poor parenting or caring skills, the primary care team is often well placed to engage positively with family members to encourage them to improve their skills and stay together. This means that steps must be taken to ensure that families are included in discussions and case conferences whenever this is feasible.

GPs frequently receive requests from social workers for patients' notes or a report on a particular patient without any form of consent or indication that the patient is aware of the information being sought. In such cases it is advisable for the GP to discuss with the social worker concerned whether it is possible and feasible to obtain consent for the information to be disclosed. When it is not possible to obtain consent, for example because this would expose a vulnerable person to risk of serious harm, the GP should consider whether the information available justifies a breach of confidentiality. GPs often express concern that their relationship of trust with families could be jeopardised if they appear to be having discussions behind patients' backs. They recognise, however, that the best interests of vulnerable parties are the paramount concern. These issues are explored in detail in Chapter 5 on confidentiality, where emphasis is placed on the sharing of such information as is necessary, relevant, and in the individual's interest, but without disregarding the person's right to confidentiality.

General practitioners' partnership agreements

In multipractice partnerships, GPs also need to consider their working relationships with other partners. It is advisable to have a formal partnership agreement that sets out clearly the rights and obligations of all the parties and for all partners to take legal, accountancy and tax advice when drawing up or entering into a partnership agreement. The BMA's General Practitioners Committee has written guidance for GPs on partnership agreements, which includes a basic framework for a medical partnership and provides advice about the points to include in a partnership agreement.[39]

In addition to the financial and management arrangements for the practice, the General Practitioners Committee's guidance recommends that the practice agreement should include a statement about the partners' obligations to each other. This should include the amount of time partners spend in the practice and the arrangements whereby they may take on commitments outside the partnership. A common area of disagreement is where one partner wishes to devote a considerable amount of time to external activities, such as committee work, conferences, or medical research. Being explicit about the amount of time that may be spent on external commitments could prove problematic for some GPs, particularly those who are keen to undertake committee or media work. It is generally better, however, that these matters are discussed and agreed in advance rather than being raised at a later stage, perhaps in a situation of conflict. The attention of the BMA has been drawn to some acrimonious disputes that have arisen between partners on issues that generally fall outside the scope of partnership agreements. This has prompted the Association to suggest that multipartner practices draw up guidelines or rules of procedure on the day to day running of practices, covering matters such as the approach to patient care, research involving patients, and the availability of chaperones for intimate examinations.

It is helpful for practices to make provision in the partnership agreement for the resolution of any disputes that may arise, for example if one partner persistently disregards agreed practice procedures or acts in a manner that could call into question the reputation of the practice. In the latter case, other doctors in the practice may be considered to have an ethical duty to take action if the wellbeing of patients or their confidence in the practice is likely to be compromised. Any member of the practice staff should be entitled to call a practice meeting to address the difficulty frankly and to attempt to resolve it in a manner that is supportive to all. When assistance is required, BMA industrial relations officers, based in the regional offices, have expertise in mediating to help parties to reach solutions that are acceptable to all involved. Depending on the nature of the problematic behaviour, advice may also be sought from defence bodies and counselling services for sick doctors, which are discussed in Chapter 21.

Doctors in general practice should also give forethought to the separation of patient lists upon the dissolution of a partnership because this is a frequent area of disagreement. When partnerships are dissolved in an atmosphere of ill will, all parties must be careful not to impugn the skill or judgment of colleagues. The GMC states that doctors must not undermine patients' trust in the care or treatment they receive, or in the judgment of those treating them, by making malicious or unfounded criticisms of colleagues.[40] Complaints about such matters sometimes arise as a result of patients seeking advice about which practice they should register with or wanting to know the reasons for a practice split. Clearly, doctors must be sensitive about discussing their colleagues, while at the same time offering a satisfactory explanation. Doctors must also not allow false information to circulate unchecked, such as rumours that a colleague is intending to retire from practice or move from the area. In this, as in all matters, patients are entitled to receive balanced advice.

Summary – working with others in primary care

- Although nurses, health visitors, and some other therapists are professionally accountable for their own actions, when they are employed by a GP, that GP retains liability for any acts and omissions under the doctrine of vicarious liability.
- Nurses and doctors in primary care often have a different perspective on a patient's problems and needs. Good communication is essential in order to develop the most appropriate care plan for the patient.
- Where other professionals are sharing premises with a GP practice it is essential that patients should understand the nature of the relationship – whether the practitioner is part of the primary care team or operating independently.
- The level of responsibility retained by GPs when they ask another person to undertake part of a patient's care depends, primarily, upon whether the task is being delegated to another person or the patient is being referred for more specialist care.
- Patients' medical records should not be available to all members of the primary care team and individual members should have access only to that information they need to know in connection with that patient's care.

Working with others in hospitals

Teamwork is also the standard model for hospital care. In the hospital healthcare team, doctors are usually responsible for the medical treatment and overall management of the patient's care. However, patients may be seen and treated by a range of doctors from different specialties as well as members of different professions, including nursing, midwifery, physiotherapy, dietetics, speech therapy, and pharmacy. In addition, increasing numbers of nurse led clinics and services are being established.

Nurse led service

In Plymouth, patients with suspected deep vein thrombosis (DVT) used to be referred by their GP to the medical assessment unit at any time of the day or night. This led to a large volume of patients attending and experiencing long delays in assessment. This system was replaced with a totally nurse led DVT service on a planned investigation unit. All patients with a suspected DVT are referred directly to the service, unless the condition is considered as an emergency out of hours, in which case the medical assessment unit is still used. The nurses have consultant support, if required, but are able to order investigations themselves and provide continuity of care. This has led to less pressure on the medical assessment unit and greater levels of patient satisfaction.[41]

As in primary care, the growing contribution, recognition, and autonomy of nurses is welcome. The aim must be to make the best use of the range of skills and resources available. Traditional concepts of the roles of doctors and nurses are increasingly being challenged as the distinction between junior doctors and experienced nurses blurs, particularly with the development of specialist nurse practitioners and nurse consultants. Some nurses, after undertaking additional training, have taken over some tasks that were previously the responsibility of junior doctors, including aspects of intravenous therapy, counselling, chronic disease management, health education and promotion, and audit. In teams with medical support, nurse practitioners have also taken an important role in the diagnosis, investigation, and treatment of minor injuries and illnesses.

Increasing numbers of conditions and procedures are covered by integrated care pathways, which describe each stage in the management of the care of patients with a particular condition, but allow scope for variation in particular cases. These involve and articulate a multidisciplinary approach to care and, as such, they can be seen to promote and facilitate effective team working in hospitals. The use of a single multidisciplinary integrated care pathway record, which is available to the patient and forms part of the patient's medical record, also leads to improved communication between the different professionals involved with providing care.[42] Another advantage of the development of integrated care pathways is the discussion and communication that takes place while they are being drawn up; this enables the views and approaches of professionals from different disciplines to be shared. In other situations, too, examples have been provided of cases in which "doctors, nurses, managers, clerical staff, porters, technicians and staff from many different areas have come together to examine the service that they provide and consider what could be improved".[43]

Multidisciplinary working in hospitals

In 2001 it was announced that the need for sickle cell admissions to Guy's and St Thomas's Hospital NHS Trust had been successfully cut by 30% over a three year period after the adoption of a multidisciplinary approach. In addition, the average length of stay in hospital dropped from over nine days to under four days. This was despite the fact that twice as many adults and children were registered with the service in 2001 than in 1998. Care was provided by a team including a specialist health psychologist, a consultant physician, two sickle cell nurse practitioners, and genetic counsellors.[44]

Many hospitals employ hospital chaplains and also have other ministers of religion available to meet patients' needs. Patients should be informed of the availability of this service and be given the option of whether to access it. Spiritual advisers do not normally need access to information about the patient's treatment in order to provide spiritual care, although, obviously, some patients are keen to discuss their prognosis and authorise disclosure (see Chapter 5, pages 186–7).

Liaison with carers and patient advocates

Advocates are increasingly available for hospital patients who are vulnerable or mentally incapacitated. These may be formally appointed by the courts, somebody may be nominated by the patient (see Chapter 3, pages 110–3), or an advocacy service may provide a volunteer who was previously unknown to the patient. Sharing information with these people is unproblematic if the patient has given his or her consent to disclosure or when the information is required by a person appointed by the court to act for the patient. In all other circumstances, however, the guiding principle should be the patient's overall best interests, bearing in mind the duty of confidentiality owed to the patient (see Chapter 5).

Doctors often liaise with people caring for those who are not able to look after themselves. As a general rule, when patients are not able to give valid consent, only information that is necessary for their care should be shared with those who need to know it.

Liaison with social care professionals and agencies

It is increasingly recognised that, if individuals are to receive the best possible care, then an integrated approach to health and social care is needed so that patients receive a "seamless service" tailored to their specific needs.[45] This includes better and more routine liaison to ensure, for example, that older patients are not left in hospital when intermediate care or additional support in their own home would better suit their needs. In September 2002, 8·9% of older patients occupying NHS acute care beds had been declared fit to leave hospital. The most common cause of delay was because patients were waiting for a placement in a nursing or residential home, or an assessment of their needs.[46] This area has been highlighted as needing improvement; legislation passed in 2003 requires local authorities in England and Wales to pay fines if the discharge of patients is delayed for reasons relating to the provision of community care services or services to carers.[47] In January 2003, guidance was issued to assist those working across the health and social care sectors in working together to meet their patients' requirements and to improve local hospital discharge policy and practice.[48] As with other situations, however, due regard should be given to confidentiality. Clinical information should be shared with other agencies only with the patient's consent or, if the patient is not competent, with those who need to know the information in order to provide care.

Summary – working with others in hospital

- Changing working practices have improved the use of available skills and resources, and must continue to do so.
- Many hospitals employ hospital chaplains and also have other ministers of religion available; patients should be informed of this.

- Spiritual advisers should be given information about the patient's treatment or care only with the individual's consent.
- Information may be shared with carers, advocates, or other agencies with the patient's consent or, if the patient is unable to consent, where it is necessary for the care of the patient.
- Within the resources available, health and social care professionals should work together to meet their patients' requirements.

Interaction between NHS and private treatment

A common enquiry to the BMA concerns the interrelationship between NHS and private care. Although the primary relationships involved are those between doctors and their patients, many doctors raise concerns about real, or perceived, conflicts of interest when they, or their colleagues, discuss private treatment with their NHS patients, or when doctors believe they are being asked to help their patient to "jump the queue". This type of enquiry is likely to become more common as the Government is increasingly buying in services from the private healthcare sector. In addition, more patients are opting to have their investigations and treatment carried out privately, either because they can be seen more quickly or because they are willing to pay for the added convenience or comfort of receiving their care in private facilities. The Department of Health has issued guidance for NHS medical staff who are also involved in private practice.[49]

Dilemmas can arise if patients choose to seek part of their treatment privately and part on the NHS. A common scenario is where a patient seeks private investigations in order to obtain an earlier diagnosis and then switches back to the NHS for any subsequent treatment. Provided patients are entitled to NHS treatment, they may opt in or out of NHS care at any stage. Patients who seek private investigations may subsequently be placed directly onto the NHS waiting list at the same position as if their consultation had been undertaken within the NHS (assuming the treatment in question is provided by the NHS).[50] Patients do not need to have a further assessment within the NHS before receiving their treatment. Some doctors are unhappy that patients who can afford to pay for private investigations are able effectively to jump the queue for treatment by reaching the waiting list earlier than those who wait for investigations and diagnosis on the NHS. Others argue that, because some people seek their investigations privately, the NHS waiting list for investigations is reduced and therefore other patients are seen more quickly. Arguably, as priority for NHS treatment is based purely on clinical need, those who have paid for their investigations privately are not able to gain any advantage over those in equal need who are already on the waiting list. Patients whose clinical need is greater may join the waiting list later, but could still receive their treatment first if they are categorised as needing urgent therapy.

When patients are referred to a specialist within the NHS it is not unusual for a doctor to provide a diagnosis and recommended care plan, but to advise that the waiting list for non-urgent treatment may be many months. Some patients may then enquire about the possibility of seeing the doctor privately. This puts doctors in a difficult position if they can be perceived as having a conflict of interest. It may be suggested, for example, that patients have been put under pressure to seek private treatment or that doctors are using their NHS consultations to promote their own private practice. It would be entirely inappropriate for any doctor to pressurise or encourage patients to transfer from NHS to private care. It is also important that doctors ensure that the information they provide about waiting times is accurate because this could influence the patient's view about seeking private treatment.

Dishonesty in financial dealings

In 2002 a consultant surgeon, working in both NHS and private hospitals, was found guilty by the GMC of serious professional misconduct and was erased from the medical register for "persistent dishonesty". Among the charges found proven against the consultant were that he had attempted to persuade patients to undertake procedures privately and provided misleading information about relevant waiting times. The doctor's incidence of self pay patients was twice that of other consultant general surgeons. He had also claimed rates of payment for procedures that were different from the appropriate rates of payment for the procedures that were actually carried out. The GMC held that his actions had been dishonest, undertaken for his own financial gain, and not in his patients' best interests.[51]

Doctors should not spend time discussing private treatment with patients during NHS consultations. However, if treatment is available but is not provided within the NHS, patients should usually be advised of this option (see Chapter 13, pages 461–2). Patients themselves, however, frequently raise questions about the availability of private treatment and views differ on how consultants should handle such direct questions. Some people argue that when patients raise the option of private treatment during an NHS consultation they should be directed back to their GP for a separate private referral. When the patient expresses a clear preference to see the same doctor privately, however, insisting on a separate referral from the GP can seem to the patient to be unnecessarily bureaucratic, as well as adding to the already heavy workload of GPs. It is for individual consultants to decide how to respond to patients' questions about private treatment within the terms agreed locally. Some consultants prefer not to discuss their private practice at all during NHS consultations and refer all enquiries to their secretaries. Consultants may briefly answer factual questions about the availability of private treatment, however, and there is no requirement for the patient to be referred back to the GP (although the GP should be kept informed of any change to the patient's care plan). A doctor in this position should make a contemporaneous note on the medical record, and inform the GP that the patient has requested information about private treatment. Patients should be informed of the option of seeing a different doctor for private treatment.

Another situation in which conflict can occur is where a patient is seeking private treatment and has asked his or her GP to issue an NHS prescription rather than paying for the medication privately. This situation is discussed in Chapter 13 (page 474).

Summary – interaction between NHS and private treatment

- Provided patients are entitled to NHS treatment, they may opt in or out of NHS care at any stage.
- If patients pay for investigations privately they may be placed directly onto the NHS waiting list for treatment according to clinical need.
- It would be entirely inappropriate for any doctor to pressurise or encourage patients to transfer from NHS to private care.
- Doctors should ensure that the information they provide about waiting times is accurate because this may influence a patient's view about seeking private treatment.
- Doctors should not spend time discussing private treatment with patients during NHS consultations, although when treatment is available but is not provided within the NHS, patients should usually be advised of this option.
- Consultants may briefly answer factual questions about private treatment and there is no requirement for the patient to be referred back to the GP.
- Patients should be informed of the option of seeing a different doctor for private treatment.

Advertising medical services

A common area of enquiry, and of disagreement between doctors, relates to the extent to which they may advertise their services to the general public. Until the late 1990s a distinction was made between GPs, who were permitted to advertise their services to the public, and specialists, who were not. From the late 1980s the BMA called for this distinction to be maintained, fearing that advertising of specialist services within the context of the existing referral system could give a false impression of greater patient choice than was actually available. To suggest that GPs would be able to refer patients to the specialist of their choice, within the NHS, was misleading and the Association was concerned that, if patients were refused a referral to the specialist of their choice, this could have a detrimental effect on the doctor–patient relationship. The BMA was also concerned that people who are ill or seeking specialist medical attention for their families can be particularly vulnerable to influence and are not in the best position to assess objectively the different services available. Patients who are seeking a GP, however, are generally healthy and able to make an informed and objective decision. As a general point, the BMA also believed that advertising by specialists would open the door to competition and consumerist attitudes that sit uneasily with the purpose of medicine. The BMA recognised, however, that this was an issue on which views were divided and that lifting the restrictions on doctors' advertising would reflect the more consumerist approach to health care within the population and in the health service itself. After consultation, the GMC decided that all doctors should be able to advertise their services, in order to provide patients with the information they need to make an informed decision. The same rules on advertising now apply to all doctors.

The GMC's guidance states that any information provided about medical services:

- must comply with the law and guidance issued by the Advertising Standards Authority
- must be factual and verifiable
- must not make unjustifiable claims about the quality of service
- must not offer guarantees of cures or exploit patients' vulnerability or lack of medical knowledge
- must not put pressure on people to use the service, for example, by arousing ill founded fear for their future health or by visiting or telephoning prospective patients.[52]

This guidance applies to all advertising, irrespective of the medium used (including information provided on the internet). Provided that the material fulfils these broad criteria, it would not breach the GMC's guidance. However, the BMA believes that, in addition, specialists should as a general rule make it clear to members of the public that they usually do not accept patients without a referral from a GP or other practitioner. The BMA believes it is important for one doctor, usually the patient's GP, to have a complete record of the individual's health care and that patients should be encouraged to discuss their healthcare needs and wishes with their GP. There are some specialties to which self referrals are accepted to be the norm, such as complementary therapies, slimming advice, infertility treatment, cosmetic surgery, and the diagnosis and treatment of sexually transmitted infections. In these cases the specialist care providers should advise patients of the benefits of keeping their GP informed of treatment and should encourage them to allow information to be shared, but confidentiality should be respected if they refuse. The GMC reminds all specialists that, if they accept patients without a referral, they should inform the patient's GP before providing treatment unless the patient objects. If the GP is not informed, the specialist is responsible for providing or arranging all necessary aftercare until another doctor agrees to take over.[53] Doctors who provide specialist services may inform GPs about their availability for private referral by sending a letter containing factual information about the service provided.

Advertising can take a number of different forms, for example formal advertisements in newspapers or magazines, a practice leaflet distributed to residents within a practice area, or an editorial or news piece in a local newspaper. Often the latter is not perceived to be advertising and inadvertent breaches of the GMC's guidance can occur. Care should be taken to ensure that this type of promotional material fulfils the criteria set out by the GMC in the same ways as other advertisements. The line between the two can sometimes become blurred, where information about a new practice or clinic is presented in the form of an article, for example, when in fact, its primary intention is to promote the service. The Advertising Standards Authority makes it clear that "marketers and publishers should make clear that advertisement features are advertisements, for example, by heading them 'advertisement feature'".[54] The purpose of doctors' advertising should be to provide factual information about the services available to enable patients to make informed decisions. For this reason the BMA has some concerns about advertising that is designed solely to promote the name of the practice or clinic without giving any factual information.

"Poaching patients"

The BMA receives occasional enquiries from GPs who believe that neighbouring practices are "poaching" their patients. Instances also arise when hospital specialists become involved in disagreements about who should manage a patient's care or when a consultant believes that a colleague has inappropriately taken over the care of a particular patient. In the past the GMC had specific guidance prohibiting doctors from poaching patients from their colleagues. This concept is now considered to be outdated and not reflective of the current emphasis on individual patient choice. Although it is clearly unacceptable for pressure to be brought to bear on patients who are registered with or under the care of one doctor to change to another, they should be free to exercise their choice about which doctor to see within the constraints imposed by the NHS. This is discussed further in Chapter 1 (pages 30–1).

Providing information to companies, firms or other organisations

Doctors who wish to offer services such as medicolegal or occupational health services to a company, firm, school, club, or association may send factual information about their qualifications and services to a suitable person in the organisation and may, where appropriate, place a factual advertisement in a relevant trade journal.

Advertising medicines

It is unlawful in the UK to advertise a prescription-only medicine to the public.[55] In the late 1990s the BMA received a number of enquiries from doctors about the boundaries between news information and advertising or promotional material. At that time, a number of articles were appearing in newspapers about clinics that were able to prescribe Viagra. The BMA took advice from the Medicines Control Agency (now replaced by the Medicines and Healthcare Products Regulatory Agency) about acceptable practice and was informed that some advertisements and news articles (which would fall within its definition of an advertisement) that mentioned or alluded to the availability of Viagra at a particular clinic may breach The Medicines (Advertising) Regulations 1994. Similar advice was issued by the Chief Medical Officer in September 2002 about the advertising of Botox.[56] In the light of this guidance, the BMA advises its members strongly against mentioning, or even alluding to, the fact that they can prescribe a particular prescription-only medicine in any material directed at the general public.

Advertising other products or services

GP practices and hospitals frequently raise money to produce patient leaflets by selling advertising space to local companies and services. In such cases, the BMA believes that the leaflet should clearly state that the practice or hospital is not endorsing the services advertised. The BMA also considers it inappropriate for leaflets to carry advertisements for products that clearly affect health adversely because this may give mixed messages to the public, despite the disclaimer regarding endorsement. Similarly, the BMA advises against advertising health related services on patient leaflets, such as for pharmacies, nursing homes, and private clinics. Despite disclaimers, such advertising could be thought to imply a recommendation of a particular service.

The BMA has concerns about doctors using their position to endorse particular goods or services and does not believe it is acceptable for them to promote or sell services, such as insurance or particular firms of solicitors, to their patients. A number of schemes have been referred to the BMA in which doctors have been offered a financial incentive to recommend a particular product or service to their patients. These types of arrangements, particularly where "per capita payments" are offered, are very likely to be interpreted as an incentive to refer people to the company; such incentives are not acceptable.[57] Not all incentives offered are financial, but the offer of free services and other benefits are equally unacceptable. Patients need to be sure that, when doctors recommend a particular product or service, they are doing so in the interests of their patients and not as a result of a financial or other incentive. Participation in such schemes is likely to breach the GMC's guidance, which states that

> you must act in your patients' best interests when making referrals and providing or arranging treatment or care. So you must not ask for or accept any inducement, gift or hospitality which may affect or be seen to affect your judgment. You should not offer such inducements to colleagues.[58]

Summary – advertising medical services

- The same rules on advertising apply to all doctors and to all media, including the internet.
- The BMA believes that specialists should, as a general rule, make it clear to members of the public that they usually do not accept patients without a referral.
- Care should be taken to ensure that promotional material and editorials giving information about medical services fulfil the criteria set out by the GMC in the same way as other advertisements.

- Material directed at the general public should not mention, or allude to, the fact that a particular prescription-only medicine can be prescribed.
- Schemes that offer incentives to doctors to recommend a particular product or service are not appropriate.

References

1   The Bristol Royal Infirmary Inquiry. *Learning from Bristol: the report of the public inquiry into children's heart surgery at the Bristol Royal Infirmary 1984–1995.* London: The Stationery Office, 2001: para 59. (Cm 5207 (I).)
2   General Medical Council. *Good medical practice.* London: GMC, 2001: para 3.
3   Leake CD, ed. *Percival's medical ethics.* Baltimore, MD: Williams and Wilkins, Baltimore, 1927:112.
4   Salvage J, Smith R. Doctors and nurses: doing it differently [editorial]. *BMJ* 2000;**320**:1019.
5   *Ibid.*
6   Nursing and Midwifery Council. *Code of professional conduct.* London: NMC, 2002.
7   General Medical Council. *Duties of a doctor.* London: GMC. This comprises a series of booklets covering a range of different issues such as confidentiality, consent, and research.
8   Nursing and Midwifery Council. *Code of professional conduct. Op cit:* para 1·3.
9   Department of Health. *The NHS plan. A plan for investment. A plan for reform.* London: The Stationery Office, 2000: para 9·5.
10 NHS Scotland. *Our national health. A plan for action, a plan for change.* Edinburgh: Scottish Executive, 2000.
11 National Assembly for Wales. *Improving health in Wales. A plan for the NHS with its partners.* Cardiff: National Assembly for Wales, 2001.
12 Davies C. Getting health professionals to work together [editorial]. *BMJ* 2000;**320**:1021–2:1021.
13 World Health Organization Study Group on Multiprofessional Education of Health Personnel. *Learning together to work together for health.* Geneva: WHO, 1988:6.
14 General Medical Council. *Good medical practice. Op cit:* para 36.
15 Nursing and Midwifery Council. *Code of professional conduct. Op cit:* para 4.
16 GMC Professional Conduct Committee hearing, 15–16 and 18–26 March 1999.
17 See discussions in: British Medical Association Health Policy and Economic Research Unit. *Teamwork in primary care.* London: BMA, 1999. British Medical Association Health Policy and Economic Research Unit. *The future healthcare workforce – discussion paper 9.* London: BMA, 2002.
18 Rubenstein L, Josephson K, Wieland GD, English P, Sayre J, Kane R. Effectiveness of a geriatric evaluation unit. *N Engl J Med* 1984;**311**:1664–70.
19 General Medical Council. *Good medical practice. Op cit:* para 37.
20 This is BMA policy. British Medical Association Annual Representative Meeting, 2000.
21 Department of Health. *Code of conduct for NHS managers.* London: DoH, 2002:3.
22 Department of Health. *Managing for excellence in the NHS.* London: DoH, 2002.
23 General Medical Council. *Management in health care – the role of doctors.* London: GMC, 1999.
24 GMC Professional Conduct Committee hearing, 18 June 1998.
25 John Roylance Appellant v General Medical Council Respondent (No. 2) [2000] 1 AC 311.
26 National Audit Office. *Inpatient and outpatient waiting in the NHS.* London: The Stationery Office, 2001: para 2·19. (HC 221.)
27 *Ibid:* paras 2·19 and 2·21.
28 National Audit Office. *Inappropriate adjustments to NHS waiting lists.* London: The Stationery Office, 2001. (HC 452.)
29· The Audit Commission. *Waiting list accuracy. Assessing the accuracy of waiting list information in NHS hospitals in England.* London: The Audit Commission, 2003.
30 Kinnersley P, Anderson E, Parry K, *et al.* Randomised controlled trial of nurse practitioner care for patients requesting "same day" consultations in primary care. *BMJ* 2000;**320**:1043–8.
31 Shum C, Humphreys A, Wheeler D, Cochrane M, Skoda S, Clement S. Nurse management of patients with minor illnesses in general practice: multicentre, randomised controlled trial. *BMJ* 2000;**320**:1038–43.
32 British Medical Association Health Policy and Economic Research Unit. *The future healthcare workforce – discussion paper 9. Op cit.*

33 General Medical Council. *Good medical practice. Op cit:* para 47.
34 Department of Health. *The NHS plan. A plan for investment. A plan for reform. Op cit.*
35 Mills SY, Budd S. *Professional organisation of complementary and alternative medicine in the United Kingdom 2000. A second report to the Department of Health.* Exeter: Exeter University Centre for Complementary Health Studies, 2000.
36 British Medical Association. *Acupuncture: efficacy, safety and practice.* Amsterdam: Harwood Academic Publishers, 2000:2.
37 *Ibid:* pp. 66–81.
38 See, for example: British Medical Association. *Complementary medicine.* Oxford: Oxford University Press, 1993. British Medical Association. *Acupuncture: efficacy, safety and practice. Op cit.*
39 General Practitioners Committee. *Partnership agreements. Guidance for GPs.* London: British Medical Association, 1999.
40 General Medical Council. *Good medical practice. Op cit:* para 35.
41 Emergency Services Collaborative. *Improvement in emergency care: case studies.* London: NHS Modernisation Agency, 2002:35–6.
42 Campbell H, Hotchkiss R, Bradshaw N, Porteous M. Integrated care pathways. *BMJ* 1998;**316**:133–7.
43 Emergency Services Collaborative. *Improvement in emergency care: case studies. Op cit:* iv.
44 Guy's and St Thomas' Hospital NHS Trust press release. *Numbers of sickle cell patients double whilst hospital admissions drop by a third.* 2001 Aug 24.
45 Department of Health. *The NHS plan. A plan for investment. A plan for reform. Op cit:* ch 7.
46 National Audit Office. *Ensuring the effective discharge of older patients from NHS acute hospitals. Executive summary.* London: The Stationery Office, 2003: paras 1–2.
47 Community Care (Delayed Discharges and etc.) Act 2003.
48 Department of Health. *Discharge from hospital: pathway, process and practice.* London: DoH, 2003.
49 Department of Health. *A code of conduct for private practice. Guidance for NHS medical staff.* London: DoH, 2003.
50 *Ibid:* para 3·22.
51 GMC Professional Conduct Committee hearing, 2–9 September 2002.
52 General Medical Council. *Good medical practice. Op cit:* paras 48–50.
53 *Ibid:* para 45.
54 Advertising Standards Authority. *The British code of advertising, sales promotion and direct marketing, 11th ed.* London: ASA, 2003: para 23·2.
55 The Medicines (Advertising) Regulations 1994, regulation 7. (SI 1994 No. 1932.)
56 Department of Health. *CMO's update 34.* London: DoH, 2002: para 2.
57 Anonymous. Guidance news. Helping doctors with real life dilemmas. *GMC News* 2002;**11**:8.
58 General Medical Council. *Good medical practice. Op cit:* para 55.

20: Public health dimensions of medical practice

The questions covered in this chapter include the following.

- To what extent may personal health information be used for public health purposes?
- How far should health promotion campaigns be enforced?
- What are the benefits and harms of population screening?
- Do target payments for immunisation raise questions about the doctor's impartiality?
- What ethical considerations should be taken into account in priority setting?
- How should the release of information about disease outbreaks be managed?

Ethics and public health medicine

Medical ethics usually focuses on the dynamics of the relationship between the individual doctor and the patient. At its centre lies the autonomy of individual patients and the need for consent before treatment can proceed. The primary duty of doctors is to the wellbeing of their patients. Public health doctors, however, do not have individual patients and their concern is with the health of entire communities or geographical areas. In aiming to distribute benefits as widely as possible across target populations, public health medicine has inevitably focused more on utilitarian justifications than on individual autonomy.

Public health aspects of medicine raise particular ethical dilemmas that have traditionally been underrepresented in the academic and professional literature. This chapter seeks to highlight important areas of interest in order to promote further debate. As well as being an emerging issue for ethical discourse, public health has also been going through a period of change in terms of how it is delivered. At the end of the twentieth century in England and Wales, for example, the majority of public health doctors moved from working in teams of three or four consultants to being single handed directors of public health in primary care trusts. These changes also introduced more multidisciplinary working in public health, such that the majority of the public health workforce is not medically qualified, and therefore the information provided in Chapter 19 will also be of relevance to those working in this field. At the same time, in England and Wales, responsibility for the infectious disease control agenda moved from local control to a new national Health Protection Agency. The full implications of these changes remain to be seen, but the dilemmas and principles guiding practice are the same, irrespective of the structure through which the service is delivered.

Many of the issues that are discussed in this chapter stem from the conflict in public health medicine between maximising the welfare of populations and respecting individual autonomy and wellbeing. Public health medicine attempts to find appropriate and legitimate solutions to balance these conflicting interests. It includes issues such as: public health interventions in the areas of health promotion, screening, and vaccination; the provision of equitable health services for the community, in terms of assessing need and commissioning services; and managing public health scares, such as disease outbreaks, including reporting incidences, contact tracing, and informing the public. Public health is not just an issue for those working in that specialty, but the work of most doctors, particularly GPs, has a public health dimension and the majority of doctors have a role to play in these endeavours. This chapter is aimed at all those whose practice has an impact on public health.

Politics and public health medicine

The goal of public health medicine is improvement of the health of populations. It includes the assessment of health and healthcare needs, the development of suitable policies to address those needs, and the commissioning, as far as possible within available resources, of suitable health services. It follows that there is an unavoidable political dimension to this branch of medicine.

Although this has always been the case, arguably the political dimensions of this role have increased. "Traditional" public health concentrated primarily on the analysis and control of microbiological sources of disease and illness. This has been augmented, and for some commentators largely replaced, by a broader focus on the social, cultural, and political foundations of health. This modern approach begins with the recognition that the sources of ill health are to be found in pathogenic social structures and emphasises the importance of socioeconomic factors in developing and sustaining good health. (This is an issue that the BMA's Board of Science and Education has considered over a number of years.[1]) The importance of this approach can clearly be seen in the increasing emphasis given to tackling health inequalities.[2]

Public health medicine is also an area in which the effects of centralised political decision making are felt very keenly. Governments impose goals or targets in relation to specific disease groups such as coronary heart disease or health related social problems, which set the framework of priorities within which public health professionals must operate. It can consequently be difficult to achieve funding for services that fall outside these broad political goals. Public health professionals must therefore accept the tensions generated by the conflict between politically unrecognised, but nevertheless genuine, health needs and the emphasis and funding given to political priorities.

Another issue often raised by public health practitioners is the question of to whom they owe responsibility[3] and how they should be held accountable to the community in whose interests they practice. This accountability is partly achieved by public scrutiny, through both the boards of commissioning bodies and the publication of annual reports and other documents relating to the health of the local community. An ethical challenge for public health practitioners, however, lies in developing methods to ascertain the acceptability and representativeness of their practice to the populations for which they are responsible.

General principles

Public health medicine should:

- address the fundamental causes of disease and the requirements for health and wellbeing, aiming to prevent adverse health outcomes
- respect the rights of individuals to the greatest extent that is compatible with protecting public health
- ensure input from all sections of the community, including those who are unable to speak for themselves
- aim to ensure that the basic resources and conditions necessary for health are available to all
- seek to prioritise interventions that favour underprivileged sections of society
- seek the best available information for carrying out its role
- provide communities with the information that is required for policy decisions and obtain the community's agreement, where appropriate, for their implementation
- act in a timely manner on available information within the resources and the mandate given
- incorporate a variety of approaches that respect the diverse beliefs and values in the community
- implement policies in a manner that most enhances the physical and social environment
- protect the confidentiality of information where appropriate.[4]

The use of health information

Public health medicine uses a large amount of health information gathered from a variety of sources, including population registers, birth notification and mortality records, disease registries, health service data banks, national and regional screening or surveillance programmes, data specifically collected through surveys and research, and medical notes. Often the data are linked together, for example information from cancer registries is linked to mortality data, to increase its potential uses. The use of these types of data is crucial to the development of public health strategies, but the usual rules of confidentiality still apply. Specific information about confidentiality and the use of personal health information is covered in Chapter 5, but the main principles that apply to the use of information for public health purposes are summarised below.

When public health doctors use data or design projects that involve data capture, the following principles should be followed.

- Wherever possible, anonymised data should be used.
- Consent should be sought for any use or disclosure of personal health information.
- Occasionally, when it is not possible to obtain consent, information may be disclosed with strict safeguards (see below).
- Where consent is sought from patients for the use of their information, they must be properly informed about the purpose and nature of its use.
- Where practitioners are not directly involved in the consent process, they should accept data only from reputable sources that have in place appropriate mechanisms for information gathering and handling.
- All processing of identifiable health data must comply with legal requirements and must be "fair and lawful".
- Disclosure should be kept to the minimum necessary to achieve the purpose.
- All patient identifiable data must be properly protected against inappropriate or inadvertent disclosure.
- All individuals who come into contact with personal health information in their work must be trained in confidentiality issues.

Where it is not possible to use anonymous information, or to obtain consent, information may be disclosed to comply with a statutory requirement (see pages 727–8) or where there is an overriding public interest (see, for example, pages 728–9). In England and Wales, disclosure is also permitted, in some circumstances, under the terms of regulations made under section 60 of the Health and Social Care Act 2001 (for more information about section 60 disclosures see Chapter 5, pages 182–3).

Section 60 exemptions for communicable diseases and other risks to public health

At the time of writing, regulations under the Health and Social Care Act have been made to permit confidential patient information to be processed, when it is not possible to obtain consent, for the following purposes:

- diagnosing communicable diseases and other risks to public health
- recognising trends in such diseases and risks
- controlling and preventing the spread of such diseases and risks
- monitoring and managing:

  - outbreaks of communicable disease
  - incidents of exposure to communicable disease
  - the delivery, efficacy, and safety of immunisation programmes
  - adverse reactions to vaccines and medicines
  - risks of infection acquired from food or the environment (including water supplies)
  - the giving of information to persons about the diagnosis of communicable disease and risks of acquiring such disease.[5]

At the time of writing, there is no equivalent provision in legislation in Scotland or Northern Ireland, and doctors in those jurisdictions should follow the advice in Chapter 5 and consider whether the public interest overrides the duty of confidentiality. They must also be prepared to justify their decisions.

Public health interventions

Health promotion

A great deal of public health activity is focused on making changes to the overall environment in which populations live. The idea of the "environment" is complex, and ranges from the quality of food, air, and water supply, through to the standard of the built environment, the control of traffic, the reduction of noise pollution, and the quality of the public service infrastructure. This is a large subject and this section considers, for illustration, two examples of this aspect of public health medicine: public health campaigns, which aim to provide information about factors that impact on individuals' lives; and water fluoridation, which aims to enhance the therapeutic benefit that individuals receive from the environment.

Health promotion campaigns

Health promotion is defined by the World Health Organization as "the process of enabling people to exert control over, and to improve, their health".[6] It is a wide ranging and well established part of the public health process, and includes public education campaigns using a variety of media, capacity building in target communities, and various forms of political advocacy.[7] Arguably, the most important goal of health promotion is to provide positive health messages that enable members of the public to make informed decisions about their health. It also has a duty to consider the cost to the public purse of health damaging behaviour and to take appropriate action to minimise it. Many health promotion campaigns, such as the antismoking campaign, have been extremely successful at getting the message across to the public, but have been less successful at bringing about the lifestyle changes required for substantive health improvements in some sections of the population. Public health involvement entails not only the provision of positive, health enhancing messages, but also, where appropriate, the suppression of messages, such as commercial advertising, that can lead to behaviour that damages health. In relation to smoking, it has also involved more coercive measures such as designated no-smoking zones and the banning of smoking on public transport and in some public places. Although such moves impinge on individual autonomy, they help to protect public health, particularly the health of children, so these moves are supported by the BMA.[8]

Although health promotion campaigns are firmly located in the tradition of public health interventions, based on ideas of the common good, they raise questions about the extent to which it is appropriate for a democratic state to legislate on matters of individual lifestyle. Providing information about healthy living allows people to make their own decisions, but enforcing such decisions, by statutory bans on smoking in public places, for example, can be considered coercive and an infringement of individual liberties.[9] Supporters of these public health interventions, however, point to the fact that individual freedoms are both dependent upon, and informed by, the social and economic environments in which they are exercised. The public, they argue, therefore require protection from aggressive commercial interests. In addition, there is a generally recognised duty imposed upon governments to protect their own populations from harm, irrespective of the choices made by individuals.

Although the general ethical arguments in favour of health promotion are persuasive, public health practitioners, having taken notice of these criticisms, have shown increased awareness of the importance of involving the public in the development and implementation of health promotion campaigns. Ultimately, the goal of health promotion activity is to make it easier and more desirable for individuals to make healthy choices.

State beneficence or individual freedom? The fluoridation of the water supply

It is now generally accepted that one of the most economic and efficient means of providing protection from dental caries, from childhood onwards, is through the fluoridation of water supplies.[10] In addition, as a public health intervention, fluoridation is a redistributive intervention, having a proportionately larger impact on the less advantaged.[11] It therefore helps to fulfil a public health duty to prioritise interventions that favour underprivileged sections of society. Furthermore, although there are health risks associated with high concentrations of fluoride, there is a considerable body of evidence to suggest that the levels of fluoride permitted in the UK are safe. In spite of this, fluoridation has proved controversial. The root of the controversy lies not in doubts about common benefit, but in concerns about harms to individuals. In particular, it raises questions about the infringement of individual autonomy, in this case about the freedom of individuals both to make decisions about the kind of water they drink and to choose whether to receive medication. Opponents of compulsory fluoridation argue that it infringes both their autonomy and their ability to make decisions on behalf of their children. These concerns were sufficiently persuasive for a Scottish court, in 1983, to recognise that "fluoride would involve an encroachment of individual rights to the extent that persons would be forced to drink a substance, fluoride, which they did not wish to drink."[12] The court held that, at that time, there was no power to add fluoride to the water and the Government subsequently legislated to give water companies that power.[13] The legislation does not, however, compel companies to fluoridate and, in spite of pressure from local health bodies, they appear reluctant to do so[14]; only around 10% of the UK's population drinks fluoridated water.[15] The BMA has, for many years, campaigned for fluoridation to be a requirement of water providers when this is requested by health authorities and trusts, following the appropriate consultation.

BMA policy on fluoridation (1998)

"That the BMA remains committed to the fluoridation of mains water supplies on the grounds of effectiveness, safety and equity and urges the Government to require that water companies fluoridate water supplies where this is formally requested by health authorities following proper consultation as required by the 1985 Water (Fluoridation) Act."[16]

Although autonomy is important, the state is also under a general duty to protect its citizens, and, given that the published research shows it to be safe and beneficial, it can clearly be argued that water fluoridation fulfils this duty. There is unambiguous evidence that fluoridation is wide ranging in its effects, benefiting all members of society collectively, but particularly those from disadvantaged sections of society.[17] Where it is not possible to respect individual choice, because there can be only one composition for the public water supply in any area, the only possible choice must be a collective one. Requirements for extensive public consultation are included in the UK legislation.

Summary – health promotion

- An important goal of public health is to provide positive health messages that enable people to make informed decisions about their health.
- There is a general duty on states to protect their own population from harm and to consider the cost to the public purse of health damaging behaviour. Some coercive measures, such as banning smoking in public places, are therefore acceptable.
- Given the clear evidence of benefit from fluoridation of the water supply, the BMA supports moves to make it compulsory for water companies to fluoridate at the request of health authorities or trusts, following proper consultation with the local community.

Population screening

Screening involves the systematic testing of a defined, usually asymptomatic, population for a specific disorder with the aim of identifying those requiring further investigation or direct medical intervention. In some respects, screening is different from other forms of health care. In ordinary healthcare practice it is the patient who approaches the health worker in search of relief or treatment for a particular disorder. With screening, however, the health service usually approaches apparently healthy individuals and invites them to undergo a test or survey from which they may derive some benefit. Clearly, in such circumstances those offering a screening programme need to be certain that there is a substantive benefit to the public health, and that it outweighs any resulting harms. According to the National Screening Committee, the

UK-wide advisory body on all aspects of screening policy, "it is unknown to find a screening programme that gives 100% benefit".[18] It is vital, therefore, that an informed judgment is made about the programme's ability to provide a net good for those being screened. Although screening in the private sector is likely to be driven by market forces, the same rigorous standards should apply.

Criteria for introducing a screening programme

There is general consensus about the basic criteria that must be fulfilled prior to the introduction of any new screening programme.[19]

- **The problem must be important.** This includes conditions that are important because they affect a relatively high proportion of the population as well as conditions that are less common but are very severe.
- **A suitable screening test should be available.** The test being used must be not only reliable but also effective at detecting the condition being sought. It must have both a high sensitivity and a high specificity, as well as a high positive predictive value (a high proportion of positive results should be true positives). A high positive predictive value is not so important if the screening test is being backed up by a "gold standard" follow up test.
- **The results must provide useful information.** There are a number of ways in which the results of screening may be useful. They may, for example:

  - permit early diagnosis followed by effective management of the condition
  - give information that would offer increased choices
  - provide information to permit planning for the future, for both the individual and the health service
  - prevent the spread of disease
  - in the case of prenatal screening, give time to prepare for the birth of a disabled child
  - permit lifestyle changes to minimise the risk of disability or disease
  - give time to adapt one's lifestyle to an impending disability.

  Screening that provides no benefit to the individuals being tested would not meet these criteria but may be helpful for planning the health needs of populations or groups.

- **The benefits must outweigh the harms.** Benefits would include the provision of curative treatment, the ability to prioritise treatment services effectively, patient wellbeing and satisfaction, and the promotion of informed decision making. These need to be balanced against any actual or perceived adverse effects, particularly those resulting from false positive or false negative results, the risks of labelling people as "sick", the social disadvantages of the information being available, and the likelihood of increased anxiety. Some form of cost–benefit analysis is also needed because, whenever different disciplines and treatments compete for limited funding, any screening programme must make good use of resources.

(Continued)

> - **Adequate provision must be made for information, counselling and privacy.** Careful consideration should be given to the provision of information about the test and its implications, and the need for and the availability of counselling. Assurances must be provided that the information obtained will remain confidential. Patients should be made aware if information will be used for planning or research purposes in an anonymised form. Information should be provided about the potential uses of the data that will be collected, including the implications for insurance and employment where appropriate.

Population screening: benefits and harms

Before a particular type of population screening is recommended, the National Screening Committee must be satisfied that the benefits outweigh the harms. There are a number of benefits that can derive from population screening (see box above), some of which, however, would clearly not be available for incompetent adults, and thus raise questions about whether they should be automatically included in such screening. However, excluding such groups could be perceived as discriminatory; individual decisions need to be made based on the efficacy of the screening for the early identification of disease. It is important that the purpose of any screening programme is clearly explained as part of the process of seeking consent, including being clear about for whose benefit it is being undertaken.

One of the known harms of screening is the raised levels of anxiety that have been reported in all forms of screening programmes including cervical, breast, and general health screening, as well as genetic screening. (For specific information on genetic screening see Chapter 9, pages 329–32.) For some people, simply receiving an invitation to participate in screening causes anxiety and some have been found to be more anxious after screening than before, regardless of the result. It should also be remembered that the motivation of those offering the screening may be different from that of the individuals who accept it. The service is provided in order to identify people who are at risk, but most individuals, believing themselves to be healthy, undertake screening for reassurance that they are not at risk. Some people therefore accept screening without properly considering the implications of receiving an unfavourable result; when they do not receive the expected result, their certainty about their health status shifts to uncertainty and this can cause considerable anxiety.[20] There is little that can be done to counter such reactions except to ensure that individuals are provided with an adequate supply of accurate information in a manner they are able to understand and are given the opportunity to discuss the information and ask questions. Undoubtedly, some of the anxieties that arise from screening are caused by a misunderstanding of the information provided, particularly about the accuracy of the test and the implications of a positive or negative result. Accurate recall of information, in all spheres of medicine, is a problem and it can therefore be helpful to supplement discussion with written material for people to take away with them.

All screening tests generate a certain number of false negatives and positives. Those managing such programmes need to aim at finding the right balance between its sensitivity (picking up a very high proportion of positive cases) and its specificity (giving a negative result in a high proportion of negative cases). This balance usually depends on the consequences of making or not making a positive finding. For example, where a positive finding would be particularly associated with anxiety or stigma, then a higher specificity is desirable. Alternatively, where the adverse consequences of a missed positive are considerable, a higher sensitivity would be preferred.

Screening tests can have four possible outcomes: true negative; false negative; true positive; false positive. People who are given a false negative or a false positive result are likely to be harmed in some way, although those with a false positive probably less so than those with a false negative, because the former will usually proceed to a definitive test, which will demonstrate that these people are free of the disease. Those with a true positive are normally regarded as enjoying a benefit, because they go on to receive treatment for the condition, but this is not always the case. For example, some true positives would not have gone on to develop the disease – it may have been a slowly developing condition and they would have died of something else – and the screening may therefore not have been beneficial.

Screening for breast cancer

In many western countries, mammography is routinely offered to women over a certain age, usually 40 or 50. The majority of medical opinion supports such screening, and roughly 1 in 160 British women who attend screening go on to be treated for breast cancer.[21] Nevertheless, a number of commentators claim that the benefits of such programmes remain uncertain.[22] They point to the risks of screening, such as false alarms that can cause long periods of anxiety. Also, because neither the screening nor the follow up tests are 100% accurate, some women will inevitably be treated for cancer when they are in fact free of it. Screening can also identify small tumours that are growing so slowly that, without treatment, the woman could live her life without ever knowing of the cancer, which would play no part in the cause of her death.

Individuals who receive a true negative result may of course enjoy the welcome benefit of reassurance. Such a result can, however, inspire a false sense of security. With breast screening, for example, a negative result indicates only that the disease was not detectable at the time of the test. For some, this may be interpreted as meaning that they are not at risk of developing the disease, which consequently prevents them from responding to early warning signs should the disease appear later. There is the additional danger that a negative test is interpreted as a "green light" to continue with unhealthy lifestyle choices. To an extent, these harms can be moderated by the provision of clear health advice at all stages of the screening process.

Summary – population screening

- Those offering screening programmes need to be certain that they offer a net benefit.
- The purpose of a screening programme, including for whose benefit it is being undertaken, needs to be clearly explained, as part of the consent process, to those who participate.
- For any screening programme, the following five criteria must be met.
  - The problem must be important.
  - A suitable screening test should be available.
  - The results must provide useful information.
  - The benefits must outweigh the harms.
  - Adequate provision must be made for information, counselling, and privacy.

Vaccination programmes

Vaccination programmes are among the most widely used and cost effective public health tools available,[23] and it is difficult to exaggerate their contribution to the improvement of both public and individual health in the years since their development. Given the benefits that these programmes have delivered, there are clearly sound utilitarian arguments for their broad deployment and for the development of robust incentives to try to ensure as wide an uptake as possible. Nevertheless, as with all health interventions, there are associated risks; for example, the swine 'flu vaccination programme in the mid-1970s was suspended because it was thought to be associated with Guillain–Barré syndrome.[24] In some respects vaccination programmes have become the victims of their own success. The mortality and morbidity associated with their target diseases have become so unusual as to fall out of popular memory, and critical attention has therefore turned on their associated risks, which are often quite minor. During the writing of this book, for example, there was intensive debate about the use of the triple vaccine to protect children against measles, mumps, and rubella (MMR). As this debate raises several important ethical issues it is used as an example on pages 714–5.

The provision of information

Immunisation is offered routinely to a variety of groups in the UK. It is not compulsory, although there is understandably a strong commitment among healthcare workers to its use. Although it is widely agreed that vaccination ordinarily provides both an individual and a communal benefit, the likelihood of any particular individual benefiting reduces as the percentage of the population vaccinated increases. This is simply because, if sufficient numbers of the population are immunised, there is a dramatic reduction in the likelihood of coming into contact with the disease. Where there is already population immunity – as is the case with a variety of common diseases in the UK – a vaccination's harms, such as side effects, are likely to be more substantial than the harm that follows from a particular individual not being vaccinated. Considered in isolation, therefore, for any particular individual living in an area with population immunity, the risk of vaccination will outweigh the benefits. This holds true only, however, if that individual remains in the community and does not, for example, travel to an area in which population immunity has not been achieved. If sufficient individuals refuse immunisation, the result can be a "tragedy of the commons"[25]: population immunity collapses and epidemics sweep through the community.

The question this raises for individual doctors is one of truth telling and the limits of patient advocacy. Should GPs who, for example, are working in places where population immunity has been achieved, inform their patients of the reduced benefits of vaccination, or do doctors' duties to the broader population outweigh the strict observance of truth telling? What would be the impact on the community if GPs offered this information, and a significant percentage started to choose not to have their children immunised? At what point would GPs have to alter the advice they give, because the area would no longer have achieved population immunity? Furthermore, do individual patients have a duty to contribute to the protection of the wider community and should they be encouraged to consider the potential costs to society of the options they choose? If patients are perceived as having wider duties, which require them to share the small risks of vaccination for the good of the overall community, do doctors have a role in drawing attention to them? These questions raise issues that need to be taken into account when assessing individual cases. Doctors should, however, answer questions honestly and should provide patients or their parents with as much information as they need to make an informed decision; this should include telling them of the disadvantages for themselves or their children, and for others within the community, if population immunity is lost.

Choice, risk, and uncertainty: the case of MMR

As the majority of immunisation programmes in the UK involve children, they also raise complex questions about the limits of the rights of parents to make healthcare choices on behalf of their children. In 1998 *The Lancet* published an article in which the authors speculated about a possible link between MMR vaccine and autism and/or inflammatory bowel disease.[26] The evidence was subsequently refuted by several studies[27] and the overwhelming evidence is that there is no proven link between MMR vaccine and autism or inflammatory bowel disease. The article was, however, widely reported in the press, sometimes in a sensationalist way, leading to notable reductions in the uptake of the vaccine, as well as an increase in those having the three vaccines separately. Taking the vaccines separately increases the risk of infection from the three diseases because the vaccinations need to be spread over a period of time. It also increases the likelihood that the course of vaccination will not be completed, thus exposing children, and the population, to risks in the future. The BMA supports the use of the MMR vaccine.

In view of the decline in uptake after the media reporting of this article, the BMA's Medical Ethics Committee considered the issues raised. These included whether it is morally acceptable for individuals to select suboptimal interventions, in this case separate vaccines, that either adversely affect the health of the community or fail to maximise it, and, should they desire such an option, whether there was any obligation on the NHS to fund it. The Committee also considered whether financial incentives to GPs to encourage the uptake of vaccines were appropriate (see pages 716–7), and whether it was morally acceptable for parents to leave their children unvaccinated, even when vaccination was in the child's best interests. Questions were also raised about the extent to which patients have a moral duty, both to contribute to the protection of the community and to explicitly consider the potential cost to society of their choices. The BMA agreed the following basic principles.

- The ethical debate over the MMR vaccine hinges on the clinical evidence. Clinical benefits and harms can be assessed by objective methods and these necessarily provide part of the basis for ethical deliberation.
- Doctors generally have a therapeutic role and are primarily concerned with the wellbeing of individual patients. However, the needs of the wider society occasionally come to the fore.
- Doctors have a duty to help patients to access the most effective treatments identified from evidence-based criteria. They also play an important role in public education.
- The Government and public health physicians have obligations to maximise public health and ensure that accurate information is provided to the public.
- Individual autonomy deserves respect up to the point at which other people are harmed, and claims based upon individual choice have to be balanced against public health needs and resource considerations.
- Parents are accountable both to society and to their children for the decisions they make on their children's behalf, and there is a limit to the risk to which parents can expose their children. Generally, however, parents are the best people to make decisions for their children and society needs strong evidence of harm before overriding their wishes.
- Individuals have duties to the broader community, and should be encouraged to consider them. However, the fulfilment of such duties can only be encouraged, it cannot be enforced.
- The concept of "risk" needs to be better communicated to, and better understood by, the public.

In addition to these broad principles, the BMA believes that patients have general rights to choose inferior treatments if they wish, both for themselves and, within reason, for their children. There is not, however, a duty on society to fund them, given that the Government has a responsibility to optimise the use of scarce public resources.

Summary – vaccination programmes

- Vaccination programmes are among the most widely used and cost effective public health tools available.
- Although vaccination programmes are highly effective, there are some attendant risks.
- Doctors should provide patients with the information needed to make an informed choice. This should include information about the disadvantages for the patient and the wider community if population immunity is lost.
- Claims based upon individual choice have to be balanced against public health needs, but patients have general rights to choose inferior treatment for themselves and, within reason, for their children.

Target payments as public health incentives

During the debate on MMR, attention was focused on the practice of doctors being offered target payments for immunisation, screening, and child health. The main concern is that doctors may be encouraged to pressurise patients to accept the intervention, fail adequately to explain the risks, or perhaps overstate the likely benefits for the individual, in order to reach their targets and qualify for the additional payment. In a 1998 article, for example, it was suggested that target payments for cervical screening encouraged doctors "to persuade all women to accept invitations to be screened and appears to place no weight on the need to give women accurate information on the risks and disadvantages to them of being screened".[28] The authors of this article went on to suggest that "one very important reason for this emphasis is the existence of targets to be achieved by all those involved in cervical screening in Britain".[29] Whether women do feel pressured to consent or not is, in some ways, immaterial because the fact that the target payments are perceived to affect the doctor's judgment could, in itself, have a negative impact on the doctor–patient relationship. If a doctor recommends a procedure without having any financial incentive to do so, patients are likely to feel more confident that they are being given balanced advice, based on the doctor's assessment of their best interests. When patients know that the doctor's income is directly affected by the number of patients undergoing the selected procedure, their trust in the doctor's impartiality is threatened. Concerns have also been expressed that doctors may be reluctant to accept new patients on to their practice lists who are unlikely to take up screening or vaccination.

The BMA shares these concerns, but is also acutely aware that immunisations and screening are extremely effective public health tools and that steps to encourage their uptake are important to the public health. The BMA has, however, called for the target payment system to be modified to reduce the risk of real or perceived pressure on patients to consent. It has suggested that women who make an informed decision to refuse cervical screening, and remove themselves from the recall arrangements, should be excluded from target payment calculations. Similarly, parents should be able to make an informed refusal of immunisation for their children and indicate a wish to be exempt from the target population. In the midst of concern about public perceptions of the objectivity of information provided about MMR, the BMA's General Practitioners Committee called for a moratorium on MMR target payments, and, at the time of writing, remains opposed to them.

Developing policies and commissioning services

Public health practitioners aim to maximise the equitable distribution of health benefits across broad populations. They gather and assess data on relevant health needs or problems and then develop appropriate strategies to respond. These strategies can then be used to approach decisions relating to prioritising, funding, planning, and commissioning health services.

Priority setting

Priority setting emerges from the clash between health needs and health resources: the former tend toward infinity, the latter are restricted. In the UK, where the NHS is committed to the universal provision of treatment on the basis of need, priority setting has traditionally been managed by waiting lists. As a result, priority setting in the NHS has tended to be implicit, rather than openly acknowledged,[30] and decisions have often appeared to be inconsistent and based upon uncertain reasoning. Nevertheless, the Government's decision to limit the availability of sildenafil (Viagra) and the creation of the National Institute for Clinical Excellence and equivalent bodies in other parts of the UK, which make decisions about priorities on the basis of clinical effectiveness, may herald a move towards more openness (see Chapter 13, pages 460–61 and 463).

This is a complex issue and a full discussion is beyond the scope of this book.[31] This section, however, provides a brief introduction to the topic and highlights a number of practical ethical considerations that need to be taken into account when considering resource allocation decisions. It seems likely that priority setting will remain an inevitable part of health care in the UK and the principal ethical challenge is to develop processes that are both equitable and transparent, and receive, as far as possible, the support of the populations they affect. The box below lists some of the factors that need to be taken into account when making decisions about priority setting.[32]

Ethical considerations for priority setting

- need
- welfare maximisation
- clinical effectiveness
- relative cost effectiveness
- equity
- individual rights
- patient choice
- communication and public involvement
- transparency and rationality of decision making.

Need

Approaches to priority setting in health care require an understanding of the healthcare needs of target populations. Although these are usually approached via health needs assessments, which aim systematically to identify unmet healthcare needs, these in turn necessarily require some prior understanding of what is meant by "need", and of the difference between "health" and "health care". On the face of it the idea of need may seem straightforward, understood as a health deficit that can benefit from an intervention. Nevertheless, on closer inspection it becomes more problematic, with perceptions of need varying according to what interventions are possible, available, and affordable.[33] The understanding of need also varies according to the definition of health employed and whether it is limited to discrete medical conditions or widened to incorporate social determinates of health and wellbeing. Variations also arise depending upon whether it is the needs of individuals or of groups that are being considered.

Welfare maximisation

At the heart of the debate about rationing lies the fundamentally utilitarian goal of managing and providing healthcare services in ways that maximise the welfare of those who are using them within the available resources.[34] Although much inevitably depends on the definition of "welfare" when resources are limited and the welfare of all persons cannot be individually maximised, attention must be shifted to maximising the welfare of the population viewed in its entirety.

Clinical effectiveness

Decisions relating to an intervention's effectiveness are based exclusively on clinical criteria (both physical and psychological), unaffected by issues of cost. A treatment is clinically effective if it alters a particular condition for the better. One treatment is more effective than another if it alters the condition more successfully or with fewer side effects or under a wider range of circumstances.[35]

Relative cost effectiveness

Cost effectiveness combines clinical efficacy and cost, with the aim of achieving the most effective use of the limited resources available. A range of measures of health benefit[36] can be used to determine cost effectiveness, but this is not a straightforward process and there are always considerable practical difficulties. Whatever measure is used, several important issues need to be addressed, including the additional length and quality of life a treatment brings, the contribution that particular treatments make to an individual's wellbeing, and the level of need of those seeking the treatment.[37]

Equity

Equity requires that like cases are treated alike, and unlike cases treated differently. This principle, when applied to health care, demands that people with the same health needs must be given an equal chance of receiving appropriate treatment of equal quality.[38] In broader public health terms it also means that the same conditions for realising good health are equally available to all members of the population. Public health practitioners need to be attentive both to discrimination and to social exclusion, which are often the result of an interplay of factors such as income, ethnicity, class, and age. Seeking equity in public health is discussed further on pages 721–2.

Individual rights

One of the ways in which the discussion of priority setting has been framed is in terms of individual rights; the nature and status of these rights have an impact on decisions about resource allocation. The notion of "rights", incorporating both substantive legal and aspirational moral entitlements, is complex and contentious. For example, the idea of rights, which prioritises individual interests, is sometimes seen as antagonistic to the central ethos of public health, which seeks to maximise communal goods.[39] The NHS is, however, required to ensure that all of its decisions are compatible with the Human Rights Act 1998 and both primary and subordinate legislation must now be interpreted in ways that are compatible with the European Convention on Human Rights.[40] The UK is also a signatory to the International Covenant on Economic, Social and Cultural Rights, which gives its citizens the right to the highest attainable standard of physical and mental health.[41]

Patient choice

There are inevitably recurrent conflicts between priority setting and patient choice. Rationing, by its nature, involves doctors and others in the hard task of denying to some patients interventions from which they could benefit because resources can be more appropriately employed elsewhere. Nevertheless, within this framework, efforts need to be made to maximise patient choice, and public health practitioners have developed a variety of methods for involving patients in decisions about their healthcare choices. These include the following.

- When research on the effectiveness of a treatment is being assessed, it is important that outcome measures important to patients are used.
- Where multiple treatments are available within the priority setting framework, patients should be encouraged to make their own choices.
- The priority setting framework should be suitably flexible to permit legitimate exceptions based on variations between patients.[42]

Communication and public involvement

Resource allocation decisions attract considerable public interest, and discussions about the criteria on which they should be based are frequently discussed in the media. Debate of these issues has prompted the identification of a "democratic deficit" in the NHS,[43] and a call for the development of new methods for involving the public in meaningful ways. Public participation in policy making is discussed on pages 722–3.

Transparency and rationality of decision making

There are seldom easy or straightforward answers to resource allocation decisions. It is essential therefore that, given their contested nature, decisions are both reasoned and transparent. When choices are based upon values rather than just facts, these should be articulated as clearly as possible, as should the process through which decisions are made.

Resource allocation – the need for transparency in decision making

In the summer of 1999, North West Lancashire Health Authority appealed against a decision in the High Court overturning its resolution to refuse funding for gender reassignment surgery for three transsexuals, A, D, and G. The health authority justified its decision on the basis that it had a statutory obligation to care for all within its area and limited resources with which to do so, requiring it to give lower priority to some medical conditions. Although its rationing policy stated that it allowed funding in exceptional cases, Lord Justice Auld said that its policy was flawed because it did not treat transsexualism as an illness. This, together with the manner of considering individual cases, amounted effectively to the operation of a blanket policy against funding gender reassignment. The appeal was dismissed.

North West Lancashire Health Authority v A, D, and G[44]

Although it is important to bear all of these ethical considerations in mind when setting priorities for the allocation of resources, it is inevitable that there will be cases in which they come into conflict. Cost effectiveness can at times work against individual need, for example, and patient choice often runs into conflict with equity. Difficult choices need to be made and must be justified with clear and transparent policies and decisions in individual cases.

Summary – priority setting

- The need for priority setting emerges from the gap between the demand for health care and the available resources.
- Priority setting is an inevitable part of healthcare provision in the UK and this should be openly acknowledged.
- Decisions must be equitable and comply with the Human Rights Act.
- Decisions must be justified with clear and transparent policies and decisions in individual cases.

Seeking equity in public health

Health inequalities arise not only through priority setting but also through the broader social, economic, and biological factors that affect health. It is therefore not enough to ensure an equitable geographical spread of services. Even if this were to be achieved, rates of uptake would still differ considerably, as would disease variations resulting from genetic and socioeconomic factors. The equity challenge for public health lies far deeper, therefore, than just the research and assessment of health problems and the commissioning of appropriate services to respond to them. It also entails an understanding of how social inequities contribute to the development and prevalence of disease, and how different population groups respond to public health initiatives. It requires the development of innovative ways to contact different communities and to present the issues in ways that are both meaningful and invite cooperation.

Coronary heart disease: a challenge to equity?

Heart disease is one of the leading causes of death in Britain, and a national service framework has been drawn up in England, which sets out a strategy for tackling it.[45] An analysis of both the epidemiology of the disease, and the rates of service uptake, however, reveal a complex variety of inequalities, such as different rates of occurrence among various population groups, and in the likelihood of different groups gaining access to primary and secondary care.[46] Geographical inequalities exist in the prevalence of the disease and the availability of services. Ethnic and gender variations also exist and there is a clear social gradient, in terms of both risk and service uptake. The risk factors for the disease itself read like a roll call of contemporary public health problems, and include poverty, diet, exercise, smoking, alcohol abuse, and genetic susceptibility; these factors impact in multiple and interdependent ways. Furthermore, unlike "traditional" public health interventions, such as improvements in sanitation, a clean water supply, and the development of vaccines, significant improvement is dependent on lifestyle changes that can be extremely difficult to bring about, particularly in the case of populations who are hard to reach.

As mentioned on page 719, the UK is a signatory to the International Covenant on Economic, Social and Cultural Rights. This commits the UK to the gradual realisation of the "right to health",[47] requiring attention to be given to the health needs of particular groups, such as women and children, as well as paying specific attention to environmental and industrial contributors to ill health. In its periodic reports to the United Nations, the UK must show that it has taken steps to address the special health needs of particular categories of the population, such as reducing its very high rate of teenage pregnancies (see Chapter 7, pages 228–9).

Public participation and involvement

In view of the conflict that can arise between individual autonomy and the common good in public health medicine (see pages 703–4), public participation takes on particular importance. Doctors working in this field have been sensitive to the charges of paternalism that have from time to time been directed at their practice, and have used a range of methods for involving populations in their work to ensure that autonomy is eroded to the minimum extent possible. Public involvement, however, requires more than just listening to representatives of "target" populations. At its best it is an ongoing dialogue and involves providing population groups with information about individual policies, the reasons for implementing them, and the desired outcomes.

Where public involvement has worked well, the public health initiatives have generally been more successful, particularly among traditionally hard to reach populations.[48] Such measures can also help to overcome the resistance some groups have shown to state initiatives and enhance the involvement of excluded groups, even though some elements of coercion may still be required, such as restrictions on smoking in public places. It is vital therefore that, before policies are introduced and services offered, a wide range of stakeholders are consulted both to inform the development of the policy and to gain the acceptance and cooperation of the local population. Achieving this is not unproblematic, however. It can be difficult, for example, to identify appropriate representatives and many of the most needy can be so disenfranchised as to be almost silent.[49] Local health professionals in both primary and secondary care have important contributions to make, as do local government and voluntary groups. Listed below are a number of methods that public health practitioners use to enhance public involvement.

Methods for public involvement

- **Public consultations:** These are an increasing feature of government activity and are used to ensure that stakeholders have an opportunity to have their voices heard in decision making processes.
- **Health panels:** These are standing panels of people who are seen to be representative of the local population. They vary in size and in the frequency with which they meet; members tend to be replaced at frequent intervals.

(Continued)

- **Citizens' juries:** These are made up of local people who sit on a jury for a specified time and debate a variety of health topics presented by health practitioners.
- **Focus groups:** These tend to comprise groups of between 6 and 12 local people and are run by a facilitator who promotes discussion on a variety of local health topics.
- **Interviews:** Individuals are selected either at random or as particularly representative and their views are sought on a variety of issues.
- **Questionnaires:** These enable the gathering of structured information from a variety of target populations.

Although public involvement in decision making should be encouraged, it does not necessarily guarantee an ethically justifiable outcome. Public priorities may be inconsistent, based upon a faulty understanding of complex issues or on individual prejudices.[50] Attempts to ascertain the public's views about healthcare priorities, for example, have shown a clear preference for the treatment of acute, life threatening diseases among children over similar treatment for older people, psychiatric services, or general health promotion. Considerable support has also been expressed for the notion that those who have contributed to their own illness, through smoking, obesity, or drinking for example, should have lower priority for treatment.[51] Such views are at odds with the general principles of equity that underpin the NHS. Although it is important to be aware of these inherent difficulties, they do not outweigh the value of such exercises and the benefits of achieving the agreement and cooperation of the local population in public health policy.

Public health policy – some classic successes and failures

Lessons can be learnt from previous attempts to introduce public health measures affecting discrete communities. A frequently quoted example of an unsuccessful campaign relates to sickle cell disease in the USA. In the 1970s, several American states passed legislation requiring black people to have genetic testing for carrier status for the disease. Little attention had been given to the provision of information, counselling, preserving confidentiality, or how to deal with sensitive inadvertent discoveries such as non-paternity. As a result, many people misunderstood the results, confusing carrier status with the disease itself, and some faced stigmatisation. Because the focus was on a particular section of the community, many felt that the screening programme was simply a method of discouraging black people from having children. As a result of these problems, the federal government subsequently offered funds for screening programmes only where they were accompanied by counselling, privacy was respected, and individuals had the right to choose whether or not to take part.

In contrast, a positive example was the introduction from the 1970s of a screening programme for Tay Sachs disease among Ashkenazi Jews in a number of countries. The initiative for the programme came from within the Jewish community itself and was combined with genetic counselling and public education. As a result there has been a significant reduction in the incidence of Tay Sachs disease because people known to be carriers have avoided having children with other carriers.

Managing public health risks

Public health management at a national level

Public health emergencies can be divided into two broad categories: infectious disease outbreaks and environmental or other disasters. In the former, the emphasis is generally on identifying the nature and source of the infection and taking appropriate steps to prevent its spread. In the latter case, the principal response is to secure the basic requirements for health and to determine immediate and future threats to the health of the community. In both cases, public health strategies may be discussed and put in place, either in response to a specific incident or in preparation for a possible future scenario. Although many policies are made at national level, the aim is to develop effective mechanisms for their implementation and to facilitate public health action at local level.

The public health response to bioterrorism: the case of smallpox

At the beginning of the twenty-first century, the potential for a terrorist attack on Britain using the smallpox virus was assessed and the question of an appropriate pre-emptive public health response, including mass immunisation, was raised. One of the difficulties with mass immunisation was that the vaccine itself carried a small risk of both harm and fatality, with a US study indicating that if more than 80 million people under the age of 30 were vaccinated, up to 200 people would die.[52] Furthermore, the vaccine could not be given to people with damaged immune systems, to pregnant women, or to sufferers from eczema. The issue turned therefore on the assessment of risk. The Government decided that, in the absence of a specific threat, it would be prudent to immunise a number of key medical and military staff. The Government also began stockpiling large quantities of the vaccine. Regional smallpox response groups were created and plans were developed to use the internet to provide doctors, who may never have encountered a case of smallpox, with information and advice on the condition.

Policy making in the face of uncertainty

In developing public health policy the usual process is to assess as accurately as possible the level and severity of risk to public health and, on the basis of that assessment, to devise a system of public protection that is proportionate to those risks. When the risk to public health is very high, even apparently draconian measures that interfere with individual human rights may be justified. If the level of risk to public health is low, such actions would not be proportionate. One of the difficulties that frequently arises in practice, however, is the lack of clear evidence on which to base accurate risk assessment. An important part of the role of those planning public health policies, therefore, is to predict, using the best information available at the time, the likely scale of the problem, so that an appropriate response can be initiated. Given that this will always be a matter of judgment, and that it is often not feasible to wait until more evidence is available, these decisions are often controversial. The Government was criticised, for example, for not taking more robust public health action in the weeks after the first UK case of severe acute respiratory syndrome (known as SARS) in March 2003.[53] Deciding what action to take and at what time is a real challenge. Those responsible for making such decisions must be willing to explain the reasons for their action, or inaction, including acknowledging areas of continuing uncertainty.

Policy making in the face of uncertainty: the case of Creutzfeldt–Jakob disease

In August 2002 a patient at Middlesborough General Hospital was unexpectedly diagnosed as suffering from Creutzfeldt–Jakob disease (CJD) after a brain biopsy. In the period between the biopsy and the diagnosis being received, the same surgical instruments were used in other patients' operations, raising the possibility that they may have been exposed to the risk of transmission of CJD, the infectious agents for which (prions) are resistant to nearly all sterilisation procedures. Worldwide, there have been a small number of cases of CJD diagnosed after the use of contaminated instruments. The Government's advisory group, the CJD Incidents Panel, advised that, of the 34 patients in Middlesborough who were subsequently operated on using the same instruments, 24 should be contacted and informed of their possible exposure, even though there is no test that could confirm their infection and there are no steps that could be taken to prevent or delay the onset of the condition if they had been infected. A subsequent independent review of the incident, carried out for the Department of Health, reported that, after ongoing assessment, it appeared that not all of the patients who were contacted were, in fact, at any real risk of exposure, and for those who were, the risk was described as "very small".[54] The review also found that, contrary to comments from the Department of Health at the time, the trust had followed the appropriate guidelines for decontamination.

Difficult questions arise when individuals are, or may have been, exposed to serious and untreatable conditions such as CJD. Whether it is appropriate to contact patients who may have been exposed in such incidents, and inform them of their possible exposure, is a complex problem. Although there is currently no treatment for CJD, they could be advised not to donate blood, organs, or tissue, and to notify the clinical team before any future surgery, in order to minimise the possible risk to others. There are, therefore, clear public health arguments for informing people, but do these potential benefits outweigh the harms to those individuals of being given the information? Given the current uncertainty about CJD and the nature of its transmission, the amount of information that can be provided is very limited. There is no test that could show for certain that the individual was exposed to the prions or has been infected. Given also the very long incubation period, which could be decades, the only information apparently healthy individuals can be given is that it is possible that they will develop an incurable and fatal disease at some stage over the next 10–30 years. This is likely to have a devastating effect on those concerned.

Although medical ethics generally promotes openness, honesty, and transparency, this does not mean that unwelcome information should be foisted on individuals when they do not, or may not, want to know it. In order to justify imposing this information on people, not for their own benefit but for the benefit of others, there needs to be a demonstrably high level of public health risk that outweighs the harms to individuals of being told. This requires a careful balancing of interests based on the most up to date scientific evidence of the level of risk. It is possible that, because of fear of future criticism, action may be taken that is not justified by the evidence of risk available at the time the decision is made. It therefore needs to be openly acknowledged that, whenever decisions are made in the face of uncertainty, it is possible that new evidence may come to light that means that, with the benefit of hindsight, different decisions would have been made.

Balancing individual autonomy and public protection

Similar conflict between individual freedoms and the common good arose in the 1980s with the AIDS epidemic. The AIDS example is instructive because it highlights the complex balance that needs to be achieved between statutory and compulsory requirements. It also illustrates the importance of gaining the confidence and cooperation of target populations, a confidence that can be destroyed by the threat of coercion. In the USA the Surgeon General and the Presidential Commission on the HIV Epidemic stressed that the protection of confidentiality was a prerequisite for the achievement of public health goals in this area.[55] Stigmatisation, marginalisation, and the possibility that those who are infected may be denied access to important social goods, are matters of concern. In addition, sensitive issues, such as sexual orientation and intravenous drug use, may be disclosed. These factors have heightened awareness of the need to protect privacy where this can be reconciled with appropriate public health measures. The successful approach to the AIDS epidemic in New Zealand (see box) clearly supports the application of a community development approach.

HIV/AIDS in New Zealand

When news of the AIDS epidemic began to spread through the New Zealand gay community, the initial response was informal and the community provided its own networking, information provision, and counselling services. As the disease spread, however, more formal strategies developed, involving a wide range of individuals and services. The key points of the campaign were the following.

- Recognition of the public health problem came from the group who were most at risk, and leadership was provided from within the community.
- Capacity building in the gay community was initiated at an early stage.
- Partnerships with key workers in the health and political arenas were developed.
- Affected groups gained representation at government advisory level – the original council included representatives of gay people, sex workers, intravenous drug users, and members of the Maori and Pacific communities.

This strategy has been highly effective for limiting the spread of HIV in New Zealand.[56]

Decisions about public health policy must be made in an open and transparent way, and information about public health strategies must be clearly and accurately presented to the public.

Summary – public health management at national level

- The level at which public health policy interferes with individual autonomy should be proportional to the extent and severity of the risk to public health.
- Policy making often requires decisions to be made in advance of clear and unequivocal evidence being available.
- Decisions about what public health action to take, and at what stage, are inevitably matters of judgment and are likely to be controversial.
- Decisions must be made on the basis of the best available evidence at the time and should be carefully explained to the public, including acknowledging areas of uncertainty.

Public health management at local level

Much public health management takes place at local level, including the implementation of national policies and, after liaison with the relevant bodies, the day to day management of public health incidents.

Infectious disease reporting

Public health legislation contains a number of powers designed to control the spread of infectious diseases.[57] This includes the power to subject individuals to compulsory medical examination, and to remove people who are suffering from a notifiable disease to hospital without their consent, or against a competent refusal if necessary, and to detain them there. Furthermore, people with notifiable diseases can be subject to certain restrictions on their movements and anyone with such a disease is not permitted to use public transport, public libraries, or public laundries.[58] Those who exercise these powers must, however, have due regard to the individual rights enshrined in the Human Rights Act.

In England and Wales, doctors are statutorily required to notify the "proper officer" of their local authority of any patient they believe to be suffering from a notifiable disease, which includes conditions such as meningitis, plague, tuberculosis, and food poisoning.[59] In Scotland, doctors are required to contact the chief administrative medical officer for the area in which the notifying doctor works. In Northern Ireland, doctors are required to notify the communicable disease surveillance centre.

Infectious disease notification: the current law in England, Wales, and Scotland

If a registered medical practitioner believes or suspects that a person he or she is attending is suffering from a notifiable disease, he or she must send to the proper officer a certificate stating:

- the name, age, and sex of the patient and the address of the premises where the patient is residing
- the disease or poisoning from which the patient is, or is suspected to be, suffering and the date, or approximate date, of its onset
- if the premises are a hospital, the day on which the patient was admitted, the address of the premises from which the patient came, and whether or not, in the opinion of the person giving the certificate, the disease or poisoning from which the patient is, or is suspected to be, suffering was contracted in the hospital.

Although consent is not required for the disclosure of this information, the doctor should nevertheless explain to the patient his or her duty to make this report.[60]

Unless consent has been obtained for wider disclosure, only the information required by the legislation should be released. In exceptional cases, the need to prevent the spread of a serious disease may constitute an overriding public interest in disclosure, such that a breach of confidentiality would be justified (see Chapter 5).

Contact tracing

Although public health legislation provides the power, in some cases, to override confidentiality in order to prevent the spread of infectious diseases, in practice it is always better to work whenever possible with the consent and cooperation of those affected. Even where statutory powers are invoked, the success of such an undertaking may ultimately depend on the cooperation of the parties involved in order to identify correctly and trace contacts who may be at risk.

With the AIDS epidemic in the early 1980s, experience showed that individuals who believed that their rights to confidentiality would be respected were more likely to come forward for testing and counselling. This led to debate, however, about both the patient's and society's duties to those who might have unknowingly been exposed to risk. The right of those at risk to be warned was therefore in conflict with sufferers' rights to confidentiality. Public health officials were keen to use established public health methods to improve knowledge about the disease, to bring about changes in individuals' risky behaviour, and to protect the population. Part of this was contact tracing, which, for libertarian opponents, represented an unwarranted intrusion into privacy with nothing to offer by way of compensation, since no treatment could be offered. Furthermore, they argued, psychological harms could be visited on large numbers of individuals by informing them of their exposure to a fatal disease for which no cure was available, even though they acknowledged that contact tracing could slow the spread of infection.

This dilemma can be particularly acute if both the infected individuals and their partners are known to the doctor or, in the context of general practice, both are registered with the same practice. In such a situation, every effort should be made to persuade infected individuals to agree to the information being shared but, if they refuse, there may be grounds for breaching confidentiality. The General Medical Council advises that "you may disclose information to a known sexual contact of a patient with HIV where you have reason to believe that the patient has not informed that person, and cannot be persuaded to do so".[61]

Summary – managing public health at local level

- The implementation of national policies and day to day management of public health emergencies are the responsibility of the local public health team.
- All doctors have a statutory obligation to provide information to an appropriate person about notifiable diseases.
- The agreement and cooperation of infected individuals should be sought, wherever possible, for both reporting notifiable diseases and contact tracing.
- If consent cannot be obtained, information to comply with statutory requirements must be provided and doctors may disclose information to a known sexual contact of a person with HIV.

The role of the media

The media can have an important role in public health medicine. Its influence and ability to contact large audiences means that it can be an extremely useful tool for disseminating a wide range of information, from general positive health messages to specific details of health risks. Media coverage can also have a negative effect, however. The MMR controversy (see pages 714–5) highlights the potential damage to public health from media generated responses drawing upon imperfect information. Although scientific papers or articles may contain carefully modulated and contextualised assessments of public health threats, there is seldom the space in the popular media to provide suitably nuanced comment. The extraction of media friendly "soundbites" in the search for good headlines can seriously distort evidence, and the likely impact of such presentation should be carefully considered.

Media impact on public health – a soap opera

Although the media is sometimes applauded for raising the profile of important health issues, at times unanticipated results ensue. In June 2002 Alma Sedgewick, a character in the soap opera 'Coronation Street', died from cervical cancer. As a result, according to researchers, an additional 14 000 cervical

(Continued)

smear tests were performed in the northwest of England, where the programme is set, an increase of 21% on the previous year.[62] Although it may be argued that this presents an example of the positive influence of the media on health education and service uptake, the reality is more complicated. Fewer than 2500 of the additional tests were on women who were either overdue or had never had a smear test before, with nearly 12 000 being unnecessary or untimely. The researchers estimated that, if this pattern was repeated across England, the storyline could have cost the NHS an additional £4 million. The large increase in the number of smear tests also led to a strain on local laboratories, with the time taken to report results increasing beyond acceptable quality assurance limits. The researchers concluded that "television programme makers should realise the power of such stories not only to achieve maximal viewing figures but also to cause fear and anxiety, as well as the consumption of scarce health care resources".[63]

When the media becomes interested in a public health issue, care must be taken to ensure that only the known facts are disclosed and discussed; speculating about possible dramatic scenarios on the basis of modest information can prove extremely damaging and should be avoided. Care should also be taken to ensure that individuals are not inadvertently identified and, wherever possible, consent should be sought. Nevertheless, there may be health benefits in providing information to the general public when it is not possible to obtain consent about an incident that affects the public health, either to warn about the risks or to provide reassurance about safety. Doctors therefore need to weigh up the benefits of informing the public against the potential risk to the confidentiality of the affected patients. Even if identifying information is not provided, factors such as general location are probably essential and can lead to identification. A case that found its way to the media in 2002, for example, was so unusual as to effectively identify the individual concerned (see below).

Confidentiality and the media – Britain's first case of rabies in a century

In the winter of 2002 a 56-year-old Scottish man contracted European bat *Lyssavirus*, a type of rabies found in several northern European countries.[64] The release of information about the case to the press raised questions about confidentiality. Once it was known, for example, that someone who worked with bats in a specific region of the UK had contracted rabies, it then became quite easy for the media to identify him. In such cases, consideration needs to be given to the extent to which apparently anonymous information can lead to identification. Furthermore, in the absence of consent, disclosure should be restricted to the minimum amount of information necessary to fulfil the aim.

The hospital informed the press that there had been a confirmed case of rabies, and also issued a statement reassuring the public that people were at risk only if they had handled bats or been bitten or scratched by them. It is not known, in this case, whether the man, or his family, were involved in decisions about disclosure to the media.

Before releasing information about public health risks to the media, it is essential to consult with the local public health department in order to assess the nature and level of risk and the need to inform the public. In some circumstances it may also be important to seek advice from press officers, communications managers, or lawyers before presenting the information to the media. For further information on confidentiality and the media see Chapter 5 (pages 187–8).

Summary – the role of the media

- The media can be extremely effective in conveying public health information.
- The effects of media involvement can be unpredictable; advice should be taken from press officers or communications managers.
- When called upon to comment in the media, it is important that doctors stick to the known facts of the case; inappropriate speculation can be damaging.
- Care must be taken to avoid inadvertent breaches of confidentiality and, wherever possible, consent should be obtained.

Looking towards the future

Media and public attention frequently focus on exciting and innovative areas of medicine, such as new advances in surgical techniques or developments in genetics, such that the potential for simple public health techniques to deliver extraordinary communal benefits sometimes goes unremarked. Vaccinations, sanitation, a clean water supply, and the recognition of the hazards of tobacco use have contributed, and continue to contribute, incalculable benefits to both the developed and the developing worlds. In the West, however, as one generation of problems has receded, others have come to fill their place.

Whereas some of the original problems, many of which still dominate the health agendas of developing countries, were amenable to simple, cost effective interventions or improvements, many of the new generation of public health issues, such as attempting to modify individual behaviour, have proved less responsive to public health initiatives. This new generation of problems include: the health effects of sedentary lifestyles and poor eating habits, alcohol and tobacco use, the effects of social disintegration such as violence and depression, the continuing consequences of social inequalities, bioterrorism, and the emergence of new drug resistant versions of older diseases. As public health professionals continue to develop methods to deal with these issues, it is likely that the ethical questions generated by the friction between state beneficence and individual autonomy, and the appropriate balance between benefits and harms, particularly for patients who are incompetent, will be subject to increased scrutiny.

Public health medicine can provide important ethical insights, insights that can easily be overlooked in the mainstream rights discourse that at times dominates discussion of health and health care. It reminds us that health is not only a private issue, but also, and inevitably, a shared undertaking.

References

1   See, for example: British Medical Association. *Housing and health: building for the future*. London: BMA, 2003. British Medical Association. *Injury prevention*. London: BMA, 2001. British Medical Association. *Growing up in Britain. Ensuring a healthy future for our children*. London: BMJ Books, 1999.

2   See, for example: Department of Health. *Saving lives: our healthier nation*. London: The Stationery Office, 1999.

3   Gostin LO. *Public health law and ethics: a reader*. Berkeley, CA: University of California Press, 2002:11.

4   Adapted from: The American Public Health Association. *Public health code of ethics*. Washington: APHA, 2002.

5   The Health Service (Control of Patient Information) Regulations 2002 s 1(a–d). (SI 2002 No. 1438.)

6   World Health Organization. *Ottawa charter for health promotion*. Geneva: WHO, 1996:1. (WHO/HPR/HEP/95.1.)

7   Nutbeam D. Effective health promotion programmes. In: Pencheon D, Guest C, Melzer D, Muir Gray JA, eds. *Oxford handbook of public health practice*. Oxford: Oxford University Press, 2002:190.

8   British Medical Association Board of Science and Medical Education and Tobacco Control Resource Centre. *Towards smoke-free public places*. London: BMA, 2002.

9   Gostin LO. *Public health law and ethics: a reader. Op cit:* p. 337.

10 Holt R, Beal J, Breach J. Ethical considerations in water fluoridation. In: Bradley P, Burls A, eds. *Ethics in public and community health*. London: Routledge, 2000:162.

11 Jones CM, Taylor GO, Whittle JG, Evans D, Trotter DP. Water fluoridation, tooth decay in five year olds, and social deprivation measured by the Jarman score: analysis of data from British dental surveys. *BMJ* 1997;**315**:514–17.

12 McColl v Strathclyde [1984] JPL 351: 354. Quoted in Montgomery J. *Health care law, 2nd ed*. New York: Oxford University Press, 2003:49.

13 Water Fluoridation Act 1985 and subsequently the Water Industry Act 1991 s87–91.

14 Holt R, *et al*. Ethical considerations in water fluoridation. In: Bradley P, *et al*. *Ethics in public and community health. Op cit:* p. 161.

15 British Medical Association. *Parliamentary briefing: safer fluoridation*. London: BMA, 2003.

16 British Medical Association Annual Representative Meeting, 1998.

17 Jones CM, *et al*. Water fluoridation, tooth decay in five year olds, and social deprivation measured by the Jarman score: analysis of data from British dental surveys. *Op cit*.

18 National Screening Committee. *First report of the National Screening Committee*. London: Department of Health, 1998:14.

19 National Screening Committee. *Second report of the UK National Screening Committee*. London: Department of Health, 2000:26–7.

20 Marteau TM. Towards an understanding of the psychological consequences of screening. In: Croyle RT, ed. *Psychosocial effects of screening for disease prevention and detection*. Oxford: Oxford University Press, 1995:187.

21 Watts G. Safe or sorry. *New Scientist* 2002;(Jun 22):34–7.

22 Gøtzsche PC. Screening for breast cancer with mammography. *Lancet* 2001;**358**:2167–8.

23 Gostin LO. *Public health law and ethics: a reader. Op cit:* pp. 377–8.

24 *Ibid:* p. 378.

25 Hardin G. The tragedy of the commons. In: Gostin LO. *Public health law and ethics: a reader. Op cit*.

26 Wakefield AJ, Murch SH, Anthony A, *et al*. Ileal-lymphoid-nodular hyperplasia, non-specific colitis, and pervasive developmental disorder in children. *Lancet* 1998;**351**:637–41.

27 See, for example: Taylor B, Miller E, Lingam R, Andrews N, Simmons A, Stowe J. Measles, mumps, and rubella vaccination and bowel problems or developmental regression in children with autism: population study. *BMJ* 2002;**324**:393–6.

28 Foster P, Anderston CM. Reaching targets in the national cervical screening programme: are current practices unethical? *J Med Ethics* 1998;**24**:151–7:153.

29 *Ibid*.

30 See: Bradley P. Application of ethical theory to rationing in health care in the UK: a move to more explicit principles. In: Bradley P, Burls A, eds. *Ethics in public and community health. Op cit*.

31 For more detailed treatments of this theme see, for example: Coulter A, Ham C. *The global challenge of health care rationing*. Maidenhead: Open University Press, 2000. Bradley P, Burls A, eds. *Ethics in public and community health. Op cit*. Griffiths S, Hope T, Reynolds J. Setting priorities in health care. In: Pencheon D, Guest C, Melzer D, Muir Gray JA, eds. *Oxford handbook of public health practice. Op cit*.

32   These reflect to some extent the experiences that emerged from the development of the Oxfordshire Health Authority's Priorities Forum. See, for example: Griffiths S. The prioritisation of health care in Oxfordshire. In: Bradley P, Burls A, eds. *Ethics in public and community health. Op cit.* Hope T, Hicks N, Reynolds DJM, Crisp R, Griffiths S. Rationing and the health authority. *BMJ* 1998;**317**:1067–9.

33   Butler J. *The ethics of health care rationing.* London: Cassell, 1999:132.

34   *Ibid*: 133.

35   Cochrane AL. *Effectiveness and efficiency.* London: The Nuffield Provincial Hospitals Trust, 1972. Quoted in: Butler J. *The ethics of health care rationing. Op cit*:32.

36   See, for example, information on quality adjusted life years (QALYs) in: Butler J. *The ethics of health care rationing. Op cit:* p. 135. See also information about disability adjusted life years (DALYs) at: http://www.healthknowledge.org.uk (accessed 29 March 2003).

37   Hope T, *et al.* Rationing and the health authority. *Op cit.*

38   Gutman A. For and against equal access to health care. In: Gostin LO. *Public health law and ethics: a reader. Op cit*:256.

39   For further discussion of these issues, see: Annas GJ. Human rights and health – the Universal Declaration of Human Rights at 50. *N Engl J Med* 1998;**339**:1777–81. Maan JM, Gostin LO, Gruskin S, Brennan T, Lazzarini Z, Fineberg H. Health and human rights. *Health Hum Rights* 1994;**1**(1):6–23. Gostin LO, ed. *Public health law and ethics: a reader. Op cit*:98–113. See also: Toebes BCA. *The right to health as a human right in international law.* Oxford: Hart, 1998.

40   For an introduction to human rights in a healthcare context, see: British Medical Association. *The impact of the Human Rights Act 1998 on medical decision making.* London: BMA, 2000.

41   The International Covenant on Economic, Social and Cultural Rights and the International Covenant on Civil and Political Rights were both adopted in 1966 and entered into force in 1976.

42   Hope T, *et al.* Rationing and the health authority. *Op cit.*

43   Jordan J, Dowswell T, Harrison S, Lilford RJ, Mort M. Health needs assessment: whose priorities? Listening to users and the public. *BMJ* 1998;**316**:1668–70.

44   North West Lancashire Health Authority v A, D and G [2000] 2 FCR 525.

45   Department of Health. *National service framework for coronary artery disease: modern standards and service models.* London: The Stationery Office, 2000.

46   See, for example: Hippisley-Cox J, Pringle M, Crown N, Meal A, Wynn A. Sex inequalities in ischaemic heart disease in general practice: cross sectional survey. *BMJ* 2001;**322**:1–5. Hippisley-Cox J, Pringle M. Inequalities in access to coronary angiography and revascularisation: the effect of deprivation and location of primary care services. *Br J Gen Pract* 2000;**50**:448–54. Vogels E, Lagro-Janssen A, van Weel C. Sex differences in cardiovascular disease: are women with low socio-economic status at high risk? *Br J Gen Pract* 1999;**49**:963–6.

47   For information about the "right to health" see: British Medical Association. *The medical profession and human rights: handbook for a changing agenda.* London: Zed Books, 2001: ch 13.

48   Pencheon D, Guest C, Melzer D, Muir Gray JA, eds. *Oxford handbook of public health practice. Op cit*:229–30.

49   For a discussion of the concept of "community", see: Heginbotham C. Return to community: the ethics of exclusion and inclusion. In: Parker M, ed. *Ethics and community in the health care professions,* London: Routledge, 1999:47–61.

50   For further discussion of these issues, see: Doyal L. The role of the public in health care rationing. *Crit Public Health* 1993;**4**:49–52. Doyal L. The moral boundaries of public and patient involvement. In: New B, ed. *Rationing. Talk and action in health care.* London: King's Fund and BMJ Publishing Group, 1997.

51   Bowling A. Health care rationing: the public's debate. *BMJ* 1996;**312**:670–4.

52   Anonymous. Key staff to get smallpox jabs. *BBC Online*, 2002 Dec 2. http://news.bbc.co.uk (accessed 4 May 2003).

53   Conservative Central Office press release. *Government must end "lethal silence on Sars".* 2003 Apr 23.

54   Kirkup B. *Incident arising in October 2002 from a patient with Creutzfeldt–Jakob disease in Middlesbrough. Report of incident review.* London: Department of Health, 2003: para 27.

55   See: Bayer R, Toomey KE. HIV prevention and the two faces of partner notification. In: Gostin LO, ed. *Public health law and ethics: a reader. Op cit.*

56   This example is quoted in: Carr J, Matheson D, Tipene-Leach D. Hard to reach populations. In: Pencheon D, Guest C, Melzer D, Muir Gray JA, eds. *Oxford handbook of public health practice. Op cit*: 230.

57   Public Health (Control of Disease) Act 1984, The Public Health (Infectious Diseases) Regulations 1988 (SI 1988 No. 1546), and the National Assistance Act 1948, in England and Wales; The Public Health (Notification of Infectious Diseases) Scotland Regulations 1988 s155 (SI 1988 No. 1550) in

Scotland; Public Health Act (Northern Ireland) 1967 and the Public Health Notifiable Diseases Order (Northern Ireland) 1989.

58 For more information about public health legislation in England and Wales see: Montgomery J. *Health care law, 2nd ed.* New York: Oxford University Press, 2003:32.

59 A complete list of notifiable diseases is available from the Health Protection Agency in England and Wales, from the Scottish Centre for Infection and Environmental Health in Scotland, and, in Northern Ireland from the Communicable Disease Surveillance Centre.

60 Public Health (Control of Diseases) Act 1984 s11.

61 General Medical Council. *Serious communicable diseases.* London: GMC, 1997: para 22.

62 Howe A, Owen Smith V, Richardson J. The impact of a television soap opera on the NHS cervical screening programme in the north west of England. *J Public Health Med* 2002;**24**:299–304.

63 Howe A, Owen Smith V, Richardson J. Television programme makers have an ethical responsibility. *BMJ* 2003;**326**:498.

64 Anonymous. Rabies confirmed in bat worker. *BBC Online*, 2002 Nov 24. http://news.bbc.co.uk (accessed 4 May 2003).

21: Reducing risk, clinical error, and poor performance

The questions covered in this chapter include the following.

- What is the role of individual doctors in minimising risk and improving quality?
- Whose job is it to ensure that stressful working conditions do not generate errors?
- What support should be available for doctors who are struggling to cope?
- What legal protection is available for doctors who "blow the whistle" on substandard care?
- What is the role of the General Medical Council (GMC) in the management of sick doctors?

Reducing error and managing risk

The main focus in this chapter is on the actions that doctors are expected to take to minimise risks of error, improve quality of care, and address indicators of potential harm. This draws together a range of issues from clinical negligence to revalidation and setting quality standards. Attention is given to both systems' failure and the difficulties of individual doctors. We begin with a brief introduction to the issues, including discussion of some of the common causes of poor practice. In particular, consideration is given to doctors' ethical obligations where they believe that either they or their colleagues may be providing substandard care. One potential reason for poor medical performance is that doctors themselves have some undiagnosed illness. Therefore, as a separate section at the end of this chapter, attention is given to doctors' health problems and some of the support mechanisms that are available.

Patient safety and quality of care are obviously key concerns for everyone involved in healthcare provision. In medicine, even quite minor mistakes can have tragic consequences for patients. Mistakes not only harm people but also undermine public trust. They are costly in terms of causing avoidable suffering, generating stress, and draining health service time and money. Medical errors demoralise staff and alarm patients. They often attract high levels of media attention, which can distort public perceptions of the relative risks and benefits of certain preventive, diagnostic, and treatment options. Highly publicised errors could adversely affect uptake of generally beneficial procedures such as screening, for example. Staff who are suspected of an error or poor performance can be suspended for lengthy periods pending investigation, leaving patients anxious and sometimes increasing colleagues' workloads. Even if exonerated in complaints' procedures, suspended staff may feel demoralised or that their career or reputation has suffered damage. All of these reasons make it vital that safety nets are in place to minimise the occurrence of mistakes and other adverse incidents.

Risks can be identified by reviewing records of complaints, claims, and adverse incident reports. Interviews with staff can also help to identify concerns, as can observation of the healthcare environment and working practices. Once identified, the problems of error and substandard care need to be addressed in several ways. These include:

- the setting and monitoring of clear quality standards
- open discussion of errors and situations in which mistakes were narrowly averted
- efforts to dismantle the blame culture to allow such discussion
- appropriate systems to try to rectify the consequences of any error
- measures to provide people who suffer harm with an explanation and appropriate compensation
- support for healthcare staff who acknowledge their own mistakes and limitations
- supportive systems for doctors and other health professionals who are themselves sick.

In this chapter, we focus particularly on the role of individual doctors in reducing errors, although brief reference is also made to some of the main organisations that monitor quality or identify poor practice.

General principles

Significant factors that contribute to common errors include inexperienced doctors undertaking decisions beyond their ability and the introduction of new procedures.[1] Doctors' primary ethical duty to patients is to provide a safe and effective standard of care. In particular, they must:

- recognise and work within the limits of their professional competence
- keep their knowledge and skills up to date throughout their working life
- observe and keep up to date with the laws and statutory codes of practice that affect their work
- take part in regular and systematic medical and clinical audit and respond appropriately to the outcomes of any review, assessment or appraisal of performance
- keep abreast of changing societal expectations
- be aware of the performance of colleagues.

Causes and categories of risk

Foreseeability and intentionality

Merry and McCall Smith point out how differing moral weight can be given to an event by the way in which it is described.[2] Saying that an "accident" has occurred implies that the event was a matter of chance for which no-one can be blamed, whereas a term such as "negligence" denotes culpability. Between the extremes of complete chance and intentional harm, there can be a variety of ways in which an individual's behaviour contributes to the risk of injury. Although the systems within which they work may also contribute to the risk of harm, individual doctors must bear responsibility for the consequences of their own deliberate risk taking behaviour. Intentionality and the foreseeability of the likelihood of things going wrong are key factors in courts deciding whether or not an event can truly be deemed an accident in the purest sense of being something that was simply not preventable. If an adverse event is foreseeable, "then there is a duty to take precautions to prevent its occurrence. A failure to do so is culpable and justifies the conclusion that what happened was not an accident".[3] Individuals, however, can reasonably be held responsible only for factors within their control and for situations in which they have some power to prevent harm occurring. "It is foreseeable that failing to supervise junior doctors will over time increase the number of harmful errors in hospital ... but in this case the onus would seem to lie primarily with others, and only partly with the junior doctors".[4]

Although the risk of clinical error and adverse incidents cannot be completely eradicated, doctors clearly have responsibilities to do all in their power to minimise the risks of individual or corporate failure. They need to be aware of the main causes of medical error and adverse incidents, including the problems that can result from continuing to practise when they themselves are sick. Mistakes also arise from doctors being unwilling to acknowledge their limitations and attempting to work beyond their knowledge base. All health professionals have a duty to audit their own performance and to participate in processes such as revalidation and appraisal. They also need to address actively any concerns that may arise about colleagues. Doctors should try to ensure that practices in their place of work include safeguards to minimise the risk of one person's mistake going undetected or harming patients, and provide appropriate support for health professionals who are still learning. Many errors are caused or compounded by a combination of factors, including poor systems of management, stressful work conditions, staff shortages, and lack of adequate time for discussion with patients or colleagues. Although individuals, or even groups of health professionals, cannot necessarily resolve such problems, they cannot ignore them but should take steps to try to have them addressed by those with the authority to do so effectively.

Inherent risks

No medical intervention is completely free of risk. Inherent risk is a product of two factors.

- Clinical interventions inevitability cause disruption. The more invasive the procedure, the more likely it is to disrupt the body's natural functions, but a procedure that is inherently risky may offer a patient a better chance of recovery. The anticipated trade-off between risk and benefit must be discussed with patients.

- The patient's personal characteristics, such as age, gender, comorbidity, and clinical condition can all affect outcomes. Lifestyle choices that result in obesity, smoking, or excessive alcohol consumption all increase patients' risks associated with anaesthesia and surgery, for example.

Inherent risks associated with clinical interventions decrease over time, although the introduction of new or more complex procedures can obviously affect such trends.[5] Reducing these kinds of risks is largely beyond the control of individual clinicians, but patients and the public generally need to be aware of these types of inherent risks when deciding on treatment options. Patients, in particular, need to know what factors within their own control could help to minimise risks for them.

Categories of risk and their management

Medical mistakes can have very tragic consequences and often there is a sense conveyed in the media and public debate that someone must be held responsible. There is a risk of individuals being blamed for events that partly reflect institutional failures or unavoidable human error. "Paradoxically, by focusing on an individual, inquiries or proceedings often fail to identify systemic deficiencies which predispose to error, or fail to protect the patient against the consequences of inevitable error".[6] Because it is unintentional, some human error is not avoidable and the responsibility for reducing it must rest in large part with those who can effect change within the system.

The BMA has suggested that the risk of errors and adverse events can be categorised in terms of five levels, or perspectives, that help to clarify the duties of individual doctors.

- Patients' perception of risk affects their willingness to accept treatment. Patients often have unrealistic expectations and the role of doctors is to help them to make informed choices and realistic assessments of the risk involved.
- The risks of individual clinical incompetence affect the nature of the doctor–patient relationship and can be a significant cause of stress to all parties concerned in treatment. Misdiagnosis is one of the commonest errors in primary care, but diagnosis in this situation is necessarily an uncertain process. It could be significantly reduced if overreferral were the norm, but this would then affect resources and lengthen waiting lists, and could transform the risks of misdiagnosis into the risks associated with waiting longer for treatment.
- Risks may be a result of systems failure. Although errors have often been perceived as the fault of individuals, they are often rooted in a series of interrelated situations and events. Systems that seem harmless can give rise to conditions in which errors are likely to occur.
- Risks may be imposed by cost constraints. Shortage of staff and other resources create pressure, reduce safety margins, and affect the capacity of healthcare systems to cope with unexpected challenges.

- Risks are inherent in clinical procedures. Even if all the other levels of risk could be eliminated, patients receiving treatment would still be subject to the inherent risks of the procedures they undergo. These vary according to factors such as gender, age, comorbidity, and lifestyle, which affect individuals' ability to cope with medical interventions and recover from them.[7]

Analysing risks in terms of these categories can help to define the means of managing them in each case. It also helps to identify whose responsibility it is to manage the different levels of risk. Clinicians are obviously accountable for their own decisions and errors, but not for the levels of risk over which they have no influence. The BMA believes that "if the distinction between different categories of risk can be made explicit, it should be possible for each party to acknowledge and bear the risks which are properly their responsibility. This bargaining process should not be left implicit".[8] Merry and McCall Smith also point out the lack of risk reduction within systems if individuals alone are blamed for errors. They draw attention to the fact that

convicting two junior doctors of manslaughter after the incorrect injection of the drug vincristine into the spinal cord failed completely to prevent the same tragedy from happening again, with two more junior doctors some years later – a mistake which has in fact been made at least ten times in British hospitals.[9]

Summary – managing risk

- Successful risk management depends on developing a culture in which mistakes and errors can be openly reported and analysed.
- Potential mistakes need to be actively sought out and addressed.
- It is inevitable that some accidents occur, but systems managers have a duty to take all reasonable steps to avoid situations of foreseeable risk or the repetition of errors.
- Responsibility for minimising risk lies with everyone, but doctors have special duties to address problems within their own direct sphere of control.

Retrospective overview

A series of relevant developments can be traced as having contributed to the interest in risk management and quality improvement in health care in the latter part of the twentieth century. Just a few of these are identified here. One focus of interest concerned the lessons to be learnt from other industries about proactively identifying and responding to potentially harmful situations and "near misses". The concept of "crew resource management" in the aviation industry, for example, provides a framework that can be relevant to health care.[10]

Learning from other professions

The concept of "crew resource management" originated in the USA in 1979 in response to efforts to deal with human error as a factor in air accidents. It focuses on the role of human factors in mistakes that occur in high risk environments. Elements include appropriate team training, simulation, interactive group debriefings, and measurement of team performance. Individuals are trained to assess their own and their peers' behaviour. This method has been applied to some healthcare situations in the USA, such as training in anaesthesia and neonatal resuscitation, but it can involve substantial expenditure in terms of training and equipment. In its discussion of this method, the BMA noted that the American experience of transposing this way of looking at error from the aviation to the medical team situation was hampered by some cultural differences between the two areas of work. Compared with aviation crews, hospital teams were more likely to favour hierarchical decision making and were less likely to believe that their performance could be compromised by fatigue. Therefore, in the BMA's view, applying useful methods developed in other spheres of work first requires a cultural shift within medicine.[11]

Widespread interest in risk management in the NHS developed in 1995, when the Clinical Negligence Scheme for Trusts was established in England by the Department of Health.[12] This put in place a national pooling arrangement for trusts to meet negligence claims after the introduction of Crown indemnity in 1990. It offered subscription discounts to trusts that had good risk management strategies in place and so provided a financial incentive to set good standards. Similar schemes were also introduced in Wales[13] and Scotland.[14] Subsequently, in the late 1990s, the concept of controls assurance was introduced as a "holistic concept based on best governance practice. It is a process designed to provide evidence that NHS organisations are doing their reasonable best ... to protect patients, staff, the public and other stakeholders against risks of all kinds".[15] Although initially concentrated on financial risks, the system was later extended to cover organisational and clinical risks, partly because these risks are often impossible to separate. It aims to provide a common framework incorporating best practice and obligatory requirements into a series of standards and criteria that must be observed. Compliance with controls assurance standards also provides financial discounts in risk pooling schemes and reinforces the incentives for trusts and commissioning bodies to manage risks as efficiently as they can.

In terms of the performance of individual doctors, the medical profession has always highly valued its independence and consistently argued that the knowledge and skill required to practise as a doctor means that people who are not medically qualified cannot adequately evaluate performance. Self regulation, therefore, has been the means to ensure good practice. Some of the major changes within the NHS in the 1990s, however, drew attention to the need for additional support for some underperforming doctors. In primary care in England and Wales, for example, new health authorities replaced district health authorities and were seen to have particular duties to support GPs through the provision of advice and training.[16] There was seen to be a need for more systematic rather than *ad hoc* arrangements to address underperformance. A subsequent White Paper emphasised the need for "clear arrangements to help identify inadequate performance by GPs"[17] and for local arrangements to support doctors whose performance gave cause for concern.

In the same period, the GMC was looking at performance issues in relation to the implementation of the Medical (Professional Performance) Act 1995, which gave the GMC new powers. It had previously been empowered to act in relation to professional misconduct or ill health, but the 1995 Act gave it new powers to investigate doctors' performance and suspend their registration or impose conditions if performance was judged to be inadequate. There was already an awareness within the profession of some problems in relation to inadequate training and poor performance, and the GMC already provided a range of clear ethical advice to doctors. Its current guidance includes advice about doctors acting within their competence and being frank with patients or their relatives about medical mistakes. (For a detailed discussion of truth telling, including acknowledgement of mistakes, see Chapter 1, pages 36–9.)

Into this situation of professional awareness of a need for change came the interim and then the 2001 final *Report of the public inquiry into children's heart surgery at the Bristol Royal Infirmary 1984–1995* (the Bristol report).[18] This highlighted a number of problems that existed to some degree throughout the NHS and medical practice generally. Since the Bristol report disclosed in a high profile way many of the problems associated with poor management, doctors' underperformance, failure to acknowledge problems, and the silencing of whistleblowers, it is worth considering it in some detail. The report also brought together much of the thinking within the profession itself about practical ways to measure and improve performance.

Cardiac surgery at Bristol

The Bristol Royal Infirmary (BRI) had been designated by the Department of Health as a "supraregional centre" for paediatric heart surgery. Together with the Bristol Royal Hospital for Sick Children, it provided care for cardiac patients, including infants and children. Parents assumed the level of care would be very good, but between 1988 and 1994 the mortality rate for children was roughly double that elsewhere in 5 out of 7 years. The high mortality could not be accounted for solely by the case mix, nor by the high risk procedures (neonatal switch and atrioventricular septal defect operations) that were carried out. Concerns about the service began to be expressed from the mid-1980s by a variety of health professionals, but the surgeons at the centre of the criticism claimed that their outcomes for paediatric cardiac surgery were equivalent to UK national results and spoke of a "campaign of vilification" against them. Even when higher mortality rates were acknowledged, it was claimed that these were due to complex procedures. By 1989, the data contained in the BRI annual reports showed "a consistent pattern of poor outcome".[19] Although the

(Continued)

reports were circulated within the BRI, no specific individual was seen as having an obligation to take action. An anaesthetist appointed in 1988 became particularly concerned about the duration of the operations and the length of time children were on bypass in comparison with other hospitals, which he concluded was affecting outcomes. He repeatedly attempted to draw attention to the mortality rates, which, by 1991, he said, were reaching crisis proportions. Dr Bolsin told the inquiry that he was rebuffed and told that he should "keep his head down".[20] Anxieties continued to be raised at many levels within the NHS and outside it. The inquiry heard, for example, that in 1992, *Private Eye* published six articles criticising the service,[21] but parents whose children were undergoing surgery were wrongly told by the senior surgeon that results at Bristol were good. Finally, in 1995 an operation performed on Joshua Loveday proved to be the catalyst for intervention when Joshua died during surgery after staff had tried to prevent the operation going ahead. A review was instituted and two of the cardiac surgeons and the trust's chief executive were found guilty of serious professional misconduct by the GMC in 1998.

The Bristol report said that its findings constituted an account of doctors who were as much victims of circumstance and of the general failings of the NHS at the time, as of individual failing.[22] The report's conclusions included the following.

- The doctors who were criticised were neither uncaring nor intending to harm.
- Although dedicated, they lacked insight and their behaviour was flawed.
- Many people had failed to communicate and work together. Leadership and teamwork were lacking.
- Management failed to intervene when necessary or listen to reasonable concerns from junior staff.
- Doctors were also caught up in poor working systems, poor organisation, and staff shortages.
- There were no agreed means of assessing quality of care.
- No systematic monitoring took place of the clinical performance of health professionals or hospitals.
- There was no independent external surveillance to review patterns of performance over time.
- A "club culture" existed in which power and control were in the hands of a few individuals.
- Open review and discussion among the staff were discouraged.
- There was no requirement for doctors to keep their skills and knowledge up to date.
- Senior doctors could introduce new techniques as they wished.

Events at the hospital raised complex issues not only of individual competence and conduct, but also of recognising the limits of acceptable variation in practice and outcomes. The results of clinical units such as the paediatric cardiac care unit obviously depend not just on surgeons but on team effort. Although the results of the operations conducted at Bristol were considerably worse than those obtained in other centres, "it is no simple matter to demonstrate that results in a relatively small series of high-risk cases are indeed beyond the limits of acceptable variation".[23] Despite the complexities involved and the well intentioned desire to help patients, the surgeons' deliberate decision to persist with the operations in the face of mounting evidence of unacceptable outcomes meant that "the actions of the doctors have the appearance of a violation rather than an error",[23] and this sparked the disciplinary proceedings taken against them by the GMC.

Steps to address concerns

As a result of a number of factors, including existing professional awareness of the need for better surveillance of standards, measures such as appraisal, continuing professional development, revalidation, accountability, agreed and published standards of clinical care, and monitoring of clinical performance were widely debated. Various institutional structures and processes to improve quality and minimise unfair discrepancies in care were introduced. The National Clinical Assessment Authority was established to consider cases of alleged poor performance (see page 756). The National Institute for Clinical Excellence advises on effective treatment options, both for existing treatments and for new initiatives (see Chapter 13, page 464). In England, a programme of evidence-based national service frameworks sets out what patients can expect to receive from the health service in major care areas or disease groups. In Scotland, the equivalent responsibilities have been devolved to the Health Technology Board for Scotland and the Scottish Intercollegiate Guidelines Network; the work of these and sister clinical assessment bodies comes under the aegis of NHS Quality Improvement Scotland. In England and Wales, the monitoring of the implementation of good quality standards is provided through the Commission for Healthcare Audit and Inspection. England also has an NHS performance assessment framework and national surveys of patient and user experience. The introduction of clinical governance, revalidation, and appraisal for doctors ensures review of doctors' skills and monitors that medical knowledge is kept up to date. In England and Wales, the National Patient Safety Agency was established to improve the safety and quality of care through the reporting and analysis of adverse incidents. It aims to promote a blame free culture that allows doctors to report incidents without fear of being reprimanded. It also encourages them to initiate preventative steps to avoid recurrence of error and help to develop coordinated learning.

Assessing the scope of the problem

In order to understand the scope of any problem, it is essential to identify precisely what is being measured. In this chapter, however, we aim to draw together several separate phenomena related to poor performance, error, or substandard care. These include the way in which work practices and conditions can make doctors more error prone, as well as the way in which doctors' own faults, failings, and illnesses can contribute to adverse incidents. Our overall aim, however, is to help practitioners to see the opportunities that they themselves have to recognise and to address potential problems.

Various definitions of underperformance exist. Common themes include:

- underperformance defined by reference to patient safety: most medical procedures include risks, but activities that put patients at unacceptable risk constitute underperformance
- poor performance defined by reference to professional conventions and good practice guidelines: performance that deviates unjustifiably from these or fails to meet explicit standards is poor performance
- underperformance defined relatively by reference to norms of ordinary good performance: anything that deviates adversely from what is normally found is underperformance.[24]

Obviously, risks to patient safety are consistently identified as indicators of poor performance, as are services that rely on outdated knowledge or fail to meet the expectations of professional colleagues or patients. It is also recognised that underperformance often involves patterns of failure rather than a single error. The inevitability of some error must be recognised and it is accepted that single incidents may not actually constitute poor performance.

Evidence of the prevalence of adverse incidents in the UK is patchy.[25] Nor is it easy to distinguish between the numbers of errors attributable to individuals and those that arise from poor work systems or a combination of factors. Nevertheless, estimates that some 10% of inpatient episodes lead to adverse incidents, and that half of these are preventable, clearly give rise to concern.[26] Less has generally been known about adverse events outside hospitals, although it has been suggested that iatrogenic injury accounts for between 5% and 36% of admissions to medical services and 11% to 13% of adult admissions to intensive care units.[27] The precise number of doctors whose performance is the subject of complaint is also unknown. In 1999 the Department of Health estimated that 6% of the senior hospital workforce in any given five year period would have performance problems.[28] It estimated that, in any given NHS hospital trust, between one and three consultants would have problems and in any given primary care trust, between three and five GPs would be in difficulty. It pointed out that between 30 and 40 preregistration or senior house officers annually are referred to postgraduate deans for serious behaviour, performance, or mental health problems.

These three broad categories – doctors' conduct, performance, and health – identify three causes of less than optimum care. They are different problems, requiring different solutions. A common factor, however, is the need for discussion to pinpoint and address the contributory factors to any mistake.

Misconduct

Negligence and substandard care may be the result of a deliberate failure to abide by professional standards. Deliberately bad or abusive conduct is not discussed here, but is covered in Chapter 1 (pages 56–7). Many of the questions raised with the BMA regarding the behaviour of doctors are not unique to the profession, but mirror concerns common in any group of people. Nevertheless, social indiscretions or misbehaviour are considered much more seriously when doctors are involved because of the potential vulnerability of some patients and the privileged access doctors have to their confidence.

Poor performance

Mistakes often arise from the inadvertent provision of substandard care by doctors who are doing their best but working in stressful or badly organised work situations. In those cases, the organisational problems need to be urgently addressed and sometimes this is simply a matter of ensuring that existing good practice guidance is implemented. Medicine has always been a stressful occupation, especially for those who have least power to influence their working conditions and workload. In 1998, for example, the BMA published a brief report on levels of work related stress among junior hospital doctors.[29] Its key findings included the following.

- Stress was implicated in illness and injury and in the deterioration of doctors' relationships at home and at work.
- Fatigue was particularly prevalent, resulting in decreased concentration, inadequate patient care, and potentially serious clinical mistakes.
- Covering for colleagues on sick leave and insufficient provision of locums contributed significantly to excessive workload.
- Demands of the workplace, including excessive workload and long hours, placed stress on doctors' personal lives.
- Junior doctors favoured informal ways of managing stress through social contact with colleagues and friends, but changes in staffing and work practices sometimes undermined access to such support.
- The professional culture prevented doctors from using formal support services.

The report concluded, however, that the majority of work related stress experienced by junior doctors could be avoided if unit managers implemented existing guidelines on staffing and locum cover. Such measures would also allow doctors to access their informal networks of peer support and reduce the costs of work related stress in terms of personal suffering, poor patient care, and medicolegal liability.

Even when not stressed or overloaded, inexperienced doctors may feel obliged to make decisions when unsupported. They may lack insight into their own limitations or feel unable to admit to other people that they are unsure. The importance of them recognising when they are out of their depth and seeking help needs to be made clear to them. Experienced nurses are often in the position of recognising that an expert opinion is needed and any professional hierarchies that may inhibit them from offering advice need to be addressed. Inadvertently poor care can also occur when experienced doctors fail to keep up to date or to ensure their mastery of new skills before they attempt procedures while unsupervised. Clear guidance and protocols about the introduction of new and complex procedures should spell out the criteria under which innovation with appropriate safeguards can be introduced (see also Chapter 14 on research and innovative treatment).

Doctors' health

A further cause of poor performance is doctors' health related problems, including addiction and other psychological difficulties. It is generally recognised that, in concentrating on patient care, doctors often overlook their own health needs. This can be a lack of insight or a response to the culture in which they work. One of the problems reported by junior doctors, but probably common to others, is the unspoken pressure for health professionals not to take sick leave when ill. "This stemmed from the expectation, inherent in the professional culture, that doctors would work through illness, with the result that doctors could end up working in a condition worse than the one they were treating".[30] The BMA has pointed out that the pressure not to take sick leave when necessary weakens doctors' ability to cope with stress, delays their recovery from illness, and can endanger patients. Nevertheless, a "culture of guilt" about taking sick leave remains and, in some circumstances, doctors also worry that being away from work increases the workload for others. These kinds of pressures, combined with deficiencies in services for sick doctors, can lead them to feel isolated and without adequate support. The BMA emphasises the importance of doctors with health problems being able to access confidential and non-judgmental sources of help. (More information on doctors' health problems is given on pages 760–5.)

Doctors exhibit higher levels of psychological disturbance than people in equivalent professional occupations.[31] Problems ranging from anxiety to depression and substance abuse affecting between 21% and 50% of the medical workforce have been reported in different surveys.[32] Throughout this book the pressures that can affect doctors' performance and their health are particularly noted, including those specifically related to acute and palliative services, and prison health care. Analysis of the work of the GMC's Health Committee indicates that 152 cases were heard against 137 doctors in 2002.[33] Of these, the health problem was solely physical in origin in only four cases; 78 had alcohol problems (21 of whom also had psychiatric problems); a further 51 had psychiatric illness without alcohol problems (although 11 of these were also abusing drugs); and 19 cases concerned drugs with no physical or psychological comorbidity. It is likely that, at any given time, there are also several hundred doctors who are being supervised under the GMC's voluntary health procedures, although these are recognised as the tip of the iceberg.

Recognising and addressing signs of problems

In order to recognise problems, it is obviously important to be aware of the standards of care required. Clinical standards may be set by specific guidelines or protocols and doctors need to demonstrate that they have good reason if they deviate from accepted best practice. On the other hand, it must also be recognised that failure to deviate when circumstances demand is also likely to be criticised. In law, the Bolam and Bolitho tests emphasise that the standards expected of doctors are those set by their peers within the specialty in question, but their decisions must also be shown to be reasonable.

The legal tests for negligence

In the 1957 case of Bolam, the High Court considered the fracture suffered by a mentally ill patient during electroconvulsive therapy. Although he had signed a consent form, the patient had not been warned of the risk of fracture, which was estimated at 1 in 10 000. Nor had he been given a muscle relaxant. He brought an action for damages for negligence. At that time there were, however, two schools of medical opinion about the management of patients undergoing electroconvulsive therapy. One favoured routinely using relaxant drugs; the other considered that such medication increased the risks for patients and so should be used only in exceptional cases. There were also differing views on whether patients should be expressly warned of the risks of fracture. The judge directed the jury that: (1) doctors were not negligent if they acted in accordance with a practice accepted as proper by a responsible body of medical opinion, even if another body of medical opinion took another view; and (2) the patient seeking to prove negligence had to show not only that the non-disclosure was negligent but also that he would not have consented to the treatment had he been informed of the risk. The effect of the case was to emphasise that doctors must be judged by the standards of care expected of professionals in that particular specialty.

Bolam v Friern Hospital Management Committee[34]

In a subsequent case, the House of Lords revisited the implications of the Bolam test when considering the brain injury suffered by Mr Bolitho. In this instance, a doctor had failed to visit this patient when requested and it was accepted that this was a breach of care. The health authority argued, however, that, even if the doctor had attended, she would not have decided to intubate the patient although this was the only action that could have prevented the brain damage. It also argued that it would have been professionally acceptable not to intubate. Initially, the trial judge expected, from a lay perspective, that intubation would have been the correct response, but the House of Lords subsequently noted that a competent body of medical opinion supported non-intubation. It adopted a revised version of the relevant test of negligence, saying not only that doctors' actions should be measured against responsible medical opinion, but also that, if the expert opinion did not stand up to logical analysis, judges could reject it. Although they found in favour of the health

(Continued)

747

authority, the Lords' decision in the Bolitho case is seen as a strong statement of law that affirms that the courts should set standards for the medical profession if medical standards are perceived to be illogical. It was acknowledged that it may only seldom be right for judges to conclude that the views of a medical expert were illogical, but that they had the right to do so.

Bolitho (administratrix of the estate of Bolitho (deceased)) v City and Hackney Health Authority[35]

The effect of these cases is to emphasise that doctors should be aware of current professional opinion within their own area of practice and that such opinion must be demonstrably logical. Consultants are not judged to be negligent if they act in accordance with the standards expected of consultants, and junior doctors must similarly comply with what is expected of their peer group.

A general practitioner may fail correctly to diagnose a patient's condition without being negligent, even though a specialist's failure to make an accurate diagnosis in the same patient would be unacceptable. Conversely, embarking on an inherently difficult procedure might be negligent if done by a general practitioner, but quite acceptable if undertaken by an experienced specialist.[36]

If, however, a doctor acts in a manner in which no reasonable practitioner in that situation would do, he or she attracts blame, and a punitive response may be called for through disciplinary procedures, the criminal courts, or civil litigation.

Failure to meet expected professional standards

In 2001 a GP was struck off the medical register after being found guilty of 42 counts of serious professional misconduct. Between 1993 and 1995, he had undertaken around 100 private liposuction operations. Although he was legally entitled to carry out such procedures as an experienced GP, he had no experience or training in surgery or anaesthesia and two patients woke up during his operations. Among the charges against him was a failure to give enough anaesthetic or to monitor a patient while she was sedated. He also failed to carry out an adequate physical examination or explain the risks of the procedure. He used a local anaesthetic when operating on another patient, although this was unsuitable for her case. Giving evidence to the GMC, the doctor acknowledged that, with hindsight, the treatment he provided fell short of what was required.[37]

Recognising problems

As mentioned above, poor performance and error can be sparked by organisational difficulties outside the control of individual doctors. Complex technological and managerial systems, centralised decision making, and competing political demands are stressful. Scarce resources coupled with high patient demand, shortage of time, and managerial systems undergoing repeated change can also impose pressure. These essentially managerial and resource problems need to be discussed with managers and others in a position to effect stability and improvement within the system. Audit of performance and outcomes can not only flag up poor performance and provide opportunities for doctors to consider positive measures to improve their skills, but also help to identify any practical obstacles to best practice. Clearly, any system of monitoring must be consistent, fair, and equitable. This is a particular concern for overseas trained doctors. It is widely accepted that overseas doctors attract higher levels of complaints, not necessarily because of lesser skills but because of factors such as cultural differences, communication difficulties, and problems of prejudice or patient expectation.[38] Transparent and well structured approaches to measuring performance should ensure consistency.

In some instances, however, the core of the problem lies with individuals rather than the system within which they work. Colleagues may be reluctant to make a judgment if an error seems an isolated act, but they need to be aware of common indicators of more deep seated performance problems.

Range of ways in which poor clinical performance is evident:

- errors or delays in diagnosis
- use of outmoded tests or treatments
- failure to act on the results of monitoring or testing
- technical errors in the performance of a procedure
- poor attitude and behaviour
- inability to work as a member of a team
- poor communication with patients.[39]

Self monitoring of performance and competence

All doctors have an ethical duty to refrain from measures in which they lack expertise and to seek advice from colleagues in instances where they are unsure of how to proceed.

Junior doctors

Junior doctors can feel particularly vulnerable to the demands and expectations of patients and colleagues. It is widely recognised that they need to gain experience, but they sometimes feel that they are expected to perform, without appropriate supervision, tasks for which they lack knowledge and expertise. In such cases, they should promptly draw the attention of senior colleagues to the situation and be ready to acknowledge when they are out of their depth. Unfortunately, there is often unspoken pressure upon them to attempt to handle difficult situations without calling upon senior staff, especially during unsocial hours. This is not acceptable and the attention of managers should be drawn to any situation in which junior doctors are insufficiently supported. BMA members can also contact their regional BMA office for advice and support. Regional offices can, for example, take up the matter with the appropriate dean or other training manager.

Unsupervised junior doctors

A 16-year-old patient with leukaemia was admitted to hospital in 1990 for his monthly treatment with cytotoxic drugs. Under the supervision of a house officer, a preregistration house officer injected vincristine (which should be given intravenously) into the patient's cerebrospinal fluid instead of methotrexate. The house officer was under the impression that he was supervising only the lumbar puncture, whereas his colleague thought that he was supervising the whole procedure. The patient died. The judge summing up in the subsequent legal case said "you could have been helped more than you were helped" and "you are good men who contrary to your normal behaviour were guilty of momentary recklessness".[40] Both doctors were convicted of manslaughter and given suspended prison sentences. The conviction was overturned on appeal. A very similar case occurred at Great Ormond Street Hospital for Children when a 12-year-old was given vincristine, but charges against the two junior doctors were withdrawn because the hospital system had contributed significantly to the error. The vincristine was wrongly sent to the operating theatre by a nurse, contrary to hospital rules, and was administered by the junior doctor after being advised by telephone by a registrar in haematology to administer the drugs that had been sent.[41]

Sometimes, even when support or advice is at hand, doctors are reluctant to call upon it in the belief that this may be seen as lack of confidence in their own judgment or as an inability to take responsibility. All doctors must recognise the limits of their knowledge and not become involved in procedures for which they lack appropriate training and adequate supervision. Inexperienced doctors have no defence if they knowingly take on tasks beyond their capability. Also, although the importance of seeking advice promptly from senior colleagues cannot be overemphasised, it is equally important to listen to other experienced staff, including nursing colleagues.

Importance of taking advice when uncertain

Two junior doctors were found guilty of manslaughter after having ignored warnings from nursing staff that a patient had become seriously ill. After a routine knee operation on a damaged ligament, the patient developed a rapid pulse, raised temperature, and low blood pressure. Toxic shock syndrome developed and, although this is a relatively uncommon condition, it was argued that the doctors should have noticed that the patient's condition was significantly abnormal and should have sought help. Winchester Crown Court heard that the doctors had been unwilling to admit that they were out of their depth and so did not promptly call a senior colleague. Nor did they take the patient's blood pressure or carry out tests. The toxic shock syndrome led to kidney failure and, by the time senior doctors were called, the patient was beyond help. He was transferred to the intensive care department but died. The doctors were sentenced to 18 months' imprisonment, suspended for 2 years.[42]

Senior hospital doctors

In hospital settings, senior doctors are frequently at the forefront of innovation. Established procedures may need to be adapted to meet unusual or unexpected demands and new technologies generate new therapeutic techniques. It is important, however, that doctors are not drawn into procedures that exceed their competence. One of the problems in the case of paediatric cardiac surgery in Bristol (see pages 741–2) was the hierarchical structure that effectively put senior doctors beyond the scope of questioning or criticism. The Bristol report emphasised the importance of clinicians being appropriately trained and directly supervised when undertaking established techniques that are new to them. When the procedure is untried, permission must be sought from a local research ethics committee.[43] Innovative therapies are discussed in detail in Chapter 14.

Importance of working within the sphere of professional competence

While examining a patient who was consulting him for advice on hormone replacement therapy, a specialist in gynaecology noticed several unsightly skin lesions. He asked the patient whether the lesions had changed or bled recently and she told him that she believed some of them had grown in size. She agreed to the gynaecologist's suggestion that they should be removed under a general anaesthetic. He gave her no warning about possible scarring. The gynaecologist carried out the procedure himself, excising nine senile keratoses from the woman's back, chest, and breasts. When the sutures were removed three days later, some of the wounds began to gape and Steristrips were applied. No follow up treatment was given. The patient developed keloid scarring and subsequently successfully sued the gynaecologist. Commenting on the case, which they defended, the Medical Protection Society emphasised the importance of doctors not acting outside their own sphere of professional practice. It also stressed that, in each case, patients should have ample opportunity to consider if the proposed treatment is necessary and in their own interests. When patients agree that they wish to have such treatment, but it is beyond the experience of the examining doctor, they should be referred to a doctor in the relevant specialty.[44]

General practitioners

In primary care, all GPs should ensure that they regularly review their own practice. Multipartner practices should have formal mechanisms set out in their practice agreements to ensure regular clinical audit and review, so that problems can be identified and resolved early. (Further information and advice about practice agreements is available from BMA regional offices.) Although such practice agreements vary, they can contain agreed mechanisms for managing problems, including addressing colleagues' failure to keep their skills up to date or ask for advice when unsure. When the problem cannot be resolved within the practice, external bodies, such as the local medical committee, may need to be involved.

The need to keep skills up to date

A GP was given a year's probation by the GMC in October 2001 when he failed to diagnose early signs of breast cancer in two women who later died of the disease. He was found guilty of serious professional misconduct after failing to refer to a specialist the two patients, who were both showing signs of breast cancer. His work had to be supervised for a year and he underwent additional training in cancer care prior to being allowed to resume unsupervised work.[45]

In general practice, there may be occasions when doctors are requested to undertake tasks for which they lack training or experience. For example, GPs may be asked to prescribe for a patient who is undergoing specialist treatment (see Chapter 13, pages 472–4) or asked to give specialised counselling. In such cases, they should refer patients to other appropriate practitioners. In the past, it was commonly the view that doctors did not require specific training in the same way as non-medically qualified practitioners for some complementary therapies, such as acupuncture. A doctor who causes injury to a patient by undertaking such therapies in the absence of proper training could face disciplinary proceedings.

The GP contract proposed in 2003 contained a quality and outcomes framework, setting evidence-based standards for clinical care, practice organisation, and patient experience. These standards were intended to be incentives to quality improvement. Practices would monitor their achievement against the standards and receive additional resources according to the standards achieved. Those resources would reflect the additional costs of providing high quality care and reward achievement. Within the system for rewarding clinical achievement was proposed a mechanism for "exception reporting", so that practices are not financially disadvantaged if patients do not comply with medical advice or treatment. The standards would reflect current research evidence and therefore adapt to new research evidence. The onus would be on practices to monitor their own standards and report to the primary care organisation in order to receive payments.

In addition to monitoring their own performance, GPs also have clear responsibilities for the safety and reliability of the staff they employ. (This is discussed in Chapter 1, pages 49–50.)

Health teams

Doctors generally work in medical and clinical teams. Responsibility for maintaining performance and for reporting "sentinel events" is therefore more than just an individual matter. All members of the team need to be alert to the possibility of unexpected error or misunderstanding. Open and cooperative teamwork, with clearly defined responsibilities and transparent and robust clinical accounting, offers the best environment in which to work towards a "no blame" culture in which patients are protected.

Unanticipated errors and the need for vigilance

Clearly, staff shortages and lack of discussion can contribute to medical errors. In January 2000, a patient was scheduled to have surgery to remove his right kidney because of a stone. After the operation had been completed, however, it was discovered that his healthy left kidney had been removed in error. The patient subsequently developed blood poisoning requiring that the diseased right kidney also be removed. He subsequently died in March 2000, five weeks after the operation. In June 2002, the surgeons were cleared of manslaughter as it was not clear that the surgery alone caused the patient's death, although it was probable that it played a part. The court heard that staff shortages at the hospital meant that the patient had not been visited by nursing staff prior to the operation and that the patient's radiographs could have been held the wrong way round when the surgeons looked at them. The case attracted considerable media attention and the consultant urologist who supervised the operation highlighted the importance of other health teams across the country learning from the publicity around the tragedy.[46]

In spite of the most assiduous attention to detail, errors can creep in to practice through no fault of health professionals. An example is the case of an elderly patient who was admitted to hospital for surgery on her right hand. That hand was correctly marked for surgery with a water soluble marker, but the patient then had to wait for several hours for the operation. She sat with her arms crossed and, as she waited, the pressure of her folded arms transferred the mark to her left arm. Fortunately, this was picked up when she was in the anaesthetic room, consent was checked, and she underwent surgery on the correct hand.[47] Such cases emphasise the importance of good communication with both patients and other members of the health team, and of robust safety checks prior to surgery.

In its guidance, the GMC suggests that teams should employ some or all of the following tools and techniques to maintain performance:

- an active and supportive approach to the professional development of each member
- the standards set by professional organisations
- recommended clinical guidelines
- detailed performance records
- internal and external medical and clinical audit
- regular review of individual members' performance
- suitable procedures for looking into complaints and avoiding unnecessary risk.[48]

Locums and out of hours services

Like all other doctors, practitioners who work as locums must ensure their own competence, but those who employ or work with them also have responsibilities for verifying the standards of their performance. The GMC advises doctors that:

If you arrange cover for your own practice, you must satisfy yourself that doctors who stand in for you have the qualifications, experience, knowledge and skills to perform the duties for which they will be responsible. Deputising doctors and locums are directly accountable to the GMC for the care of patients while on duty.[49]

The GMC has noted a reluctance on behalf of employers to try to resolve serious problems with underperforming locums.[50] Clearly, responding to poor performance by locum doctors can be problematic because there is seldom an ongoing relationship with a single employer, but problems cannot be ignored simply because the doctor is on a short term contract. If the problems are unresolved, the doctor may well move on and pose a threat to patient safety elsewhere. (A case example of this is given in Chapter 1, page 56.) If it is not possible to resolve problems with locums through standard local procedures it may be necessary to contact the GMC directly for advice on how to proceed. Doctors employing locums whose performance is the subject of serious doubt should bear in mind that they have a responsibility to inform the locum agency. It may also be advisable to contact the Regional Director of Public Health to discuss the possibility of issuing an alert letter (see page 756). The Department of Health has issued guidance on employing locum doctors that emphasises the need for employers to be assured of the standing and competence of locum doctors before they are appointed, and to use only those locum agencies that have reliable quality control systems in place.[51] Furthermore, a 1999 Audit Commission study into the use of locum doctors recommended the establishment of a national performance review and accreditation system for locums.[52]

Summary – maintaining one's own performance

- All doctors must ensure that they both recognise and work within their limitations.
- Junior doctors should refuse to undertake without appropriate support procedures for which they are not properly qualified if called upon to do so by senior colleagues.
- All doctors should take extreme care when embarking on medical procedures or providing advice in specialties outside their own area of expertise.

Addressing poor performance by colleagues

When doctors experience difficulties, early intervention is generally beneficial both for the doctor and for patients. Undoubtedly, there is reluctance to criticise or to report struggling colleagues, but inactivity helps nobody. When problems occur, early action is advisable. Having said that, however, although isolated mistakes may be obvious, an awareness of patterns of medical malpractice or error takes time to develop.

Doctors who have concerns about the performance of colleagues or about the impact of substandard services on patient care may need to gather information to establish the facts. Nevertheless, they need to be aware of patient confidentiality. The BMA advises candour and truth telling, but first it is important to ascertain the basic facts (see Chapter 1, pages 37–9). Unless they are currently treating the patient, doctors do not have rights of access to the patient's records. Where possible, they should discuss their concerns with those in authority so that a formal audit of the necessary information can be carried out.

Health professionals have an obligation to act if patient safety or standards of care are compromised. Hospital doctors should notify their trust or other employer. A written record of the nature of the problems and the steps to remedy them should be kept. In a profession as complex and at times as unpredictable as medicine, some disagreements inevitably arise. Whenever possible, doctors should discuss the matter with senior or experienced colleagues before deciding on a course of action. Further advice is available from the medical indemnity organisations.

Using local procedures

Problems should be addressed as early as possible, either through informal discussion with the person concerned or through local mechanisms. Professional etiquette has traditionally suggested that problems should be sorted out privately and informally. This conforms with good practice because it is generally preferable to try to attend to problems as close as possible to their source. Local policies and procedures for dealing with underperformance vary, as do the exact roles and responsibilities of the individuals involved, but every trust, health board, local medical committee, general practice, and primary care trust should have its own procedures. Occupational health services, where they exist, can also be an invaluable source of advice, both for those with problems themselves and those concerned about the performance of colleagues. The GMC says that, where there is a pattern of poor practice which, if continued, would put patients at risk, immediate steps must be taken. The people who need to be involved may include:

- within trusts and health boards: the chairman, chief executive, medical director, clinical director, director of public health, and director of primary care
- within local medical committees: the chairman and secretary
- within general practices: the senior or executive partner
- occupational health services where available.

When the doctor whose practice is raising questions is in a training post, it may also be necessary to contact the postgraduate dean or the director of postgraduate general practice education. In some instances, the regional or local director of public health may be able to offer general advice and may consider taking over the inquiry. When the problem is one of clinical performance, the relevant Royal College, specialist association, the National Clinical Assessment Authority (NCAA; see below) or, in Scotland, NHS Quality Improvement Scotland, may also be able to provide advice. When problems cannot be solved at a local level by talking to the doctor concerned and to other colleagues or management, it is essential to consider further alternatives.

The National Clinical Assessment Authority

At the beginning of 2001, the Government established the NCAA in England and Wales. (At the time of writing, negotiations are also under way to extend NCAA services to Northern Ireland.) In Scotland, an external clinical advisory service provides some of the functions of the NCAA. Since January 2003, NHS Quality Improvement Scotland has coordinated the work of Scotland's clinical effectiveness organisations. The NCAA provides a performance assessment and support service to which a doctor can be rapidly referred, when concerns about his or her performance can be assessed and appropriate solutions devised. The main concern of the NCAA is with the practice of an individual within a team and clinical setting, not the fitness of the doctor to remain on the GMC register.

When local procedures have proved ineffective, employers can refer a doctor to the NCAA, which initiates an assessment of the doctor's clinical practice. The NCAA is an advisory body and the employer or trust remains responsible for resolving the problem at all stages. Doctors undergoing assessment by the NCAA have to give a binding undertaking not to practise in the NHS or private sector other than in their main place of NHS employment until the NCAA assessment is complete. The NCAA has no statutory powers, although in exceptional circumstances it can make a direct referral to the GMC or to the Commission for Health Audit and Inspection set up by the Health Act 1999 to assure, monitor, and improve the quality of clinical care in England and Wales. The NCAA normally accepts referrals from the senior person responsible for managing poor performance in the particular healthcare organisation. Nevertheless, when there is a clear and immediate danger to patients that cannot be resolved locally, referral to the GMC remains the appropriate course of action.

Alert letters

When an employee is not being assessed by the NCAA and an employer considers that that person could place patients or staff at serious risk of harm, the employer can consider making a request to the Regional Director of Public Health for the issue of an "alert letter". If the Director of Public Health considers it appropriate, an alert letter, drawing the attention of potential employers to problems associated with the doctor or health professional concerned will be cascaded to all NHS bodies. In almost all cases in which an alert letter is issued, referral should be made to the individual's regulatory body.[53]

Involving the GMC

Ultimate responsibility for investigating and monitoring the behaviour and performance of registered doctors lies with the GMC. In the first instance, the matter can be discussed with the GMC without necessarily revealing the identity of the doctor concerned and advice can be sought. It may, however, be necessary formally to refer the matter to the GMC for further action.

Whistleblowing

In cases in which it is essential to draw attention to dangerous practice or substandard conditions, health professionals who have exhausted local remedies may consider raising the issues more widely. In July 1999 the Public Interest Disclosure Act 1998 came into force in England, Wales, and Scotland. This legislation is designed to encourage people to raise concerns about malpractice in the workplace by protecting whistleblowers in a variety of circumstances. In Northern Ireland, some of the features of this legislation are covered by the Public Interest Disclosure (Northern Ireland) Order 1998. These regulations apply to people at work who raise concerns about crime, civil offences (including negligence), danger to health and safety, or any attempt to cover these up. They apply whether or not the information is confidential and extends to malpractice occurring overseas. The legislation also applies to "trainees" and is therefore relevant to medical students who are undertaking clinical training. It protects whistleblowers who disclose information "in good faith" to a manager or employer. Within the NHS, disclosure in good faith direct to the Department of Health is protected in the same way as internal disclosure. The provision of information to the police, media, or MPs, for example, is protected, as long as this is "reasonable", not made for personal gain, and meets three conditions:

- whistleblowers reasonably believe they would be victimised if they raised the matter internally or with a prescribed regulator
- they believe a cover-up is likely and there is no prescribed regulator
- they have already raised the matter internally or with a prescribed regulator.

If, as a result of their activities, whistleblowers are victimised, they can bring a claim to an employment tribunal for compensation. If sacked, they can apply for an interim order to keep their job. So-called "gagging clauses" in employment contracts are void insofar as they conflict with the legislation. As a separate issue, the terms and conditions of hospital doctors also contain a provision allowing them "without prior consent of the employing authority, to publish books or articles and to deliver any lecture or speak", including on matters relating to their hospital service.[54] Further advice on whistleblowing can be obtained from BMA regional offices or support organisations, such as Public Concern at Work, which provides free advice and assistance to individuals who are concerned about apparent danger or malpractice in the workplace.

Summary – identifying and addressing poor performance of colleagues

- Identifying poor performance can be complex and the causes multifactorial.
- Clarifying the facts may involve discussion with the doctor concerned and with colleagues.
- Local procedures should be the first avenue to be tried.

- A formal audit or investigation may be required if problems cannot be resolved informally.
- The BMA, the GMC, and the medical protection organisations can all offer advice.
- The public interest disclosure legislation can protect whistleblowers who have followed appropriate procedures and acted in good faith.

Dealing with the consequences of poor performance

Acknowledging error

One of the potential consequences of error or poor performance is the risk of harm to patients. The importance of talking to them and providing a full explanation of the facts and their implications is discussed in Chapter 1. People who have suffered harm need to be able to obtain appropriate help and compensation. For this they need access to information about precisely what has occurred. Clearly, it is important to verify the facts and ensure that the patient is supported if the information is likely to be distressing. Who should tell patients of past errors or substandard care is a matter to be decided within the relevant health team.

Preventing repetition

Understanding why a mistake has occurred is important in efforts to prevent recurrence. The current emphasis within the profession is to attempt to change the culture in which medicine is practised in order to identify the facts rather than attribute blame. This focus also recognises that the system, rather than the individual, is sometimes a significant factor in the occurrence of errors. Maximum disclosure can be encouraged only if individuals feel able to discuss openly their uncertainties or "near misses" as well as actual errors. Recognising this fact, all information supplied to the National Patient Safety Agency (see page 743) through its national reporting system are anonymous and reports made outside this system are confidential.[55] It has been suggested, however, that in practice it is often difficult for doctors who are reporting untoward incidents to conceal their identity.[56]

Writing references

When doctors are asked to write references for colleagues it is important that they give an honest and factual appraisal of performance. Glowing references should not be given in order to encourage the mobility of underperforming colleagues. In its guidelines, *Good medical practice*, the GMC states "you must be honest and objective when appraising or assessing the performance of any doctor including those you have supervised or trained. Patients may be put at risk if you describe as competent someone who has not reached or maintained a satisfactory standard of practice".[57]

The importance of writing truthful references

In 1994 a consultant anaesthetist was found guilty of serious professional misconduct by the GMC. The doctor had been asked by a colleague for advice about the professional performance of a locum doctor in order to write a reference. In its ruling the GMC found that the anaesthetist in question had failed to provide information that the locum had been involved in a very serious incident that was the subject of a pending inquiry. In its determination, the GMC made the following observation.

Doctors who have reason to believe that a colleague's conduct or professional performance poses a danger to patients, must act to ensure patient safety. Before taking action in such a situation, doctors should do their best to establish the facts. Where there is doubt, it is unethical for a doctor to give a reference about a colleague, particularly if it may result in the employment of that doctor elsewhere. References about colleagues must be carefully considered; comments made in them must be justifiable, offered in good faith, and intended to promote the best interests of patients.[58]

A changing culture

One of the positive things to emerge from the Bristol report was the acknowledgement that efforts needed to be made to abolish the "culture of blame" that had grown up within the NHS, and which has contributed to a reluctance to talk openly about adverse events and underperformance. There are clear indications that considerable change has occurred, as was seen in the detailed responses to the Bristol report published by many medical bodies, incorporating practical suggestions and advice.[59] As the report pointed out, a concern for safety can flourish only in an open and non-punitive environment in which health professionals talk about adverse events and "sentinel events".[60] The report also emphasised that, for this to take place, everyone, including patients, must accept that some errors inevitably happen. Appraisal, clinical audit, and revalidation have led to more open and regular discussion of adverse events, and make it less likely that serious errors or bad practice can go undetected. Institutional changes are reinforcing this cultural shift and some of the main ones, such as the National Patient Safety Agency, have already been noted earlier in the chapter (see page 743).

Changing role of the GMC

At the time of writing, the GMC's fitness to practise procedures are undergoing fundamental change. Traditionally, the GMC's statutory interest in underperforming doctors has focused on the three main causes of underperformance discussed above: conduct, performance, and health. In future, investigation will be carried out under the supervision of a GMC committee, followed by an adjudication procedure focusing on whether or not the doctor's fitness to practise is impaired to a degree justifying suspension of registration. As well as the current options of no action, imposing conditions, suspension, or erasure, the GMC will have the additional option of issuing a formal warning to the doctor. The formal separation of the investigatory function from the adjudication is a significant change resulting from the implementation of the Human Rights Act 1998. Separate procedures will deal with cases involving criminal convictions, conduct, health, performance, and referrals or convictions from other professional regulatory bodies, such as those overseas. Details of the procedures followed by the GMC are available directly from the GMC or accessible via its website. Informal advice is also available.

Appraisal and revalidation

At the time of writing, appraisal is still in its infancy among hospital doctors and being introduced for GPs. At the same time, one of the medical profession's most ambitious responses to the problem of underperformance is the development of revalidation. This has been described as an important part of individual doctors' contracts with society and as "at the core of the GMC's renewed contract with the public and the profession".[61] By this process, doctors periodically demonstrate to the GMC that their clinical skills are up to date and they are fit to practise. Successful completion of revalidation is a prerequisite for doctors' continued licence to practise. The GMC has traditionally been dependent on patients or employers contacting it with concerns about the performance of individual doctors. Automatic review through revalidation assesses the proficiency of all doctors in the UK. Nevertheless, when there are concerns about individual doctors' performance and local mechanisms cannot resolve the matter, the GMC should be contacted.

Addressing doctors' health problems

Risks to doctors' health

Doctors are routinely exposed to serious health risks in the course of their work, ranging from exposure to infection, to needlestick injuries, and attacks by violent or mentally ill patients. In addition, they may be subject to health and safety problems associated with their routine working patterns. In 1999 and 2000, for example, the BMA published reports analysing the health effects of factors such as long hours, sleep disturbance, workload pressures, dealing with organisational change, and coping with patients' suffering.[62] Among the effects of such pressures are burnout, suicide, alcohol abuse (among male doctors, mortality from cirrhosis is three times greater than in the general population[63]), excessive smoking, and early retirement. The pressures were also perceived by doctors as having a detrimental effect on patient care, ranging from stress causing a general lowering of standards to irritability with patients and serious clinical mistakes.[64] The solutions were seen to include flexible employment practices, better access to appropriately trained locum cover, encouragement of uptake of annual and study leave, and increased participation of staff in decision making and work policies. Also seen to be vitally important were better support for staff, and a culture in which they feel valued and receive positive feedback.

Personal responsibility

All doctors have a responsibility to ensure that their health does not adversely affect the care that they provide to patients. Circumstances arise, however, particularly in cases of mental health and addictive illness, in which the individual's insight into the need for help and treatment is diminished. In such circumstances, a doctor's close colleagues have a duty to take action, in the interests of both patient care and the doctor's health. Intervention should be seen as an ethical responsibility and also as a caring act. Not to intervene inevitably leads to a deterioration in the doctor's health, and, ultimately, in performance.

As previously mentioned, however, there is a cultural expectation within medicine that doctors do not expect themselves or their colleagues to be sick. Only a third of junior doctors register with a GP.[65] Doctors are often reluctant to acknowledge illness because of the pressure this puts on colleagues. Furthermore, the need to portray a healthy image, combined with unease about adopting the role of a patient and worries about confidentiality, can lead doctors to take responsibility for their own care. There is considerable evidence to suggest that this is particularly true of mental disorder.[66] The hazards of self diagnosis are many, but of particular concern are the lack of medical notes, the temptation to extend oneself beyond one's competence, and the ever present possibility of denial. The GMC emphasises that, other than in an emergency, doctors should avoid treating themselves or their close family.[67] This issue is discussed further in Chapter 1 (pages 53–4) and Chapter 13 (page 478).

The BMA stresses the importance of all doctors being registered with a GP and acting promptly on any early warning signs, especially when they have a suspicion that their health is affecting their performance. They should discuss the matter at the earliest possible opportunity with their GP and informal or "corridor" consultations should be avoided. (The BMA has issued a guidance note on the treatment of doctors as patients.[68])

Responsibilities of colleagues

Clearly, where other health professionals believe a doctor to be putting patients at risk, they need to take action. This sometimes happens when doctors fail to realise how serious their health problems are and colleagues need to intervene. Doctors themselves have a professional duty to take steps to protect patients from risk of harm posed by other health professionals. The GMC states:

If you have grounds to believe that a doctor or other healthcare professional may be putting patients at risk, you must give an honest explanation of your concerns to an appropriate person from the employing authority, such as the medical director, nursing director or chief executive, or the director of public health, or an officer of your local medical committee, following any procedures set by the employer. If there are no appropriate local systems or local systems cannot resolve the problem, and you remain concerned about the safety of patients, you should inform the relevant regulatory body. If you are not sure what to do, discuss your concerns with an impartial colleague or contact your defence body, a professional organisation or the GMC for advice. [69]

The mechanisms available for addressing poor performance by colleagues are set out on pages 754–8.

Confidentiality

Health professionals who are ill are entitled to the same confidentiality as other patients. Doctors, particularly those suffering from mental health and addictive problems, are often reluctant to seek medical advice owing to concerns about levels of confidentiality in the "small world" of the medical profession.[70] These fears are not entirely unfounded. It may be difficult for doctors who are caring for other doctors as patients to avoid conflicts of interest when patient care is compromised; this is especially relevant in the dual responsibility that occupational health physicians have when involved in the care of a sick doctor. It is obviously extremely regrettable if the confidentiality owed to a patient who happens to be a doctor is overlooked. Concerns about confidentiality act as barriers to a doctor seeking help. "Out of area" referrals can be arranged as a solution to this problem; indeed, the Department of Health supports the concept of out of area consultations for NHS staff and it is often particularly helpful for psychiatric consultations.[71]

As with other patients, however, doctors' rights to confidentiality are not absolute and action needs to be taken when they pose a threat to other people. Wherever possible, this should be discussed by the treating doctor with the patient prior to disclosure being made to other people.

Mental illness

The three most common disorders for doctors (depression, anxiety, and alcoholism) are readily treatable with a wide range of effective therapies.[72] Problems can arise, however, when doctors have little knowledge about how to access appropriate and confidential services for themselves, or are worried about the prospect of disclosure. This emphasises again the importance of all health professionals being registered with their own GP and being able to ask for an out of area referral.

It is worth pointing out that doctors who are referred to the GMC and suffering from mental illness or addiction can, under appropriate circumstances, continue to practise if they follow an agreed treatment regimen and are suitably supervised. The fact that a health or addiction problem is referred to the GMC does not automatically mean that doctors are unable to practise. Where it is judged that they do not present a risk to patients, they may well be able to continue to do so. Characteristically, the loss of professional abilities occurs late in the progress of addictive disease, and an addicted doctor is not necessarily performing at a level that is harmful to patient care. On the other hand, it is essential that doctors who suspect or know that they have a health or addiction problem do not rely on their own judgment of their ability to continue working, but seek expert assessment.

Dealing with addiction

More than two thirds of the cases considered by the GMC's Health Committee in 2002 involved the misuse of drugs or alcohol.[73] It has been estimated that approximately 1 in 15 UK doctors is likely to suffer from some form of dependence.[74] Doctors who misuse alcohol are often also taking other drugs. Junior doctors and nurses may be among the first to recognise such problems in senior colleagues, but they may be reluctant to take action for fear of damaging their career or because of the sense of loyalty owed to a mentor.[75] The GMC emphasises, however, the duty of all doctors to prevent risks to patients, including those arising from the ill health of colleagues.[76] Once in treatment, doctors generally do very well. Early recognition and treatment considerably increase the chances of successful rehabilitation.

Addiction is a primary disease that is progressive, and which is managed most effectively through abstinence-based treatment. It attracts stigma, both from society and from the profession, although alcohol addiction is sometimes overly tolerated. It should not be seen as a sign of weakness or failure, but rather as a clinical problem requiring appropriate management. Experience in the USA and Canada has shown that, with a structured approach to treatment, using intervention, residential care, and long term monitoring and support, doctors have extremely good outcomes, and most are able to return to safe and effective clinical practice.[77] Support mechanisms need to be available to help them. Experience in the UK suggests that a combination of effective treatment followed by peer support is the most successful approach to ensuring long term recovery, and therefore a safe return to patient care.

Guidance for doctors suffering from infectious conditions

Many organisations have issued advice on the question of doctors suffering from conditions such as hepatitis B or HIV infection.[78] It is imperative, both in the public interest and for doctors' own care, that expert advice is sought from a consultant in occupational health, infectious diseases, or public health if doctors suspect they may have a serious communicable condition. Specialist advice should be sought on the extent to which they should limit their professional practice in order to protect their patients, and on whether they should inform their current, previous, or any prospective employer. Doctors must act upon the advice given. In some circumstances, this means they must not practise or must limit their practice in certain ways. No doctors should continue in clinical practice merely on the basis of their own assessment of the risk to patients. When doctors become aware that they may have exposed past patients to a risk of infection, they must follow the advice of specialists in regard to appropriate procedures regarding notification of those people.

If doctors treat colleagues who have a serious communicable disease, but refuse suitably to modify their professional practice, this should be reported to an appropriate body. Wherever possible, the doctor concerned should be informed before information is passed on to an employer or regulatory body. Among the individuals and bodies to contact are the trust's occupational health physician, the local medical committee, the local or regional director of public health, or the GMC. If necessary, the GMC can take action to limit the practice of such doctors or to suspend their registration. Examining doctors may conceivably have a legal liability if they take no steps to prevent a doctor who is medically unfit from practising. When doctors have become infected in the course of their work and are unable to continue practising, this does not mean that their skills need to be lost. They should be helped to retrain or to work in areas in which they do not present a risk to patients.

Employment and pre-employment health checks

In 2002–2003, there were a series of UK consultations and guidance documents about the public health management of some communicable diseases. Some of these focused on the management of diseases such as hepatitis C in the public at large,[79] but others concentrated on the health risks to patients from NHS staff who are suffering from a communicable disease. In 2001 an expert group was established to assess the potential health risks posed to patients from health workers new to the NHS and infected with serious communicable diseases. Following its recommendations, in September 2002, the Scottish Executive consulted on a range of changes regarding health workers who are infected with bloodborne viruses.[80] It issued new advice on patient notification when a health worker is found to be HIV infected, concluding that it is not necessary to notify every patient who has undergone an exposure-prone procedure carried out by an infected health worker because of the low risk of transmission and the anxiety associated with being notified.

In January 2003 it was proposed that all new healthcare workers must have standard health clearance, involving being free from tuberculosis, with immunisation where appropriate, and to be offered immunisation against hepatitis B.[81] In addition, it was proposed that all new healthcare workers who would be performing exposure-prone procedures must be shown to be free from hepatitis B, hepatitis C, and HIV, as well as from tuberculosis, before appointment or commencement of training. It was emphasised that the proposals were not intended to prevent health professionals with bloodborne viruses from working in the NHS, but to restrict them to clinical areas in which their condition would not pose a risk to patients.

In its response to these proposals, the BMA emphasised that any such testing must be backed by appropriate confidential occupational health and careers advice as well as counselling. The stress and anxiety of being tested should not be underestimated and extra support should be available. Robust arrangements need to be in place for doctors who test positive. The Association also pointed out that there are practical difficulties associated with the screening of healthcare workers because a constant programme of testing would be needed to ensure that infection did not develop after the individual took up employment. It noted that patient safety could be assured only if healthcare workers were to be encouraged to accept testing whenever they were potentially exposed to infection, such as when they sustained a needlestick injury. Encouragement for testing should include plans for infection management and treatment.

The Association also called for clear guidance for medical schools and information for medical students on how to protect themselves against infection, the tests available, and the range of careers that would not involve exposure-prone procedures. It considered that students should be encouraged to be tested for a serious communicable disease if they have concerns or feel that they may have been exposed to infection. To discover infection with a serious communicable disease prior to embarking on a chosen specialty has considerable ramifications on career plans. Early diagnosis of hepatitis B or hepatitis C as a medical student allows for treatment and possible clearance of the disease, still giving the individual an opportunity to pursue a career that involves exposure-prone procedures.

The GMC, in its guidance *Student health and conduct*, states:

Subject to meeting a University's regulations, anyone can graduate provided that they meet all the outcomes and curriculum requirements in *Tomorrow's doctors*. The view of the GMC is that students with a wide range of disabilities or health conditions can achieve the prescribed standards of knowledge, skills, attitudes and behaviour. Each case is different and has to be viewed on its merits. The safety of the public must always take priority.[82]

Summary – maintaining health and safety

All doctors:

- have a responsibility to ensure that their health does not affect patient care
- should avoid self treatment and "corridor consultations"
- should be registered with their own GP
- are entitled to the same strict rules of confidentiality as other patients
- have a responsibility to ensure that they are protected from infectious diseases
- should seek and follow advice from a suitably qualified practitioner if they may have been exposed to a serious communicable disease.

Charging colleagues

The BMA's ethics department receives occasional enquiries relating to charging professional colleagues and their dependants. This is a matter of etiquette, not ethics. The BMA generally supports the tradition of not charging colleagues for medical treatment. When doctors intend to charge, it is strongly recommended that this be made very clear before beginning treatment.

Support and advice services

A range of advisory and support schemes are available, including local initiatives and national programmes.

The Staffordshire GPs' support scheme

Many of the stresses imposed on doctors stem from factors, such as workload, which are not within their control. They may need to work with colleagues and managers to deal with the problems. The Staffordshire primary care support scheme is an example of how doctors' stress can begin to be approached, although such schemes are not seen as providing comprehensive answers. The scheme began in 1994 to provide help for any GP in Staffordshire who felt under stress or in distress. It was initially funded by the then Family Health Services Authority. Information was circulated by means of booklets providing contact numbers. Depression and stress are the main triggers prompting GPs to use the service and an average of 10 use it each year. Consultations involve a skill mix, including GPs, psychologists, psychiatrists, psychotherapists, and counsellors specialised in careers, relationships, and substance abuse. In addition, the scheme runs stress management courses and issues workbooks and cassettes about dealing with pressure and stress.[83]

The National Counselling Service for Sick Doctors is a confidential independent service supported by the Royal Colleges, the Joint Consultants Committee, the BMA, and other medical professional bodies. The service started in 1985 and since then has been asked to help a large number of doctors whose health is causing concern to colleagues, often because the doctor is not taking steps to deal with the problem. In addition, about a quarter of the calls received come from doctors seeking help for themselves, outside the geographical area of their own practice.

The Sick Doctors Trust aims to identify and assist doctors who are suffering from the effects of addiction to alcohol, drugs, or a combination of both. It operates a 24 hour national helpline and can arrange prompt assessment with a view to admission to an appropriate centre for treatment. It can also provide advocacy and support for doctors involved in proceedings before the GMC or the civil courts. It works closely with the British Doctors and Dentists Group, which, through a network of regional meetings, provides support to recovering health professionals.

Clinician's Health, Intervention, Treatment and Support (known as CHITS)[84] is a confederation established by the medical, dental, pharmaceutical and veterinary professions to argue for specific programmes to help health professionals who are affected by alcohol or drug misuse.

Support is available from a variety of sources, such as the Doctors' Support Network and the BMA's own counselling service. Recognising that this variety of provision was itself a barrier to a doctor being able to identify the appropriate avenue of help, the BMA has established a new department, "doctors for doctors", which will provide expert guidance, through the BMA's regional services, to members whose employment or performance may be undermined by illness.[85]

References

1   Weingart SN, Wilson RMcL, Gibberd RW, Harrison B. Epidemiology of medical error. *BMJ* 2000;**320**:774–7.
2   Merry A, McCall Smith A. *Errors, medicine and the law*. Cambridge: Cambridge University Press, 2001:27.
3   *Ibid:* p. 28.
4   *Ibid:* p. 29.
5   British Medical Association. *Patient safety and clinical risk*. London: BMA, 2002:24.
6   Merry A, *et al. Errors, medicine and the law. Op cit:* p. 2.
7   British Medical Association. *Patient safety and clinical risk. Op cit:* p. 9.
8   *Ibid.*
9   Merry A, *et al. Errors, medicine and the law. Op cit:* p. 2.
10 British Medical Association. *Patient safety and clinical risk. Op cit:* p. 13.
11 *Ibid.*
12 NHS Executive. *Clinical negligence scheme for trusts (CNST)*. Leeds: Department of Health, 1995. (EL(95)40.)
13 Information about the Welsh Risk Pool and clinical negligence arrangements for Wales were set out in: Welsh Office. *Insurance in the NHS – employers'/public liability and miscellaneous risk pooling*. Cardiff: Welsh Office, 2000. (WHC(2000)04.)
14 In Scotland, the scheme was known as the Clinical Negligence and Other Risks Indemnity Scheme. Information was provided in: Scottish Executive Health Department. *Clinical negligence and other risks indemnity scheme (CNORIS)*. Edinburgh: SEHD, 2000. (NHS MEL(2000)18.)
15 NHS Executive. *Governance in the new NHS: controls assurance statements 1999–2000, risk management and organisational controls*. Leeds: NHSE, 1999. (HSC 1999/123.)
16 Department of Health. *Towards a primary care led NHS*. London: DoH, 1994. (EL(94)79.)
17 Department of Health. *Primary care: delivering the future*. London: HMSO, 1996.
18 The Bristol Royal Infirmary Inquiry. *Learning from Bristol: the report of the public inquiry into children's heart surgery at the Bristol Royal Infirmary 1984–1995*. London: The Stationery Office, 2001. (Cm 5207 (II).)
19 *Ibid:* p. 136.
20 *Ibid:* p. 138.
21 *Ibid:* p. 141.
22 *Ibid:* p. 1.
23 Merry A, *et al. Errors, medicine and the law. Op cit:* p. 26.
24 Such measures are discussed in: Rotherham G, Martin D, Joesbury H, Mathers N. *Measures to assist GPs whose performance gives cause for concern*. Sheffield: Sheffield University School of Health and Related Research (ScHARR), 1997:12.
25 British Medical Association. *Patient safety and clinical risk. Op cit:* p. 5.
26 Department of Health. *An organisation with a memory. Report of an expert group on learning from adverse events in the NHS*. London: DoH, 2000. Vincent C, Neale G, Woloshynowych M. Adverse events in British hospitals: preliminary retrospective record review. *BMJ* 2001;**322**:517–19.
27 Weingart SN, *et al.* Epidemiology of medical error. *Op cit.* Also discussed in: British Medical Association. *Patient safety and clinical risk. Op cit:* p. 5.
28 Department of Health. *Supporting doctors, protecting patients: a consultation paper on preventing, recognising and dealing with poor clinical performance of doctors in the NHS in England*. London: DoH, 1999: para 2·4.
29 British Medical Association. *Work-related stress among junior doctors*. London: BMA, 1998.
30 *Ibid:* p. 8.
31 Williams S, Michie S, Pattani S. *Improving the health of the NHS workforce. Report of the partnership on the health of the NHS workforce*. London: Nuffield Trust, 1998.

32   *Ibid.*
33   General Medical Council. *Fitness to practise statistics for 2002 [Council paper].* London: GMC, 2003:Annex E.
34   Bolam v Friern Hospital Management Committee [1957] 2 All ER 118.
35   Bolitho (administratrix of the estate of Bolitho (deceased)) v City and Hackney Health Authority [1997] 4 All ER 771. This is discussed in: Montgomery J. *Health care law, 2nd ed.* New York: Oxford University Press, 2002.
36   Montgomery J. *Health care law, 2nd ed. Op cit:*177.
37   GMC Professional Conduct Committee hearing, 20–23 August 2001.
38   Department of Health. *Maintaining medical excellence: review of guidance on doctors' performance.* London: DoH, 1995.
39   Department of Health. *Supporting doctors, protecting patients: a consultation paper on preventing, recognising and dealing with poor clinical performance of doctors in the NHS in England. Op cit:* para 2·1.
40   Merry A, *et al. Errors, medicine and the law. Op cit:* pp. 18–19.
41   *Ibid:* p. 19.
42   Anonymous. Guilty doctors spared jail. *BBC Online,* 2003 Apr 11. http://news.bbc.co.uk (accessed 28 May 2003).
43   The Bristol Royal Infirmary Inquiry. *Learning from Bristol: the report of the public inquiry into children's heart surgery at the Bristol Royal Infirmary 1984–1995. Op cit:* p. 15.
44   Medical Protection Society. Act within the limits of your expertise. *UK Casebook* 1999;**13**:12.
45   GMC Professional Conduct Committee hearing, 16–17 October 2001.
46   Anonymous. Kidney death doctors face probe. *BBC Online,* 2002 Jun 26. http://news.bbc.co.uk (accessed 28 May 2003).
47   Butler M, Belcher HJCR. [Minerva]. *BMJ* 2002;**325**:1182.
48   General Medical Council. *Maintaining good medical practice.* London: GMC, 1998:8.
49   *Ibid:* p. 14.
50   *Ibid:* p. 13.
51   NHS Executive. *Code of practice in the appointment and employment of HCHS locum doctors.* London: DoH, 1997.
52   Audit Commission. *Cover story – the use of locum doctors in NHS trusts.* London: Audit Commission, 1999. See also: Commission for Health Improvement. *Employing locum consultants – matters arising from the employment of Dr Elwood.* London: CHI, 2000.
53   For more information about alert letters, see: Department of Health. *The issue of alert letters for health professionals in England.* London: DoH, 2002. (HSC 2002/011.)
54   Department of Health. *National Health Service hospital and dental staff and doctors in public health medicine and the community health service (England and Wales).* London: DoH, 2002: para 330.
55   National Patient Safety Agency. *Questions and answers.* http://www.npsa.nhs.uk (accessed 5 June 2003).
56   Merry A, *et al. Errors, medicine and the law. Op cit:* p. 34.
57   General Medical Council. *Good medical practice.* London: GMC, 2001: para 13.
58   GMC Professional Conduct Committee hearing, 14–18 March 1994.
59   See, for example: The Senate of Surgery for Great Britain and Ireland. *The Senate of Surgery response to the report of the public inquiry into children's heart surgery at the Bristol Royal Infirmary 1984–1995.* London: Royal College of Surgeons, 2001.
60   The Bristol Royal Infirmary Inquiry. *Learning from Bristol: the report of the public inquiry into children's heart surgery at the Bristol Royal Infirmary 1984–1995. Op cit:* p. 16.
61   Anonymous. Insight into revalidation. *GMC News* 2003;**17**:1.
62   British Medical Association. *Health and safety problems associated with doctors' working patterns.* London: BMA, 1999. British Medical Association. *Work-related stress among senior doctors.* London: BMA, 2000.
63   Office of Population Censuses and Surveys, Health and Safety Executive. *Occupational health. Decennial supplement.* London: HMSO, 1995:72.
64   British Medical Association. *Work-related stress among senior doctors. Op cit:* p. 11.
65   Department of Health. *Supporting doctors, protecting patients: a consultation paper on preventing, recognising and dealing with poor clinical performance of doctors in the NHS in England. Op cit:* para 2·44.
66   See, for example: Davis M. The doctor with psychiatric problems. In: O'Hagan J, Richards J, eds. *In sickness and in health.* Wellington: Doctors' Health Advisory Service, 1997.
67   General Medical Council. *Doctors should not treat themselves or their families.* London: GMC, 1998.
68   British Medical Association. *Ethical responsibilities involved in treating doctor-patients.* London: BMA, 1995.
69   General Medical Council. *Good medical practice. Op cit:* para 27.

70 See, for example: Cupples M, Terry B, Sibbett C, Thompson W. The sick general practitioner's dilemma – to work or not to work. *BMJ* 2002;**324**:s139–40.
71 Bennett L. The next steps. *BMJ* 2003;**326**:s103.
72 *Ibid.*
73 General Medical Council. *Fitness to practise statistics for 2002 [Council paper]. Op cit.*
74 British Medical Association, Academy of Royal Colleges, Medical Council on Alcoholism, Medical Defence Union, Medical Protection Society, Society of Occupational Medicine. *The misuse of alcohol and other drugs by doctors.* London: BMA, 1998:3.
75 *Ibid:* p. 4.
76 General Medical Council. The duties of a doctor registered with the General Medical Council. In: General Medical Council. *Good medical practice.* London: GMC, 2001.
77 Talbott GD, Gallegos KV, Wilson PO, Porter TL. The Medical Association of Georgia's impaired physicians program: review of the first 1000 physicians. *JAMA* 1987;**257**:2927–30.
78 General Medical Council. *Serious communicable diseases.* London: GMC, 1997. The Senate of Surgery for Great Britain and Ireland. *Blood borne viruses and their implications for surgical practice and training.* London: Royal College of Surgeons of England, 1998. UK Health Departments. *Guidance for clinical health care workers: protection against infection with blood-borne viruses: recommendations of the expert advisory group on AIDS and the advisory group on hepatitis.* London: DoH, 1998. Scottish Executive Health Department. *Hepatitis C infected health care workers.* Edinburgh: SEHD, 2002. (NHS HDL (2002) 75.)
79 Department of Health. *Hepatitis C strategy for England.* London: DoH, 2002.
80 Scottish Executive Health Department. *HIV infected health care workers: consultation on guidance on the management of HIV infected health care workers and patient notification.* Edinburgh: SEHD, 2002.
81 Department of Health. *Health clearance for serious communicable diseases: new health care workers.* London: DoH, 2003. National Assembly for Wales. *Health clearance for serious communicable diseases: new health care workers.* Cardiff: National Assembly for Wales, 2003. Department of Health, Social Services and Public Safety. *Health clearance for health care workers for serious communicable diseases.* Belfast: DHSSPS, 2003. At the time of writing Scotland is also planning to consult on this issue.
82 General Medical Council. *Student health and conduct: guidance for universities and medical students.* London: GMC, 2002.
83 Chambers R. Supporting GPs. *BMJ* 2003;**326**:s100.
84 Fowlie DG. Have you heard about … CHITS. *BMJ* 2003;**326**:s99.
85 Wilks M, Freeman A. "Doctors in difficulty": a way forward? *BMJ* 2003;**326**:s99.

Appendix a

The Hippocratic Oath

The methods and details of medical practice change with the passage of time and the advance of knowledge. Many fundamental principles of professional behaviour have, however, remained unaltered throughout the recorded history of medicine. The Hippocratic Oath was probably written in the fifth century BC and was intended to be affirmed by each doctor on entry to the medical profession. In translation (this by Francis Adams, London, 1849) it reads as follows.

I swear by Apollo the physician, and Aesculapius and Health, and All-heal, and all the gods and goddesses, that, according to my ability and judgement, I will keep this Oath and this stipulation – to reckon him who taught me this Art equally dear to me as my parents, to share my substance with him, and relieve his necessities if required; to look upon his offspring in the same footing as my own brothers, and to teach them this Art, if they shall wish to learn it, without fee or stipulation; and that by precept, lecture and every other mode of instruction, I will impart a knowledge of the Art to my own sons, and those of my teachers, and to disciples bound by a stipulation and oath according to the law of medicine, but to none other. I will follow that system of regimen which, according to my ability and judgement, I consider for the benefit of my patients, and abstain from whatever is deleterious and mischievous. I will give no deadly medicine to anyone if asked, nor suggest any such counsel; and in like manner I will not give to a woman a pessary to produce abortion. With purity and with holiness I will pass my life and practise my Art. I will not cut persons labouring under the stone, but will leave this to be done by men who are practitioners of this work. Into whatever houses I enter, I will go into them for the benefit of the sick, and will abstain from every voluntary act of mischief and corruption; and, further, from the seduction of females, or males, of freemen or slaves. Whatever, in connection with my professional practice, not in connection with it, I see or hear, in the life of men, which ought not to be spoken of abroad, I will not divulge, as reckoning that all such should be kept secret. While I continue to keep this Oath unviolated, may it be granted to me to enjoy life and the practice of the Art, respected by all men, in all times. But should I trespass and violate this Oath, may the reverse be my lot.

Appendix b

Declaration of Geneva

Adopted by the 2nd General Assembly of the World Medical Association, Geneva, Switzerland, September 1948

and amended by the 22nd World Medical Assembly, Sydney, Australia, August 1968

and the 35th World Medical Assembly, Venice, Italy, October 1983

and the 46th WMA General Assembly, Stockholm, Sweden, September 1994

AT THE TIME OF BEING ADMITTED AS A MEMBER OF THE MEDICAL PROFESSION:

I SOLEMNLY PLEDGE myself to consecrate my life to the service of humanity;

I WILL GIVE to my teachers the respect and gratitude which is their due;

I WILL PRACTISE my profession with conscience and dignity;

THE HEALTH OF MY PATIENT will be my first consideration;

I WILL RESPECT the secrets which are confided in me, even after the patient has died;

I WILL MAINTAIN by all the means in my power, the honour and the noble traditions of the medical profession;

MY COLLEAGUES will be my sisters and brothers;

I WILL NOT PERMIT considerations of age, disease or disability, creed, ethnic origin, gender, nationality, political affiliation, race, sexual orientation, or social standing to intervene between my duty and my patient;

I WILL MAINTAIN the utmost respect for human life from its beginning even under threat and I will not use my medical knowledge contrary to the laws of humanity;

I MAKE THESE PROMISES solemnly, freely and upon my honour.

Index

Abbreviations: CAM, complementary and alternative medicine; GP, General Practitioner; NHS, National Health Service; PAS, physician assisted suicide.

rabies, media and individual
identification 730
rape
serious crime and disclosure of
information 190, 193
victim examination 638–9
recordings
anonymised 207
see also anonymous information
audio 50–1, 209
children 206
consultations/appointments
by doctors 51
by patients 50–1
covert *see* surveillance cameras
GMC advice 46–7, 205–6
identifiable 206–7
for teaching, audit or research 206, 209
incapacitated patients 206, 208
medicolegal 46, 206
not needing consent for use 207
photographs 198, 207–8
prompt recordings importance 200
published material 206
summary 209
video recordings *see* video recordings
references, for colleagues 49–50, 758, 759
referral
duty of care 30
receiving payment for 48
refugees *see* asylum seekers
refusal
doctors to accept patients 29
information receiving 35–6, 80–1
treatment *see* treatment refusal
Regional Director of Public Health,
colleagues poor performance and alert
letters 754, 756
Regulation of Investigatory Powers Act
(2000) 47
relatives
child restraint, decision making and
support 149
consent on behalf of incapacitated
adults 99
of deceased patients
access to information proposals 438
asking about organ and tissue
donation 554
coping with loss 416–17
family linkage studies 429
genetic test information 429
grief 417
information disclosure on 437–8

information refusal 445
method of confirming death
and anxiety 440
parentage testing 429
postmortem information 425, 431
resolving tensions between 444–5
responsibilities of doctors 423–4
retention of material and 443, 523, 524
sensitivity and terminology for
handling 411–13
see also deceased persons
emergency care setting 553–4
see also accident and emergency
(A&E) departments; emergency
care
incapacitated patients
life-prolonging treatment 357–8
providing reassurance 109–10
research and innovative treatment
508, 553–4
see also incapacitated (incompetent)
patients
information
terminal illness diagnosis of patient
370, 372
translation of 77
live organ donation 91
support for, dying patients 384–5
unduly influenced by 83–4
withheld information 35
see also parents
religion
circumcision (male), request for
prohibited 150–1
Jehovah's Witnesses and blood products
see Jehovah's Witnesses, blood
products refusal
parental non-consent to abortion 245
Renal Association, living donor kidney
transplantation 93
renal failure, living donation 90
Report of the Committee on the Ethics
of Gene Therapy, germ cell gene
therapy 345
reproduction
assisted *see* assisted reproduction
autonomy 225–6
continuing dilemma of ethics 265
general principles 225
legal rights
fetus 225, 227
women 226–7
nature of ethics 224–5
negative and positive rights 226–7